T0213361

"Dr. Volpe has produced an excellent work in the field of informatics where the intersection of clinical pathways, technology, change management, and psychology cohabitate. Everyone interested in this field should read the appropriate chapters so that they are comfortable with this comprehensive field."

— **Sam Amifar**, MD, MS, ABP-CI,
CMIO, CIO The Brooklyn Hospital Center

"This text presents a multi-disciplinary view of health informatics, offering perspectives to help us better understand the successes, challenges, as well as opportunities towards a more equitable healthcare system that prioritizes patient care and public health."

— **Vibhuti Arya**, PharmD, MPH, FAPhA | Curating Brave Spaces
Global Lead, Gender Equity and Diversity Workforce Development
International Pharmaceutical Federation (FIP)
Professor, St. John's University

"*Health Informatics*: *Multidisciplinary Approaches for Current and Future Professionals* is essential reading for policy makers, doctors, administrators and frontline healthcare workers. The book illustrates that deep *integration* by and between all aspects of care delivery, including IT, employee training and education, finance, and clinical practice will produce improved health outcomes and reduced costs."

— **John August**, Program Director, Partners Program,
ILR Scheinman Institute, ILR School, Cornell University

"Thank you Dr. Volpe and co-authors for investing in this multi-disciplinary book that sheds a bright light on the opportunity and challenges of health informatics. Managed care organizations, health care delivery systems and community health workers can all benefit from understanding the new world of shared decision making, digital connection and use of data to drive meaningful insights and findings, while protecting patient privacy and promoting equity."

— **Susan Beane**, MD, FACP, Executive Medical Director,
Healthfirst Partnerships – Medical Outcomes

"Dr. Volpe is highly regarded not only for his extensive expertise working at the intersection of clinical care and informatics, but also as a student of the art and science of the field – an expert who readily identifies and learns from the insights of leaders across disciplines who are making change, every day. The result is this uniquely valuable compendium that will serve as the go-to resource for those seeking to understand all aspects health informatics to make care better, more efficient, and more effective."

— **Amy Boutwell**, MD, MPP, Founder and President,
Collaborative Healthcare Strategies

"As health care advances, there is more patient data in different platforms ranging from providers to insurance plans. The need for timely patient data exchange and integration is even more imperative to achieve a holistic picture of the patient from the realms of medical, behavioral health and social determinants of health services. This welcome edition brings together the many disciplines and perspectives to enhance the understanding of the many opportunities that informatics and health IT play towards transforming patient care and population health."

— **Peggy Chan**, MPH, former NYS DOH DSRIP Director

"This book eclipses many others with the expansiveness of the contributions from so many accomplished authors. The foundation of 21st century healthcare is the use of effective and ethical use of informatics. The space has moved from niche to center stage – it is in this context that the next innovators in technology and patient care will find their opportunity."

— **Joseph Conte**, PhD, CPHQ, Executive Director, Staten
Island Performing Provider System

"Dr. Volpe has created perhaps the first truly comprehensive book on health informatics in print. Its breadth of coverage is truly inspiring. It should become a required text for the rapidly increasing number of online, hybrid and in-person Masters' Degrees programs in health informatics becoming available both to recent college graduates and established professionals."

— **James B. Couch**, MD, JD, FACPE
Interim Director, MS in Health Administration Degree Program,
Fordham University

"True wellness innovation requires the recruitment of multi-disciplinary participants. This book breaks the mold with examples from healthcare and other professionals who have leveraged informatics to better the lives of their constituents."

— **Jason Helgerson**, Founder and CEO, Helgerson Solutions Group LLC

"I am saying nothing new when I say, 'healthcare is complicated' Dr. Salvatore Volpe has assembled a team of many of America's best-versed experts from a variety of disciplines and made complex, technical issues of today's healthcare easy to understand. Not only informative, but a road map for developing best of class healthcare practices. A must read of healthcare leaders, present and future."

— **Russ Jones**, Executive Advisor, Felix Global

"Whether for management of a global pandemic at the population level or treating individual patients in a high stake, fast-paced emergency department, the urgent imperative for better collection, analysis, and availability of actionable health data is abundantly clear. Through this valuable text, Dr. Volpe and his co-authors empower healthcare professionals to be catalysts and leaders equipped to create the robust, reliable, and interoperable health informatics processes and tools so urgently needed by patients, clinicians, and policymakers."

— **Steven J. Stack**, MD, MBA, FACEP

"An interprofessional owner's manual on health informatics for all health care providers! Educators must embrace the notion that the future of health care lies in encouraging technology and innovations and this book will benefit future nursing professionals to be practice ready when they graduate. Just what we need in higher education."

— **Patricia A. Tooker**, RN,DNP, Dean, Evelyn L. Spiro School of Nursing Wagner College

"Information technology (IT) has revolutionized healthcare over the last decade and promises to transform healthcare for the foreseeable future. How can we harness an IT-enabled approach to address future health care challenges? How can IT be leveraged to prevent the next pandemic and for surveillance of other epidemics? How will IT rectify the inequities already present in the healthcare system? These are the questions at the core of this remarkable book. *Health Informatics* is required reading for anyone who plans on changing the future of healthcare. A must read for everyone!"

— **Angelo Volandes**, MD, President, ACP Decisions;
Faculty, Harvard Medical School and Massachusetts General Hospital
— **Aretha Delight Davis**, MD, JD, ACP Decisions,
Co-Founder/Chief Executive Officer

"Dr. Volpe makes an inspiring case for combining the principles of computer and information science with life sciences research, health professions, education, public health and patient care by recruiting a broad network of contributors to the field of Health Information Technologies. This book is a mind expander. *Health Informatics* will make you think differently about the future of healthcare and how multidisciplinary teams come together to help those in need."

— **Aiyemobisi Williams**, Co-founder, *Massive Change Network,* and Co-host and Creator of
Health2049, a podcast about the future of health

"Advances in health information technology (IT) have impacted the healthcare stakeholders, especially during the COVID-19 pandemic. This book is a must-read for healthcare leaders who are helping endorse the development of cutting-edge health IT and integrating it into clinical practice! The book brings into focus strategic health IT opportunities for care improvements, enhancement of preventative care, optimization of patient care quality and outcomes, reduction of cost, and maintenance of provider and patient satisfaction, and more. It is a fantastic resource for current and future healthcare professionals!"

— **Aleksandra Zagorin**, DNP, MA, AGPCNP-BC, RN,
Maimonides Medical Center Department of Medicine and Geriatrics,
Clinical Advisor and Scholar, NYU Hartford Institute for Geriatric Nursing,
Director of Undergraduate Studies and Associate Professor,
Evelyn L. Spiro School of Nursing, Wagner College

Health Informatics

Multidisciplinary Approaches for Current and Future Professionals

Health Informatics

Multidisciplinary Approaches for Current and Future Professionals

Salvatore Volpe,

MD, FAAP, FACP ABP-CI, FHIMSS, CHCQM

Foreword by Dr. Paul Grundy

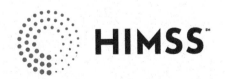

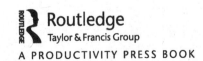

A PRODUCTIVITY PRESS BOOK

First published 2022
by Routledge
605 Third Avenue, New York, NY 10158

and by Routledge
2 Park Square, Milton Park, Abingdon, Oxon, OX14 4RN

Routledge is an imprint of the Taylor & Francis Group, an informa business

ISBN: 978-1-138-39088-1 (hbk)
ISBN: 978-1-032-20774-2 (pbk)
ISBN: 978-0-429-42310-9 (ebk)

DOI: 10.4324/9780429423109

Typeset in Adobe Garamond Pro
by Apex CoVantage, LLC

Dedication

Tribute to Dr. Kenneth Ong

Several of the authors that are fortunate to know Ken pay tribute to him in this section. Ken has been a friend and mentor for many years to those that have benefited from collaborations with him. His understated manner belies his breadth of achievements. Many of us have been fortunate to have been taken under his wing. In particular, the HIMSS NYS Chapter benefited by his wisdom, humor, and volunteerism. With his assistance, the HIMSS NYS Chapter was recognized as a leader in program development and fostering of new relationships. He invited many of us to contribute to his book, Medical Informatics, An Executive Primer which has been a well-recognized reference. I will always remember his humility and his willingness to treat "junior" members of a project with respect.

– Salvatore Volpe, MD

Ken is an educator and a truly transformational physician health IT (HIT) leader. With his in-depth knowledge of clinical workflows, he played an important role in the early days of Electronic Health Record implementation ensuring seamless transition from paper medical records and minimal clinician burn-out. His three editions of Medical Informatics Primer are a true testament of bringing in all the HIT champions together, collating wisdom and resulting as one of the best sellers of HIT publications till date. His legacy will be continued in this new guide as we move in to digital transformation of next generation health care services.

– Jitendra Barmecha MD, MPH, SFHM, FACP

I first met Ken about 25 years ago when clinical informatics was a new idea and physician IT leaders were rare. Ken and I started meeting over dinner and drinks, sharing stories, advice, and sorrows as we each tried to build the case for EHRs in our respective institutions. As we found more like-minded souls to attend our dinners, we decided to give ourselves a name, Medical Informatics New York, or MINY. Ken was the glue that brought us together. Soon we were lecturing together and the lectures begat the book. Because of pioneers like Ken, we now have scores of peers, international professional societies, and journals. When I think of the handful of people who shaped our field nationally and positively influence my own career, Ken is at the top. We have all accomplished more because of his kindness, generosity, creativity, and boundless energy.

– Curtis Cole

I met Ken Ong back in 2013 when I was putting together a coalition of hospitals for a digital health accelerator in New York State. I was struck by how someone at such a senior level at a hospital was so interested in helping emerging entrepreneurs succeed in health tech and navigate the complex mess that healthcare is. Ken served as a champion for health tech, for innovation in

New York State, and helped many including me in their career. I wish Ken well in his retirement and thank him for his mentorship and hope to pay forward his kindness and wisdom.

– Anuj Desai

Ken Ong is a brilliant thinker and an inspiring mentor. We first met when he approached me to write a chapter on Patient Engagement for the 3rd edition of Medical Informatics. *Through the process of writing the chapter, Ken was invariably encouraging and supportive, all while providing thoughtful and insightful feedback. During the process, Ken and I became friends as well as colleagues. Post publication of the book, Ken continued his role as mentor by suggesting me for speaking opportunities and even recommending me as a candidate for the North American HIMSS Board. While my candidacy was ultimately unsuccessful, Ken provided guidance and support through the whole process. Ken was wise about Healthcare IT and Medical Informatics, but even wiser about what it means to be a supportive and encouraging human.*

– Jan Oldenburg

When asked to write a homage to the editor of the first three editions of this text, I quipped that the accolades are going to require a much larger book.
Dr. Ken mentored so many in the realms of academia, informatics, and personal lives. Florence Nightingale wrote about multiplicity, mentoring to extend her work far and wide. In many respects, Dr. Ken is the Florence Nightingale of medical informatics, with apprentices making the world a better place through healthcare technology.
As an educator, his true satisfaction in teaching was in seeing students' achievements. By that standard, Dr. Ken held an outstanding record. He provided me with academic guidance and then the honor of serving on my PhD committee. As a guest lecturer in my classes, he helped guide students on their path toward becoming emerging informatics professions. To connect with them, he described his humble entry into healthcare as a nurse's aide.
As an informaticist, he integrated research and best practices into information systems for the betterment of population health. His innovative work markedly improved healthcare delivery, the effects of which extend beyond his vast documented body of work.
He relished how legislation such as Health Information Technology for Economic and Clinical Health (HITECH) and the Affordable Care Act could extend quality healthcare to the masses and responded to their passages like a kid on Christmas morning. Although a technology aficionado, he truly rejoiced in seeing collaborative efforts serving the greater good of humanity. He imparted a moral obligation to use skills and talent to advance healthcare delivery, a lesson that has shaped my personal and professional aspirations.
In retirement, I gave Dr. Ken a few guitar lessons. He used his newfound skills to regularly perform at senior centers. He used music as therapy for those afflicted with dementia and participated in fundraisers. We even performed together and rocked the joint.
The world of healthcare informatics owes a debt of gratitude to industry pioneers such as Dr. Ken Ong. I'm glad to have crossed paths and gained a mentor, teacher, boss, editor, PhD committee member, fellow musician, and friend.

– Keith Weiner

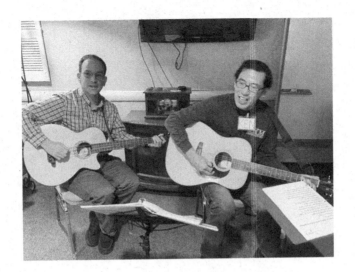

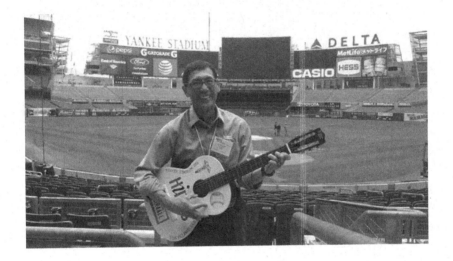

Contents

About the Editor

Salvatore Volpe, MD, FAAP, FACP, ABP-CI, FHIMSS, CHCQM, has achieved board certification in pediatrics, internal medicine, geriatrics and clinical informatics and he currently serves as the Chief Medical Officer working closely with the IT staff at the Staten Island Performing Provider System (SI PPS). The SI PPS is an alliance of clinical and social service providers focused on improving the quality of care and overall health for Staten Island's Medicaid and uninsured populations, which include more than 180,000 Staten Island residents, and was the highest performing group under the New York State Department of Health's Delivery System Reform Incentive Payment (DSRIP) program.

His practice was the first solo practice in the United States to achieve Level 3 2011 NCQA Patient Centered Medical Home Recognition. In addition to running a solo primary care practice for 30 years, Dr. Volpe has had many leadership roles outside the office. He served as physician champion for the NYC Department of Health and Mental Hygiene Primary Care Information Project (NYC DOH MH PCIP); president of Healthcare Information and Management Systems Society New York State (HIMSS NYS); president of the Richmond County Medical Society (RCMS); chairman of the HIT Committee for the Medical Society of the State of New York (MSSNY) and Richmond County; member of the board of directors of the New York eHealth Collaborative (NYeC); and member of the board of the Medical Liability Mutual Insurance Company.

Learning from others and sharing this knowledge has been another important aspect of his professional career. He has been invited to speak on health and technology topics locally and nationally. In addition to contributing to numerous journals, Dr. Volpe was a contributor for the PCMH chapter for the second and third editions of *Medical Informatics: An Executive Primer.*

Dr. Volpe and his practice have been recognized by many organizations. For work with the geriatric population and informatics, they were presented the Island Peer Review Organization (IPRO) Quality Award and SUNY Downstate Medical School Geriatrics Medicine Award. Their focus on PCMH was acknowledged by the Patient-Centered Primary Care Collaborative (PCPCC) with the Patient-Centered Medical Home Practice (PCMH) Award. Due to the innovations introduced by Dr. Volpe and his executive board at HIMSS NYS, he was honored with the Chapter Leader of the Year Award.

Dr. Volpe received his bachelor of arts from Columbia University, his medical degree from SUNY Downstate and completed a combined pediatrics and internal medicine residency at Staten University Hospital (now a member of the NorthWell Health Network).

About the Contributors

Daniel J. Barchi, MEM, is Senior Vice President and Chief Information Officer of NewYork–Presbyterian, one of the largest healthcare providers in the United States and the university hospitals of Columbia and Cornell. He leads 2,000 technology, pharmacy, informatics, artificial intelligence, and telemedicine specialists who deliver the tools, data, and medicine that physicians and nurses use to deliver acute care and manage population health.

Daniel previously led healthcare technology as CIO at Yale and earlier as CIO of the Carilion Health System. He was president of the Carilion Biomedical Institute and Director of Technology for MCI WorldCom. Daniel graduated from Annapolis, began his career as a US Naval officer at sea, and was awarded the Navy Commendation Medal for leadership and the Southeast Asia Service Medal for Iraq operations in the Red Sea.

Jitendra Barmecha, MD, MPH, SFHM, FACP, is Chief Information Officer and Senior Vice President of Information Technology and Clinical Engineering for St. Barnabas Health System (SBH). He leads IT and analytics strategy for population health management for SBH, which is a leading DSRIP Performing Provider System in the Bronx. His team is responsible for managing and upgrading the technical infrastructure, ensuring clinical IT systems, and patient monitoring devices are well integrated in the EHR.

As a senior executive team member of SBH's COVID-19 pandemic command center, Dr. Barmecha has been instrumental in providing technology, telecommunication, biomedical engineering, clinical, and public health knowledge and resources to the emergency response effort. As telehealth became a necessity during the pandemic, he contributed to the publication of telehealth manuals for both the American Medical Association and the American College of Physicians.

Dr. Barmecha holds numerous board and committee leadership positions, including serving as chair of the Digital and Telehealth Advisory Board of the American College of Physicians and an executive member of the New York eHealth Collaborative's Physician Advisory Group. He is a fellow of the American College of Physicians and a governor of the New York State chapter, as well as a senior fellow of the Society of Hospital Medicine.

In addition to IT leadership, Dr. Barmecha continues his passion for bedside patient care as a hospitalist. He enjoys teaching clinical staff and medical students, and he routinely lectures on healthcare management, technology, digital medicine, innovation, and health policy.

Nancy J. Beale, MSN, RN-BC, As a healthcare professional for 35 years, Nancy's experience spans clinical operations, vendor perspective, consulting, and IT operations. While at NYU Langone Health, Nancy led a team of 250 people, and growing award-winning talent to achieve HIMSS 6, HIMSS 7, HIMSS Davies Award, and several innovation partnerships. As an IT executive, she served as a leader in the successful development and execution of the clinical IT strategy for the health system, as well as the clinical IT strategy and execution to support merger and acquisition activity of the health system. Her work also included forming an offshore partnership with a vendor in India for operational IT support services and oversight of onshore clinical help desk operations. In her role as vice president, Nancy provided leadership and guidance over the clinical systems team in the clinical IT implementation of a new and fully digital hospital in Manhattan. Her work is nationally recognized and award winning, recognized as the 2019 HIMSS-ANI Nursing Informatics Leader of the year.

Nancy holds a master's in nursing with an emphasis in health systems and healthcare informatics. She is board certified in nursing informatics and currently a PhD candidate at the University of Wisconsin–Madison focused on clinical technology adoption with a minor in human factors and design thinking. As a doctoral student, Nancy led a team of design students to win first place in the 2019 Medline Innovation Challenge across multiple universities to redesign patient gowns and surgical masks.

As a clinician, Nancy worked across the continuum of care including long-term care, acute care medical and surgical, inpatient obstetrics/labor and delivery, and ambulatory care. The majority of her clinical years in direct care were spent in the specialty of perinatal nursing. Nancy has held a variety of positions from staff nurse, mentor, and educator to manager and director in clinical roles. Since leaving direct patient care in 2002, Nancy has held a variety of roles in healthcare IT, including clinical lead of software implementation, program director, executive consultant, senior director, and vice president. From 1998 to 2003 she served in leadership roles in the Wisconsin Region of the Association of Women's Health and Neonatal Nursing. She is the current co-chair of the Alliance of Nursing Informatics and chair-elect for the Midwest Nursing Research Society–Health Systems, Policy & Informatics research interest group. Nancy has served in policy roles for both the Alliance of Nursing Informatics and the Nursing Knowledge Big Data workgroup. She is also one of two nurses serving on the national DaVinci Clinical Advisory Committee. Nancy holds additional membership in AONL, ACHE, AMIA, ANA, ANIA, AWHONN, HIMSS, MNRS, and Sigma Theta Tau. Nancy has worked with national healthcare leaders implementing technologies. Nancy's work has included partnerships with IT, vendors, nursing, physicians, and allied health providers. She has provided systems strategy, configuration, and clinical transformation guidance as well as collaborative oversight and integration with revenue cycle systems and operations. Her blend of experience has provided a rich background in the role of an executive in healthcare IT and clinical informatics. Nancy's desire to impact change in healthcare as a lifelong learner, along with her professional experiences have positioned her well as an advisor for strategic systems leadership.

Patricia Bomba, MD, MACP, FRCP, a nationally and internationally recognized palliative care/end-of-life expert, served as vice president and senior medical director of geriatrics and palliative care at Excellus BlueCross BlueShield (BCBS). Dr. Bomba founded the New York Medical Orders for Life-Sustaining Treatment (MOLST) and eMOLST programs. At the request of the commissioner of the New York State Department of Health, she developed and served as chair of the MOLST Statewide Implementation Team. Prior to working at Excellus BCBS, Dr. Bomba spent four years in academic medicine and nearly two decades in private practice focused on the care of frail older adults and patients with multiple co-morbidities.

She is a founding member of National POLST, serves on the Leadership Council and the Executive Committee of the Plenary Assembly, and chairs the Public Policy Committee. She served on the Institute of Medicine's Committee that produced *Dying in America: Improving Quality and Honoring Individual Preferences Near the End of Life*, the NASEM Roundtable on Quality Care for People with Serious Illness; NCQA's Geriatric Measurement Advisory Panel (GMAP); and the Medical Society of the State of New York Ethics Committee.

Dr. Bomba is author of several articles on issues related to advance care planning, palliative care, elder abuse, and end-of-life concerns. She has spoken extensively regionally, statewide, nationally and internationally to professionals, community groups, and professional organizations on issues related to advance care planning, MOLST, palliative care, pain management, elder abuse, and other geriatric topics. Dr. Bomba earned a bachelor's degree from Immaculata College and graduated from the University of Virginia School of Medicine. She completed her residency in internal medicine at the University of Rochester. Dr. Bomba is board certified in internal medicine, with added qualifications in geriatric medicine. She attended the Executive Development Program at the Wharton Business School.

Anne L. Burns, BSPharm, RPh, PhD, is Vice President, Professional Affairs, at the American Pharmacists Association (APhA). She is responsible for the association's strategic initiatives focused on advancing pharmacists' patient care services in team-based care delivery models, as well as payment for pharmacists' services, collaboration with other healthcare practitioners, and healthcare quality. She leads the association's practice initiatives on pain management and the opioid crisis, and also works on AphA's medication management, health IT, medication safety, and credentialing and privileging programs. She has served on many medication management, quality, and prescription drug misuse and abuse advisory councils. She currently serves on the board of directors for the Pharmacy Quality Alliance and the Council for Credentialing in Pharmacy, the national advisory board for the National Rx Drug Abuse and Heroin Summit, and is Chair of the Pharmacy HIT Collaborative Workgroup on Professional Service Claims and Codes. Ms. Burns joined AphA in 1997. Prior to AphA, she served on the faculty at The Ohio State University (OSU) College of Pharmacy. She received her BS in pharmacy from OSU and completed the Wharton Executive Management Program for Pharmacy Leaders.

Whende M. Carroll, MSN, RN-BC, FHIMSS, has been a registered nurse for 25 years, serving in leadership roles in quality improvement and clinical effectiveness at Catholic Health Initiatives and nursing informatics at KenSci, Inc., an artificial intelligence (AI) solutions start-up for providers and health plans. She currently works at Contigo Health and directs informatics transformations and clinical IT optimization. Whende aims to optimize patient quality, safety, and outcomes and to impact data-driven digital technologies for innovative patient care delivery solutions. As a nursing and big data advocate, she has a proven track record of working in advanced analytics, existing and emerging technologies, and developing innovative processes, models, and products. Whende aims to drive Quadruple Aim goals, promote health equity, and reduce health disparities in her digital health initiatives work. She has demonstrated experience in leading critical projects and programs in multi-facility healthcare systems and ambulatory, non-profit, vendor, and start-up environments.

Whende is also the founder of Nurse Evolution, a health IT information hub established to educate nurses about using emerging technologies, advanced data analytics, and innovation strategies to optimize people's and populations' health and improve the nurse experience. Whende serves as the Chair of the Nursing Knowledge: Big Data Science Policy and Advocacy Workgroup and is a member of the North America Healthcare Information and Management Systems Society (HIMSS) Nursing Informatics Committee. She has authored numerous papers on AI and nursing. She is the co-author and editor of the American Journal of Nursing award-winning textbook *Emerging Technologies for Nurses: Implications for Practice.* Whende is currently a senior editor at the *Online Journal of Nursing Informatics*, for which she regularly writes about big data–enabled emerging technologies.

Adam D. Cheriff, MD, is the Chief Medical Information Officer and Chief of Clinical Operations for the Weill Cornell Physician Organization. In addition to managing the implementation and support of Weill Cornell's shared ambulatory electronic health record and practice management system, Dr. Cheriff is responsible for Weill Cornell's data warehouse, data dictionary, online physician directory, and patient portal.

As Chief of Clinical Operations, Dr. Cheriff focuses on process improvement around capacity planning, patient access, and digital engagement. He has maintained an active internal medicine practice while overseeing clinical operations for Weill Cornell Medicine. Dr. Cheriff's interests and expertise include clinical system usability, interoperability standards, provider productivity, and process improvement. His research efforts have centered around measuring the effects of the EHR on provider productivity, medication prescribing accuracy and safety, and reduction of administrative waste in provider-payer interactions.

Joshua R. Cohen, J.D., is a founding member of the law firm DeCorato Cohen Sheehan & Federico, LLP. He has been representing physicians, hospitals, and healthcare professionals for over 30 years. He has devoted his practice to innovative strategies on the cutting edge of law, including health informatics and technology. A frequent author and lecturer, he shares knowledge and experience on complex health litigation and risk management.

Mr. Cohen is a past president of the New York State Medical Defense Bar Association and was the chairperson for the Association of the Bar of the City of New York Committee on Medical Malpractice. He is listed in *Who's Who in American Law* and is A.V. Peer Review rated by Martindale-Hubbell, its top rating. He is also a fellow of the Litigation Counsel of America, an invitation-only honorary society representing less than one half of one percent of American lawyers. He is the Secretary of the Health Law section of the International Association of Lawyers.

Curtis L. Cole, MD, is the Assistant Vice Provost and Chief Information Officer for Weill Cornell Medical College (WCM), where he is also the Frances and John L. Loeb Associate Professor of Libraries and Information Technology and an Associate Professor of Clinical Medicine and Population Health Sciences. After medical school at Cornell and residency at the then New York Hospital, he was a Clinical Investigator in Medical Informatics. He has led the implementation of several EMR systems and WCM's TruData terminology server. As CIO, Dr. Cole is also responsible for the other core information systems that support research, education, and administration at the college. His current work focuses on the secondary use of clinical data for research and education. He is active mentoring students at WCM and CornellTech in the development of new health information technologies.

Anuj Desai, MBA, is a healthcare business development executive with 21 years of experience focused on health information technology (HIT). Anuj is a strategic thinker with an extensive network of senior-level relationships at healthcare providers, payers, pharma, startups, and within the investor community. Anuj is a resourceful leader who builds high performance teams that deliver results and thrives in the development of new partnerships that lead to growth. Named by AlleyWatch as one the top 100 Tech Influencers in New York City and a member of the prestigious Crain's New York Business "40 under 40" class, he sits on multiple industry advisory boards and advises tech startups in areas related to policy, interoperability, and innovation.

Currently, Anuj is the Vice President of Business Development at Change Healthcare, driving strategic partnerships across the business. Previously he was the VP of Corporate Business Development at Allscripts and VP Market Development at New York eHealth Collaborative (NYeC).

He led the New York Digital Health Accelerator program for health tech startups selling to large healthcare providers and the largest health tech conference in the region, the NyeC Digital Health Conference.

As an industry thought leader, Anuj is a frequent public speaker and has spoken at many industry conferences on topics related to innovation, interoperability, value-based care, policy, and entrepreneurship. He has appeared in many journals, magazines, and broadcast media. Anuj has also been the recipient of multiple industry recognitions, including 2013 Modern Healthcare "Up and Comers" and 2015 MedTech Boston "40 Under 40" Healthcare Innovators.

Anuj holds an MBA degree from the University of Maryland and a bachelor of science degree in biotechnology from Rutgers University.

Nathan Donnelly, MS, brings deep knowledge across a broad range of critical healthcare issues, value-based care, delivery system reform, strategic planning, finance, and health disparities. He has served as senior vice president, Policy and Analysis, at the New York eHealth Collaborative (NYeC), where he led the policy, analytics, financial modeling, data governance, clinical informatics, and strategy with the chief executive officer for the organization and the Statewide Health Information Network for New York (SHIN-NY).

His portfolio also includes leading and supporting multidisciplinary teams with analyses at Manatt Health and the Healthcare Association of New York State (HANYS). His data science experience involves large healthcare data sets, including claims, electronic health records, and social data, to advise on design, methodology, strategy, policy, finance, and business planning.

John Easter BS Pharm, RPh, PhD, joined the UNC Eshelman School of Pharmacy in January 2016 as a Professor of the Practice and Director, Center for Medication Optimization (CMO). CMO conducts applied research that implements and evaluates medication optimization interventions to inform value-based payment models. Jon also directs the US healthcare course and leads the pharmacy practice domain within the global PharmAlliance collaboration. Jon previously spent 19 years at GlaxoSmithKline (GSK), where he led a health policy team focused on quality measurement and medication management policy development. Jon has a BS in pharmacy from the University of Georgia and is a registered pharmacist.

J. Travis Gossey, MD, MS, MPH, practices internal medicine in New York City. He also serves as the Associate Chief Medical Information Officer for Weill Cornell Medicine. As part of this role, he advances ambulatory areas of the electronic medical record system, health information exchange and interoperability, telemedicine, and the patient digital experience including the patient portal. He has been active in informatics since 2005.

Thomas R. Gray, Esq., is a 1997 cum laude graduate of Albany Law School, admitted to practice in New York state and federal courts. Mr. Gray began his legal career representing defendants in civil litigation and ultimately complex civil litigation including labor law, products liability and medical malpractice. He has represented his clients through trial to verdict and argued in the Appellate Division.

In 2003 Mr. Gray joined the law firm that is now Fager Amsler Keller & Schoppmann, LLP, opening the Latham office to expand legal services to MLMIC and its insureds. While at FAK&S, he represented physicians, dentists, hospitals, and other healthcare providers in medical malpractice and professional licensing matters and provided legal counsel on risk management and health law issues.

Mr. Gray joined MLMIC Services, Inc. in 2014, overseeing upstate claims operations from the Latham office. He currently holds the position of Senior Vice President of Risk Management, working toward positive patient outcome through the identification and mitigation of risk in all healthcare settings.

Valerie Grey, MA, is Senior Vice Chancellor for Academic Health & Hospital Affairs for the State University of New York (SUNY) system where she works with campus and health sciences leaders to establish, lead and support the development of the strategic direction of SUNY hospitals, medical centers, College of Optometry and Veterans Home.

Previously, she was Chief Executive Officer for the New York eHealth Collaborative (NYeC), a nonprofit organization dedicated to advancing care, improving patient outcomes, and lowering costs in New York State by leading the state's public health information network, the Statewide Health Information Network for New York (SHIN-NY), one of the largest in the country. Val also serves on numerous state and national committees focused on improving healthcare delivery, including the ONC's Federal Health Information Technology Advisory Committee (HITAC).

Prior to joining NYeC, Val served as Executive Vice President for Policy at the Healthcare Association of New York State (HANYS). She has also spent many years in public service including the NYS Assembly, Comptroller's office, State Education Department, Department of Health and Governor's office. Val holds a Master's degree in Economics from SUNY Albany.

Ray Hess, FHIMSS, RRT, MSA, is Director of Data Analytics for Penn Medicine, the University of Pennsylvania Health System, in Philadelphia. Ray has over 40 years of healthcare experience. His information management and process improvement experience includes having overseen business intelligence for 18 years, health information management for 6 years, and workflow automation/clinical decision support efforts for 10 years. He is a Six Sigma Green Belt. His clinical experience includes 10 years in patient care and rehabilitation, and he has administrative experience from managing cardiology services for 4 years. He holds a master's degree in healthcare administration from West Chester University. Hess has addressed audiences throughout the United States and internationally and has published multiple articles and book chapters. Hess is a fellow of HIMSS and is involved in multiple HIMSS communities and projects. He currently oversees data analytics and healthcare information exchange for Penn Medicine.

Ye Hoffman, MS, CPHIMS, leads the Advisory Board's Quality Reporting Roundtable team. She provides strategic guidance to health system executives on the complex and evolving landscape of federal health IT and quality reporting requirements. Her areas of expertise include the CMS Quality Payment Program and Promoting Interoperability program, as well as the ONC health IT certification program and information blocking provision. She specializes in health informatics, quality reporting, interoperability, regulatory analysis, and IT project management. Prior to joining the Advisory Board, Ye served as IT project manager and business data analyst at the Fred Hutchinson Cancer Research Center. Ye earned a master of science from Northwestern University's Feinberg School of Medicine in health informatics and is a certified professional in Healthcare Information & Management Systems (CPHIMS).

Mary Ann Kliethermes, BS Pharm, Pharm. D., FAPhA, FCIOM, received a BS in pharmacy from the University of Michigan in 1977 and her doctor of pharmacy from the Philadelphia College of Pharmacy and Science in 1981. Her career includes clinical practice and management in hospital, home infusion, ambulatory practice, and academia. Her current position is Director of Medication Safety and Quality at the American Society of Health-System Pharmacists. Her expertise is in pharmacist reimbursement, medication optimization, safety, and quality attainment associated pharmacist services, particularly in new healthcare models and value-based payment systems.

She has served as chair of the Section of Ambulatory Care for ASHP, represented ASHP at the Joint Commission Ambulatory Professional and Technical Advisory Group, the Care Transitions Work Group of the PCPI, and the Ambulatory Patient Safety Technical Advisory Panel for ASPE/HHS. She has served as chair of the executive committee and board member, and on numerous committees for the Pharmacy Quality Alliance (PQA). She is past chair for the AphA PCMH/ACO SIG. Mary Ann has been awarded Pharmacist of the Year, Shining Star Award, and the Amy Lodolce Mentorship Award from ICHP, the Distinguished Service Award and Distinguished Leadership in Health-System Pharmacy Practice from ASHP, CCP Outstanding Faculty Award, and the Daniel B. Smith Practice Excellence Award from AphA.

Naomi Levinthal, MA, MS, CPHIMS, is a 15-year health information technology (IT) and medical informatics professional. Today she serves as Vice President with AVIA, the nation's leading digital transformation partner for healthcare organizations. AVIA provides unique market intelligence, proven collaborative tools across a network of 50+ leading health systems, and results-based consulting to help solve healthcare's biggest strategic challenges. At AVIA, Naomi leads AVIA's strategic partnerships business and product strategy. Previously, Naomi served as Managing Director at the Advisory Board Company for their health IT research programs serving the C-suite of hospitals and health systems and physician practices throughout the United States and overseas. Her areas of expertise are health informatics, quality reporting, digital health and innovation. Naomi received an MS from Northwestern University's Feinberg School of Medicine in Health Informatics and an MA from Loyola University Chicago, and she is a certified professional in Healthcare Information & Management Systems (CPHIMS).

Virginia Lorenzi, MS, CPHIMS, has been working in health IT for over 30 years with vendor, consulting, provider, and faculty experience. She is currently a Senior Technical Architect at NewYork–Presbyterian Hospital, where she advises on regulatory programs and interoperability and is on the faculty at Columbia University where she helps with workforce and FHIR efforts and serves as Program Director for the Certification of Professional Achievement in Health IT. She has deep experience in interoperability and standards, including over 26 years of active involvement in HL7. She is active in New York HIMSS and enjoys the community it offers to her as well as to students and early careerists in the field.

Owen Moss, MPH, is the Director of Healthcare Delivery at CDPHP in Albany, NY. He's been at the organization for over eight years and helps operationalize CDPHP's healthcare delivery strategy. He specializes in healthcare policy, primary care and specialty value-based reimbursement models and healthcare business operations. He began his career at Booz Allen Hamilton, driving quality improvement and innovation efforts for large federal healthcare agencies. He is currently completing his master's in public health at the Yale School of Public Health. He graduated from Williams College with a BA in Political Economy. He lives just south of Albany with his wife, Julia, and their son, William.

David Mou, MD, MBA, David is a psychiatrist, healthcare executive, and serial entrepreneur. He serves as the Director of MGH Psychiatry's Innovation Council. David is the Chief Medical Officer of Cerebral, one of the largest tele-health companies that has provided high quality mental healthcare to more than 300,000 patients across all 50 states. Cerebral also works with pharmaceutical companies to pioneer decentralized clinical trials, for which David serves as Principal Investigator. Previously, David was President, Co-founder and Chief Medical Officer of Valera Health, a telehealth company that reduced unnecessary hospitalizations for patients with serious mental illness. David is on faculty at Harvard Medical School, where he has conducted research on how digital technologies can help better predict and prevent suicidal behaviors. He has been named 'Top 10 under 35 for Healthcare' by LinkedIn, as well as '40 under 40' for healthcare innovation by MedTech Boston. David graduated from Harvard College with a degree in neurobiology and earned his MD MBA from Harvard Medical School and Harvard Business School. His writings have appeared in the New England Journal of Medicine and Stat.

Sameer Malhotra, MD, MA, is the Senior Director of Clinical Informatics at Regeneron Pharmaceuticals, where he leads initiatives on clinical and genomic data integration and development of analytical platforms for research. Previously, he was the medical director of Informatics at Weill Cornell Medicine, where for over 12 years he implemented, optimized, and integrated health IT systems for patient care. He has extensively worked on clinical decision support (CDS) systems and radiology IT systems and nurtured the first integration of genomic data into the organization's electronic health record. He continues to maintain a faculty appointment in the Departments of Medicine and Population Health Sciences at Weill Cornell. Dr. Malhotra provides patient care as a hospitalist at NewYork–Presbyterian Hospital. He teaches, mentors students and directs courses on health informatics in the master's and executive MBA programs at WCM.

Mary Roth McClurg, Pharm.D., MHS, is Professor and Executive Vice Dean-Chief Academic Officer at the UNC Eshelman School of Pharmacy. Roth McClurg practiced for 12 years as a clinical pharmacist in primary care practice within the VA Health System and in the interdisciplinary geriatric clinic within the Department of Geriatrics at UNC Healthcare, providing direct patient care as part of an interprofessional care team. Roth McClurg has focused her research efforts on advancing comprehensive medication management and the role of the clinical pharmacist as an integral member of the primary care team, with the goal of optimizing medication use and improving care in patients with multiple chronic diseases. Roth McClurg is a fellow of the American College of Clinical Pharmacy.

Dr. Parag Mehta, MD, FACP, is the Senior Vice Chairman of the Department of Medicine at NewYork–Presbyterian Brooklyn Methodist Hospital. He is also the Chief Medical Information Officer (CMIO) and an associate professor of Clinical Medicine at Weil Medical College.

He is board certified in internal medicine, hospital medicine, and hospice and palliative care medicine. He is also certified in health information technology and artificial intelligence in business. He is board certified in OB-GYN from India.

Dr. Mehta is passionate about teaching and has been awarded the Best Teacher and Best Research Mentor Awards on numerous occasions. He is a strong advocate of resident education, patient safety, and quality improvement. As CMIO, he strives to use technology to improve workflow, reduce the cognitive burden, and improve physician well-being. As a wellness champion from ACP, he believes in bringing back the joy in medicine. He actively participates locally and nationally in advocacy efforts for the patient before paperwork. He led the team to achieve the HIMSS7 level at his organization. He can find simple and creative new solutions to complex problems by applying his clinical acumen and analytical thinking skills.

He is an energetic leader who is active with several organizations like the American College of Physicians, Medical State Society of New York, and American Medical Association. He has received numerous honors and awards.

He has an unquenchable thirst for knowledge, and he is on an endless quest to learn new ideas. With his years of experience as a clinician, administrator, and teacher, he takes the utmost pride in training many young and enthusiastic physicians. He feels privileged to have made a difference in the lives of his many patients.

Holly Miller, MD, MBA, FHIMSS. For over 10 years, Dr. Miller has been the Chief Medical Officer of MedAllies, a company that leverages HIT and clinical practice transformation to improve healthcare value. MedAllies operates one of the leading Health Information Service Provider (HISP) networks in support of interoperability. At MedAllies, Dr. Miller provides operational, tactical, and strategic collaborative leadership.

Dr. Miller is currently a co-chair or member of many Health Information Technology (HIT) interoperability–related committees and workgroups engaged in enhancing healthcare value. These include committees within the following organizations: Carequality; DaVinci; HL7; CMS: PACIO; ONC and Integrating the Healthcare Enterprise (IHE): 360X; DirectTrust; NCQA; HIMSS; and KLAS. She continues to be a frequent speaker at national conferences.

Dr. Miller was formerly a vice president and the CMIO of University Hospitals and Health Systems (UH), a community-based system with more than 150 locations, seven wholly-owned and four affiliated hospitals throughout Northern Ohio. Prior to joining UH, she worked as an HIT Managing Director for the Cleveland Clinic, where she also maintained a clinical practice in general internal medicine. She has been active in healthcare informatics research and has been a co-investigator on multiple grants.

As a member of HIMSS since 1999, Dr. Miller is a past vice chair of the HIMSS Board and a past inaugural member of the HIMSS World Wide Board. Her past roles within HIMSS also included being a physician leader of the HIMSS/AMDIS Physician Community and serving as the board liaison to HIMSS Europe for four years. She was also active in a variety of previous S&I ONC committees and other state and government HIT committees.

Rick A. Moore PhD, FACHE, FHIMSS, CPHIMS, CISM, CCSFP, PMP. As NCQA's Chief Information Officer, Rick Moore is responsible for the vision and strategic direction of the Information Services, Information Technology and Information Products. The National Committee for Quality Assurance (NCQA) is a private, 501(c)(3) not-for-profit organization dedicated to improving healthcare quality. Since its founding in 1990, NCQA has been a central figure in driving improvement throughout the healthcare system, helping to elevate the issue of healthcare quality to the top of the national agenda.

Prior to joining NCQA in 2008, Rick was the director of health informatics at the National Association of Children's Hospitals, where he led the development of information services and products for over 200 member hospitals. He has also served the Office of the Secretary of Health Affairs at the Department of Defense, where he led the development of electronic health record (EHR) systems and was awarded the Information Technology Officer of the Year of the Joint Medical Information Systems Office in 2004.

William D. Myhre, MPA, (American University), has 30 years' experience in human resources leadership of non-profit organizations. His expertise is transforming human resources via mergers, new government programs, and consulting and governmental lobbying and testimony.

Recent recognitions include the President's Medal, College of Staten Island; an Award from the Richmond County Medical Society; and National Fund for Workforce Solutions: Emerging Champion of the Front Line Workforce.

Katie Orem, MPH, Katie Orem is the geriatrics and palliative care program manager at Excellus BlueCross BlueShield and the eMOLST administrator for New York State. She has worked on New York's MOLST program for more than ten years. She supports the expansion and evaluation of advance care planning, palliative care and end-of-life care initiatives internally, across New York State and nationally. She has assisted many organizations in improving their advance care planning and MOLST processes, complying with New York State Public Health Law, and implementing eMOLST.

Katie is a member of the New York State MOLST Team's Executive Committee, the National POLST Technology Committee and New York's National Healthcare Decisions Day Committee.

Katie graduated with her Master's in Public Health from the Yale School of Public Health, with a concentration in Health Policy & Administration. She received her undergraduate education at Cornell University and earned a BS in Biology & Society with a concentration in Community & Public Health.

Jan Oldenburg, FHIMSS, is the principal in Participatory Health Consulting, where she advises start-ups and healthcare organizations regarding the evolving digital health landscape. Jan is passionate about making healthcare more engaging, more convenient, and more healing for patients, especially through incorporating appropriate digital technologies. Ms. Oldenburg has focused on digital transformation in healthcare for more than 20 years. Her experience includes leadership roles in several advisory firms, including EY and her current role. She has also served as the vice president of patient and physician engagement in Aetna's ACO organization and held senior leadership roles at HealthPartners and in Kaiser Permanente's Digital Services Group. Through these roles, she has engaged with organizations from every aspect of healthcare.

She is the principal editor of *Participatory Healthcare: A Person-Centered Approach to Transforming Healthcare* (2016) and *Engage! Transforming Healthcare through Digital Patient Engagement* (2013). Ms. Oldenburg also authored chapters in the third edition of *Medical Informatics* and a chapter in *The Journey Never Ends*. She is a board member of the Society for Participatory Medicine and the former co-chair of the HIMSS Connected Health Committee. She currently cochairs an HL7 Committee writing a white paper on patient-contributed data. Ms. Oldenburg is also a member of the Patient Advocacy & Ethics Group for the Datavant COVID-19 Research Database. Ms. Oldenburg tweets @janoldenburg.

Anantachai (Tony) Panjamapirom, PhD, MBA, CPHIMS, is an independent consultant in healthcare management and health information technology. He was a research director with the Health Care Information Technology Advisory and Quality Reporting Roundtable research programs at the Advisory Board Company. He led strategic and best practice research, served as a subject matter expert, and provided policy analysis, strategic and operational guidance in support of hospital and health system executives. His principal areas of expertise included CMS quality reporting programs (e.g., Promoting Interoperability, Quality Payment Program, MACRA), value-based payment models, IT performance management, and IT implications in accountable care environment. He is a certified professional in Healthcare Information and Management Systems (CPHIMS).

Paul Quigley, MBA, is the CEO/CTO/co-founder of www.Liberado.io, a Wyoming-based start-up digital asset custody solution-as-a-service (SaaS) platform designed to support merchant, bank, and credit union partnerships. Paul is a serial entrepreneur with leadership, strategic, operating, and technical experience in eight start-up companies, one IPO, and two private exits. He has domestic and international experience in more than 20 high-growth and complex turn-around environments across several industries, including banking and healthcare. He was an early adopter (2012) of the blockchain and the use cases for interoperability, cryptocurrency, and identity management.

Paul spent more than 10 years at the international consulting firms of Ernst & Young and Accenture as a senior manager in their emerging technology practices. He was a founding member of the International Blockchain Lab for Philips Healthcare in the Netherlands, examining the global impact of Blockchain across all of Philips' product lines. He is presently a member of several Hyperledger (Linux Foundation) workgroups.

Paul is an Adjunct Professor at Harvard University's Graduate School of Arts and Sciences and co-teaches a graduate course about disruptive innovation, blockchain, and artificial Intelligence (ME-4508).

Paul recently completed a term as a governor-appointed (2018–2019) member for the Colorado Council for the Advancement of Blockchain Technology, which brought new legislation to Colorado for Open Blockchain/Utility Token/Virtual Currency Money Transmitter Exemption Bills to Colorado. He speaks regionally, nationally, and internationally (World Economic Forum) on the uses of blockchain in banking, financial services, and identity.

He was an active participant in the Wyoming Blockchain Coalition and helped bring 13 landmark pieces of legislation into Wyoming, and into the United States for an open blockchain, the definition of a utility token and SPDI (Special Purpose Depository Institution). This legislation has been adopted across more than 17 other states. This legislation is creating new space and a stable legal framework for digital asset innovation.

Paul is an honors graduate of the Massachusetts Institute of Technology (MIT) Fintech/Blockchain Certificate Program, has an MBA in entrepreneurship and finance from the F. W. Olin Graduate School of Business, Babson College, and is an honors graduate of Northeastern University, College of Health Sciences.

He earned a PhD in health services administration, an MBA from the University of Alabama at Birmingham (UAB), and an MS in information and communication sciences from Ball State University. He has published research articles in academic journals (e.g., *Health Care Management Review, Preventive Medicine, Journal of General Internal Medicine*, and *Studies in Health Technology and Informatics*) and presented at a number of conferences (e.g., Healthcare Information and Management Systems Society, Academy of Management, American Medical Informatics Association, and Academy Health).

Michael Renzi, DO, joined CDPHP in 2019 as medical director for population health development, and currently serves as president of healthcare delivery. As a fervent proponent of aligned member payer-provider value, Dr. Renzi leads CDPHP in network development, sustainable MLR, reproducible five-star quality and next-generation care delivery. Additionally, Dr. Renzi oversees CDPHP technology, analytics, and clinical data aggregation.

Dr. Renzi received his bachelor's degree at Lafayette College and earned his doctor of osteopathic medicine degree at Philadelphia College of Osteopathic Medicine. He spent 25 years as a primary care internist while developing several multi-specialty physician groups. Over the last

15 years, Dr. Renzi pioneered and built population health ventures with the sole intent of aligning payment and value for everyone who finances, delivers, and receives medical care.

For Dr. Renzi, the best part about working for CDPHP is the single-focus, matrixed, and collaborative culture that extends from the boardroom to the mailroom: provide members what they need.

Teresa Rufin, MPH, is a Program Manager at Valera Health. Prior to Valera, she worked as a behavioral health researcher at Columbia University Medical Center. She received her master's in public health in health policy at the Harvard T. H. Chan School of Public Health and holds an AB in psychology from Princeton University.

Chang-Hui Shen, PhD, is a professor and Chair of Biology at the College of Staten Island, City University of New York. He is also affiliated with the Graduate Center and Institute of Macromolecular Assemblies, City University of New York. Dr. Shen completed his doctorate at the University of Edinburgh (UK).

He previously was a visiting fellow of the National Institutes of Health (USA) before taking a position at the College of Staten Island. Dr. Shen's research interests lie in the area of the regulation of gene expression, with an emphasis on the roles of epigenetic factors and transcription factors in gene activation. He also pursues topics such as the regulation of programmed cell death through major cellular signal transduction pathways, as well as the use of next generation sequencing in microbiome and genomic analysis. He supervises the Medical Laboratory Science program at the College of Staten Island and works closely with hospitals to provide clinical training for medical laboratory science students. Recently, he is funded to establish the CSI Genomic Facility for NGS training and genomic research.

Marie Smith, PharmD, FNAP, is the Henry A. Palmer Endowed Professorship of Community Pharmacy Practice and, Assistant Dean for Practice and Public Policy Partnerships at the University of Connecticut School of Pharmacy. In 2013, she served as senior adviser to the CMS Innovation Center (CMMI) in Baltimore, MD, to develop a national strategy and implementation plan to integrate pharmacist-provided medication management services in the Comprehensive Primary Care Initiative. Dr. Smith has worked with multiple state-level and national healthcare reform policymakers and stakeholders to address healthcare delivery issues that involve medication management programs, patient safety, performance measures, health information technology, and integration of clinical pharmacists in advanced primary care practices (workforce development).

Prior to joining the Uconn School of Pharmacy faculty, Dr. Smith was vice president, e-strategy and integration, at Aventis Pharmaceuticals, and was on the senior management staff at the American Society of Heath-System Pharmacists, where she led business development, publishing and software development teams. Dr. Smith is a graduate of the University of Connecticut and Medical College of Virginia Schools of Pharmacy, and completed a hospital pharmacy residency at Thomas Jefferson University Hospital in Philadelphia. In addition, she completed a Fellowship in Change Management at Johns Hopkins University and post-graduate work in global leadership executive education at the Wharton School (University of Pennsylvania) and INSEAD (France).

Daniel M. Stein, MD, PhD, is the Associate Chief Information Officer at Memorial Sloan Kettering Cancer Center. He leads the Tech Incubation team, which aims to transform cancer care through experimentation with new technologies in a variety of breakthrough domains. Dr. Stein has over a decade of research, teaching, and operational experience in clinical informatics, primarily working with clinician- and patient-facing systems with a focus on supporting safe, effective, and collaborative care. He mentors and teaches graduate students as Adjunct Assistant Professor and "Clinical Innovator in Residence" at Cornell Tech, and as Assistant Professor of Healthcare Policy and Research at Weill Cornell Medicine.

Victoria L. Tiase, PhD, RN-BC, FAMIA, FAAN, is a nurse, informatician, and researcher. She is the Director of Research Science in the Value Institute at NewYork–Presbyterian Hospital and is an Assistant Professor in Health Informatics at Weill Cornell Medicine. She supports a range of clinical information technology projects related to patient engagement and is passionate about the integration of patient generated health data into clinical workflows.

Dr. Tiase serves on the steering committee for the Alliance for Nursing Informatics and is the current Chair of the HIMSS Nursing Informatics Committee. She also serves on the boards of AMIA, NODE.Health, and the CARIN Alliance. She was appointed to the National Academy of Medicine's Future of Nursing 2030 Committee to envision the nurse's role using technology to tackle disparities, promote health equity, and create healthier communities. She completed her BSN at the University of Virginia, her MSN at Columbia University, and her PhD from the University of Utah.

Troy Trygstad, PharmD, MBA, PhD, is the Executive Director of CPESN USA, a clinically integrated network of community-based pharmacy networks that endeavors to improve the quality and effectiveness of enhanced services provided by participating pharmacies and align them with the workflows and payment reform incentives of physicians, their support staff, and other healthcare providers. He also serves as the Vice President of Pharmacy Provider Partnerships for Community Care of North Carolina, an organization providing wrap-around population health management supports for nearly 2,000 primary care practices.

Troy possesses over 20 years of experience with multidisciplinary care teams and intervention development under alternative payment and support models. He was the project director for a Center for multi-year Medicare and Medicaid Innovation Award that tested new models of payment and pharmacy connectivity to primary care providers. Troy co-founded the Pharmacy Home Project in 2007 and a web application to accompany that combined more than 50 different medical list contexts into a single portal utilized by multiple care team members and care managers, including pharmacists in multiple settings of care.

Troy proudly practices in a community pharmacy setting on nights and weekends and served recently as a board member for the American Pharmacists Association Foundation and the Pharmacy Quality Alliance, as well as editor in chief of *Pharmacy Times*. Troy received doctor of pharmacy and master's in business administration degrees from Drake University and a PhD in pharmaceutical outcomes and policy from the University of North Carolina at Chapel Hill.

Thomas Tsang, MD, MPH, is the CEO and co-founder of Valera Health, a telehealth organization providing personalized team-based clinical care. His prior experiences include working as CMO of the largest FQHC network for Asian Americans, CMO at Merck's Digital Service/Solutions division, and medical director at ONC/HHS rolling out aspects of the Affordable Care Act. He was a congressional staffer on the Ways and Means Committee and helped draft legislation for the ACA and also a senior advisor to the governor of Hawaii on value-based.

Salvatore G. Volpe, MA, is a medical student at SUNY Downstate College of Medicine pursuing an MD degree. He earned his MA in biomedical informatics from Columbia University, where he also received his BA in neuroscience with a concentration in computer science.

His areas of research include interoperability, quality improvement, user-interface design, patient-centered technologies, and health equity. Salvatore's graduate studies culminated in a thesis project developing a pipeline for transforming clinical trial data using Fast Healthcare Interoperability Resources (FHIR) protocols and standardized according to the Observational Medical Outcomes Partnership Common Data Model (OMOP CDM) for integration into translational research endeavors and clinical decision support. He has developed mobile applications for clinical and public use in collaboration with University of Colorado Anschultz, Cliexa, and the New York Health Artificial Intelligence Society. Salvatore has published research on COVID-19 in *Nature Communications* and has presented his research at the American Medical Informatics Association Annual Symposium.

When he isn't trying to become a medical multi-hyphenate, Salvatore is an avid musician and composer. He has written and produced songs for short films, stage plays, and full-length musicals.

Keith Weiner, PhD, RN-BC, is a cybersecurity professional, researcher, and professor with 20 years of informatics experience including a decade in information security leadership positions.

He serves on several boards and committees in an effort to help improve health through informatics.

He is also a fellow of the New York Academy of Medicine and active member of HIMSS.

Keith continues to present at research and industry conferences. A contributing author of several textbooks and publications, he has also served on an editorial board and peer reviewer for scientific journals.

In his spare time, Keith plays several musical instruments and is constantly exploring new technologies.

Foreword

Data will do for the healthcare team minds what imaging and x-rays have done for eyes make it clear. Data/health informatics will for the first time allow us to have a plan for every patient and clearly see that plan with ease. Health Informatics: A Comprehensive Guide with Multidisciplinary Approaches is targeted at the expanded participating in the care of patients: nurses, pharmacists, physicians, attorneys, geneticists, public health workers, healthcare executives, programmers and so many more as the family of healthcare expands This is the read you will not but down from the prospective college and graduate students who would like to "make a difference" to the clinician in her 30th year of practice.

Health Informatics brings together healthcare-generated information with technology for the purpose of advancing the quadruple aim of Improved Patient Experience, Better Outcomes, Lower Costs, and Improved Clinical Experience. Written by experts who lived it, Health Informatics: A Comprehensive Guide with Multidisciplinary Approaches provides a comprehensive introduction to key concepts that are vital to healthcare informatics including electronic health records (EHRs), ethics, data and information, privacy and security, research, and future trends. Real-world examples and case studies are used throughout the text to illustrate the concepts.

Dr. Paul Grundy is an American physician known as the "godfather" of the Patient Centered Medical Home. He was named a member of the Institute of Medicine and recipient of the Barbara Starfield Primary Care Leadership Award and the 2012 National Committee for Quality Assurance (NCQA) Quality Award. Dr. Grundy served as IBM's Global Director of Healthcare Transformation and Chief Medical Officer of IBM's Healthcare and Life Science Industry.

Dr. Paul Grundy

Acknowledgements

Since this is not the Oscars where a musical "hook," often brings this section to close, I would like to take a few moments to acknowledge some of the key figures that formed me as person, physician and informaticist.

I must begin with my parents, Gino and Maria Volpe. The two hardest working and caring individuals that I have been blessed to have known. Despite being immigrants with limited education, they successfully faced many challenges and were known in the community as the "go to people." They taught me how to be a loving brother and father and by extension a physician. For a physician who does not love, is just a technician.

Rachel Volpe, my wife, has been my partner in many endeavors and is truly a blessed mother to our sons. She sets the standard for volunteerism in our home.

My sons, Gino and Salvatore. These two wonderful young men sometimes wondered why Papa wasn't around but supported Rachel and me in our mission to serve the community as they have done themselves. Gino, as a young but astute child would often ask if the people we met in the neighborhood were my friends. Yes, patients who would become lifelong friends.

Dr. Francis Giordano, a true mentor and friend for most of my life.

Dr. Edward Wagner created the well-known and widely used Chronic Care Model, and over the course of his career, he has worked to support high-functioning primary care teams to meet the quadruple aim: better care experiences, better population health, lower cost, and happier staff.

Dr. Paul Grundy, "Godfather of the Patient-Centered Medical Home," has spent four decades focused on population health that is built on a platform of a healing relationship of trust in primary care.

Dr. William Hersh who accepted me in his AMIA-OHSU 10x10 Program over 15 years ago and encouraged and assisted many of us to become informaticists through all his academic endeavors.

Dr. Farzad Mostashari and Mat Kendall who gave this solo practice doc a chance to participate in one of the greatest health information technology transformations in NYC while still caring for my patients.

Dr. Kenneth Ong who invited me and several of our current authors to contribute to his book and who has been a friend and mentor for many years.

Dr. Joseph Conte and the team at the Staten Island Performing Providers System who have created an environment that fostered excellence in the pursuit of improving the quality of life for our fellow Staten Islanders.

My fellow authors who despite the toll taken upon them and their families by COVID-19 persevered in their day jobs while providing us with informative chapters that give us the tools to address the gaps in healthcare delivery while helping us prepare for the next health crisis.

Last but not least, Kristine Mednansky our Senior Editor at Taylor and Francis for her encouragement and guidance in the creation of this book.

Introduction

According to the American Medical Informatics Association (AMIA), "Biomedical and health informatics applies principles of computer and information science to the advancement of life sciences research, health professions education, public health, and patient care. This multidisciplinary and integrative field focuses on health information technologies (HIT), and involves the computer, cognitive, and social sciences."[1] According to the Healthcare Information and Management Systems Society (HIMSS), "health IT is interprofessional by nature and must be reflected in education and training."[2]

The COVID-19 pandemic has made us aware of the strengths and weakness of our healthcare system and society. One of the healthcare system's strengths was the health information technology infrastructure in some regions that permitted more effective exchange of patient information. This was particularly critical as patients were transferred between non-affiliated healthcare systems and often to locations that were not originally designed for healthcare, such as convention centers. Other types of information were also exchanged. Specifications for personal protective equipment and even ventilators were freely shared so that garage factories could produce what was needed using 3-D printers and other means.

Many people from different professions came together to offer their services to help those in need.

This book is a clarion call for those that want to continue this tradition. Whether you are in high school, college, or graduate school, or at the patient's bedside or your work desk (virtual or otherwise), let this book open your eyes to the opportunities. We are calling out to all who are looking to make a difference in the general well-being and health of their communities. The authors and their chapters represent a wide spectrum of professions: attorneys, behavioral health experts, business development experts, chief information officers, chief medical officers, chief nursing information officers, consumer advocates, cryptographic experts, futurists, geneticists, informaticists, managed care executives, nurses, pharmacists, physicians, public health professionals, software developer, systems security officers, and workforce experts.

Join and help us grow our team – this book is just the beginning!

1. See https://www.amia.org/fact-sheets/what-informatics
2. See *Understanding Health Informatics Core Competencies*, by Johannes Thye, MA, faculty of Business Management and Social Sciences, University of Applied Sciences Osnabrück, Germany; consortium member of the EU*US eHealth Work Project, https://www.himss.org/resources/health-informatics

Chapter 1

The Value of Health IT

Nancy J. Beale, MSN, RN-BC

Contents

As the model of healthcare in the United States shifts from a volume-based model into a value-based model, operationalizing the concepts and tenets of a value-based model can be challenging. Pursuant to this transformational change, significant investments in health and information technology continue to soar to meet the demands of quantifying value. In early 2020, global healthcare technology spending was projected to hit $4 trillion by 2021 (Park 2020). Since the start of the pandemic, many systems have shifted strategy and adjusted budgets to ensure their systems could remain viable (Drees 2021). Despite these adjustments, organizations across the globe continue to invest significant resources with an aim toward enhanced clinical and financial outcomes.

Measuring Value

The Health Information Management Systems Society (HIMSS) maturity models were designed as vendor agnostic roadmaps to convey a vision of desired outcomes realized with technology in healthcare. These maturity models have evolved to include analytics (AMAM), continuity of care (CCMM), clinically integrated supply outcomes (CISOM), digital imaging adoption

DOI: 10.4324/9780429423109-1

(Saxena et al. 2018), electronic medal records (EMRAM), infrastructure (INFRAM), and out-patient medical record adoption (O-EMRAM) (HIMSS 2017). Each of these models includes eight stages and acknowledges the unique requirements for the specified area of focus, providing guidance and measures to measure and advance an organization's progress toward achieving the greatest value from technology. Many examples can be found among organizations across the globe that have achieved measures of success through the various HIMSS maturity and adoption models (HIMSS 2017). These successes range from cost savings to improved patient outcomes and error reduction.

Health IT as a Strategic Asset

The view of technology by healthcare executives is shifting from a cost center to a strategic asset, as healthcare organizations leverage the advanced capabilities that technology can enable. Technology has been successfully demonstrated by many organizations to enhance patient and financial outcomes, improve efficiencies, and enhance patient and clinician satisfaction. Leading organizations align technology plans with organizational strategic plans. With a clear vision of both horizontal and vertical transparency for the organization, NYU Langone Health executed that vision, leveraging data to manage the organization on the basis of metrics and benchmarks (Haseltine 2019). Foundational use of technology to create accessible, actionable, and integrated data laid the groundwork for transformational change at this organization. Aligning technology with the strategic plan of the organization enabled NYU Langone Health to integrate and share data across the health system, significantly improving quality, safety, efficiency, and financial stability. In the span of a decade, combining organizational strategy and management with technology enhanced capabilities, the NYU Langone Health moved from the bottom third in national quality and safety to one of the top two academic health systems in the country (Haseltine 2019). While not entirely unique, the NYU Langone Health success story is a leading example of how to realize the value of health IT as a strategic asset.

Technology Enabled Care

In the midst of a pandemic, technology has quickly taken an expedited step forward, with telehealth center stage. In Wuhan, China the novel coronavirus disease (Covid-19) surfaced at the end of 2019. Prior to the Covid-19 pandemic, the implementation and adoption of telehealth was minimal among most healthcare organizations across the globe. In the United States, there were reimbursement and regulatory barriers as well as fundamental infrastructure gaps for some healthcare organizations. Relaxation of these regulations as well as reimbursement for telehealth services allowed rapid expansion of telehealth services for those with programs in place. For others, the lack of broadband or smartphone access as well as gaps in basic digital skills remain barriers to successful telehealth implementation and adoption. Beyond the pandemic, there is a significant push in healthcare to enhance access to telehealth as a standard of care. The use of telehealth has been identified as a significant strategy to enhance access to care, particularly in rural areas that may be remote from an emergency department or urgent care (Khairat et al. 2019) (See chapter 28 Telemedicine and Beyond).

The role of Health Information Exchange (HIE) became increasingly important and also challenging during the early days of the pandemic. As patients were moving because of the pandemic, in many cases triaged from one facility to another, it was challenging to access health information.

Pre-existing regulations around privacy at both the state and local levels presented a significant barrier to the creation of ad hoc systems of care and dissemination of information about a patient's infectious status across state lines amid a mobile population (Lenert and McSwain 2020). The technological capabilities exist; however, regulation and policies must align. (See chapter 15: Health Information Exchange: An Overview & New York State's Model).

Never before has day-to-day knowledge of data been shared across the globe at every level and at the speed with which the Covid-19 data and statistics have been shared. Data is the currency enabled by technology. Data are being shared daily about testing, infections, and vaccinations. This profound use and consumption of data by scientists, healthcare professionals, and consumers has thrust the importance of data, data quality, and analytics to the fore.

Examining Success Stories and Incentives

The Health Information Technology for Economic and Clinical Health (HITECH) Act was signed into law in 2009 with an aim to accelerate electronic health record implementation and meaningful use in US health systems. Billions of dollars in incentive payments were created to encourage health systems to adopt electronic health records by 2016. The Meaningful Use (MU) program defined the criteria to receive incentive payments (Technology 2013). Outcomes from the MU program have shown an overall increase in adoption of electronic health records and health-care IT across the United States; however, disparities in adoption and access to technology remain in rural areas and other underserved settings (Mack et al. 2016). The HIMSS maturity models were designed as a vendor-neutral methodology to align and support the industry best practices. Each of the maturity models has eight levels, ranging from Stage 0 at the lowest level to Stage 7 at the highest level. More than a decade after inception, the HIMSS analytics database shows that more than 65% of healthcare facilities have advanced their capabilities to an EMRAM Stage 5 or greater since inception in 2005. Yet, some have predicted that a considerable number of hospitals will not be able to achieve Stage 7 by 2035 (Kharrazi et al. 2018). Those organizations achieving Stage 7 EMRAM have met the required criteria, which includes a complete EMR, an external HIE, data analytics, governance, and disaster recovery, as well as privacy and security measures in place (HIMSS 2017). While achieving Stage 7 may seem daunting and expensive, results have demonstrated that implementing these technologies makes a difference.

Maturity Model Exemplars. Rush University Medical Center demonstrated an improvement to clinical workflow through the integration of predictive models to identify patients most likely to leave the emergency department without being seen (LWBS) by a practitioner. This initiative led to a reduction of LWBS in the emergency department from 3.83% to 1.25%, gaining approximately $1.5 million in revenue per year as a result (HIMSS Analytics 2019). This technology intervention used the HIMSS Analytics Adoption Model for Analytics Maturity (AMAM) to achieve increased efficiencies, enhanced quality, and improved patient satisfaction.

Davies Awards

The HIMSS Nicholas E. Davies Award of Excellence was first introduced in 1994, recognizing outstanding achievement by organizations that utilize health information and technology to improve clinical outcomes and drive operational and financial value (HIMSS 2021). In more than 25 years of recognizing organizations for demonstrating sustainable improvements using healthcare technology, organizations continue to find innovative strategies to leverage technology tools, improve care quality, and maximize savings. The case studies of Davies Award winners are numerous and demonstrate a variety of strategies that organizations are using to realize the value of healthcare IT.

Multiple organizations have submitted HIMSS award-winning use cases demonstrating a variety of strategies to combat the opioid crisis. Strategies and solutions ranged from configuration and workflow changes to identify patients with high risk of addition to connections between the electronic health record (EHR) and multiple state prescription drug monitoring programs (PDMP). Mercy Health in Ohio and Yale New Haven Health in Connecticut are organizations that leveraged the electronic health record to impact the clinical treatment of patients, effectively reducing the overall opioid prescription rate. Through the development of tools, analytics, and workflow modifications to improve and measure opioid-prescribing behavior, these organizations were able to leverage technology and realize enhanced healthcare value. Through the use of these tools, this organization was able to realize significant improvements in one year, including a 43% reduction in the number of acute opioid orders prescribed with more than a seven-day prescription.

Patient Engagement

The patient's journey begins long before they step into a healthcare facility. Organizations are beginning to implement integrated mobile health (mhealth) technologies that leverage geolocating to enable directions to the facility. Mhealth solutions are also used to engage patients before their visit to complete tasks like verifying information, reviewing instructions, or answering questionnaires to prepare for their appointment. Some mobile platforms are also connecting patient devices to upload their health data such as blood pressure, weight, or glucometer readings to their medical record, enabling patients as true partners in their care. The consumer is playing a growing role in defining how they want to experience healthcare. Patients want access to their health information and to be partners in their care.

In the acute care space, there are a growing number of technology platforms aimed at patient engagement. These platforms have a variety of integrations that can combine access to multiple functions, such as the patient's record, information about the care team, patient education, meal ordering, integrative health, and patient entertainment, among others. (See chapter 2 Patient Engagement).

The Value of Informatics

It is only once the technology is in place that we can begin to realize value; that value can only be realized with the knowledge and skill of the informatics team, which will bring about that return on investment and value realization. Having a well-qualified team that includes not only skilled technologists but also knowledgeable clinical informaticists is essential. In addition to holding critical knowledge that about clinical workflow, clinical informaticists play an integral role in design, implementation, training, and optimization, each of which impacts patient safety. Design of decision support, use of artificial intelligence, and design of algorithms that can improve outcomes and health equity requires knowledgeable clinical informaticists (Veinot, Ancker, and Bakken 2019).

Clinical Informatics Executive Roles

In 2010, the chief medical information officer (CMIO) role was considered an emerging position in US health systems, with few identifying this role in their organizational chart (Stanley 2010).

In 2021, most major US health systems have identified the work of informatics as highly interprofessional, with a need for governance structures, adequate resources from the clinical professions (medicine, nursing, pharmacy, etc.), and role-based competencies (Collins, Alexander, and Moss 2015). The chief nursing informatics officer (CNIO) role has evolved similarly to the CMIO role over time, with a growing number of organizations employing the role of CNIO. These key executive clinical IT roles are important interprofessional partners that contribute to the quality and safety of an organization, guiding clinical technology strategy and practice (Collins, Alexander, and Moss 2015). The chief clinical information officer (Kannry and Fridsma 2016) role encompasses the CMIO and CNIO roles as well as other clinical informatics executive roles. This role was introduced in 2016 and is supported by the American Medical Informatics Association (Kannry and Fridsma 2016) in acknowledgment of the professionalization of the informatics field and the rise in leadership positions that recognize the importance of informatics (Kannry and Fridsma 2016). Clinical informatics leadership plays a critical role in successful governance, implementation, and support of a clinical technology plan that will yield value.

The Value Equation

Technology alone will not provide value in healthcare. People, process, and technology are integral pieces of a larger and more complex puzzle that must be carefully aligned to realize the value of technology in healthcare. EHR and other health technology software vendors are shifting to sociotechnical systems models to design and implement software (Carayon and Salwei 2021). In the Systems Engineering Initiative for Patient Safety (SEIPS) model 2.0, the concepts of configuration, engagement, and adaptation are incorporated into the original SEIPS model, consisting of the main principles of systems orientation, person-centeredness, and design-driven improvements (Holden et al. 2013). A continued evolution of this framework, SEIPS 3.0 includes enhancements to reflect the patient journey and the distributed nature of care over time and space (Carayon et al. 2020). The use of design-thinking and sociotechnical approaches to healthcare technology design, implementation, and optimization will continue to be substantial factors in value realization for the future.

About the Author

Nancy J. Beale, MSN, RN-BC, As a healthcare professional for 35 years, Nancy's experience spans clinical operations, vendor perspective, consulting, and IT operations. While at NYU Langone Health, Nancy led a team of 250 people, and growing award-winning talent to achieve HIMSS 6, HIMSS 7, HIMSS Davies Award, and several innovation partnerships. As an IT executive, she served as a leader in the successful development and execution of the clinical IT strategy for the health system, as well as the clinical IT strategy and execution to support merger and acquisition activity of the health system. Her work also included forming an offshore partnership with a vendor in India for operational IT support services and oversight of onshore clinical help desk operations. In her role as vice president, Nancy provided leadership and guidance over the clinical systems team in the clinical IT implementation of a new and fully digital hospital in Manhattan. Her work is nationally recognized and award winning, recognized as the 2019 HIMSS-ANI Nursing Informatics Leader of the year.

Nancy holds a master's in nursing with an emphasis in health systems and healthcare informatics. She is board certified in nursing informatics and currently a PhD candidate at the University of Wisconsin–Madison focused on clinical technology adoption with a minor in human factors and design thinking. As a doctoral student, Nancy led a team of design students to win first place in the 2019 Medline Innovation Challenge across multiple universities to redesign patient gowns and surgical masks.

As a clinician, Nancy worked across the continuum of care including long-term care, acute care medical and surgical, inpatient obstetrics/labor and delivery, and ambulatory care. The majority of her clinical years in direct care were spent in the specialty of perinatal nursing. Nancy has held a variety of positions from staff nurse, mentor, and educator to manager and director in clinical roles. Since leaving direct patient care in 2002, Nancy has held a variety of roles in healthcare IT, including clinical lead of software implementation, program director, executive consultant, senior director, and vice president. From 1998 to 2003 she served in leadership roles in the Wisconsin Region of the Association of Women's Health and Neonatal Nursing. She is the current co-chair of the Alliance of Nursing Informatics and chair-elect for the Midwest Nursing Research Society–Health Systems, Policy & Informatics research interest group. Nancy has served in policy roles for both the Alliance of Nursing Informatics and the Nursing Knowledge Big Data workgroup. She is also one of two nurses serving on the national DaVinci Clinical Advisory Committee. Nancy holds additional membership in AONL, ACHE, AMIA, ANA, ANIA, AWHONN, HIMSS, MNRS, and Sigma Theta Tau. Nancy has worked with national healthcare leaders implementing technologies. Nancy's work has included partnerships with IT, vendors, nursing, physicians, and allied health providers. She has provided systems strategy, configuration, and clinical transformation guidance as well as collaborative oversight and integration with revenue cycle systems and operations. Her blend of experience has provided a rich background in the role of an executive in healthcare IT and clinical informatics. Nancy's desire to impact change in healthcare as a lifelong learner, along with her professional experiences have positioned her well as an advisor for strategic systems leadership. (The author has elected to list all the references used for the chapter at the end without direct in-text citation).

References

Analytics, HIMSS. 2017. "STAGE 7 SPOTLIGHT mercy health: 50% Reduction in opioid prescriptions." *HIMSS*, accessed May 26. https://www.himssanalytics.org/news/stage-7-spotlight-mercy-health-50-reduction-opioid-prescriptions.

Analytics, HIMSS. 2019. "STAGE 7 SPOTLIGHT RUMC: Improving the clinical workflow." *HIMSS*, accessed May 26. https://www.himssanalytics.org/news/stage-7-spotlight-rumc-improving-clinical-workflow.

Carayon, P., A. Wooldridge, P. Hoonakker, A. S. Hundt, and M. M. Kelly. 2020. "SEIPS 3.0: Human-centered design of the patient journey for patient safety." *Applied Ergonomics* 84:103033. doi:10.1016/j.apergo.2019.103033.

Carayon, P., and M. E. Salwei. 2021. "Moving toward a sociotechnical systems approach to continuous health information technology design: The path forward for improving electronic health record usability and reducing clinician burnout." *Journal of the American Medical Informatics Association* 28 (5):1026–1028. doi:10.1093/jamia/ocab002.

Collins, Sarah A., Dana Alexander, and Jacqueline Moss. 2015. "Nursing domain of CI governance: Recommendations for health IT adoption and optimization." *Journal of the American Medical Informatics Association* 22 (3):697–706. doi:10.1093/jamia/ocu001.

Drees, J. 2021. "IT budget spend: Where hospital CIOs are focusing in 2021." *Becker's*, accessed May 22. https://www.beckershospitalreview.com/healthcare-information-technology/it-budget-spend-where-hospital-cios-are-focusing-in-2021.html.

Haseltine, William A. 2019. *World class: A story of adversity, transformation, and success at NYU Langone Health*. First edition. New York: Fast Company Press.

HIMSS. 2017. "Electronic medical record adoption model." *HIMSS*, accessed January 27, 2021. https://www.himssanalytics.org/emram.

HIMSS. 2021. "HIMSS Davies Award of Excellence." *Health Information Management Systems Society*, accessed May 26. https://www.himss.org/what-we-do-opportunities/davies-award-excellence.

Holden, R. J., P. Carayon, A. P. Gurses, P. Hoonakker, A. S. Hundt, A. A. Ozok, and A. J. Rivera-Rodriguez. 2013. "SEIPS 2.0: A human factors framework for studying and improving the work of healthcare professionals and patients." *Ergonomics* 56 (11):1669–1686. doi:10.1080/00140139.2013.838643.

Kannry, Joseph, MD, Chair, AMIA Task Force on CCIO Knowledge, Education, and Skillset Requirements, and Doug Fridsma, MD, PhD, FACP, FACMI, President and CEO, AMIA. 2016. "The chief clinical informatics officer (CCIO)." *Journal of the American Medical Informatics Association* 23 (2):435–435. doi:10.1093/jamia/ocw034.

Khairat, Saif, Timothy Haithcoat, Songzi Liu, Tanzila Zaman, Barbara Edson, Robert Gianforcaro, and Chi-Ren Shyu. 2019. "Advancing health equity and access using telemedicine: A geospatial assessment." *Journal of the American Medical Informatics Association* 26 (8–9):796–805. doi:10.1093/jamia/ocz108.

Kharrazi, H., C. P. Gonzalez, K. B. Lowe, T. R. Huerta, and E. W. Ford. 2018. "Forecasting the maturation of electronic health record functions among US hospitals: Retrospective analysis and predictive model." *Journal of Medical Internet Research* 20 (8):e10458. doi:10.2196/10458.

Lenert, Leslie, and Brooke Yeager McSwain. 2020. "Balancing health privacy, health information exchange, and research in the context of the COVID-19 pandemic." *Journal of the American Medical Informatics Association* 27 (6):963–966. doi:10.1093/jamia/ocaa039.

Mack, D., S. Zhang, M. Douglas, C. Sow, H. Strothers, and G. Rust. 2016. "Disparities in primary care EHR adoption rates." *Journal of Health Care for the Poor and Underserved* 27 (1):327–338. doi:10.1353/hpu.2016.0016.

Park, A. 2020. "IT spending to hit $3.9T in 2020: 4 things to know." *Becker's Health IT*, accessed May 10. https://www.beckershospitalreview.com/healthcare-information-technology/it-spending-to-hit-3-9t-in-2020-4-things-to-know.html.

Saxena, K., R. Diamond, R. F. Conant, T. H. Mitchell, I. G. Gallopyn, and K. E. Yakimow. 2018. "Provider adoption of speech recognition and its impact on satisfaction, documentation quality, efficiency, and cost in an inpatient EHR." *AMIA Summits on Translational Science Proceedings* 2017:186–195.

Stanley, D. 2010. "The evolution of the CMIO role. Interview by Mark Hagland." *Healthcare Informatics* 27 (11):45–46.

Technology, Office of the National Coordinator for Health Information. 2013. What is meaningful use? edited by U.S. Department of Health and Human Services: Healthit.gov.

Veinot, T. C., J. S. Ancker, and S. Bakken. 2019. "Health informatics and health equity: Improving our reach and impact." *Journal of the American Medical Informatics Association* 26 (8–9):689–695. doi:10.1093/jamia/ocz132.

Chapter 2

Personal Health Engagement

Jan Oldenburg, FHIMSS

Contents

Introduction

"Nothing about us without us" and "give me my DaM data"[1] are mantras of the e-patient movement. Their power lies in the acknowledgment that health is owned by the patient; that health, treatment, recovery, and even billing are things that the healthcare ecosystem needs to do *with* patients, not *to* them.

Personal health engagement entails the recognition that health is intensely personal and is a critical dimension of people's whole lives, not limited to their role as patients within the healthcare system. This perspective allows us to move from a "patient engagement" perspective, which primarily refers to people in their role as patients, to look more broadly at what it means to be engaged with your own health as well as the health of your family, friends, and community. In this chapter, we will explore personal health engagement and how digital tools support people in

DOI: 10.4324/9780429423109-2

9

the many dimensions of health. Because much of the available research is still focused on "patient engagement" – the way people interact within the healthcare system – we will talk both about "personal health engagement" *and* "patient engagement."

Many factors are converging today to force changes in the healthcare system, but four have special impact on consumers' attitudes and perspectives about health, healthcare, and technology:

- The rise of consumerism and personal empowerment in our society as a whole means that individuals are coming to their healthcare experiences expecting to be treated and cared for as individuals and partners.
- Ubiquitous access to technology and digital tools creates expectations that the convenient digital capabilities people use elsewhere in their everyday lives will be available to them to manage their health.
- Consumers in the US pay an increasing part of their healthcare costs, which means that individuals expect to be able to research prices, understand ahead of time what treatments will cost, receive timely, clear, and straightforward bills, and pay in convenient ways.
- Improvements in sensors, wearable devices, apps, and at-home monitoring tools create the opportunity to integrate information about an individual's health and behavior between visits into care and treatment. While there is still conflicting data about the effectiveness of these devices in helping people better manage their health, the opportunity and potential are significant.

All of these elements are driving change that can be a key lever in healthcare transformation. Wise health systems are paying attention, looking for ways they can support consumers, build loyalty, and lower costs by providing technology and services that better serve consumers.

In healthcare, we have traditionally assessed a person's level of engagement based primarily on whether he/she is compliant with the plan of care that we've created. We have taught people that their role in relation to the healthcare system is to be passive and obedient. But the ideal of "compliant" patients is shifting as we realize that patients are demanding more control over and participation in their health choices. Today many consumers expect a measure of control even when they are patients in the healthcare system. They expect to be treated as valued customers or partners who have a say in what happens. They expect digital tools to make interacting with the healthcare system easier. They may even choose self-service, telehealth, or peer support rather than or in addition to consulting a traditional doctor in a traditional setting. Healthcare systems must address these new consumer expectations and behaviors in order to create satisfying experiences.

The healthcare system is responding to these changes, albeit slowly. The Center for Advancing Health published a definition of patient engagement in 2011 as part of their "Engaging Behavior Framework." They defined patient engagement as follows:

> Actions individuals must take to obtain the greatest benefit from the health care services available to them. This definition focuses on behaviors of individuals relative to their health care that are critical and proximal to health outcomes, rather than the actions of professionals or policies of institutions. *Engagement is not synonymous with compliance.* Compliance means an individual obeys a directive from a health care provider. Engagement signifies that a person is involved in a process through which he or she harmonizes robust information and professional advice with his or her own needs, preferences and abilities in order to prevent, manage, and cure disease.[2]

We have modified that definition to incorporate *personal* health engagement as follows:

> Personal health engagement signifies that a person is involved in a process through which they harmonize robust information, professional advice, and tools available to them with their own needs, preferences, and abilities in order to live healthily and prevent, manage and cure disease as an individual, caregiver, patient, and community member.

The modified definition highlights the fact that a personal health engagement is not limited to choices about treatment options in the context of existing professional care relationships. It also includes choices about where to get care, what care team the person wants, and the lifestyle choices and options that impact a person's health.[3]

Personal health engagement is significant because when individuals take responsibility for their care, all dimensions of the triple aim of healthcare are affected in positive ways:

- ■ Improving the individual experience of care (including quality and satisfaction)
- ■ Improving the health of populations
- ■ Reducing the per capita costs of care for populations[4]

In 2014, an article in the *Annals of Family Medicine* suggested that the triple aim should be expanded to be the quadruple aim, with "care team wellbeing" as the fourth aim.[5] Many healthcare institutions have adopted some version of this expanded definition, though they may refer to it as "joy in work" or "improved clinical experience" rather than "care team wellbeing." Others have made the fourth aim "health equity." In the military, the fourth aim is "readiness." IHI cautions that in adding a fourth aim, institutions must remember that the triple aim is really one goal with three components; in adding a fourth aim, it's important to remember that the focus still needs to be on patients. [6] In this chapter, we will refer to the fourth aim as "care team wellbeing," as patient care, engagement, and experience suffer when the care team is struggling. We'll highlight the impact that personal health tools are having across all dimensions of healthcare. We will also discuss the issues that are impeding the progress and adoption of health IT tools that support individuals.

Current State of Personal Health IT

For years, consumers and patients have been saying they are interested in having access to their own healthcare data in a consolidated form as well as the ability to email their doctors and see their doctors' notes – the capabilities offered by most patient portals. Many people also use sensors, apps, and tools to communicate with their doctors and track their own health. When surveyed, people indicate high interest in digital capabilities that will help them manage their health.

Yet, many Americans don't access their health data even when it is available. As of 2017, 52% of Americans had been offered access to their health records through a portal, and a little over half of those individuals actually looked at their records – 28% of Americans.[7] In 2018, the overall percentage of Americans who looked at their records rose to 33%,[8] rising further to 40% in 2019.[9] Practices that tightly integrate portal use with other aspects of care tend to have higher portal registration rates. Kaiser Permanente and Group Health Cooperative are examples of this tight integration, and both boast health portal enrollment of over 70% of members.[10] Fewer people access their hospital records than their ambulatory records. A November 2019 study, using data from 2016–2017, found that only about 10% of hospital patients accessed their records – even fewer in underserved communities.[11] These results are echoed in a study published in 2018 from University of Iowa Hospitals and Clinics.[12]

This behavior regarding patient portals contrasts with consumer adoption of other online tools. In 2018, 80% of American consumers used mobile banking tools at least nine days a month – and the percentage of people banking electronically is even higher when you include web-based tools.[13] Almost 70% of Americans shopped online in 2018,[14] and 82% of Americans got at least some of their news digitally.[15] These levels of adoption of digital tools significantly outpace adoption in healthcare. We'll explore some of the reasons for the slower pace of adoption in healthcare later in the chapter.

The use of digital health tools, specifically portals, is generally correlated to higher socio-economic status. Socio-economic status has a greater impact on health portal use among Blacks and Hispanics than among Caucasians.[16] Other research "indicates that nonusers are more likely to be male and age 65 or older, have less than a college degree, not be employed, live in a rural location, be on Medicaid, and not have a regular provider." Importantly, factors that correlated to lower health portal enrollment also lowered the likelihood that portal use was even discussed with patients.[17] Data from ONC indicates that doctors are more likely to recommend the portal to wealthier and more highly educated individuals.[18] This differential is likely to exacerbate the digital divide in portal use.

A 2019 meta-study looked at more than 100 studies that documented disparities in health portal use among vulnerable populations in order to understand what interventions best address the disparities. The authors identified a variety of interventions that matter, including increasing the usability of portals, assigning videos to be viewed via portals, and providing support/training to patients to increase their understanding of how to use them. Addressing health literacy for all patients is likely to also impact disparities in portal use: "Interventions to improve awareness of the portal and eHealth literacy skills of patients and further integration of the patient portal in normal care are needed to increase use and potential benefits for patients."[19] One of the study's important conclusions is that both one-on-one and organizational-level interventions contribute to reducing disparities in portal use.

One of the initiatives that has shown success in getting people to use their online portals is the open notes initiative, which provides patients with access to their physician's notes. Although the uptake rates on patients invited to view their notes were not significantly different than portal uptake in general, open notes seemed to be particularly useful in helping underserved populations take control of their health. A study exploring these issues looked at six potential benefits from patients reading their notes: feeling in control, preparing for visits, remembering the plan of care, taking care of health, making the most of visits, and having an active role. They reported the following outcomes:

> Black patients were more likely than white patients to rate note reading as very important for 5 of the 6 benefits and patients aged 45 years or older rated it very important for 4 of the benefits compared with those aged 18 to 24 years. Those who usually spoke a language other than English at home were more likely than English speakers to use notes to make the most of visits, remember the plan of care, and prepare for visits. Patients with the fewest years of education and Hispanic patients were more likely than others to cite note reading as very important for remembering the care plan and preparing for visits. Patients who read a greater number of notes were more likely to cite reading notes as very important for all 6 benefits.[20]

People also use wearable devices, smartphone applications, and social media to engage with their health outside of the constraints of the healthcare system. A Gallup poll conducted in November of 2019 showed that about a third of Americans have used a fitness tracker or mobile app to track their health now or in the past. In the same survey, about 75% of current or past users of wearable fitness trackers found them very (30%) or somewhat helpful (46%). About 82% of those who used health apps found them very (29%) or somewhat helpful (53%).[21] The poll also found that adults under 55 were almost twice as likely to have used digital health tools as adults aged 55 and older.

Deloitte has been tracking consumer attitudes about health since 2011. In their 2018 survey, 42% of individuals reported using digital tools for measuring health and fitness goals, up from 17% in 2013.[22] Similarly, a 2018 study across Canada showed that about two-thirds of adults tracked at least one health metric regularly and about a quarter used digital tools to do so. Of those who used digital tools, 68% said that the smart digital devices allowed them to maintain or improve their health condition and 66% said the tools helped them to be better informed about their health in general.[23]

The news about apps and wearables is not universally good, however. There were 400 million downloads of medical apps in 2018, up 15% from 2016; health and wellness app downloads also grew during that period.[24] Despite the plethora of digital health and wellness apps (400,000+ at last count),[25] only about 50% of health apps are downloaded more than 500 times, and most (70%) are kept on people's phones less than 90 days.[26] Most health apps receive fewer than 10,000 downloads.[27]

Accenture has been tracking use digital health annually for five years. For the first time, the 2020 survey, conducted in 2019, showed reductions in the use of apps and trackers to manage health.

> Use of mobile devices and applications fell from nearly half (48%) using these tools in 2018 to only 35% in 2020. Use of wearable technology – for instance, devices that collect health data such as fitness and vitals – has decreased from 33% in 2018 to just 18% in 2020.[28]

These are decidedly mixed signals. There is evidence that digital health tools can positively impact health outcomes, healthcare costs, and patient/physician relationships. There's also evidence that to realize their promise, digital tools need to be improved. They need to be more intuitive, more convenient, and better integrated into healthcare systems, and must deliver better and more actionable insights. Consumers also want to be able to trust that the tools incorporate strong privacy protections and consumer choice about access to their data as part of their underlying infrastructure.

Personal Health IT Regulatory Background

Providing patients with electronic access to their records was fueled by the adoption of Meaningful Use requirements in 2010 as part of the Health Information Technology for Economic and Clinical Health (HITECH) Act passed in 2009.[29] The associated rule-making, focused on providing patients with electronic access to their data, amplified existing HIPAA rules. The process was influenced in part by the testimony of e-patients such as Dave deBronkart, who testified to the Meaningful Use Workgroup's HIT Policy Committee as well as the Adoption and Certification Workgroup,[30] and Regina Holiday, who testified to the National Committee on Vital Health

Statistics.[31] The Meaningful Use requirements called for physicians to provide timely access to any records held electronically. In addition, the rules required qualifying organizations to enable patients "to **view online, download and transmit** their health information." Initial Meaningful Use rules also required healthcare organizations to demonstrate the ability to "use **secure electronic messaging to communicate with patients** on relevant health information." The initial Stage 1 and 2 rules required organizations both to provide access as a condition of MU certification and also to show that a rising percentage of patients were actually using the tools.

Healthcare organizations and associations pushed back on the requirement to demonstrate that patients were actually using the tools. They argued that it was unfair for them to be held accountable for choices their patients made and suggested that it was difficult to increase adoption as quickly as the rules required. In 2016, as part of Stage 3 Meaningful Use provisions, the requirement was changed so that qualifying organizations only had to demonstrate that "at least one unique patient" could access their health information electronically.[32] In changing the rule, CMS stated that the reduction would, "allow providers additional time to determine the best ways to educate patients on the importance of accessing their health care information, and assist them to access their health information electronically."[33]

In 2016, Meaningful Use Stage 3 transitioned into the MIPS program under the Medicare Access and CHIP Reauthorization Act of 2015 (MACRA). The requirements for patient access were adopted into the MIPS program. While the "one patient" requirement was maintained, the requirement for patients or caregivers to "view, download, and transmit" their health information evolved to include the ability for patients to obtain their data through an Application Programming Interface (API) using an application of their choice. The 2020 rules assign significant weight to patient access.[34] CMS stated that the emphasis was appropriate:

> We believe that the emphasis placed on the Provide Patients Electronic Access to their Health Information measure through the redistribution of points reflects our emphasis on patient engagement in their health care and patient's electronic access of their health information through the use of APIs.

They further state that this redistribution "allows for health IT solutions that encourage adoption and innovation."[35] (See Chapter 6.)

The 2020 MIPS requirements include the following requirement, unchanged from 2019:

> The patient (or the patient-authorized representative) is provided timely access to view online, download, and transmit his or her health information; and the MIPS eligible clinician ensures the patient's health information is available for the patient (or patient authorized representative) to access using any application of their choice that is configured to meet the technical specifications of the Application Programming Interface (API) in the MIPS eligible clinician's CEHRT.[36]

Further specifications require that the information must be made available to patients within four business days of the information being available to the clinician. They also specify that providers must send or answer at least one secure direct message with one unique patient and collect patient-generated health data from one unique patient.[37] Qualifying providers must also identify patient-specific education materials for at least one patient and provide the materials electronically.

Seema Verma, Administrator of the Centers for Medicare and Medicaid Services (CMS); Alex Azar, Secretary of Health and Human Services (HHS); and Dr. Donald Rucker, national coordinator for health IT (ONC) joined forces to make sure that the policy infrastructure supports the ability of patients to access their own data using tools of their choice. Those commitments are realized in two final rules released in March 2020 through HHS. These rules provide the regulatory framework for the 21st Century Cures Act, which was passed in 2016: [38]

- The ONC Final Rule establishes new rules to prevent information blocking practices by providers, developers of certified Health Information Technology, and Health Information Exchanges. It is intended to realize the vision set forth in the 21st Century Cures Act. In addition, the rule establishes requirements for secure, standards-based application programming interfaces (APIs). It requires provider organizations to provide patients with the ability to access those APIs using whatever application they choose. Significantly, the rules spell out that providers must include access to both structured and unstructured data via the API, and that patients should be able to gain access at no cost. The unstructured data addressed by the requirement explicitly includes clinical notes and patient goals. This rule establishes Fast Interoperability Resources (FHIR) as the standard for APIs and sets up the United States Core Data for Interoperability (USCDI) as the standard set of data resources for interchange, clarifying the standards that will govern the path forward.
- The CMS Interoperability and Patient Access final rule requires health plans to share claims data electronically with patients via the patient access API.

Both rules are intended to unleash a flood of innovation by eliminating information blocking and encouraging the development of health apps that use API data in new and creative ways.

These rules are not without controversy. Organizations such as Epic Systems Corporation and several major health systems pushed back against the proposed rules, suggesting that they won't adequately protect patient data.[39] Secretary Alex Azar summarized the reaction to this in prepared remarks at the ONC Summit: "Providers should be able to use health IT tools to provide the best care for patients without excessive cost or technical barriers. . . . Unfortunately, some industry stakeholders are defending the balkanized, outdated status quo."[40] In the final rule, CMS noted that its scope doesn't include governance of applications and pointed to the FDA as the appropriate body for protecting the ways that third-party apps use patient data.

The standards for API access and information exchange broaden the amount of information available to patients, caregivers, and app developers. If knowledge is power, the unequal distribution of knowledge in healthcare has been one of the things that has kept patients at a disadvantage when interacting with their doctors. Providing direct access to clinical records and the ability to choose what tools you use to access your data is a key step in recalibrating the balance of power between patients and their doctors.

The Link Between Use of Digital Tools and Health Activation

There is no single perfect study showing that use of digital tools directly raises consumers' activation and engagement regarding their health. Nonetheless, emerging research highlights strong correlations between use of digital tools and health engagement rates.[41,42]

Terminology use in this area is confusing: patient activation is conflated with both patient engagement and patient empowerment. And, while there are linkages between the three terms, they are not identical.[43] In general, patient engagement is an umbrella term. Patient activation is a measure of individual attitudes about their responsibility for their health and is a subset of patient engagement. Patient empowerment is associated with engagement. As described later, there is a way to measure activation, but there are no similarly researched measures for engagement or empowerment.

Judith Hibbard, PhD, developed the Patient Activation Measure (PAM) as a way to measure differences in individual levels of activation about health. Since its inception in 2004, the measure has been used in a wide variety of studies that show that more highly activated patients, as measured by the PAM score, correlate to better healthcare outcomes, lower costs, and higher satisfaction with the healthcare system.[44] Qualitative research suggests that patients who are highly activated view themselves as working in partnership with professionals, whereas patients who are at low levels of activation view their role as one of compliance.

The PAM measure does not directly measure engagement with health tools, although studies using the PAM score have shown that higher activation levels are correlated to the likelihood of using digital tools. Dr. Hibbard's research indicates that providers were 30% more likely to recommend the use of a patient portal to highly activated patients compared to patients at low levels of activation. Among the patients whose providers recommended use of the patient portal, highly activated patients were 20% more likely to act upon the offer than less activated patients.[45]

Several studies showcase the emerging linkages between use of digital tools and health activation. A 2016 study from Oschner found that use of a digital tool for remotely monitoring high blood pressure impacted both health outcomes and PAM scores, although it was not entirely clear what was the causal element. The group monitored with the digital tool had more than twice the improvement in blood pressure control than the usual care group (71% vs 31%). PAM scores in the digital control group also rose, with the most significant rise coming from people who started the experiment in low activation categories.[46]

Another study from the University of Pennsylvania Health System showed that patient portal use had a significant positive impact on patient adherence to preventive measures, but a negligible impact on chronic disease management.[47] A meta-study reviewed outcomes from 170 papers on digital health. It showed that "overall, 88.8% (151/170) of studies showed positive impact on patient behavior and 82.9% (141/170) reported high levels of improvement in patient engagement."[48] Another meta-study showed that patient portal use impacted a wide range of "patient psycho-behavioral outcomes, such as health knowledge, self-efficacy, decision making, medication adherence, and preventive service use," but did not conclusively affect health outcomes.[49]

Other studies show that there can be impacts on both patient engagement and outcomes from patient portal use. A 2015 study of veterans with HIV showed that

> the use of electronic personal health records was associated with significantly higher levels of patient activation and levels of patient satisfaction for getting timely appointments, care, and information. ePHR was also associated with greater proportions of undetectable plasma HIV-1 viral loads, of knowledge of current CD4 count, and of knowledge of current viral load.[50]

A Canadian study found that diabetic portal users had improved glycemic control vs a control group.[51] Kaiser Permanente compared portal users who received nudges regarding preventive care via the portal to those who didn't receive nudges. Those who received the nudges showed increased completion of necessary preventive care.[52] Similarly, a recent study showed that a wireless home monitoring program actually seemed to "potentiate" changes in PAM scores and associated reductions in blood pressure, drinking, and smoking behaviors.[53]

Some organizations have expressed fears that direct release of lab results to patients would increase anxiety. UPMC conducted a study focused on the impact of lab tests directly released through a patient portal, which included interviews with patients who had viewed an abnormal PAP release or any HBA1C test through the portal. More than 80% of users felt the lab test results were very useful, and 70% felt access to their data on the portal made the information more useful to them. Those who viewed an abnormal result felt that interpretation by the physician and access to education about it would have helped them.[54] These results mirror the results of an earlier study conducted by Kaiser Permanente regarding lab results release. In that study, patients reported feeling satisfied (72%), appreciative (68%), and calm (65%) after viewing their lab test results via a portal.[55]

At least one study tested the impact of an in-patient portal on PAM scores. The researchers found that access to the portal improved PAM scores in meaningful ways. They also uncovered a number of barriers to use that offer guidance on effective ways of implementing in-patient portals.[56]

Not all studies showed as much effectiveness. One 2016 study showed no improvement in PAM scores through focused use of a personal health portal for cardiac patients.[57] A Finnish study found no significant impact on patient activation from the introduction of a patient portal. The researchers noted, however, that their portal didn't include some features that may have been important to activation enhancement, specifically interactive, condition-specific education and patient-generated health data.[58]

The variations in outcomes make it difficult to assess the effect of digital tools on patient activation, empowerment, and self-efficacy. It is not easy to separate issues caused by poorly designed tools and poorly structured implementations from the impact of the tools themselves. This is a fast-growing area of study, and we expect that further research will reveal the features that make digital tools most effective in increasing patient activation, feelings of empowerment, and self-efficacy regarding health.

Health Information Seeking

The most common digital health activity is searching for health information on the internet. By any measure, this should be considered engagement, as it speaks to individuals looking for information about their own or someone else's health status. There's a deep connection between a person's health literacy – the ability to understand and make decisions about care and treatment – and engagement with their health. The extent of searches for health information can be read as an indicator of a deep hunger to understand health, wellness, and illness.

Susannah Fox reported in January of 2014 on a Pew Internet Survey that found

> seven-in-ten (72%) adult internet users say they have searched online for information about a range of health issues, the most popular being specific diseases and treatments. One in four (26%) adult internet users say they have read or watched someone else's health experience about health or medical issues in the past 12 months.[59]

Use of the internet for finding health information hasn't gone away in the years since that Pew Internet study. Google Health Chief Dr. David Feinberg said in 2019 that about 7% of all Google searches are health related. To provide perspective, this equates to about 70,000 searches *a minute* or *a billion* health inquiries a day. [60]

A meta-study from 2017 reviewed six years of studies of health information-seeking behavior on the internet and in social media settings. The study authors note that consumers have different needs for health information, which drive different behaviors. They urged further study on how to help consumers find reliable information that addresses their in-the-moment information needs.[61] A four-year study of health information-seeking behavior published in 2017 showed the percentage of adults who used the internet as their first source of information on medical or health issues was high and rising compared to all other channels for health information. The other sources included family/friend/coworker, healthcare professional, and traditional media. All of them were under 15% of the population and the percentages didn't change throughout the four-year period. In contrast, the internet was cited as their first source by 43% in the first year, rising to 47% in the fourth year (See citations list; Figure 2.1).[62]

We've always been aware that people get information and referrals about medical issues from friends and neighbors "over the back fence." We now see that propensity amplified by online tools in virtual communities, as social media is also an important part of the way people seek health information online. Consumers use social channels to become educated on health issues, to critique the care they get, and to manage both acute and chronic illness.

In the Pew Internet study just cited, Ms. Fox notes that one of the enduring findings of the Pew Research Center is that health search is social – more than half of all health searches online are performed on behalf of someone else, even by people with multiple chronic conditions.[58] Health is social in other ways as well. An analysis of 32 years of data from the Framingham study demonstrated that obesity is contagious. A person's likelihood to become obese increased by 57% if he or she had a friend who became obese during a given interval.[62] Similarly, research from 2017 shows that exercise is also socially contagious – for both good and ill.[63] Online social networks use this relationship impact on health to support health behavior changes.[64]

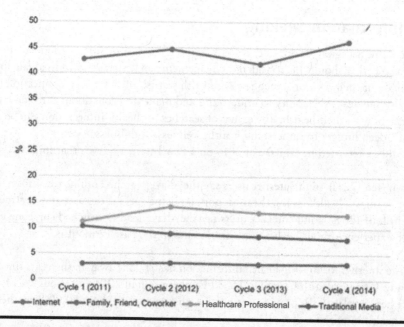

Figure 2.1　Health information seeking behavior

People use the internet to find other patients like them in order to learn from other people's coping skills and to seek understanding, reassurance, and social support. In 2010, Pew Research found that one in four people with a chronic condition went online to find others with similar issues.[65] It is likely that the number has increased rather than decreased in the years since that study, although current research on adult behaviors is sparse. Research from 2018 on teens and young adults found that two in five young people between 14 and 22 years old have gone online looking for peers with health conditions like theirs. A full 84% of those teens and young adults found someone similar to them. Of those who found peer support online for a health condition, 91% say their last experience with an online peer was somewhat or very helpful. [66]

A recent WEGO Health study found that 91% of users who were part of a patient community said that the community impacted their health decisions.[67] In 2016, researchers created a Facebook group for liver transplant patients and families. At the end of the nine-month study, 95% of survey respondents said that joining the group had a positive impact on their care and 97% said their main motivation for joining was to provide or receive support from other patients.[68] A meta-study from 2016 also found that online peer interactions about health conditions positively impact how individuals self-manage their conditions. The study also found that the social support provided in online groups meets a need that is hard to address offline.[69]

Peer support seems to be effective not just as a way of increasing coping and self-management skills, but also as an aid to behavior change. Peer support has been demonstrated to be effective in everything from smoking cessation to diabetes management and weight loss. A meta-analysis published in February of 2014 concluded, "This review offers preliminary evidence that social networking-based health interventions may be effective in changing behavior."[70] In 2019, a study indicated that participation in an online community positively impacted individual PAM scores, with the greatest amount of change in PAM scores occurring among the least-activated patients.[71]

There is reason to be concerned that people may find inappropriate, false, or misleading health information online, or be unduly influenced by ads offered in conjunction with health information. We are all familiar with the way that anti-vaccination activists have flooded the internet with misinformation about the harms of vaccination, with troubling impacts to overall vaccination rates. Similar misinformation can be found for cancer, stem cell treatments, and a host of other health concerns. Tech companies have not been especially helpful in managing misinformation that proliferates on their platforms.

There is reason for hope, however. A 2016 study rated health information exchanged in 25 threads across several sites (Reddit, Mumsnet, and Patient). Their ratings found that the information exchanged was likely to be of reasonably high quality by a factor of 4 to 1. Even lower quality information was unlikely to lead readers to act inappropriately.[72] This aligns with results from earlier studies. A 2006 study showed that only 10 out of 4600 posts in an online breast cancer community were inaccurate or misleading. Of those ten misleading posts, seven were found and corrected within an average of 4½ hours.[73] A 2009 study found that information posted in an online diabetes forum closely aligned with clinical guidelines.[74] Trained and alert community moderators can help keep the knowledge of the community accurate and on track.[75]

If we are going to preserve online environments as a source for social engagement with health, we also need to address the privacy and security of each individual's information. Accenture found this year that concerns are growing about the privacy of health information, including health information posted on private social support sites.[26] Andrea Downing and Fred Trotter found bugs in Facebook's private group settings that enabled sensitive information to be accessed by third parties.[76] Issues such as these reduce trust and usage of social media sites as vehicles for individuals to share their personal health stories and receive support.

The behavior of health information seekers online gives reason for optimism about the desire people have for reliable and curated information to support their health journeys. New models directly involve consumers in research design and information development. Applications are newly focused on delivering personalized and targeted education. In addition, organizations are exploring how to deliver peer support that is more secure and perhaps better curated. All of these developments offer hope that the journey to health literacy can be enhanced as a critical component of patient engagement.

Patient and Consumer Engagement Impact All Dimensions of the Quadruple Aim

Patient activation and engagement matter because they affect all dimensions of the quadruple aim. Digital tools can increase convenience for patients and their families while improving the quality of care, the cost of care, the experience of care, and even the wellbeing of the care team.

Digital Health Engagement Impact on Quality

As more people gain access to their records via digital means, evidence is emerging that such access has a positive impact on quality and outcomes. We discussed earlier how access to digital records has been shown to increase health activation, including self-efficacy and self-management. In addition, there are specific indications that digital patient engagement increases the quality of care.

ONC found that one in ten people who accessed their medical record found an error of some sort.[77] Information from someone else's records can be mixed into your chart or simple typographical or transcription errors can lead to misinformation.[78] One expert estimates that 70% of Americans have some incorrect information in their medical record,[79] and another study found that 70% of medication errors were not caught before the patient received the prescription.[80]

Open notes can be particularly helpful in addressing medical record errors. A retrospective study on three health systems that had implemented open notes before 2014 found that more than 98% of patients felt access to their notes was a good thing. Patients rated note reading as very important for helping take care of their health (73%), feeling in control of their care (79%), and remembering their plan of care (66%).[81] When open notes patients were provided with a feedback tool, about 7% used it to contact their doctors. Nearly 30% of those contacts were to correct a medical error.[82] When patients help correct their data, it can make care safer.

Earlier studies showed that after 16 months, a quarter of patients who used online records were up to date on their preventive care – double the rate of non-users.[83] Several Kaiser Permanente studies also indicate correlations between portal use and improved outcomes. A study published in 2014, funded by the National Institutes of Health, concluded that diabetic Kaiser Permanente members who used only online tools to refill their medications were more likely to be cooperative with their medication regimen with associated positive outcomes.[84] Another retrospective Kaiser Permanente study noted that children whose parents used Kaiser's online portal were 2.5 times more likely to attend all well child visits.[85] A third Kaiser Permanente study published in *HealthAffairs* indicated that diabetic patients who used the portal to securely message their physicians had higher HEDIS scores than non-users.[86]

When digital tools are used effectively, they can increase the partnership between patients and their clinicians while contributing to positive health outcomes. We believe that improved partnership between patients and their clinicians can also improve the wellbeing of the care team by increasing the opportunities for authentic interactions in the service of healing.

A team at Sloan Kettering developed a digital tool that enabled cancer patients to report on their symptoms. Those using the tool to work with their care team reported significant improvements in quality of life. They also lived an average of five months longer than those who were in the "usual care" group.[87] The Sloan Kettering team's aim was to improve communication and symptom management. The study team was surprised by the results as they hadn't anticipated that improving these elements might affect survival time.

The Cardiac High Acuity Monitoring Program (CHAMP) tool enabled at Children's Mercy Hospital in Kansas City, Missouri, provides another example of the way digital technologies can increase the partnership between physicians and families. It is used to monitor babies with Hypoplastic Left Heart Syndrome (HLHS). The condition is rare and complex, with a mortality rate of about 25%. Usual care required parents to check vital signs at home, then phone that information to the hospital weekly. With the CHAMP system, parents report results of at-home vital signs daily and the entries are available to the hospital care team in minutes. As a result, the hospital care team is able to spot and address emerging problems quickly. Since they started using CHAMP, Children's Mercy has had a 100% survival rate. They've also seen the cost of treating these children lowered as a result of the tool.[88,89]

Another interesting intervention started as part of an IT Challenge Grant awarded by the ONC to Indiana Health Information Technology in 2011. The project focused on a small group of patients who had undergone cardiac surgery. Each individual was trained on the NoMore-Clipboard PHR application, and their PAM scores were assessed both before and after they used the portal. Michael Mirro, MD, a cardiac electrophysiologist at Parkview Physicians Group and medical director at Parkview Research Center, noted that "we could demonstrate in that study that patients were more engaged in their care, but also that some of their intermediate outcomes were improved, such as their LDL cholesterol and hemoglobin A1c."[90] Since 2011, Dr. Mirro has expanded his use of patient portals to enable cardiac patients to monitor data from their Implanted Cardioverter Defibrillators (ICDs). His outcomes have continued to demonstrate that doing so leads to better activation and feelings of control on the part of patients. In this example, patients become partners with their doctors by sharing data that enables both parties to enhance cardiac management. This approach reinforces the position of patients like Hugo Campos, who has advocated for years that he should have access to the data from his ICD. He says, "It's my body, my life, my health. Why shouldn't I have access to do as I please with this data?"[91]

The #NightScout community is another example of a collaboration approach by patients and caregivers who created tools to use data from Continuous Blood Glucose (CGM) monitors to improve diabetes managing.[92] Having access to CGM data enabled the group to design a variety of useful tools, ranging from remote monitoring of glucose readings (especially helpful for parents of diabetic children) to a continuous loop artificial pancreas.[93] Their efforts are being watched by the FDA and medical device companies alike as they demonstrate what care for diabetes will look like in the next future.

The ability to reach out to your provider online as well as the potential to get reminders, information, and encouragement from your provider between visits may positively impact a person's sense of being known, as well as provide a sense of the caring and abiding presence of the physician. The TeleVox Healthy World study, "Technology Beyond the Exam Room," reported that

of the 66 percent of patients who have received a voicemail, text or email from a healthcare provider, many reported a variety of positive outcomes. Fifty-one percent reported feeling more valued as a patient, 35 percent said digital communication improved their opinion of their provider, and 34 percent reported feeling more certain about visiting that healthcare provider again.[94]

All of these factors highlight the impact that patient engagement can have on the quality of care and the development of healing partnerships between patients and providers. Effective deployment of digital tools leads to more continuous interactions between patients and their care teams, which we think of as connected care. Improved access to information and improved communication channels seem to impact medical outcomes as well as patients' sense of control and empowerment. Advances in remote monitoring and telehealth are both suited to improving these ongoing connections between care teams and patients if they are done in ways that are sensitive to improving agency for patients.

Digital Health Engagement Impact on Cost

The holy grail of healthcare has been the hope that engaged and activated patients will take better care of themselves, delaying the progression of disease and reducing the cost of care. There are three specific ways that digital health tools help reduce overall healthcare costs. The first is that these tools lower medical costs by improving health outcomes. The second is that they lower costs by increasing self-service and automating services, which improves efficiency and reduces staffing costs. The third is that they enable consumers to take cost, quality, and efficacy into account in their healthcare buying decisions.

Several meta-studies of digital health interventions for prevention and treatment in cardiac care found that the majority of the interventions were clinically and cost-effective ways to reduce cardiac events.[95,96]

In addition to clinical advantages, self-service features such as appointment scheduling, online prescription refill requests, pre-visit registration capabilities, and online bill payment programs can save health systems money while increasing patient satisfaction. Other industries have introduced self-service tools over the past two decades, often finding that the shift from full service to self-service reduces costs by a factor of 10:1. When consumers can complete activities online at a time that is convenient for them, their satisfaction levels generally increase. When patients manage services themselves that previously required staff, healthcare systems reduce costs.

Health economists and health plans have been working on benefit designs that support and nudge consumers to make wise as well as cost-conscious decisions regarding medical care by taking into account consumer spending behaviors. In part as a consequence of this work, the last ten years have seen a significant rise in the amount consumers pay for their healthcare. These cost increases, intended to give consumers "skin in the game" in relation to their healthcare costs, have not been accompanied by corresponding increases in education or clarity about costs. Instead, the rising share of cost has too often meant that Americans put off needed care even if they have insurance.[97] A Commonwealth study found that

the share of continuously insured adults with high deductibles has tripled, rising from 3 percent in 2003 to 11 percent in 2014. Half (51%) of underinsured adults reported problems with medical bills or debt and more than two of five (44%) reported not getting needed care because of cost.[98]

In this environment, nearly 68% of the people who filed for bankruptcy in 2016 cited medical debt as a contributor – and those individuals were two or three times more likely to have skipped needed care and medications.[99] The percentage of bankruptcies due to healthcare costs was still 67% in a Harvard study from 2019.[100]

Although consumers bear a higher percentage of healthcare costs and are interested in spending their money wisely, it is difficult for them to make cost-conscious health decisions. One reason is the lack of easily available (and comparable) information about cost. Another is that consumers tend to use the cost of medical services as a proxy for their quality.[101] This equation, which works effectively in most purchasing decisions, does not work very well in healthcare, where there are wide variations in the cost and quality of specific procedures, where appropriate care may mean less rather than more intervention, and positive consumer experiences may not be the same as the best clinical care. To obtain the expected benefits of creating a consumer marketplace in healthcare, we need to do the following things:

- Provide consumers with a straightforward way to understand the relationship between cost and quality
- Enable cost estimation and cost transparency tools that fully reflect individual variations in both plan design and treatment effectiveness
- Reduce the impact of intermediaries that make it more difficult to understand the direct cost of consumer choices[102]

Consumers also want more understanding of what they should pay and more convenient ways to pay healthcare bills. This is no easy feat in a situation where provider and hospital bills come on monthly cycles while claims are resolved as they are submitted. Determining what is actually due and what is appropriate to pay can be time-consuming and confusing – especially in the middle of a healthcare crisis or its aftermath. Instamed's ninth annual survey on healthcare costs, published in 2019, highlighted a confusing and frustrating scene for consumers: 70% of consumers were confused by their medical bills and explanation of benefits (EOBs), 56% of consumers wouldn't be able to pay medical bill over $1000, and 93% of consumers had been surprised by a medical bill.[103]

Tools that help consumers understand and reconcile bills with claims would significantly reduce the stress of handling healthcare financials for many consumers. United Health Group employed Instamed to enable consumers to pay providers what is owed after claims adjudication directly from the myuhc.com website, eliminating confusion about what is owed to whom.[104]

With a larger percentage of their revenue coming from consumers rather than payers, healthcare systems must increase payment convenience both to reduce the cost of collections and to improve consumer satisfaction. Consumers that have a bad billing experience are far more likely to rate the overall experience of care as poor, giving health systems another reason for paying attention to offering convenient and clear payment options.[105] Many consumers, faced with bearing more cost for healthcare, need payment plans to allow them to pay high deductibles over time. Healthcare institutions can employ financing services that offer consumers low or no-interest loans for healthcare expenses as long as they pay on time, with the further benefit that providers get payments nearly immediately.[106]

Healthcare systems that offer convenient, online ways to predict costs, pay bills, finance the cost of care, and eliminate surprise medical bills will find it is justified by a boost in consumer satisfaction as well as a rise in payments collected.

Digital Health Engagement Linked to Satisfaction and Loyalty

Access to digital tools is only one dimension of the overall patient experience, albeit an emerging and important one. Organizations that understand the importance of focusing on providing seamless care centered on helping and supporting patients and families are well positioned to build both trust and loyalty. The Medicare Stars program, the JD Powers annual health rankings, and focus on net promoter scores mean health plans are paying more attention to consumer satisfaction. At the same time, patient satisfaction is a factor in the payment infrastructure for CMS programs, which adds reasons for providers to focus attention on consumer and patient satisfaction and loyalty. It is hard to impact patient and consumer health behaviors – digitally or otherwise – if you have high turnover rates.

Convenience and digital access build loyalty and "stickiness" by increasing the perceived cost of switching providers or plans.[107] The impact of these loyalty features is multidimensional. Patients who feel loyal and value convenience are more likely to stay inside the system for care, enabling better care coordination and reducing duplicative tests and procedures. Fee-for-value models of care put providers at risk for the care of their population of patients, wherever the patients get care. Building loyalty via enhancing convenience is one of the ways to support this requirement. "If we're not able to limit [leakage], it makes it harder to . . . manage the entire population to the best of our capabilities," says Reinhold Llerena, MD, medical director of Arlington Heights, Illinois-based Alexian Brothers Accountable Care Organization, a Medicare Shared Savings ACO."[108] Regardless of payment models, leakage impacts an organization's bottom line. In 2018, Fibroblast found that over 40% of healthcare executives say they're losing 10% or more of annual revenues due to leakage, 19% are losing over 20%, and 23% don't know how much they are losing due to leakage.[109]

Consumers increasingly consider the digital experience in selecting doctors. In October 2019, Cedar sponsored a survey that focused on the impact that digital administrative tools, such as online bill pay, access to insurance information, digital pre-appointment forms, and digital bill delivery have on how patients choose providers. They found that 41% of consumers overall and 61% of consumers 18–24 – the healthiest and least costly consumers – said they'd leave their provider over a bad digital experience. This contrasts to only 21% in people over 66 who said they would leave over a bad digital experience.[110] In the same survey, 20% of patients had already switched providers because of a poor digital experience. Losing younger patients because of a bad digital experience risks income from those patients over their whole lifetime, not to mention the ability to impact their health behaviors when they are young.

Accenture's 2019 Digital Health Consumer survey found similar results. Their survey asked consumers, "If you were choosing a new provider or adding an additional provider, would being able to use the following electronic capabilities make it more likely you would choose that provider?"[111] In response, the following percentages of consumers said the capability would influence their decision:

- Request prescription refills electronically – 77%
- Receive reminders via email or text message, when it is time for preventive or follow-up care – 70%
- Communicate with your provider through secure email – 69%
- Book/change/cancel appointments online – 68%
- Use remote or telemonitoring devices to monitor and record your own health indicators – 53%
- Communicate with your provider through video conferencing – 49%

The responses to each of these questions were at least 10% points higher than in Accenture's 2016 survey. The survey found that younger consumers were significantly more likely to be influenced in their choice of physicians by access to digital tools than their elders.

Accenture's 2020 Digital Health Consumer Survey found that 26% of consumers surveyed said they were likely to switch providers for high-quality digital services. Half of surveyed consumers also said a bad digital experience with a provider ruins the whole experience, while 39% said a good digital experience has a "major influence" on their overall experience with a provider.[26]

There are many opportunities for health systems to benefit from these correlations. Expanding use of self-scheduling, online bill payment, virtual visits, and electronic prescription refill are some of the early wins for healthcare, but their use could be expanded further. Adding the ability for patients or caregivers to confirm health and coverage information ahead of time rather than while sitting in the waiting room is also a promising capability that offers convenience to customers while reducing costs for consumers. Using telehealth to address smaller health concerns also adds convenience for consumers and expedites care both for the patients and the practice. Dr. Susan Kressly (@kiddrsue) reported in a conference panel and on Twitter that her clinic gives preferential treatment to those who complete forms online by taking them directly back to the exam room; one result is that the visit can begin with the patient's questions, rather than the doctor's. Other opportunities to build loyalty include interacting with patients between visits and providing upgraded apps and portals using API services to extract data from health records and personalize interactions with patients. All of these features not only satisfy consumer's need for convenience but also remove barriers to care. They also tend to raise the cost of switching providers, a benefit to health systems in their quest to build loyalty.

Mobile Capabilities

Mobile phone apps, especially when combined with sensors and medical devices, offer great promise for improving consumers' engagement with their health. In 2019, at least 81% of US adults had a smartphone and 96% had a cell phone.[112] These percentages are very similar among whites, Hispanics, and Blacks. Home broadband capabilities are not as evenly distributed, as rural Americans and lower income households are less likely to have high-speed broadband capabilities at home.[113] Baby Boomers are one of the fastest growing segments in the online space and even in the Silent Generation, 40% own smartphones.[114] With the widespread availability of significant computing power in the palm of your hand comes the opportunity to extend healthcare capabilities into daily lives and daily routines in ways that are engaging and also help people actually achieve their health goals.

Part of the promise of mobile technologies for healthcare is that people carry their mobiles with them almost all the time – including 62% of parents and 39% of children who sleep with their phone near their bed so as not to miss updates during the night.[115] The things that make smartphones addictive also make them potent allies for behavior change. As Predrag Klasnja and Wanda Prat note in "Healthcare in the Pocket: Mapping the Space of Mobile-Phone Health Interventions" there are four reasons that smart phones offer such promise as behavior change tools: [116]

1. Increasingly, everyone has a mobile phone
2. People keep their phones near them most of the time, which makes them useful for health-related reminders and interventions

3. They are very personal devices, which may increase acceptance of interventions delivered through them

4. Sophisticated devices incorporate information about a person's context, which means they can deliver messages that are timely, personalized, and contextually appropriate

Consumers, application developers, health plans, and providers alike are exploring ways to use mobile devices to help individuals monitor and manage their health and perform health-related tasks. Among the simplest interventions are text-based alerts and reminders. Consumers can sign up for texts that remind them to refill prescriptions, prepare for an upcoming appointment, or provide positive messages about health goals. A recent meta-study highlighted the effectiveness of simple text messaging in changing behaviors for a wide range of health conditions that included weight loss, smoking cessation, and medication adherence.[117]

Many health systems venture into the mobile space by providing web portal capabilities on mobile phones. Having the capabilities available while mobile seems to improve overall digital access. Kaiser Permanente, an early leader in the digital space, noted in its 2018 Annual Report that "more than half of all member and patient interactions are now conducted online. In 2018, 64% of all visits to kp.org were from mobile devices – nearly 199 million visits."[118] As organizations begin making APIs available as required by the new regulations, consumer choices for how to get their data and what to do with it will expand.

Health systems and startups alike are also exploring ways to use mobile devices to stay connected with people about their health during the 90% of time when individuals are not interacting directly with the health system. They are sending encouragement about healthy behaviors, providing timely information and updates, and exchanging data that can keep someone out of the hospital or help them achieve health goals.

There are indications that well-designed apps are helpful in addressing people's health and data needs. Some of those outcomes have already been discussed in the section on quality and cost. In this section, we'll explore the elements that lead to effective mobile capabilities for supporting consumers in managing their health and healthcare.

Stanford researchers recently studied smartphone interventions for the impact on step counts as part of the MyHeart Counts Cardiovascular Health Study. Four different smartphone interventions were tested. The study demonstrated that all four interventions had a significant impact on users' daily activity levels – at least in the short term.[119] Other studies reinforce the concept that activity trackers can help people increase physical activity and sustain exercise programs.[120] There's also evidence that users with diabetes and hypertension who used activity trackers were more likely to also be adherent to their medication regimen, although the reasons for the correlation were not entirely clear.[121] Users of diet and exercise apps also report that the apps supported changes in behavior necessary for achieving their goals.[122]

The issue of user abandonment of wearables and sensors has been widely reported, and researchers are just beginning to study associated behaviors. It appears that signs predicting the likelihood of future abandonment of such tools show up in the first 30 days of use – and early interventions can help people get and stay engaged. Further research is needed to understand the interplay of personality, app capabilities, and perceived tool usefulness to better understand how to build effective and sustainable apps to support healthy behaviors.

In designing health apps to support behavior change, we can learn from the RAMP framework described by game designer Andrzej Marczewski, which focuses on fostering intrinsic motivation:[123]

- **Relatedness** – meaningful connection to others; a sense of belonging
- **Autonomy** – behavior as an expression of self; the freedom to make decisions independently
- **Mastery** – the process of mastering a new skill; progressing toward a goal
- **Purpose** – desire to add value to a cause larger than themselves

Other suggestions on ways to foster long-term engagement for healthy behaviors include:

- Create checking habits that can keep users aware of how they are doing in relation to the action they want to change
- Increase "social translucence" by making a users' behavior available to others and by making the person aware that others can see their behaviors
- Supporting action by suggesting things that people can take action on immediately[124]

Increasingly, it seems clear that success in creating digital tools that support health behaviors lies not in the channel (web, mobile, or social) as much as the way media is combined to create rich, engaging, and in-the-moment experiences. This is the process of engineering teachable moments that are personal, relevant, convenient, and contextual. In the future, we are likely to see interesting options that involve social capabilities delivered on multiple platforms seamlessly. They will allow users to interact with whatever channel is most convenient for them at any given time. We are also likely to see capabilities that incorporate symptom tracking, social support, direct access to personal clinical information, personalized education, predictive insights, and competition. Applications with these intertwined elements are already emerging, especially in apps that incorporate game-playing technologies.

Gamification is defined by Merriam Webster as "the process of adding games or game-like elements to something (as a task) so as to encourage participation." While the concept has been around for some time, the word is a product of the digital age. When applied in healthcare, it represents the process of using appealing (and potentially addicting) techniques from the world of games, such as badges, points, or competitions, to help people get engaged with their health – and even to help them change unhealthy behaviors. Not everyone is motivated in the same way, but incorporating game-like elements can have desirable effects when applied to health: motivation, participation, a sense of mastery, and a sense of community.

Although many healthcare programs and tools currently incorporate gamification elements, few use them effectively. A 2017 PWC survey found that 63% of employer wellness programs incorporated some sort of gamification elements, and another 24% of employers were interested in adding gamification elements.[125] A 2016 study looked at 1680 "top rated" (by revenue and downloads) health apps and found that 4% included gamification elements. Of the programs that included gamification elements, only a few used them in accordance with core behavioral health principles such as empathy, meeting people where they are, incorporating their goals and motivations, and solving for key actions.[126]

Jane McGonigal is a gamification expert and the Director of Games Research and Development at the Institute for the Future in Palo Alto, California. She created a game to help herself heal from a traumatic brain injury – and then turned it into a tool for anyone. Her game, SuperBetter, had the highest score in a study of apps that incorporated health behavior change principles.[127] Bernadette O'Keefe highlights why game principles should be incorporated into behavior change and recovery programs:

> McGonigal describes three innate strengths that help us improve and bring about behavior change: we are stronger than we know, we're surrounded by allies and

supporters, and we are the heroes of our own story. These strengths underpin player agency and empowerment, elements central to success.[128]

The concept of effectively embedding game-playing in healthcare apps is promising enough that has seen considerable industry investment. Pharma Astellas, in conjunction with two Japanese universities, is building a lab to test gamification tactics.[129] Insurers made significant bets on gamification in the 2010–2014 time period, but focus on these initiatives seems to have faded. One of the exceptions is Wellvolution, launched by Blue Shield of California in 2009, first for its own employees, then enabled for all members in 2014. Wellvolution incorporates a wellbeing score that can be measured over time, a daily challenge, and the ability to ask friends and family for support.[130] Wellvolution has evolved into Wellvolution Next with a new platform from Solera Health launched in 2019. It is an active and vital part of the Blue Cross of California ecosystem.[131] One of its points of differentiation is that it only offers apps whose outcomes have been verified.

Aetna recently announced a partnership with Apple, using a co-developed app called Attain. The program enables users to "earn back" the price of an Apple Watch through healthy activities. The program is personalized based on users' health data and will provide user-specific daily and weekly activity goals. The Attain app will also include gamification elements where users can earn points for actions that improve their overall health and wellbeing, such as getting more sleep, increasing mindfulness, and improving nutrition.[132]

In addition to appropriate use of game-playing elements, app developers are increasingly grounding their capabilities in sound behavioral economics principles. Simple behavioral economics modifications can increase the effectiveness of gamification elements, such as using opt-out rather than opt-in enrollment, using social networks to support care, and harnessing the power of loss aversion.[133] Incorporating broader behavioral economic principles in game design, as described in "The Top 5 Behavioural Economics Principles for Designers," can increase both the effectiveness and the stickiness of apps.[134]

Designers are also paying more attention to behavioral health principles as they design their apps. Grounding reinforcement and design in motivational theory can help people work toward their goals more effectively.[135] BJ Fogg is one of the pioneers of this movement. He's researched what works in persuasive design and how to create an ethical framework for its use. The principles he framed are explicated in *A Behavior Model for Persuasive Design*.[136] Hundreds of designers and healthcare executives have attended his boot camp at Stanford to learn how to apply the principles in designing more effective apps and digital tools.

Mark Aloia is a clinical psychologist who studies sleep apnea. His team at Philips Respironics used principles of behavioral motivation to design SleepMapper, later renamed as DreamMapper. It is an app that engages CPAP users in their own care with personalized insights and motivation. Several retrospective studies by Philips as well as an external study using a control group showed that app users were significantly more likely to wear their CPAPs consistently, use them longer on a nightly basis, and reach clinical levels of adherence by 90 days than those who did not use the app.[137,138,139]

We are likely to see more and better digital tools emerging in the near term as it becomes second nature to designers to embed gamification, behavioral economics, and behavioral motivation principles into apps.[140] To be successful, apps need to incorporate strategies that are known to positively impact behavior change, engagement, and stickiness: social support, competition, ability to track achievements over time, personalized rewards, and fun.

Why Aren't People Adopting Digital Healthcare Tools Faster?

Many factors come into play in understanding consumer patterns of digital health adoption. We touched on both barriers and success stories earlier in this chapter. Some adoption issues can be traced back to health systems that have either been slow to incorporate digital tools or have not embedded them effectively in workflow and clinical practice. Other adoption issues are linked to consumer behavior. To unpack this complex dynamic, we need to look at the factors that impact adoption.

Consumers are frustrated by the proliferation of health portals. The average person has at least five medical providers; people with chronic conditions average 14 different physicians. Many Americans have a different portal for each doctor they visit. Each of those portals has a different logon requirement, a different user experience, and only a slice of their health data. Just keeping track of portals and logons is a chore; using them to make sense of your overall health in a comprehensive way can be daunting.[141] The recently adopted HHS rules prohibiting information blocking and requiring healthcare organizations to provide clinical data via APIs will eventually allow consumers to aggregate their health data in one location, alleviating some of these frustrations.

In addition, many healthcare organizations have taken a minimalist approach to their portals. Examples of minimalist approaches include:

- Offering minimal health record information on the portal or requiring patients to ask for their health data to be posted
- Not providing contextual education about the health data provided on the portal, leaving patients to search elsewhere for explanations and meaning
- Not responding to patient messages in a timely fashion – or at all – or having medical assistants respond with generic responses that force consumers to call or make appointments to get their questions answered
- Failing to display abnormal lab test results, pathology reports, and physician notes
- Failing to incorporate convenience features such as cost estimates, bill pay options, appointment management, and pre-visit forms completion
- Not encouraging portal sign-up and use

Providers who encourage patients to sign up for and use their portal show increased rates of use. One study showed a full 63% of patients did so after the provider encouraged them compared to 38% who signed up without physician encouragement.[142] This highlights the ways that personal interactions and medical team behaviors can impact consumers.

The general framework of patient portals hasn't changed significantly since their introduction. It's more than time to make portals more dynamic and useful. Improvements we'd like to see in 3.0 portals include:

- Longitudinal health information that summarizes information from multiple providers and shows conditions, medications, labs on a timeline
- Seamless integration of patient-generated health data (PGHD) with classic clinical data to offer a continuous profile of a person's health
- Predictive capabilities that offer personalized risk profiles and recommendations rather than static information

- Data presented in visually appealing ways
- Seamless integration with virtual care
- Data combined in more useful ways, such as showing the impact of air pollution or pollen levels on an asthma patient's symptoms or medication use or medication refill data correlated to a patient's hospitalizations

For example, for individuals with multiple chronic conditions, it might be helpful to be able to see medication lists organized by what drugs treat what conditions. Several organizations have suggested revamping the display of lab test results to make the display more intuitive and meaningful, as Wired did in a 2010 redesign.[143] An individualized dashboard could summarize the actions the person should be taking and highlight information to which they need to pay attention.

There are similar issues in the world of apps and sensors. Far too few apps incorporate sound clinical, behavior change, behavioral economics, and user-centered design principles in their design and execution. Many are designed and implemented with little understanding of patient/caregiver needs or the healthcare environment. Fewer still have been the subject of rigorous analysis that incorporates assessment of outcomes along with an assessment of the tool's usability and usefulness.

A 2019 white paper outlines a credible approach for validating digital health tools, recognizing varying degrees of clinical risk and the associated levels of evaluation rigor required.[144] It will likely require a widely adopted evaluation system such as the one outlined to help providers determine what approaches to adopt and recommend while enabling consumers to make purchasing decisions with confidence. As more and better ways to measure and rate app effectiveness emerge, high ratings will begin to have an impact on the choices consumers make and will reduce confusion in the market. A future where apps are routinely prescribed as "digital therapeutics" relies on high quality comparative evaluations.

The Future of Personal Health Engagement

This chapter presents a mixed view of the future of personal health engagement using digital tools. Although the potential is great, far too many implementations fall short. Despite this, consumers continue to press for convenient, engaging technology in healthcare that matches or exceeds capabilities they are using in the rest of their lives. To meet and exceed consumer expectations, health insurers, health systems, and technology developers will need to focus on making digital tools accessible, engaging, convenient, effective, and fun.

Looking forward, we make the following predictions about personal health engagement:

- **Healthcare value and cost transparency.** Consumers' rising share of cost continues to drive attention to cost transparency in healthcare. Improved tools will help consumers become more effective in shopping for healthcare services. If we are lucky, apps will help users make choices about cost in the context of value and outcomes. Fueled with up-to-date data and personalized to understand the person's insurance coverage and health issues, tools will emerge to help consumers make personal choices that are congruent with their values and their pocketbooks.
- **Personal health analytics.** Analytic tools that enable a deeper understanding of patterns of disease and causality, combined with gene sequencing and self-tracking, will enable individuals to obtain timely and personalized perspectives on their health. Tools that enable

accurate measurement of the calories in food and drink, as well as improved sensors and wearables that can measure caloric expenditure and location, will help guide behavior with deeply personal insights. When those insights are provided in sensitive ways that recognize who the person is and what motivates him/her, new tools will help people make and sustain changes. With these capabilities will come far more attention to consumers' rights to choose what data is shared with whom – as well as more opportunities to trade privacy for increased privileges such as lower costs or better access.

■ **Interconnected care.** Changes in healthcare incentives and financing are already leading to more seamless care for patients in all of their healthcare interactions. This trend will accelerate, fueled by the rise in consolidated community data and quality measures that reward systems that get it right. Consumers will also benefit from changes that allow them to get more care at home, supported by virtual visits, remote monitoring, community support, and enhanced self-monitoring tools. The same motivators will also enable more seamless, multi-channel, and interconnected care management programs, where clinical and patient-generated information is available to and shared between patients, caregivers, physicians, nurses, health coaches, and insurers – all focused on supporting individuals most appropriately in managing health and disease.

■ **Convenience.** Payers and providers will find themselves competing on who offers the most convenient and frictionless experience. This will affect the channels available to consumers to engage with the health system and the quality and quantity of do-it-yourself healthcare applications. We hope it will drive further innovation around virtual medicine capabilities to benefit consumers and reduce the cost care.

■ **Attitude and culture change.** Individuals, health systems, providers, employers, and insurers all are going through a gradual but inevitable change in perspective from viewing individuals as passive recipients of instructions and knowledge to partners in wellness, treatment, and care. This shift from paternalism to independence will have the long-term effect of helping people take responsibility for their health and healthcare. In addition, the bright line we have drawn between wellness and illness will fade, making it easier to understand the continuum between health and disease.

Conclusion

Although it is clear that people have good intentions about their health – perennial favorite New Year's resolutions are to lose weight, exercise more, eat healthier, stop smoking, and manage stress better – most of us don't do very well at sustaining those resolutions over time.[145] Many people wear tracking devices only for a short period of time, or engage with health games and activities sporadically in activities and programs designed to improve their health.

Rather than seeing the short-term nature of these engagements as a sign that people don't want to engage around their health, we should take hope from them. They indicate a hunger on the part of consumers to be more aware of their health and a belief that changes could make a significant difference in helping them live happier and healthier lives. What they also indicate is that we have not completely "cracked the code" on what helps people make and sustain behavior change to live happier and healthier lives.

New research is helping us better understand the science of motivation and change and how to create applications and digital tools that help us in make such changes while eliciting support (and participation) from friends and family. Digital tools that help us to understand our health, track health activities, and engage with the health system are increasingly available and getting better at providing interactions that raise people's knowledge and sense of empowerment. Interconnected data and interconnected systems raise the potential for understanding one's health over time and providing everyone – family, friends, care team members, health plans, life sciences companies – with more complete information to support each individual's personal health goals.

Personal health engagement continues to emerge as an agent of transformation both for individuals and for the healthcare system as a whole.

About the Author

Jan Oldenburg, FHIMSS, is the principal in Participatory Health Consulting, where she advises start-ups and healthcare organizations regarding the evolving digital health landscape. Jan is passionate about making healthcare more engaging, more convenient, and more healing for patients, especially through incorporating appropriate digital technologies. Ms. Oldenburg has focused on digital transformation in healthcare for more than 20 years. Her experience includes leadership roles in several advisory firms, including EY and her current role. She has also served as the vice president of patient and physician engagement in Aetna's ACO organization and held senior leadership roles at HealthPartners and in Kaiser Permanente's Digital Services Group. Through these roles, she has engaged with organizations from every aspect of healthcare.

She is the principal editor of *Participatory Healthcare: A Person-Centered Approach to Transforming Healthcare* (2016) and *Engage! Transforming Healthcare through Digital Patient Engagement* (2013). Ms. Oldenburg also authored chapters in the third edition of *Medical Informatics* and a chapter in *The Journey Never Ends*. She is a board member of the Society for Participatory Medicine and the former co-chair of the HIMSS Connected Health Committee. She currently cochairs an HL7 Committee writing a white paper on patient-contributed data. Ms. Oldenburg is also a member of the Patient Advocacy & Ethics Group for the Datavant COVID-19 Research Database. Ms. Oldenburg tweets @janoldenburg.

Notes

1. deBronkart, D. "Gimme My DaM Data:" The Video, the Story, the Next Speech. September 2012. https://www.epatientdave.com/2012/08/27/gimme-my-dam-data-the-story-the-video-the-next-speech/
2. Grumman J, Holmes-Rovner M, French ME et al. *Patient Engagement Behavior Framework: What Is Patient Engagement?* March 2010. Available at: https://web.archive.org/web/20120120150821/http://www.cfah.org/pdfs/CFAH_Engagement_Behavior_Framework_current.pdf (Accessed March 2020)
3. Bailo L, Guiddi P, Vergani L, Marton G, Pravettoni G. The Patient Perspective: Investigating Patient Empowerment Enablers and Barriers Within the Oncological Care Process. *Ecancermedicalscience.* March 28, 2019;13:912. doi:10.3332/ecancer.2019.912. Available at: https://www.ncbi.nlm.nih.gov/pmc/articles/PMC6467453/ (Accessed March 2020)
4. Berwick D, Nolan T, Whittington J. *The Triple Aim: Care, Health, and Cost, Health Affairs.* May 2008. Available at: http://content.healthaffairs.org/content/27/3/759.full (Accessed March 2020).
5. Bodenheimer T, Sinsky C. From Triple to Quadruple Aim: Care of the Patient Requires Care of the Provider. *Ann Fam Med.* November 2014. Available at: https://www.ncbi.nlm.nih.gov/pmc/articles/PMC4226781/#__ffn_sectitle (Accessed May 2020)
6. Feeley D. The Triple Aim or the Quadruple Aim? Four Points to Help Set Your Strategy. November 2017. Available at: http://www.ihi.org/communities/blogs/the-triple-aim-or-the-quadruple-aim-four-points-to-help-set-your-strategy (Accessed March 2020)

7. Patel V, Johnson C. Individuals' Use of Online Medical Records and Technology for Health Needs. April 2018. Available at: https://www.healthit.gov/sites/default/files/page/2018-03/HINTS-2017-Consumer-Data-Brief-3.21.18.pdf (Accessed March 2020)

8. Patel V, Johnson C. Trends in Individuals' Access, Viewing and Use of Online Medical Records and Other Technology for Health Needs: 2017–2018. May 2019. Available at: https://www.healthit.gov/sites/default/files/page/2019-05/Trends-in-Individuals-Access-Viewing-and-Use-of-Online-Medical-Records-and-Other-Technology-for-Health-Needs-2017-2018.pdf (Accessed March 2020)

9. Pifer R. Patient Use of Digital Tools, 3rd-Party Apps to Access Health Records Rises in 2019. *Healthcare Dive*. January 2020. Available at: https://www.healthcaredive.com/news/patient-use-of-digital-tools-3rd-party-apps-to-access-health-records-rises/571147/ (Accessed March 2020)

10. Baldwin J, Singh H, Sittig D, Giardina T. Patient Portals and Health Apps: Pitfalls, Promises, and What One Might Learn From the Other. Healthcare. September 2016. Available at: https://doi.org/10.1016/j.hjdsi.2016.08.004 (Accessed March 2020)

11. Lin S, Lyles C, Sakar U, Adler-Milstein J. Are Patients Electronically Accessing Their Medical Records? Evidence from National Hospital Data. *Health Affairs*. November 2019. Available at: https://www.healthaffairs.org/doi/abs/10.1377/hlthaff.2018.05437 (Accessed March 2020)

12. Oest S, Hightower M, Krasowski, M. Activation and Utilization of an Electronic Health Record Patient Portal at an Academic Medical Center – Impact of Patient Demographics and Geographic Location. January 2018. Available at: https://www.ncbi.nlm.nih.gov/pmc/articles/PMC6172938/ (Accessed March 2020)

13. Bombardier J. Mobile Banking One of Top Three Most Used Apps by Americans, 2018 Citi Mobile Banking Study Reveals. April 2018. Available at: https://www.multivu.com/players/English/8313051-citi-mobile-banking-study-2018/ (Accessed March 2020)

14. Fishel B. NPR/Marist Poll: Amazon Is a Colossus in a Nation of Shoppers. May 2018. Available at: https://www.npr.org/about-npr/617470695/npr-marist-poll-amazon-is-a-colossus-in-a-nation-of-shoppers (Accessed March 2020)

15. Pew Research. 2018 Pew Research Center's American Trends Panel. August 2018. Available at: https://www.journalism.org/wp-content/uploads/sites/8/2018/09/PJ_2018.09.10_social-media-news_TOPLINE.pdf (Accessed March 2020)

16. Senecal C, Widmer RJ, Bailey K, Lerman LO, Lerman A. Usage of a Digital Health Workplace Intervention Based on Socioeconomic Environment and Race: Retrospective Secondary Cross-Sectional Study. *J Med Internet Res* April 2018;20(4):e145. Available at: https://www.jmir.org/2018/4/e145/ (Accessed March 2020)

17. Landi H. Who Isn't Using Patient Portals? New Study Sheds Light on Portal Use. December 2018. Available at: https://www.hcinnovationgroup.com/population-health-management/news/13030963/who-isnt-using-patient-portals-new-study-sheds-light-on-portal-use (Accessed March 2020)

18. Patel V, Johnson C. Trends in Individuals' Access, Viewing and Use of Online Medical Records and Other Technology for Health Needs: 2017–2018 May 2019. Available at: https://www.healthit.gov/sites/default/files/page/2019-05/Trends-in-Individuals-Access-Viewing-and-Use-of-Online-Medical-Records-and-Other-Technology-for-Health-Needs-2017-2018.pdf (Accessed March 2020)

19. Hoogenbosch B, Postma J, de Man-van Ginkel J, Tiemessen N, van Delden J, Os-Medendorp H. Use and the Users of a Patient Portal: Cross-Sectional Study, September 2018. *J Med Internet Res*. Available at: https://www.jmir.org/2018/9/e262/?utm_source=TrendMD&utm_medium=cpc&utm_campaign=JMIR_TrendMD_0 (Accessed March 2020)

20. Walker J, Leveille S, Bell S, Chimowitz H, Dong Z, Elmore JG, Fernandez L, Fossa A, Gerard M, Fitzgerald P, Harcourt K, Jackson S, Payne TH, Perez J, Shucard H, Stametz R, DesRoches C, Delbanco T. OpenNotes After 7 Years: Patient Experiences with Ongoing Access to Their Clinicians' Outpatient Visit Notes. *J Med Internet Res*. May 2019. Available at: https://www.jmir.org/2019/5/e13876/ (Accessed March 2020)

21. McCarthy J. One in Five U.S. Adults Use Health Apps, Wearable Trackers. December 2019. Available at: https://news.gallup.com/poll/269096/one-five-adults-health-apps-wearable-trackers.aspx (Accessed March 2020)

22. Betts D, Korenda L. Inside the Patient Journey: Three Key Touch Points for Consumer Engagement Strategies. September 2018. Available at: https://www2.deloitte.com/us/en/insights/industry/health-care/patient-engagement-health-care-consumer-survey.html (Accessed March 2020)

23. Paré G, Leaver C, Bourget C. Diffusion of the Digital Health Self-Tracking Movement in Canada: Results of a National Survey. *J Med Internet Res*. May 2018. Available at: https://www.ncbi.nlm.nih.gov/pmc/articles/PMC5956159/ (Accessed March 2020)

24. Sydow L. Medical Apps Transform How Patients Receive Medical Care. April 2019. Available at: https://www.appannie.com/en/insights/market-data/medical-apps-transform-patient-care/ (Accessed March 2020)

25. IQVIA Institute. The Growing Value of Digital Health. November 2017. Available at: https://www.iqvia.com/insights/the-iqvia-institute/reports/the-growing-value-of-digital-health (Accessed March 2020)

26. Birnbaum F, Lewis D, Rosen RK, Ranney ML. Patient Engagement and the Design of Digital Health. *Acad Emerg Med*. June 2015. Available at: https://www.ncbi.nlm.nih.gov/pmc/articles/PMC4674428/ (Accessed March 2020)

27. Georgiou M. Developing a Healthcare App in 2020: What Do Patients Really Want? January 2020. Available at: https://www.imaginovation.net/blog/developing-a-mobile-health-app-what-patients-really-want/ (Accessed March 2020)

28. Safavi K, Kalis B. Why Is Consumer Digital Health Adoption Stalling? March 2020. Available at: https://www.accenture.com/us-en/insights/health/why-consumer-digital-health-adoption-stalling (Accessed March 2020)

29. CMS.gov. HITECH Act Enforcement Interim Final Rule. October 2009. Available at: https://www.hhs.gov/hipaa/for-professionals/special-topics/hitech-act-enforcement-interim-final-rule/index.html#:~:text=The%20Health%20Information%20Technology%20for,use%20of%20health%20information%20technology. (Accessed March 2020.)

30. deBronkart, D. Let Patients Help. We Are the Ultimate Motivated Stakeholders. Testimony Before the Meaningful Use Workgroup HIT Policy Committee. April 2010. https://participatorymedicine.org/epatients/wp-content/uploads/sites/3/2010/04/2f-deBronkart-MU-WG-testimony-4-20-10.pdf (Accessed May 2020)

31. Holiday R. Testimony to NCVHS. May 2010. https://participatorymedicine.org/epatients/2012/03/regina-hollidays-testimony-at-ncvhs.html (Accessed May 2020)

32. CMS.gov. Stage 3 Program Requirements for Eligible Hospitals, CAHs and Dual-Eligible Hospitals Attesting to CMS. April 2018. Available at: https://www.cms.gov/Regulations-and-Guidance/Legislation/EHRIncentivePrograms/Stage3_RequieEH (Accessed March 2020)

33. CY 2017 Hospital Outpatient PPS Policy Changes and Payment Rates and Ambulatory Surgical Center Payment System Policy Changes and Payment Rates CMS-1656-P. Fed Regist. November 2016. Available at: https://www.federalregister.gov/documents/2016/11/14/2016-26515/medicare-program-hospital-outpatient-prospective-payment-and-ambulatory-surgical-center-payment (Accessed March 2020)

34. CMS.gov. 2020 Medicare Promoting Interoperability Program Overview Fact Sheet. August 2019. Available at: https://www.cms.gov/Regulations-and-Guidance/Legislation/EHRIncentivePrograms/Downloads/Medicare_FactSheetFY2020.pdf (Accessed March 2020)

35. CY 2020 Revisions to Payment Policies Under the Physician Fee Schedule and Other Changes to Part B Payment Policies; Medicare Shared Savings Program Requirements; Medicaid Promoting Interoperability Program Requirements for Eligible Professionals. Centers for Medicare & Medicaid Services (CMS), HHS. Fed Regist. 84 FR 62568. November 2019. Available at: https://federalregister.gov/d/2019-24086 (Accessed March 2020)

36. CMS.Gov. Quality Payment Program Explore Measures and Activities: 2019 Promoting Interoperability. Available at: https://qpp.cms.gov/mips/explore-measures/promoting-interoperability?py=2019#measures (Accessed March 2020)

37. CMS.gov. Medicare Program; Merit-Based Incentive Payment System (MIPS) and Alternative Payment Model (APM) Incentive Under the Physician Fee Schedule, and Criteria for Physician-Focused Payment Models. Centers for Medicare & Medicaid Services (CMS0. November 2016. Fed Regist.

81 FR 77008 Available at: https://www.federalregister.gov/documents/2016/11/04/2016-25240/medicare-program-merit-based-incentive-payment-system-mips-and-alternative-payment-model-apm#p-2831 (Accessed March 2020)

38. HealthIT.gov. 21st Century Cures Act: Interoperability, Information Blocking, and the ONC Health IT Certification Program. Department of Health and Human Services (HHS). 45 CFR Parts 170 and 171. December 2016. Available at: https://www.healthit.gov/sites/default/files/cures/2020-03/ONC_Cures_Act_Final_Rule_03092020.pdf (Accessed March 2020)

39. Farr C. Epic's CEO Is Urging Hospital Customers to Oppose Rules That Would Make It Easier to Share Medical Info. January 2020. Available at: https://www.cnbc.com/2020/01/22/epic-ceo-sends-letter-urging-hospitals-to-oppose-hhs-data-sharing-rule.html (Accessed March 2020)

40. Inserro A. HHS Stands Behind Final Rules on Interoperability of Patient Data. February 2020. AJMC. Available at: https://www.ajmc.com/conferences/academyhealth-nhpc-hdp-2020/hhs-stands-behind-final-rules-on-interoperability-of-patient-data (Accessed March 2020)

41. Henry S, Shen E, Ahuja A, Gould M, Kantar M. The Online Personal Action Plan: A Tool to Transform Patient-Enabled Preventive and Chronic Care. January 2016. AJPM. Available at: https://www.ajpmonline.org/article/S0749-3797%2815%2900780-1/abstract (Accessed March 2020)

42. Thakkar J, Kurup R, Laba T. Mobile Telephone Text Messaging for Medication Adherence in Chronic Disease: A Meta-Analysis. March 2016. JAMA. Available at: https://jamanetwork.com/journals/jamainternalmedicine/fullarticle/2484905 (Accessed March 2020)

43. Risling T, Martinez J, Young J, Thorp-Froslie N. Evaluating Patient Empowerment in Association with eHealth Technology: Scoping Review. September 2017. *J Med Internet Reg*. Available at: https://www.jmir.org/2017/9/e329/ (Accessed March 2020)

44. Insignia Health. Research Studies Using Patient Activation Measure (PAM) Available at: https://www.insigniahealth.com/research/archive/ (Accessed March 2020)

45. Hibbard J, Sacks R, Overton V. When Seeing the Same Physician, Highly Activated Patients Have Better Care Experiences Than Less Activated Patients. December 2013. Available at: https://pubmed.ncbi.nlm.nih.gov/23836747/ (Accessed March 2020)

46. Milani R, Lavie C, Bober R, Milani A, Ventura H. Improving Hypertension Control and Patient Engagement Using Digital Tools. January 2017. *Am J Med*. Available at: https://www.amjmed.com/article/S0002-9343(16)30844-0/pdf (Accessed March 2020)

47. Huang J, Chen Y, Landis J, Mahoney K. Difference Between Users and Nonusers of a Patient Portal in Health Behaviors and Outcomes: Retrospective Cohort Study. October 2019. *J Med Internet Res*. Available at: https://www.jmir.org/2019/10/e13146?utm_source=TrendMD&utm_medium=cpc&utm_campaign=JMIR_TrendMD_0 (Accessed March 2020)

48. Sawesi S, Rashrash M, Phalakornkule K, Carpenter J, Jones J. The Impact of Information Technology on Patient Engagement and Health Behavior Change: A Systematic Review of the Literature. January–March 2016. *J Med Internet Res*. Available at: https://www.ncbi.nlm.nih.gov/pmc/articles/PMC4742621/ (Accessed March 2020)

49. Han H, Gleason K, Sun C, Miller H, Kang S, Chow S, Anderson R, Nagy P, Bauer T. Using Patient Portals to Improve Patient Outcomes: Systematic Review. June 2019. *J Med Internet Res Human Factors*. Available at: https://humanfactors.jmir.org/2019/4/e15038/ (Accessed March 2020)

50. Crouch PB, Rose CD, Johnson M, Janson SL. 2015. A Pilot Study to Evaluate the Magnitude of Association of the Use of Electronic Personal Health Records with Patient Activation and Empowerment in HIV-Infected Veterans. March 2015. *PeerJ*. Available at: https://peerj.com/articles/852/ (Accessed March 2020)

51. Lau M, Campbell H, Tang T, Thompson D, Elliott T. Impact of Patient Use of an Online Patient Portal on Diabetes Outcomes. February 2014. *Pub Med*. Available at: https://pubmed.ncbi.nlm.nih.gov/24485208/ (Accessed March 2020)

52. Davis J. Kaiser: Online Tools Increase Likelihood Patients Will Receive Preventative Care. February 2016. *Healthcare IT News*. Available at: https://www.healthcareitnews.com/news/kaiser-online-tools-increase-likelihood-patients-will-receive-preventative-care (Accessed March 2020)

53. Kim J, Wineinger N, Steinhubl S. The Influence of Wireless Self-Monitoring Program on the Relationship Between Patient Activation and Health Behaviors, Medication Adherence, and Blood Pressure

Levels in Hypertensive Patients: A Substudy of a Randomized Controlled Trial. *J Med Internet Res.* June 2016. Available at: https://www.jmir.org/2016/6/e116/ (Accessed March 2020)

54. Pillemer F, Price R, Paone S, Martich G, Albert S, Haidari L, Updike G, Rudin R, Liu D, Mehrotra A. Direct Release of Test Results to Patients Increases Patient Engagement and Utilization of Care. *PLoS One.* June 2016. Available at: https://journals.plos.org/plosone/article?id=10.1371/journal.pone.0154743 (Accessed March 2020)

55. Available at: https://participatorymedicine.org/journal/evidence/research/2013/10/03/viewing-laboratory-test-results-online-patients-actions-and-reactions/ (Accessed March 2020)

56. Christensen K, Sue V. Viewing Laboratory Test Results Online: Patients' Actions and Reactions. *J Soc Particip Med.* October 2013. Available at: https://www.ncbi.nlm.nih.gov/pmc/articles/PMC6670280/ (Accessed March 2020)

57. Toscos T, Daley C, Heral L, Doshi R, Chen Y, Eckert G, Plant R, Mirro M. Impact of Electronic Personal Health Record Use on Engagement and Intermediate Health Outcomes Among Cardiac Patients: A Quasi-Experimental Study January 2016. *J Am Med Inform Assoc.* Available at: https://www.ncbi.nlm.nih.gov/pubmed/26912538?dopt=Abstract (Accessed March 2020)

58. Riippa I, Linna M, Rönkkö I. The Effect of a Patient Portal with Electronic Messaging on Patient Activation Among Chronically Ill Patients: Controlled Before-and-After Study. *J Med Internet Res.* November 2014. Available at: https://www.ncbi.nlm.nih.gov/pmc/articles/PMC4260064/ (Accessed March 2020)

59. Fox S. The Social Life of Health Information. January 2014. Available at: http://www.pewresearch.org/fact-tank/2014/01/15/the-social-life-of-health-information/ (Accessed March 2020)

60. Murphy M. Dr Google Will See You Now: Search Giant Wants to Cash in on Your Medical Queries. March 2019. Available at: https://www.telegraph.co.uk/technology/2019/03/10/google-sifting-one-billion-health-questions-day/ (Accessed March 2020)

61. Zhao Y, Zhang J. Consumer Health Information Seeking in Social Media: A Literature Review. *Health Information and Libraries Journal.* December 2017. Available at: https://onlinelibrary.wiley.com/doi/full/10.1111/hir.12192 (Accessed March 2020)

62. Christakis N, Fowler J. The Spread of Obesity in a Large Social Network Over 32 Years. July 2007. Available at: http://www.nejm.org/doi/full/10.1056/NEJMsa066082 (Accessed March 2020).

63. Available at: https://www.nature.com/articles/ncomms14753 (Accessed March 2020)

64. Ball K, Jeffery R, Abbott G, et al. Is Healthy Behavior Contagious: Associations of Social Norms with Physical Activity and Healthy Eating. July 2010. Available at: https://ijbnpa.biomedcentral.com/articles/10.1186/1479-5868-7-86 (Accessed March 2020)

65. Fox S. Peer-to-Peer Health Care. February 2011. Available at: https://www.pewresearch.org/internet/2011/02/28/peer-to-peer-health-care-2/ (Accessed March 2020)

66. Fox S. Peer Health Advice Among Teens and Young Adults. August 2018. Available at: https://susannahfox.com/2018/08/06/peer-health-advice-among-teens-and-young-adults/ (Accessed March 2020)

67. Netolicky L. Role of Patient Influencers: How do Patients Truly Share Information? 2017 Available at: https://tglv8lyxesoiyue1wzi0cmgt-wpengine.netdna-ssl.com/wp-content/uploads/2017/05/PT-2-WEGO-Health-Solutions_BIS_sharing-behavior.pdf (Accessed March 2020)

68. Dhar V, Kim Y, Graff J, Dick L, Harris J, Shah S. Benefit of Social Media on Patient Engagement and Satisfaction: Results of a 9-Month, Qualitative Pilot Study Using Facebook. *Surgery.* November 2017. Available at: https://www.surgjournal.com/article/S0039-6060(17)30717-1/fulltext (Accessed March 2020)

69. Allen C, Vassilev I, Rogers A. Long-Term Condition Self-Management Support in Online Communities: A Meta-Synthesis of Qualitative Papers. *J Med Internet Res.* March 2018. Available at: https://www.ncbi.nlm.nih.gov/pmc/articles/PMC4807245/ (Accessed March 2020)

70. Maher C, Lewis L, Ferrar K. Are Health Behavior Change Interventions That Use Online Social Networks Effective? A Systematic Review. February 2014. Available at: https://www.jmir.org/2014/2/e40/ (Accessed March 2020).

71. Costello R, Anand A, Evans M, Dixon W. Associations Between Engagement with an Online Health Community and Changes in Patient Activation and Health Care Utilization: Longitudinal Web-Based Survey. *J Med Internet Res.* August 2019. Available at: https://www.jmir.org/2019/8/e13477/ (Accessed March 2020)

72. Cole J, Watkins K. Health Advice from Internet Discussion Forums: How Bad Is Dangerous? *J Med Internet Res*. June 2016. Available at: https://www.jmir.org/2016/1/e4/ (Accessed March 2020)

73. Accuracy and Self Correction of Information Received from an Internet Breast Cancer List: Content Analysis. April 2016. BMJ. Available at: https://www.ncbi.nlm.nih.gov/pmc/articles/PMC1444809/ (Accessed March 2020)

74. Hoffman-Goetz L, Donelle L, Thomson MD. Clinical Guidelines About Diabetes and the Accuracy of Peer Information in an Unmoderated Online Health Forum for Retired Persons. *Inform Health Soc Care*. March 2009. Available at: https://pubmed.ncbi.nlm.nih.gov/19412842/ (Accessed March 2020)

75. Vydiswaran, V, Reddy, M. Identifying Peer Experts in Online Health Forums. *BMC Med Inform Decis Mak*. April 2019. Available at: https://doi.org/10.1186/s12911-019-0782-3 (Accessed March 2020)

76. Prior R. This Breast Cancer Advocate Says She Discovered a Facebook Flaw That put the Health Data of Millions at Risk. March 2020. Available at: https://www.cnn.com/2020/02/29/health/andrea-downing-facebook-data-breach-wellness-trnd/index.html (Accessed March 2020)

77. Patel V, Johnson C. Individuals' Use of Online Medical Records and Technology for Health Needs. *Office of the National Coordinator of Health IT*. April 2018. Available at: https://www.healthit.gov/sites/default/files/page/2018-03/HINTS-2017-Consumer-Data-Brief-3.21.18.pdf (Accessed March 2020)

78. Graham J. Check Your Medical Records for Dangerous Errors. November 2018. Available at: https://khn.org/news/check-your-medical-records-for-dangerous-errors/ (Accessed March 2020)

79. Farr, C. This Patient's Medical Record Said She'd Given Birth Twice – in Fact, She'd Never Been Pregnant. December 2018. Available at: https://www.cnbc.com/2018/12/09/medical-record-errors-common-hard-to-fix.html?utm_source=newsletter&utm_medium=email&utm_campaign=newsletter_axiosvitals&stream=top (Accessed March 2020)

80. Lawes S, Grissinger M. Pennsylvania Patient Safety Authority. Medication Errors Attributed to Health Information Technology. March 2017. Available at: http://patientsafety.pa.gov/ADVISORIES/Pages/201703_HITmed.aspx (Accessed March 2020)

81. Walker J, Leveille S, Bell S, Chimowitz H, Dong Z, Elmore J, Fernandez L, Fossa A, Gerard M, Fitzgerald P, Harcourt K, Jackson S, Payne T, Perez J, Shucard H, Stametz R, DesRoches C, Delbanco T. OpenNotes After 7 Years: Patient Experiences with Ongoing Access to Their Clinicians' Outpatient Visit Notes. May 2019. *J Med Internet Res*. Available at: https://www.jmir.org/2019/5/e13876/#Body (Accessed March 2020)

82. Sigall K Bell, Roanne Mejilla, Melissa Anselmo, Jonathan D Darer, Joann G Elmore, Suzanne Leveille, Long Ngo, James D Ralston, Tom Delbanco, Jan Walker. When Doctors Share Visit Notes with Patients: A Study of Patient and Doctor Perceptions of Documentation Errors, Safety Opportunities and the Patient – Doctor Relationship. *BMJ*. June 2016. Available at: https://qualitysafety.bmj.com/content/26/4/262 (Accessed March 2020)

83. Krist AH, Woolf SH, Rothemich SF, et al. Interactive Preventive Health Record to Enhance Delivery of Recommended Care: A Randomized Trial. *Ann Fam Med* 2012;10(4):312–319. Available at: http://www.annfammed.org/content/10/4/312.figures-only (Accessed March 2020)

84. Sarkar U, Lyles C, Parker M. Use of the Refill Function Through an Online Patient Portal Is Associated with Improved Adherence to Statins in an Integrated Health System. May 2014. Available at: http://journals.lww.com/lww-medicalcare/Fulltext/2014/05000/Use_of_the_Refill_Function_Through_an_Online.12.aspx (Accessed March 2020).

85. Tom J, Chen C, Zhou Y. Personal Health Record Use and Association with Immunizations and Well-Child Care Visits Recommendations. January 2014; Available at: http://download.journals.elsevierhealth.com/pdfs/journals/0022-3476/PIIS0022347613010743.pdf (Accessed March 2020).

86. Zhou Y, Kanter M, Wang J, et al. Improved Quality at Kaiser Permanente Through e-mail Between Physicians and Patients. *Health Aff (Millwood)* 2010;29(7):1370–1375. Available at: https://pubmed.ncbi.nlm.nih.gov/20606190/ (Accessed March 2020)

87. Roth A. Online Symptom-Monitoring Tool Improves Survival for Those Undergoing Chemotherapy for Metastatic Cancer. June 2017. Available at: https://www.mskcc.org/blog/asco17-online-symptom-monitoring-tool-improves-survival-those-undergoing-chemotherapy-metastatic (Accessed March 2020)

88. Shirali G, Erickson L, Apperson J, Goggin K, Williams D, Reid K, Bradley-Ewing A, Tucker D, Bingler M, Spertus J, Rabbitt L, Stroup R. Harnessing Teams and Technology to Improve Outcomes in

Infants with Single Ventricle. *Cardiovascular Quality and Outcomes.* May 2016. Available at: https://www.ahajournals.org/doi/full/10.1161/CIRCOUTCOMES.115.002452 (Accessed March 2020)

89. Children's Mercy App Brings Doctors Home, Virtually, with Babies Born with Heart Disease. July 2016. Available at: https://news.microsoft.com/transform/childrens-mercy-app-brings-doctors-home-virtually-with-babies-born-with-heart-disease/ (Accessed March 2020)

90. Donnell, J. CASE STUDY: An HIE-Populated Personal Health Record for Cardiac Revascularization Patients. May 2014. Available at: https://www.nomoreclipboard.com/providers/info/case-study-an-hie-populated-personal-health-record-for-cardiac-revascularization-patients/ (Accessed March 2020).

91. Standen A. Patients Crusade for Access to Their Medical Device Data. May 2012. Available at: https://www.npr.org/sections/health-shots/2012/05/28/153706099/patients-crusade-for-access-to-their-medical-device-data (Accessed March 2020)

92. Daley C, Toscos T, Mirro M. Data Integration and Interoperability for Patient-Centered Remote Monitoring of Cardiovascular Implantable Electronic Devices. March 2019. Bioengineering. Available at: https://www.mdpi.com/2306-5354/6/1/25/htm (Accessed March 2020)

93. Lee J. Patient as Expert, Maker, and Collaborator: Nightscout. October 2014. Available at: https://medium.com/@joyclee/patient-as-expert-maker-and-collaborator-nightscout-42ba1ce2f24d

94. Available at: Zimmerman, S. Technology Beyond the Exam Room. April 2013. Available at: https://www.televox.com/downloads/technology_beyond_exam_room.pdf (Accessed March 2020).

95. Widmer RJ, Collins NM, Collins CS, West CP, Lerman LO, Lerman A. Health Interventions for the Prevention of Cardiovascular Disease: A Systematic Review and Meta-Analysis. April 2015. *Mayo Clin Proc* 2015;90(4):469–480. Available at: https://pubmed.ncbi.nlm.nih.gov/25841251/ (Accessed March 2020)

96. Jiang X, Ming W, You J. The Cost-Effectiveness of Digital Health Interventions on the Management of Cardiovascular Diseases: Systematic Review. *J Med Internet Res.* June 2019. Available at: https://www.jmir.org/2019/6/e13166/ (Accessed March 2020)

97. Brot-Goldberg Z, Chandra A, Handel B, Kolstad J. What Does a Deductible Do? The Impact of Cost-Sharing on Health Care Prices, Quantities, and Spending Dynamics. *Quarterly Journal of Economics.* April 2017. Available at: https://academic.oup.com/qje/article-abstract/132/3/1261/3769421?redirectedFrom=fulltext (Accessed March 2020)

98. Collins S, Rasmussen P, Beutel S, Doty M. The Problem of Underinsurance and How Rising Deductibles Will Make It Worse. May 2015. Available at: https://www.commonwealthfund.org/publications/issue-briefs/2015/may/problem-underinsurance-and-how-rising-deductibles-will-make-it?redirect_source=/publications/issue-briefs/2015/may/problem-of-underinsurance (Accessed March 2020)

99. Himmelstein D, Lawless R, Thorne D, Foohey P, Woolhandler S. Medical Bankruptcy: Still Common Despite the Affordable Care Act. March 2019. *American Journal of Public Health.* Available at: https://ajph.aphapublications.org/doi/10.2105/AJPH.2018.304901 (Accessed March 2020)

100. Konish L. This Is the Real Reason Most Americans File for Bankruptcy. February 2019. Available at: https://www.cnbc.com/2019/02/11/this-is-the-real-reason-most-americans-file-for-bankruptcy.html (Accessed March 2020)

101. American Institutes for Research. Lessons Learned: Consumer Beliefs and Use of Information About Health Care Cost, Resource Use, and Value. October 2012. Available at: https://www.rwjf.org/en/library/research/2012/10/consumer-beliefs-and-use-of-information-about-health-care-cost-.html (Accessed March 2020).

102. Starc A. Four Ways to Improve the Efficiency of US Healthcare Markets. December 2017. Available at: https://insight.kellogg.northwestern.edu/article/4-ways-to-improve-the-efficiency-of-u-s-health-care-markets (Accessed March 2020)

103. Instamed. Trends in Healthcare Payments Ninth Annual Report: 2018. April 2019. Available at: https://www.instamed.com/white-papers/trends-healthcare-payments-report-2018/?creative=356235550077&keyword=instamed&matchtype=b&network=g&device=c&gclid=Cj0KCQiA4sjyBRC5ARIsAEHsELG3zbQ3E1WLzDwp3pzAySnXzFbw_AezfYV71FnCI1OxDdHPoRz_TZcaAmlgEALw_wcB (Accessed March 2020)

104. Instamed. UnitedHealthcare Enables Consumers to Pay Medical Bills Online. August 2013. Available at: https://www.instamed.com/news-and-events/unitedhealthcares-new-online-service-lets-consumers-pay-their-medical-bills-online-and-better-manage-health-care-expenses/ (Accessed March 2020)

105. Transunion. Survey: Providers Fall Short of Meeting Growing Patient Demand for Greater Health-care Cost Transparency. June 2014. Available at: https://www.globenewswire.com/news-release/2014/06/23/962947/0/en/TransUnion-Survey-Providers-Fall-Short-of-Meeting-Growing-Patient-Demand-for-Greater-Healthcare-Cost-Transparency.html (Accessed March 2020)

106. DeLeonardo J. CareCredit and Medical Group Management Association (MGMA) Partner to Address Rising Cost of Medical Care. October 2019. Available at: https://www.carecredit.com/press release/carecredit-mgma-partnership (Accessed March 2020)

107. Buell R, Campbell D, Frei F. Are Self-Service Customers Satisfied or Stuck? May 2009; Available at: https://www.hbs.edu/faculty/Pages/item.aspx?num=40014 (Accessed March 2020).

108. Punke, H. Reducing ACO Patient Leakage Begins with Education. September 2013. Available at: https://www.beckershospitalreview.com/accountable-care-organizations/reducing-aco-patient-leakage-begins-with-education.html (Accessed March 2020).

109. Sage Growth Partners, Fibroblast. Leakage: A New Survey Highlights High Costs, Limited Control. October 2018. Available at: https://fibroblast.com/wp-content/uploads/2018/10/Patient-Leakage-A-new-survey-highlights-high-costs-limited-control-October-2018-1.pdf (Accessed March 2020)

110. Landi H. 60% of Younger Patients Will Switch Healthcare Providers Over a Poor Digital Experience: Survey. October 2019. Available at: https://www.fiercehealthcare.com/tech/60-younger-patients-will-switch-healthcare-providers-over-a-poor-digital-experience-survey (Accessed March 2020)

111. Safavi K, Webb K, Kalis B. Accenture's 2019 Digital Health Consumer Survey: US Results. February 2019. Available at: https://www.accenture.com/_acnmedia/pdf-94/accenture-2019-digital-health-consumer-survey.pdf (Accessed March 2020)

112. Pew Research Center. Mobile Fact Sheet. June 2019. Available at: https://www.pewresearch.org/internet/fact-sheet/mobile/ (Accessed March 2020)

113. Anderson M, Kumar M. Digital Divide Persists Even as Lower-Income Americans Make Gains in Tech Adoption. May 2019. Available at: https://www.pewresearch.org/fact-tank/2019/05/07/digital-divide-persists-even-as-lower-income-americans-make-gains-in-tech-adoption/ (Accessed March 2020)

114. Vogels E. Millennials Stand Out for Their Technology Use, but Older Generations also Embrace Digital Life. September 2019. Available at: https://www.pewresearch.org/fact-tank/2019/09/09/us-generations-technology-use/ (Accessed March 2020)

115. Smith A. The Best (and Worst) of Mobile Connectivity. November 2012. Available at: https://www.pewresearch.org/internet/2012/11/30/the-best-and-worst-of-mobile-connectivity/ (Accessed March 2020).

116. Klasnja P, Pratt W. Healthcare in the Pocket: Mapping the Space of Mobile-Phone Health Interventions. *J Biomed Inform*. February 2012. Available at: https://pubmed.ncbi.nlm.nih.gov/21925288/ (Accessed March 2020).

117. Hall AK, Cole-Lewis H, Bernhardt JM. Mobile Text Messaging for Health: A Systematic Review of Reviews. *Annual Review of Public Health* 2015 March;36:393–415. DOI: 10.1146/annurev-publhealth-031914–122855. March 2015. Available at: http://europepmc.org/article/MED/25785892 (Accessed March 2020)

118. Tyson B, Sewell G. Kaiser Permanente 2018 Annual Report. December 2018. Available at: https://healthy.kaiserpermanente.org/static/health/annual_reports/kp_annualreport_2018/ (Accessed March 2020)

119. Shcherbina A, Hershman S, Lazzeroni L, King A, O'Sullivan J, Hekler E. The Effect of Digital Physical Activity Interventions on Daily Step Count: A Randomised Controlled Crossover Substudy of the MyHeart Counts Cardiovascular Health Study. *The Lancet Digital Health*. October 2019. Available at: https://www.thelancet.com/journals/landig/article/PIIS2589-7500(19)30129-3/fulltext#%20 (Accessed March 2020)

120. Brickwood KJ, Watson G, O'Brien J, Williams AD. Consumer-Based Wearable Activity Trackers Increase Physical Activity Participation: Systematic Review and Meta-Analysis. *JMIR Mhealth Uhealth* 2019;7(4):e11819. August 2018. Available at: https://mhealth.jmir.org/2019/4/e11819/ (Accessed March 2020)

121. Quisel T, Foschini L, Zbikowski SM, Juusola JL. The Association Between Medication Adherence for Chronic Conditions and Digital Health Activity Tracking: Retrospective Analysis. *J Med Internet Res* 2019;21(3):e11486. March 2019. Available at: https://www.jmir.org/2019/3/e11486/ (Accessed March 2020)

122. West JH, Belvedere LM, Andreasen R, Frandsen C, Hall PC, Crookston BT. Controlling Your "App"etite: How Diet and Nutrition-Related Mobile Apps Lead to Behavior Change. *JMIR Mhealth Uhealth* 2017;5(7):e95. July 2017. Available at: https://mhealth.jmir.org/2017/7/e95/ (Accessed March 2020)

123. Marczewski A. The Intrinsic Motivation Ramp. October 2017. Available at: https://www.gamified.uk/gamification-framework/the-intrinsic-motivation-ramp/ (Accessed March 2020)

124. Karapanos E. Sustaining User Engagement with Behavior-Change Tools. *ACM Interactions*. August 2015. Available at: https://interactions.acm.org/archive/view/july-august-2015/sustaining-user-engagement-with-behavior-change-tools (Accessed March 2020)

125. Gniewek B, Mansur G, Antonelli K, Atkinson D, Rubin J. PWC Health & Well-Being Touchstone Survey Results. June 2017. Available at: https://www.pwc.com/us/en/hr-management/publications/assets/pwc-touchstone-2017.pdf (Accessed March 2020)

126. Surve S. Embracing the Science of Behavior Change. Relationships Are Fuel for Motivation and Behavior Change (Both Positive and Negative). Motivations, Triggers and Ease of Action Are Keys to Enabling Behavior Change. May 2018. Available at: https://healthrosetta.org/education/swatee-surve-embracing-the-science-of-behavior-change/ (Accessed March 2020)

127. Payne HE, Moxley VB, MacDonald E. Health Behavior Theory in Physical Activity Game Apps: A Content Analysis. *JMIR Serious Games* 2015;3(2):e4. Published 2015 July 13. doi:10.2196/games.4187. Jul 2015. Available at: https://www.ncbi.nlm.nih.gov/pmc/articles/PMC4526993/ (Accessed March 2020)

128. Keefe B. Gamification in Healthcare – Let's Play! March 2016. Available at: https://blog.centerforinnovation.mayo.edu/2016/03/25/gamification-in-healthcare-lets-play/ (Accessed March 2020)

129. Sandle T. New Digital Healthcare Solutions Using Gamification Tested Out. *Digital Journal*. August 2019. Available at: http://www.digitaljournal.com/life/health/new-digital-healthcare-solutions-using-gamification-tested-out/article/555966 (Accessed March 2020)

130. Pai A. Two Blues Discuss Healthy Behavior Change, Rewards, Loss Aversion, and Regret Theory. *Mobihealthnews*. July 2013. Available at: https://www.mobihealthnews.com/24129/two-blues-discuss-healthy-behavior-change-rewards-loss-aversion-and-regret-theory (Accessed March 2020).

131. Kalousek A. More Than Half of California's Top 10 Health Conditions Can Be Treated with ZERO Negative Side Effects. October 2018. Available at: https://news.blueshieldca.com/2018/10/03/well volution-10-year (Accessed March 2020)

132. Landi H. Aetna Launching New Apple Watch App to Gather Health Data, Reward Healthy Behavior. *FierceHealthcare*. January 2019. Available at: https://www.fiercehealthcare.com/tech/aetna-launching-new-apple-watch-app-to-gather-health-data-reward-healthy-behavior (Accessed March 2020)

133. Patel M, Change S, Volpp K. Improving Health Care by Gamifying It. *HBR*. May 2019. Available at: https://hbr.org/2019/05/improving-health-care-by-gamifying-it (Accessed March 2020)

134. Schruder K. The Top 5 Behavioural Economics Principles for Designers. February 2018. Available at: https://uxplanet.org/the-top-5-behavioural-economics-principles-for-designers-ea22a16a4020 (Accessed March 2020)

135. Deloitte Consulting. Closing the Wellness Gap: Fusing Mobile Technologies with Behavioral Science to Improve Health Outcomes December 2016. Available at: https://www2.deloitte.com/us/en/insights/focus/behavioral-economics/improving-health-outcomes-mobile-health-care.html (Accessed March 2020)

136. Fogg BJ. A Behavior Model for Persuasive Design. April 2009. Available at: https://www.mebook.se/images/page_file/38/Fogg%20Behavior%20Model.pdf (Accessed March 2020)

137. Hardy W, Powers J, Jasko J, Stitt C, Lotz G, Aloia M. SleepMapper a Mobile Application and Website to Engage Sleep Apnea Patients in PAP Therapy and Improve Adherence to Treatment. 2014. Available at: https://www.semanticscholar.org/paper/SleepMapper-A-mobile-application-and-website-to-in-Hardy-Powers/3cbeda2376f13a46af19b096ecf4c44c4e1b2d60 (Accessed March 2020)

138. Hardy, W, Powers J, Jasko J, Stitt C, Lotz G, Alois M. A Mobile Application and Website to Engage Sleep Apnea Patients in PAP Therapy and Improve Adherence to Treatment. Available at: http://alliednlassets.s3.amazonaws.com/rt-mrkt/phlprp-dm-1611/PR_DreamMapperWhitePaperV2-Final.pdf Accessed March 2020)

139. Hostler JM, Sheikh KL, Andrada TF, Khramtsov A, Holley PR, Holley AB. A Mobile, Web-Based System Can Improve Positive Airway Pressure Adherence. *J Sleep Res* 2017;26(2):139–146. doi:10.1111/jsr.12476. December 2016. Available at: https://pubmed.ncbi.nlm.nih.gov/27933667/ (Accessed March 2020)

140. Mesko B. The Top 15 Examples of Gamification in Healthcare. *Medical Futurist*. July 2017. Available at: https://medicalfuturist.com/top-examples-of-gamification-in-healthcare/ (Accessed March 2020)

141. Murphy-Abdouch K, Dolezel D, McLeod A. Patient Access to Personal Health Information: An Analysis of the Consumer's Perspective Perspectives. Summer 2017. Available at: https://perspectives.ahima.org/patient-accesstophi/ (Accessed March 2020)

142. Crotty BH, Winn AN, Asan, O. Clinician Encouragement and Online Health Record Usage. *J Gen Intern Med* July 2019;34:2345–2347. Available at: https://link.springer.com/article/10.1007%2Fs11606-019-05162-9 (Accessed March 2020)

143. Leckart S. The Blood Test Gets a Makeover. *Wired*. November 2010. Available at: https://www.wired.com/2010/11/ff_bloodwork/ (Accessed March 2020)

144. Mathews S, McShea M, Hanley C, Ravitz A, Labrique A, Cohen A. Digital Health: A Path to Validation. *npj Digital Medicine* 2, Article number: 38 (2019). Available at: https://www.researchgate.net/publication/333065524_Digital_health_a_path_to_validation (Accessed March 2020)

145. Ballard J. Exercising More and Saving Money Are the Most Popular 2020 New Year's Resolutions. *YouGov*. January 2020. Available at: https://today.yougov.com/topics/lifestyle/articles-reports/2020/01/02/new-years-resolutions-2020-health-finance (Accessed March 2020)

Chapter 3

Fostering Innovation in Health IT

Anuj Desai, MBA

Contents

DOI: 10.4324/9780429423109-3

Introduction

Unlike banking, travel, and consumer goods, the health IT market historically has not been a fertile area for dynamic innovation. Until the advent of the personal computer and the Internet, disparate market players displayed a marked reluctance to embrace innovative health IT solutions.

Through most of the latter part of the 20th century, health IT innovation was limited to major medical centers or commercial enterprises that targeted the healthcare industry. Both entities had to fight an uphill battle against the prevalent healthcare market culture, which shunned work-flow innovation. This culture results, to a large extent, from doctors' medical training experience, which resembles an apprenticeship leading to entry to the medical guild. After being subjected to years of rigorous and often rigid medical training, many healthcare practitioners emerge determined to do things their own way, rather than being directed by any authority.

At hospitals fortunate enough to possess advanced IT resources, chief information officers (CIOs) historically were compelled to give highest priority to customized systems that reflected the desires of administrative and physician leadership. These needs were driven by the ever-changing healthcare regulatory/reimbursement environment, as well as dynamic advances in clinical care. IT management tried to be responsive, often creating multidisciplinary information systems committees with membership drawn from the administrative, financial, and clinical ranks to set priorities and deadlines. Often, however, the demands were so numerous and the IT resources so thin that the most frequently heard response from IT was "We can't do that" or "We will eventually get to that."

Meanwhile, commercial corporates, recognizing the opportunity to capitalize on the lucrative healthcare market, created and marketed centralized shared systems based on time-sharing technologies and, later, standalone systems running on minicomputers installed at hospital sites. Initially focused on revenue cycle management, the systems eventually began to address clinical workflow challenges like order entry/reporting and ancillary department management. Enterprising companies had to contend with the notoriously long sales cycles and significant regulatory burdens indigenous to the healthcare market, both of which exerted a drag on rapid innovation.

Luckily, the advent of personal computers and the unprecedented adoption of the Internet have utterly altered the landscape. No longer will innovation be held hostage to the business plans and sales cycles of "big iron" health IT companies. No longer will hospital administrators or doctors need to queue up outside the IT department's front door, only to be told to "come back when I have finished my other priorities." Today, healthcare apps of real value can be created by entrepreneurs possessing a disruptive idea, access to some funding, and an understanding of healthcare workflow.

Even the most useful, clever, and innovative app will not see the light of day unless adopted by providers in the rendering of healthcare. Healthcare culture has not yet changed all that much.

The entrenched channels, long sales cycles, and significant regulatory burden in health care are at odds with the volume-driven model of rapid start-up development . . . the risk-averse culture of health care and a lack of proven revenue models . . . can make pilots and early revenue difficult to obtain.[1]

All of this highlights the need for healthcare technology innovators to carefully balance the competing interests of varying stakeholders and seek opportunities to establish relationships with key providers who control much of the funding being sought by innovators. Innovators need to understand the necessary steps and stages in growing a successful health IT business that is dynamic, sustainable, and responsive to its market.

Key Trends in Health IT That Drive Innovation

Policy Initiatives Drive Adoption of Health IT

As the first decade of the 21st century came to a close, the need for health IT innovation intensified. Key to the adoption of health IT were specific legislative actions. With the passage of the American Recovery and Reinvestment Act of 2009 (ARRA), Congress authorized funding for providers adopting EHR systems. The next year, Congress passed the Patient Protection and Affordable Care Act (PPACA), which created new programs like accountable care organizations (ACOs), charged to align various healthcare market stakeholders and provide them with incentives for quality care.

These congressional actions spurred the development of new IT solutions. Even though EHR vendors invested heavily in newer technology, they could not keep up with the high market demand. Customers and investors wanted new, innovative solutions that would best meet government requirements.

21st Century Cures

Most hospitals and physician practices have now adopted EHRs, but the transition from paper has not been easy on providers. Providers have struggled with overly burdensome documentation requirements and software has not been optimized to their workflow. There have been additional concerns around the lack of interoperability between health IT software that prohibit true care coordination. Patients have struggled to get access to their own data, and entrepreneurs have been limited in the ways they can access health information to develop more intuitive software.

The 21st Century Cures Act was signed December 13, 2016, by President Obama.[2] This bipartisan bill is one of the most important pieces of legislation to advance health IT. While the bill is largely known to help fund efforts such as precision medicine, it contains some provisions to improve healthcare IT – most notably, in relation to nationwide interoperability and information blocking. Certain sections are focused on "improving quality of care for patients," with interoperability a main concern. It also places strong emphasis on providing patients access to their electronic health information in a way that is "easy to understand, secure and updated automatically."

The Cures Act[2] is focused on health IT in four important areas: requiring the development and promotion of modern APIs to unleash valuable clinical data, developing mechanisms to prevent information blocking, driving interoperability across networks, and working with the Centers for Medicare and Medicaid Services (CMS) to create a strategy for reducing administrative and reporting burden among clinicians.

Importantly, the Cures Act builds on the 2015 edition of ONC's health IT certification criteria by calling for the development of modern APIs that do not require "special effort" to access and use.[2] The bill promotes the use of FHIR[2] (Fast Healthcare Interoperability Resources) APIs, which is a developer-friendly way of representing clinical data. The modern FHIR APIs replace clunky legacy standards that required custom development and have enabled new types of software companies that do not have a legacy in health information technology to innovate for some of healthcare's problems.

There are over 100 regional health information exchanges (RHIOs) and multiple national level organizations that support exchange of health information. There is still limited connectivity across these information exchanges, state to state, and region to region. This connectivity has been hampered by varying state policies such as opt in vs opt out consent laws, difference in standards, and governance issues. This has limited how providers and patients can get access to vital health information. The Cures Act calls on ONC to develop or support a trusted exchange framework and common agreement to address policies and practices between health information networks.[2] The final trusted exchange framework will set common principles, terms, and conditions that facilitate trust between disparate health information networks.[2] It will seek to scale interoperability nationwide. This means patients who have received care from multiple doctors and hospitals should have their medical history electronically accessible on demand by any other treating provider in a network that signed the Common Agreement.[2]

Perhaps the most important health IT provisions of the 21st Century Cures Act has to do with the information blocking.[2] For years, providers, patients, and developers have struggled to get access to vital healthcare information from health IT systems. While many times the blame has been put on lack of interoperability, many times the issue is in fact that an actor simply does not want to share data. This can be true of health IT vendors that do not want to share with a competing system, a provider that does not want to share with a payer, and vice-versa. Or a health system that chooses not to share data with a competing health system even though a patient shows up for care in both health systems. The information blocking provision of the Cures Act addresses actions that can impede the flow of electronic health information, or its use to improve health and the delivery of care. The prohibition against information blocking applies to healthcare providers, health IT developers, exchanges, and networks. The Cures Act also permits substantial penalties for information blocking.[2]

Value-Based Care Programs Drive Demand for New Solutions

An area that has seen significant activity is the drive toward value-based care (VBC). Unlike pay-for-performance, where providers are paid based on the amount of healthcare services they deliver, VBC is a healthcare delivery model in which providers are paid based on patient health outcomes. The "value" is derived by measuring health outcomes against the cost of delivering the outcomes. There are a myriad of government-led VBC programs for large and small providers that have had mixed levels of success at both the federal and state level, including bundled payments, Merit Based Incentive Payment Systems (MIPS), Medicare ACOs, Medicaid programs, and Comprehensive Primary Care Plus (CPC+).[1]

Common to all VBC programs is the need for new solutions to help providers remain profitable and deliver quality patient care under these programs. Providers have been ill equipped to manage the variety of programs offered. Providers must make investments that focus on patient-centric care while advancing data and analytics capabilities. Key areas of focus for providers include care coordination, analytics, and patient engagement. Care coordination refers to the ability to access data and care across the care continuum, both inside and outside of a providers' network. Analytics is a broad area encompassing population health and the ability to mine different types of data to make more informed decisions related to what works for VBC programs. Finally, patient engagement refers to the solutions that enable the patient to become a partner in their care. The entrepreneurship community has latched onto the needs for new solutions, and unsurprisingly, investments in digital health are greatest in VBC opportunity areas.

Telehealth Is Mainstream

One of the areas of digital health that has seen the most adoption is telehealth. Telehealth is focused on virtual care in which a provider is accessible through a remote consultation. According to the telehealth vendor AmericanWell, more than 75% of hospitals are using or implementing a telehealth program and 22% of all physicians have used telehealth to see patients, up 340% from 2015.[3] Employers are increasingly incorporating telehealth services into their benefits packages as healthcare costs rise. Companies may also view telehealth as an effective means to offer new kinds of treatments. For example, according to the National Business Group on Health's survey,[3] 13% of large employers will introduce mental/behavioral and diabetes management telehealth services in 2019, a reflection of the growing perception that telehealth can help companies address gaps in their healthcare coverage. Policy also supports telehealth.[3] The Centers for Medicare and Medicaid Services (CMS) have been granting telehealth waivers to a group of Medicare Accountable Care Organizations (Next Gen ACOs). Twenty-six states have adopted laws requiring insurers to reimburse telehealth visits, and more states are considering legislation.[3]

Social Determinants of Health Focuses on All Factors Affecting Patients

As government programs such as Medicaid try to drive improved outcomes for patients of all socioeconomic status, it is becoming increasingly clear that nonmedical factors can affect a person's overall health and health outcomes. The majority of factors that materially impact a person's health occur outside of the doctor's office, and yet most of the annual U.S. healthcare spend is still incurred in the clinical setting. As defined by the World Health Organization (WHO), Social Determinants of Health (SDoH) are "the conditions in which people are born, grow, live, work and age. These circumstances are shaped by the distribution of money, power and resources at global, national and local levels."[4] SDoH aims to aggregate information from social service providers; public health resources, including information from family and social support; economic stability sources; food banks; community safety; and education, among other resources, to drive an action plan that works for a particular patient. Innovative companies that have emerged as seizing this opportunity include CityBlock Health, which was formed by Google, Healthify, and UniteUs.

New Technologies Like Artificial Intelligence Have Come Mainstream

Advancements in artificial intelligence (AI) are helping to drive new insights and opportunities in digital health by predicting outcomes and identifying patterns. AI in healthcare is the use of complex algorithms and software to emulate human cognition in the analysis of complicated medical data without direct input.[5] AI includes Natural Language Processing (NLP) and translation, pattern recognition, visual perception, and decision making. Machine Learning (ML) involves the development of computational approaches to automatically make sense of data – this technology leverages the insight that learning is a dynamic process, made possible through examples and experiences as opposed to pre-defined rules.[5] Like a human, a machine can retain information and become smarter over time. Unlike a human, a machine is not susceptible to sleep deprivation, distractions, information overload, and short-term memory loss – that is where this powerful technology becomes exciting.

The implementation of AI in healthcare has been limited to date due to factors such as high capital required for initial deployment, difficulties in deployment, reluctance by healthcare practitioners to adopt new technologies that potentially could reduce the workforce, and ambiguous privacy and security regulations.

According to TM Capital,[5] which has profiled a number of initiatives focused on artificial intelligence, there are many use cases of AI technology being evaluated and implemented across healthcare, including intelligent diagnostics, patient and provider data management, advanced analytics for drug discovery processes, medical devices and robotics, and home health using AI. Investments from major tech companies and investors have led to an increase in the deployment of potential use cases across all of healthcare.

Health APIs

One conversation topic that is constantly discussed at digital health industry events is the idea of data silos. The real potential for health data, many people believe, will come when it can be combined with other data and integrated into other apps and platforms, rather than being locked away wherever it was originally collected.

This is increasingly being done through application programming interfaces, or APIs, which are offered by consumer companies such as Fitbit and Apple, but also EHRs such as Allscripts and administrative clearinghouses such as Change Healthcare. APIs are also being used in high-profile platforms looking to create an integrated user experience for the variety of digital health app available services, such as Kaiser Permanente's Interchange or RunKeeper's Health Graph.

The now-defunct patient health information hubs Google Health and Microsoft HealthVault both made APIs an important part of their strategy as early as 2008. But, back then, they were arguably too early for the space and were not able to find many API-ready partners with which to integrate. Perhaps the biggest move forward for health APIs came in June 2018, when Apple launched its Apple its health records API to developers.[6] Apple began its rollout by forming relationships with over 500 hospitals and ambulatory providers to provide access for patients to access their healthcare data on their phones, but later opened up access to all healthcare providers.[6] Apple enabled an ecosystem of app developers to build solutions leveraging that data to better manage medications, enable better disease management, help facilitate research, and track health conditions, and formed partnerships with major tech vendors.

Three Stages of Health IT Innovation

Any successful health IT innovation solution goes through three distinct stages of development: concept, seed funding/start-up, and scale.

Concept Stage

At this stage, a small group of entrepreneurs or an individual develop(s) a business idea addressing a significant issue in healthcare. The founder begins to conduct research to assess product features, likely demand, benefit to stakeholders, cost to develop/deploy, and potential customers.

Seed Funding/Start-Up Stage

At this stage, the entrepreneurs may raise funds from friends and family, as well as angel and venture capitalist (VC) investors, enabling them to build an innovative product in preparation for market introduction. By running pilot programs with carefully selected beta customers, innovators can gain valuable insights that yield product improvements, enabling an optimal fit to market needs. This enables their products to be provided to early adopters for initial market introduction. At minimum, innovators must put into place all of the basic accounting, operations, client services, marketing and sales processes, channel strategies, and resources needed for a successful market introduction, along with identifying first adopters, size of market, pricing, anticipated revenue, sales approaches, and profitability.

Scale Stage

Here, the entrepreneur drives toward profitability, focusing on the milestones to reach to break even before investing to achieve a dominant position in their market. The innovator develops solid sales strategies, with paying clients generating revenue. In addition, the innovator may engage with VCs for Series B and later funding to further grow their business capabilities. The focus is on building out robust businesses, enabling market development and the addition of new customers. The companies have developed marketing/sales/support/distribution strategies and are focusing on strategic partners who can help them scale at a rapid pace.

Innovation Targeted at Concept Stage Companies

At the first stage, innovators can avail themselves of hackathons and challenges. A hackathon or code-a-thon is an event in which developers and designers collaborate intensively on software projects. Hackathons typically last one or several days. Some hackathons are intended simply for educational or social purposes, although in many cases, the goal is to create usable software that could be spun out into a product.

NYC BigApps is an example of a successful hackathon. NYC BigApps is an annual competition sponsored by the New York City Economic Development Corporation that provides programmers, developers, designers, and entrepreneurs with access to municipal data sets to build technologic products that address civic issues affecting New York City (NYC).[7] Programming teams compete for up to $100,000 in cash prizes. Through the NYC Open Data portal and other private and nonprofit data sources, contestants have access to more than 1,000 data sets and application programming interfaces (APIs).[7] Examples of available data include healthy living, weekly traffic updates, schedules of citywide events, property sales records, catalogs of restaurant inspections, and geographic data about the location of school and voting districts. The contest is part of a broader NYC effort to increase government transparency and encourage entrepreneurship.[7]

A healthcare challenge is a project in which multidisciplinary teams are tasked with building technology solutions that address issues identified by a sponsoring organization, such as a non-profit, foundation, or for-profit company. Often, these are held as part of conferences or stand-alone events geared to digital health app development. Prizes are typically awarded to the team with the best app.

Innovation Targeted at the Seed Funding and Start-Up Stage

As companies move into the next stage of innovation (seed funding and start-up), they are eligible to participate in incubator or accelerator programs. Whereas incubators usually provide space, work resources, management, and mentoring to assist companies to create prototype products that can qualify for seed money, accelerators generally look for companies that can benefit from a blend of mentoring, funding, and market relationships that will prepare them to go to market.[8]

The origin of the accelerator model can be attributed to the 2005 launch of the first accelerator, called "Y Combinator" (YC).[8] The former cofounder and CEO of Viaweb, Paul Graham, founded YC with the strategy that making small investments in large number of start-ups, typically $125,000 in exchange for between 2% and 10% equity, would result in more successes than investing in only a few.[8] The start-ups in the program move to Silicon Valley for three months to get access to a co-working space and mentors from the business community, and work intensively on their pitches for investors. The conclusion of the program is a demo day in which they pitch their business plans to a group of outside investors with the hope that the pitch will turn into subsequent VC investment. Since 2005, YC has invested in over 2,000 start-ups that have a combined market cap of over $100 billion, including highly successful companies such as Reddit, Dropbox, Airbnb, Codeacademy, and Stripe.[8] Following the success of YC, other notable tech accelerators emerged as well.

There are four models of health accelerators: commercial seed accelerators, market-led programs, virtual networks, and university-affiliated accelerators (See Table 3.1).

1. **Commercial seed accelerators.** These accelerators leverage the successful YC model and offer capital, guidance, access to mentors, and a demo day for investors. These accelerators are typically aimed at very early stage companies who may be at the idea stage or have a beta product. The program length is typically 3–4 months and provides from $20,000 to $100,000 in return for an average of 65% equity. Successful commercial seed accelerators include Rock Health, HealthBox, BluePrint Health, Dreamit Health, and Tech Wildcatters.

2. **Market-led programs.** The newly emerging model of market-led programs is being created by customers and economic development organizations looking for particular types of innovation in specific focus areas. The New York Digital Health Innovation Lab is an example. This program was created with a focus on healthcare providers who are looking to adapt new technologies. Market-led programs typically are longer than commercial seed accelerators, offer more investment capital, and take less equity stake (~2%). The focus of these programs is often on economic development in addition to commercial success of the companies.

Table 3.1 Types of Accelerator Models

	Commercial Seed	*Market-Led*	*Virtual Networks*	*University-Affiliated*
Structure	3–5 months, demo day, 2 classes per year, up to 10 companies per class	5–9 months, demo day, 2 classes per year, up to 10 companies per class; location-specific job creation requirements	36-month program; up to 100 start-ups per year	6-month program; demo day, 2 classes per year, 10 companies per class
Capital	$20,000; 6% equity	$100,000–$300,000; 2.5% equity; funding for pilots	No direct funding; program receives 2–10% equity over 3 years	$5,000 stipend per founder, no equity stake
Focus	Concept to early stage health tech companies	Late-seed to growth-stage health tech companies focused on needs of particular customers	Seed to Series B health tech companies	Concept to Series B health tech companies and biotech
Market Ties	Academic institutions, pharma, health plans, corporate sponsors	Healthcare providers, pharma, health plans strategic investors, corporate sponsors, economic development, government	Corporate sponsorships, health plans, government	University-affiliated, corporate sponsors
Examples	Rock Health, HealthBox, BluePrint Health, Dreamit Health, Tech Wildcatters, SAP Foundry	Texas Medical Center Accelerator (TMCx), Jlabs, New York Digital Health Innovation Lab, Plug and Play Tech Center	StartUp Health, Mass Challenge	StartX Med, Georgia Tech Health @ei2, StartupUCLA

3. **Virtual networks.** StartUp Health is an example of a virtual network model. This program provides its network members with access to business connections, virtual collaboration, and quarterly CEO summits.[9] The program typically does not provide any direct capital to companies, but takes a small equity stake in each company over a three-year period.[9] StartUp Health focuses on CEOs, whom they term "Healthcare Transformers." The vision of StartUp Health is to invest in 1,000 companies over 10 years.[9] The organization has also formed strategic partnerships with a number of corporate sponsors.

4. **University-affiliated accelerators.** The structure of university-led accelerators is similar to commercial seed accelerators, but often they do not take as much equity from the entrepreneurs involved. The most notable university-affiliated accelerator is StartXMed, which is affiliated with Stanford University. However, some commercial seed accelerators have also

formed strategic relationships with universities. For example, Dreamit Health has formed a strategic relationship with Drexel University and Johns Hopkins, while Rock Health has formed a strategic partnership with the University of California San Francisco (UCSF). Thus, the categories have become somewhat blurred.

Public–Private Sector Initiatives

There are several public–private sector initiatives focusing on helping start-ups find ways to fix healthcare problems faced by government entities. These initiatives typically provide seed funding, office space, and mentorships to civic start-ups. One example is **Code for America** (San Francisco). Code for America,[10] the technology world's equivalent of the Peace Corps, provides seed funding, office space, and mentorship to civic start-ups. It aims at helping early stage start-up companies focused on civic issues get the financial, strategic, and operational support they need to succeed. Start-ups receive 200+ hours of mentorship from industry leaders, pitch to numerous government officials, and gain access to civic tech investors and sales leads. There is a four-month residency and a demo day.[10]

International Sponsored Programs Driving

Innovation in Health IT

Health IT innovation is not just a focus within the United States; internationally sponsored programs have been developed that seek to drive the same types of goals, such as fostering entrepreneurship and job creation, and driving the open use of health data. These programs work with batches of start-ups to prepare them for marketing their digital health products in the local and international market. Examples include:

- **European Connected Health Alliance (ECH)** (Europe). The European Connected Health Alliance[11] is a nonprofit organization focused primarily on the European Union countries to support and promote the wider adoption of healthcare products, services, applications, and innovation. The Alliance has membership that includes corporates, foundations, academia, and government members and is seen as the primary convener of these disparate organizations within the region.
- **Dubai Futures Accelerators.** The Dubai Futures Accelerators is an imitative that was the vision of UAE Vice President, Prime Minister, and Ruler of Dubai Sheikh Mohammed bin Rashid Al Maktoum and created by the Dubai Futures Foundation.[12] It is set up as a nine-week program that forges partnerships with government entities and private sector organizations from Dubai with start-ups from around the world to co-create and solve named challenges.[12] Arguably one of the most global programs for emerging companies, the program has focused on specific challenges laid out by government organizations, and start-ups solve these needs. The government works with the company to form pilots that eventually may lead to broad enterprise sales.
- **Station F** (France). Station F is a business incubator in Paris that claims to be the world's largest business incubator.[13] Station F is located in an unused rail station, is home to over 1,000 start-ups, and offers incubator programs from large firms such as Facebook, Microsoft,

and L'Oréal. While it has been endorsed by the French government, Station F is an initiative owned by Xavier Niel, the founder of telecom company Iliad. According to Pitchbook, Station F has contributed to a boom in venture funding in France from €1.6 billion in 2015 to €2.5 billion in 2019.[13]

Innovation Targeted at the Scale Stage

Once it reaches the scale stage, a company has proved the value of its portfolio of products, has a strong management team and sustainable funding, and has achieved successful adoption. It must continue to innovate to stay ahead of the market, and it must pull together a mix of resource talent, strategic and tactical plans, and effective marketing and sales so as to achieve a market leading position. Companies that have achieved a certain level of scale and adoption are often on the lookout for potential exit opportunities. These options can range from taking in additional funding to allow for growth and ability to scale, strategic partnerships with larger companies that bring in additional capital and new opportunities, to a potential sale of the business for a healthy multiple to provide management and investors a return.

Digital Health Investment Continues to Grow

Digital health investment activity has grown from something overlooked by investors into a strong focus of the investment community. According to Rock Health,[14] which measures the level of investments in digital health, nearly one in ten venture dollars invested in the United States has been put toward digital health. In 2019, 359 digital health start-ups in the United States raised $7.4 billion from over 625 investors. According to a report by Rock Health, the amount of investment in digital health has increased from $1.1 billion in 2011 to $7.4 billion in 2019, while the number of deals increased from a low of 92 in 2011 to 374 deals in 2019.[14]

Digital Health IPOs

Following a number of years with little to no IPO activity in digital health solution areas, 2019 resulted in 15 companies going public. According to Pitchbook, IPOs produced $7.7 billion of the cumulative $14.7 billion in healthtech VC exit value.[15] The most notable digital health IPOs have included Health Catalyst, Phreesia, One Medical Group, Livongo, Peloton, and Change Healthcare.[15] Digital health is more and more attractive to the public market because of a combination of strong product offerings and increasing revenues driven by macro trends around health and wellness in markets with large growth potential.[15]

Large Corporates Enter Digital Health Through M&A

In addition to digital health IPOs, with the rise of venture investments, there has also been considerable mergers and acquisition (M&A) activity within digital health. Strategic investors made up of large corporates in particular have been paying a hefty premium for digital health companies, as they understand digital health companies need access to distribution channels and proven expertise, particularly in the consumerization of healthcare to succeed. These acquisitions have contributed to higher than normal valuations of digital health companies.

Some notable acquisitions in recent years in digital health include:

■ **Roche acquires Flatiron Health.**[16] Swiss Pharmaceutical company Roche acquired oncology EHR software firm Flatiron Health in 2019 for $1.9 billion, a company in which it previously had an investment.[16] Flatiron captures and normalizes oncology data from multiple data sources to generate valuable real-world evidence that can be used to draw unique insights. This notable acquisition of a relatively small tech firm emphasizes the importance of pharma investing in tech and the value of clinical data generated at the point of care.

■ **Dassault Systèmes acquires Medidata.**[17] Cloud-based clinical trial SaaS Medidata was acquired by French 3-D and product lifecycle management specialist Dassault Systèmes for a hefty $5.8 billion in June 2019.[17]

■ **Amazon acquires PillPack.**[18] Amazon took a big leap into the pharmacy space with its $753 million acquisition in 2018 of PillPack.[18] Pillpack offers an online pharmacy for patients to get access to bundles of their medication in an easy to use pack. Key to the deal is PillPack's relationships with distributors.

■ **Google acquires Fitbit.**[19] Google acquired fitness and wellness tracker company Fitbit for $2.1 billion in 2019. Google makes software that powers smartwatches but does not have health trackers in its portfolio. Potentially more importantly, Google gains the health data and insights into the 28 million active users that Fitbit has.[19]

Sustaining Innovation

To sustain the innovation initiated by entrepreneurs, many companies need access to additional capital. The venture capital (VC) industry is often the source of this funding. VC investment is money given to an entrepreneur or start-up business by a venture capital firm at an early stage in the company's development, with the hopes that the firm will receive a large return on its investment. Some of the world's largest companies, including Starbucks, Home Depot, Whole Foods, Apple, Microsoft, and others were originally backed by VC investors. While the 2009 Health Information Technology for Economic and Clinical Health (HITECH) Act helped launch the sector through its $17 billion allocation toward the adoption of meaningful use of health IT, private investments in the sector have continued to rise with increasing EHR adoption.

Funding Innovation

As a company graduates from the concept stage into the start-up phase and beyond, it is important to seek the counsel of an expert financial adviser to identify the appropriate means of gaining access to capital. Some of the most prevalent funding sources for start-ups include:

■ **Friends and family.** Many very early stage start-ups gather some initial seed funding from friends and family to survive on until the business raises additional capital.

■ **Small Business Innovation Research (SBIR) grants**[20] **or SBA loans.** The U.S. government has created grant programs and loans for small businesses to succeed. The Small Business Association[21] (SBA) has taken a keen look at health technology and is actively looking to fund high-potential businesses that will create jobs and solve big healthcare issues. For more information, see www.sbir.gov and www.sba.gov.

- **Angel investors.** Angel investors[22] are individuals or groups that invest their own money in early stage companies. Often, these are high net worth individuals who are looking to take a small part of an emerging business. More information is available at http://www.angelcapitalassociation.org/.
- **VC investors and strategic investors.** By far the most active group of investors is traditional VC firms. Many new entrants who previously focused on biotech deals are now entering the health technology space. Corporate venture capital groups typically led by pharma and tech firms have created funds that often offer better terms than traditional VCs.
- **Organic growth.** This funding comes from growth of the business based on sales alone, thus obviating the need to raise external funds. Organic growth can be a viable option if a business has enough dollars from the founders or backers to succeed. However, the pace of growth may not be satisfying enough, and the company may need additional capital in order to scale.

The Role of the Mentor

At the concept and start-up stages, a strategy for success for a start-up is to work with multiple mentors. Mentors can assist an early stage start-up in several different ways, including validating product concepts, identifying unmet needs, advising on leadership decisions, and assisting with business development and identification of customers, investors, and partners, to name just a few. For a mentor, access to cutting-edge innovation, an opportunity to share their insights and learning, and networking with other industry partners are often motivations for getting involved. Mentors may seek compensation in the form of payment or equity share in the company, although often mentors work with start-ups gratis, as they see it as a way of giving back to the community.

It is important for an early stage company to recognize that it can't solve every problem on its own and, instead, should work with many different types of mentors, as each provides a different set of capabilities. Some different types of mentors include:

- **Entrepreneur mentors.** These mentors are successful CEOs of businesses that may be in the same industry as the start-up or in different industries. These leaders can provide valuable insights into what has worked and what has not, guidance on scaling a business and raising capital, and strategic insights into product strategy. These relationships can often lead to new business development partnership opportunities. Seed and later stage accelerators work with this mentor group as a core part of their program.
- **Corporate mentors.** Large companies are often interested in working with early stage companies to identify new innovations and to seek potential pilot opportunities that can lead to investments. Often, corporate development executives at large companies, including tech firms, pharma, insurance companies, and consulting firms, are very well connected and able to assist start-ups in identifying strategic partners. Also, these firms may be interested in funding pilots for start-ups.
- **Customer mentors.** One of the most important types of mentors are customer mentors. For an early stage start-up, it is critical to identify a potential customer who is willing to provide candid feedback on product development and validate the market need the start-up is trying to fulfill. Often, start-ups focus on sales and not on the important mentorship aspect of this relationship. By collaboratively working with a customer, especially for business-to-business (B2B) companies, start-ups can maximize the benefits received and may even gain

a reference client that will vouch for the company and its credibility. In return for their time, customers may seek advisory board representation, discounts on product fees, or equity stakes.

Case Study: The New York Digital Health Innovation Lab

A prime example of a successful digital health accelerator that promotes innovation is the New York Digital Health Innovation Lab, a program run by the New York eHealth Collaborative (NYeC) in conjunction with the Partnership Fund of New York.

New York State is a national leader in healthcare. The third most populous state in the United States, New York's healthcare community comprises more than 230 hospitals, 60,000 physicians, and 19.5 million consumers of health services.[23] New York has pioneered numerous innovations in healthcare delivery, including insurance market reforms and regulatory approaches that long predated the country's recent adoption of comparable strategies under comprehensive healthcare reform.

In recent years, New York has taken unprecedented steps to improve both the quality and efficiency of healthcare delivery, making substantial investments in health IT and undertaking a broad range of other regional/local and private sector initiatives to improve health services through IT.

Since 2006, the New York State (NYS) Department of Health has invested over $840 million toward the adoption of health IT in the state.[23] This funding has led to significant adoption of EHRs across the state and the formation of 11 regional health information organizations (RHIOs), which have consolidated into seven Qualified Entities or QEs. These QEs, with the appropriate patient consent, have the capacity to share medical information between healthcare providers in their region.[23] Connecting all of these QEs or regional health information exchange organizations (HIE) is the Statewide Health Information Network of New York (SHIN-NY), which manages the technology platform that connects the QEs and enables the statewide sharing of data such as lab results, radiology reports, electronic health records, and more.[23]

New York Is a National Center of Tech Innovation

New York has a strong technology community with access to many resources that can be leveraged by early stage companies to thrive. New York is already the hub of the financial technology, digital media, and VC industries. Beginning with Google's move to NYC in 2003, the strong growth of tech start-ups has made NYC host to many of the most important Silicon Valley companies, including Facebook and Yahoo. From 2007 to 2012, more than 11,000 new IT jobs were created in NYC, up 28.7%, from 41,100 to 52,900.[24] Former Mayor Michael Bloomberg recently expanded the "We Are Made in NY" initiative to include IT companies, with more than 900 tech start-ups currently hiring for over 3,000 jobs.[24] NYC is also unrivaled in the density of major healthcare organizations and hospitals. More than 80% of its hospitals use EHR systems, up 200% since 2008. More than half of doctors and other eligible providers also use EHRs, leading to more healthcare data available to developers than ever before.[25]

All of this has created a tremendous opportunity for NYeC to work with the emerging health technology industry to establish New York as the hub of health IT innovation. Health IT entrepreneurs highlight as key impediments such issues as a lack of access to potential customers, misunderstanding of health policy issues, and lack of a support network to engage with other entrepreneurs and healthcare leaders facing similar challenges. Healthcare providers have cited the lack of awareness of new applications and the lack of time and staff to engage with the healthcare entrepreneurial community.

Partnering to Create the NY Digital Health Innovation Lab

The New York Digital Health Innovation Lab[25] was developed by New York eHealth Collaborative (NYeC) with the Partnership Fund for New York City to stimulate a new marketplace and create the next generation of healthcare tools, while positioning New York as a hub of health IT innovation. The nine-month program, modeled after the Partnership Fund's successful Fintech Innovation Lab for emerging financial start-ups, provides companies with mentorship and feedback from senior executives as their potential customers.[25] Geared toward early and growth-stage digital health companies, the accelerator program supports the development of cutting-edge technology products focused on care coordination, patient engagement, analytics, and workflow improvement for healthcare providers.

Innovation Objectives of the Innovation Lab

With the advent of the Patient Protection and Affordable Care Act of 2010 (PPACA) and other healthcare reform activities, innovative solutions are critical to support the complex needs of patients and providers, as well as the changing healthcare market. The accelerator program is well positioned to facilitate and support the development of technology solutions to champion new payment and service delivery models, including ACOs, Shared Savings, and Bundled Payment programs spearheaded by CMS and the NYS Department of Health.

With the strong shift in incentives and payment models, providers in New York and across the country are being forced to review their workflow, seeking new tools to better coordinate care. Typically, providers ask their EHR vendors to provide these tools. An EHR system can help physicians manage their patients within a practice, hospital, or system; providers currently need to share data across systems to support entirely new models of care.

Providers are demanding innovative tools, particularly in the areas of care coordination and patient engagement. Care coordination refers to collaborative care solutions that reflect the continuum of information regarding a patient. Patient engagement refers to personal health management solutions that facilitate better healthcare decisions and help improve care management communications between the provider and/or family members.

Through partnerships between the providers and the technology companies, the Accelerator Program fosters the creation of products that meet the needs of the providers by facilitating timely communication and providing coordinated and integrated care to improve the lives of patients. The accelerator is unique in that it provides the tech companies accepted into the program direct access to customers and product development feedback from senior-level executives of leading healthcare provider organizations in New York. It is through this partnership between the tech companies and providers that the accelerator is able to successfully stimulate growth of an ecosystem in which new IT tools and new jobs are created. The accelerator is at the heart of NYeC's approach toward growing a vital digital health ecosystem in the state.

The accelerator delivered solid results. "After graduating from the program, alumni companies raised more than $390 million, participated in over 50 pilots and created nearly 400 jobs."[26]

The program received significant accolades from many leading experts in the health IT industry. The California Healthcare Foundation called the accelerator one of the most successful accelerator models in the country, in light of the financial and strategic ties that have already been forged.[27] The Rotman School of Management in Canada ranked the accelerator number one in the world among 21 similar programs. Their ranking was based on ten different criteria, including access to customers, investors, government, and support for innovation. Todd Park, former chief technology officer (CTO) of the United States, has said that this program is the one that other states should seek to emulate.[25]

Conclusion

The time is ripe for innovation across the health IT space. Government initiatives, commercial interests, and consumer needs are aligning and are all pointing to an era of explosive opportunity for digital health entrepreneurship. Mobile devices and Internet access are ubiquitous and are being universally adopted. Fitness, wellness, care collaboration, telemedicine, patient engagement, "the Internet of Everything," big data, small data, predictive analytics – each of these areas is attracting innovators and investors in unprecedented numbers. And there is no end in sight.

Innovators who wish to succeed in the digital health market should be mindful of the following points:

- One doesn't have to be a healthcare expert to build an app that will be useful in the market space. If you have an idea that works well in another market and have reason to believe it is applicable to healthcare, validate it with healthcare experts and make it happen.
- The best start-ups are built around a team of founders possessing the requisite business, marketing, and tech development skills necessary for early success.
- Take advantage of the plethora of incubators, code-a-thons, hackathons, accelerators, and other programs that are rapidly spreading across the globe. They can provide you with the funds, space, and market exposure so immeasurably valuable to a start-up enterprise.
- Look for funding beyond the familiar friends-and-family sources. Angel investors and VCs are actively seeking "the next big thing" in healthcare. Attend conferences where they congregate and network, network, network.
- Actively seek mentors, both healthcare subject matter experts and leaders of companies that stand out as successful in the market. Their advice and counsel will be invaluable and save you the trouble of learning through your own (inevitable) mistakes.
- Read everything you can get your hands on about digital health and stay on top of the latest developments in this most dynamic industry. Clients want to deal with innovators who understand their market and can teach them something they do not already know.
- Above all, enjoy yourself and allow yourself the satisfaction that derives from doing something that tangibly improves the health of your fellow humans.

About the Author

Anuj Desai, MBA, is a healthcare business development executive with 21 years of experience focused on health information technology (HIT). Anuj is a strategic thinker with an extensive network of senior-level relationships at healthcare providers, payers, pharma, startups, and within the investor community. Anuj is a resourceful leader who builds high performance teams that deliver results and thrives in the development of new partnerships that lead to growth. Named by

AlleyWatch as one the top 100 Tech Influencers in New York City and a member of the prestigious Crain's New York Business "40 under 40" class, he sits on multiple industry advisory boards and advises tech startups in areas related to policy, interoperability, and innovation.

Currently, Anuj is the Vice President of Business Development at Change Healthcare, driving strategic partnerships across the business. Previously he was the VP of Corporate Business Development at Allscripts and VP Market Development at New York eHealth Collaborative (NYeC). He led the New York Digital Health Accelerator program for health tech startups selling to large healthcare providers and the largest health tech conference in the region, the NyeC Digital Health Conference.

As an industry thought leader, Anuj is a frequent public speaker and has spoken at many industry conferences on topics related to innovation, interoperability, value-based care, policy, and entrepreneurship. He has appeared in many journals, magazines, and broadcast media. Anuj has also been the recipient of multiple industry recognitions, including 2013 Modern Healthcare "Up and Comers" and 2015 MedTech Boston "40 Under 40" Healthcare Innovators.

Anuj holds an MBA degree from the University of Maryland and a bachelor of science degree in biotechnology from Rutgers University.

References

1. Don Rucker. Achieving the Interoperability Promise of 21st Century Cures. June 19, 2018. The Health Affairs Blog. Accessed February 15, 2020.
2. NEJM Catalyst. What Is Value-Based Healthcare? January 1, 2017.
3. Meg Bryant. Physician Telehealth Use Up 340% Since 2015, Survey Finds. April 17, 2019. Healthcaredive.com. Accessed February 15, 2020.
4. https://www.who.int/social_determinants/en/. Accessed February 15, 2020.
5. TM Capital Industry Spotlight. The Next Generation of Medicine: Artificial Intelligence and Machine Learning. www.tmcapital.com/healthcare. Accessed February 15, 2020.
6. Dave Muio. Apple Health Records Now Available to All US Providers with Compatible EHRs. June 28, 2019. Accessed January 10, 2020.
7. www.nycbigapps.com. Accessed February 6, 2020.
8. https://www.ycombinator.com/. Accessed January 10, 2021.
9. https://www.startuphealth.com/. Accessed January 10, 2021.
10. http://codeforamerica.org/. Accessed February 6, 2020.
11. http://www.echalliance.com/. Accessed February 6, 2020.
12. https://dubaifutureaccelerators.com/en/. Accessed February 15, 2020.
13. Leah Hodson. Station F: A Symbol of France's Startup Ambitions. 2019. https://pitchbook.com/news/articles/station-f-a-symbol-of-frances-startup-ambitions. Accessed February 15, 2020.
14. Sean Day and Elena Gambon. In 2019, Digital Health Celebrated Six IPOs as Venture Investment Edged Off Record Highs. Rock Health. Accessed February 15, 2020.
15. Peter Barlas. 2019 Is the Year of the Digital Health IPO, but Will It Last? *MedCity News*. August 25, 2019.
16. Reenita Das. The Flatiron Health Acquisition Is a Shot in the Arm for Roche's Oncology Real-World Evidence Needs. February 26, 2018. Forbes Magazine.
17. Nathan Eddy. Medidata Acquired by Dassault Systèmes for $5.8 Billion. June 13, 2019. Healthcare IT News.
18. Christina Farr. The Inside Story of Why Amazon Bought PillPack in Its Effort to Crack the $500 Billion Prescription Market. May 13, 2019. CNBC.
19. Brent Rose. Everything You Need to Know About Google Buying Fitbit. November 18, 2019. Outside Magazine.

20. www.sbir.gov. Accessed February 6, 2020.

21. www.sba.gov. Accessed February 6, 2020.

22. http://www.angelcapitalassociation.org/. Accessed February 6, 2020.

23. www.nyehealth.org. Accessed February 6, 2020.

24. New Tech City. Center for an Urban Future. May 2012. https://nycfuture.org/pdf/New_Tech_City.pdf. Accessed January 26, 2015.

25. https://digitalhealth.nyc/. Accessed February 6, 2020.

26. Greenhouse Effect: How Accelerators Are Seeding Digital Health Innovation. California Healthcare Foundation. 2013. http://www.chcf.org/~/media/MEDIA%20LIBRARY%20Files/PDF/G/PDF%20GreenhouseSeedingDigitalHealth.pdf. Accessed January 26, 2015.

27. https://partnershipfundnyc.org/programs/new-york-digital-health-innovation-lab/. Accessed January 10, 2021.

28. Priyamvada Mathur. 21 Charts Showing Current Trends in US Venture Capital. July 24, 2019. Pitchbook.

Chapter 4

Ambulatory Systems
Electronic Health Records

Curtis L. Cole, MD, Adam D. Cheriff, MD,
J. Travis Gossey, MD, MS, MPH, Sameer Malhotra,
MD, MA, and Daniel M. Stein, MD, PhD

Contents

DOI: 10.4324/9780429423109-4

Introduction

The ambulatory electronic health record (AEHR) as a distinct entity is evolving due to the evolution of more integrated EHRs that combine with inpatient systems. Similarly, over the past several decades, various specialty, acute care, ancillary, and ambulatory systems have advanced individually and also converged. But inpatient and outpatient care are still largely distinct and typically paid for by different payment systems. Whether unified across specialties, AEHRs, especially for primary care, are typically the closest approximation of the patient's archetype of "my chart": a cradle-to-grave record of a patient's healthy growth, sickness, recovery, and aging.

Increasingly, a representation of this vernacular "chart" is emerging, either through large multi-functioned EHRs or the aggregation of data from disparate systems through sophisticated interfaces and information exchange between providers or within the patient's own computer. This reflects technological advancement, organizational changes within healthcare, and evolving reimbursement methods. Aggregation may improve access to data across the continuum of care, but it also creates new problems of how to sort and organize so much information to prevent data overload, alert fatigue, and a very different kind of provider inefficiency than was the challenge faced by AEHR pioneers decades ago.

In this chapter, we review the key features of the AEHR as they have evolved and discuss some of the remaining challenges facing the designers of future AEHRs. We begin with practice management because, other than the nature of technology itself, healthcare reimbursement methods remain a core driver of how AEHRs are structured. We then discuss the fundamental clinical features such as order entry, documentation, results review, messaging, and decision support. Next, we discuss reporting and analytics where the increasing quantity and quality of data captured in the AEHR can be leveraged to improve care delivery, outcomes, and the AEHR itself. To achieve an integrated view of the patient and a longitudinal time perspective, data integration is required. We review this in the context of the AEHR as well as the role of niche systems. We touch on patient engagement as an increasingly important aspect of the AEHR, though this is also addressed in other chapters of this text. We end with a discussion of the cost and value of the AEHR, a topic that has evolved from a defensive justification to a more mature analysis of clinical and business value.

Practice Management Systems

It is widely accepted that administrative complexity is an important driver of healthcare costs.[1,2] Ambulatory practice management systems (PMS) supply the tools to manage patient flow and the revenue cycle. These are the operational and financial sides of the same coin. The PMS is the outpatient cousin to inpatient ADT (admit discharge transfer) and patient accounting systems. While many providers have implemented some form of a PMS in the absence of an EHR, tight integration between the administrative and clinical functions is becoming increasingly necessary to ensure maximum productivity and revenue cycle efficiency.

While the key functions of a mature PMS are patient registration, scheduling, and billing, full-featured practice management systems provide many more features. Some provide scanning and document management capabilities. Some manage paper charts in ways analogous to a hospital information management (HIM) system. Many have sophisticated materials management capabilities, which are particularly important in specialties where expensive medications or equipment are used. The best systems support data interchange with payers as well as patients.

Registration

Whether you view the PMS through an operations or a financial lens, the business begins with patient identification. From this starting point, the divergence with inpatient systems begins. The concept of "registration" is very different between the inpatient and outpatient worlds. The conceptual difference is permanence. The ambulatory world treats registration as a persistent beginning of a lifetime record. Patients see their doctors over and over, but they only register once; they reasonably expect their doctor to remember them. In the inpatient world, registration is the beginning of a finite stay and is repeated with each admission. Inpatient EMRs typically maintain demographics across stays, but in many systems, the patient's chart is broken up by hospital admission rather than being a continuous record.

From a systems perspective, the difference is the combination of three related functions: identification, registration, and scheduling. Patient identification is increasingly the realm of specialized systems known as the electronic master patient index (EMPI). These systems contain a database with a small amount of identity and demographic data about every patient in their dominion. The job of the EMPI is to make sure that each patient has only one set of data, even across multiple systems, specialties, locations, and institutions.

Almost all PMSs have some built in EMPI functionality. Large PMSs tend to have more sophisticated functionality. For example, advanced EMPI systems can make use of complex algorithms to evaluate and weigh dozens of patient characteristics on a transactional basis to determine possible identity matches. A key factor for PMS selection is to make sure this functionality is sophisticated enough to meet organizational needs *or* that the system is capable of integration with an external EMPI, which is increasingly the preference of large organizations. With the advent of wide-scale health information exchanges, the ability to link patients across centers is both harder and more important, especially given that systems try to match patients in external systems in an automated fashion before patients arrive for encounters.

The details of patient identification can seem tedious, particularly to those who fail to grasp their importance – but ignore them at your peril. The ambulatory world can be deceptively simple in this regard. If you view each practice independently, it may be easy to keep a few thousand patients straight without a large number of duplicates. But when you combine practices or try to combine data from patients across practices or locations, you quickly realize that the ambulatory world is very large indeed. The lack of a single universal patient identifier makes matching logic more critical. The well-documented failures and risks of using Social Security numbers (SSNs) make the task ahead look even more challenging.[3,4] Inadequate or improperly implemented EMPIs can lead to duplicate records or inappropriately merged patient records within clinical and administrative systems. These identity problems are not rare and can impede productivity, compromise revenue cycle efficiency, and introduce significant patient safety risks.[5]

Congress has banned the government from creating a national patient identifier,[1] leaving it to each provider to calculate unique identities across shared patients.[6,7,8] One particularly disturbing

---

[1] As of this writing, federal agencies are once again examining the problem of creating a national patient identifier. See https://www.federalregister.gov/documents/2019/03/04/2019-02200/medicare-and-medicaid-programs-patient-protection-and-affordable-care-act-interoperability-and#p-489

Table 4.1 Ethnic Bias in Duplicate Names

Same First and Last Name	Same First and Last Name and Same Date of Birth
JOSE RODRIGUEZ	TAYLOR LI
MARIA RODRIGUEZ	ELVIRA VLASICH
MARIA GONZALEZ	JEFFREY XU
MARIA GARCIA	MARY GRAVES
JOSE PEREZ	CYNTHIA MCMANUS
JOSE RIVERA	RONNI FINK
JOSE GARCIA	MARTIN HARTY
JUAN RODRIGUEZ	ANTHONY REYES
MARIA PEREZ	STAVROS ZAFIRIS
JOSE HERNANDEZ	RICHARD KEINER
JOSE MARTINEZ	JOSEPH BUCCINO
JOSE GONZALEZ	MARY SINCOVICH
LUIS RODRIGUEZ	ROBERT VELASQUEZ
MARIA MARTINEZ	FATHIMUNIS BEEGUM
CARMEN RODRIGUEZ	ANTHONY MEGNATH

Note: An ethnic bias in duplicate names is evident by examining the most commonly repeated names. These data were taken from our institutional EMPI in 2019 with more than 12 million patients. These are the most frequent names where the first name and the last name are the same or the first and last name plus the date of birth are the same.

aspect of this decision is that the negative impact of this inefficiency is not equally distributed across society because of the different frequency of names among various ethnic groups. See Table 4.1.

Once the patient is identified, the formal registration can begin. This involves the collection of more detailed patient demographics, including insurance coverage information, emergency contacts, customer service information such as contact preferences, and similar non-clinical information. In the most sophisticated PMSs, insurance eligibility verification may occur at this step in an EDI (electronic data interchange) transaction analogous to a retailer validating a credit card. Practice management systems are often connected to large clearinghouses for these eligibility queries.

Failure to completely and accurately collect all necessary registration information can have profound consequences in subsequent workflows. A failure to standardize data storage conventions can lead to patient misidentification. Incomplete or inaccurate contact information can delay clinical communications between providers and patients. Perhaps most commonly, registrations fail to accurately record patient insurance coverage attributes. This can lead to claim denials, time-consuming follow-up by both providers and patients, and ultimately lost revenue for rendered services.

Scheduling

In the inpatient world, the next step in the workflow is bed management. In the ambulatory environment, the analogous critical next step is the scheduling of clinical services. Because patients are admitted to the hospital at a particular point in time, scheduling is inherent in the admission process. For the ambulatory patient, all future encounters will key off the original registration (generally with registration data confirmation and/or necessary updates), and the schedule is the focus of subsequent patient interactions.

Because the process of scheduling is so tightly linked with registration, it is not surprising that many clinical scheduling systems are integrated with registration systems within the PMS. There are a few key qualities of ambulatory scheduling that differentiate the various systems available on the market. Perhaps the most important is how they differ from non-clinical scheduling systems such as Microsoft Outlook or Google Calendar, which for clarity are referred to here as calendaring systems.

Calendaring systems have been (and continue to be) used to schedule patient visits/services in the ambulatory context, though this is increasingly less common with the adoption of the EHR. The main distinction between a scheduling system and a calendaring system is the linkage to the patient record. In a typical business calendaring system, the user cannot quickly locate a whole history of a given patient's appointments or sort them by type. The appointment is usually encoded as free text, whereas in a clinical scheduling system the appointment is linked in a computable manner with a specific patient already registered in the database.

Clinical schedules are also linked to billing transactions. This is critical from the financial perspective, as the majority of medical service charges are linked to specific encounters. One of the first interventions in a typical revenue cycle enhancement program is to match charges against the schedule. This is a manual process with a calendaring system, but it can be made into an automated "missing charge report" in a clinical scheduling product.

Clinical scheduling systems typically allow for complex templates and rules to maximize patient flow and appointment availability. Supported concepts such as appointment type, waitlists, recurring visits, pre-visit instructions, and multidisciplinary care will have variable importance in different practices and specialties. For example, patients on specific chemotherapy protocols or physical therapy routines can be extremely complicated to schedule. Sophisticated clinical scheduling systems can offer appropriate searching algorithms and decision support that can span visits or include specific resource availability.

Resource linking is particularly critical in procedural areas. For example, in specialties with endoscopes, the availability of the scope itself and the time needed for sterilization must be accounted for by the scheduling system to maximize throughput. A decision support rule may alert a radiology scheduler regarding total radiation dose. Similar issues exist for many other procedures like oncology infusions, dialysis, and physical therapy. Linkage to materials management systems may also be important for inventory and cost controls.

In academic environments, there are complex regulatory rules affecting scheduling that must be accounted for to allow compliant billing. For example, the 1969 CMS IL372 supervision regulations require that primary care supervisors oversee no more than four residents at a given time.[9] Without that ratio, supervisors cannot bill for their supervision. Similarly, patients may be part of a clinical trial protocol, and therefore communication regarding a research visit with a clinical trials management system may be important.

Increasingly, the most sophisticated ambulatory practices are providing online access to self-directed scheduling. Frequently, online scheduling is offered via patient-facing health portals that are tightly integrated with the EHR or PMS. One of the most commonly used application programming interfaces (APIs) supported by modern EHRs allows for accessing provider schedule slot availability and appointment booking. This has enabled online scheduling capabilities from institutional physician directories and third-party websites. Stand-alone consumer services such as ZocDoc (www.zocdoc.com) have gained popularity by offering patients the ability to directly schedule appointments with participating providers.

Though offering online access for self-directed scheduling isn't extremely technically complex, there are workflow challenges to its implementation. Particularly for highly sub-specialized medical service, patients can't know about complex business rules that might factor into the assignment of the correct resources, appointment duration, or even service provider. Further, the need to properly address managed care pre-certifications and medical necessity rules also can impede the delivery of this popular convenience. Though providers have historically been guarded about offering patients direct scheduling access, adoption has increased as consumers increasingly demand online scheduling capabilities.

Check-in and Patient Tracking

Automated check-in is an increasingly common PMS feature. This can be done online at home in the patient portal or in the waiting room in an airport-like kiosk or tablet. Typically, demographics and financial data are verified. Insurance cards can be scanned and patient photos added to the chart. Some practices also add questionnaires that may be standard clinical instruments or start the physician note with patient-entered data regarding the present illness, family history, medications, and the like.

Some form of a patient tracking system is often implemented in conjunction with PMSs to track all aspects of clinical workflow and patient throughput. Some systems can parse a variety of wait times such as time to room, time in room, time with registered nurse, and time with doctor. Some systems use radio frequency identification (RFID) or other technologies to automate patient tracking, though that is hardly mainstream. When used well, these tools provide practice administrators and clinicians the necessary data to optimize patient flow, maximize resource utilization, and improve patient satisfaction.

Billing and Collections

The core of most PMSs is the financial component. The tools needed to manage billing and accounts receivable are enormously varied due to the wide variety of reimbursement rules and methods throughout the country. The majority of PMSs are optimized for the traditional reimbursement model within the United States: fee-for-service. Generally speaking, providers are paid a negotiated or (in the case of government payer) determined fee for specific procedures or services on the basis of justifying diagnoses. The PMS must allow for efficient charge capture, generation of medical service claims to payers, and mechanisms for follow-up and resolution of accounts receivable.

Within ambulatory systems, the focus is generally on professional fee billing rather than facilities fee billing, which is an important factor in the inpatient setting. While facility and professional fee billing are increasingly happening concurrently within single enterprise billing systems, historically distinct systems were used to manage facility and professional fee billing. One important (and possibly counterintuitive) needed feature this may imply is for the *ambulatory* PMS to support *inpatient* professional billing. Physicians who see inpatients and do not bill "globally," or through the hospital, send their bills from their office. Therefore, certain types of integration with the inpatient system, such as an admission, discharge, and transfer (ADT) interface, may be desirable for this purpose.

Virtually all PMSs have the ability to transact with partner entities via electronic data interchange (EDI) standards. The HIPAA EDI transaction set governs system communication formats for electronic eligibility queries, claims submission, status checks, and remittance.[10] Ambiguity in operating rules and implementation standards have made system integration complicated and expensive. Many PMS vendors partner with EDI clearinghouse vendors to simplify their own EDI communication. This way providers only need to communicate with one company, which communicates with all the payers on their behalf. Conversely, the payers only need to communicate with a few clearinghouses rather than thousands of providers. In theory, maturation of internet standards and security, further refinement of operating rules, and regulatory pressure may simplify system integration and facilitate some degree of disintermediation.

Charge Capture

Today's financial systems put increasing emphasis on capturing data as early in the encounter as possible. Prior to widespread adoption of EHRs, charge capture was often done as a separate step from clinical documentation. Current Procedural Technology (CPT) and International Statistical Classification (ICD) diagnosis codes were often captured via specialty-specific, paper-based "superbills" and then manually transcribed into the billing system. Gradually, the process of charge capture moved into the electronic realm. In the past two decades, some practices have started using mobile devices like smartphones to capture charges. These systems may be stand-alone or integrated with a PMS or clinical system. Regardless of the platform, these systems offer another way to eliminate paper encounter forms and capture data more accurately and directly into the billing system.

With more widespread adoption of the EHR, charge capture has become more integrated into the clinical workflow at the point of care. CPT and ICD codes are now captured as part of routine clinical documentation within the EHR. This information can then be interfaced to a separate PMS or directly provide the content to the billing functions for those EHR platforms that have integrated practice management capabilities. A major step that has facilitated clinician charge capture is the trend towards embedding clinician-friendly terminology to document procedures and diagnoses. Because these clinician-friendly interface terms are mapped to reference terminologies such as CPT or ICD-10, providers can easily capture clinical intent while still supplying the necessary administrative billing codes.

The shift from back office to point-of-care charge capture can provide significant opportunities to decrease costs and enhance revenue. The elimination of charge-entry clerks and certified professional coders is a potential opportunity to decrease labor costs. Further return on investment (ROI) from these systems stems from a possible reduction in lost charges and reduced service-to-posting lag. Charge capture within the EHR also affords the opportunity to deploy financial decision support in real time, such as medical necessity rules or level of service calculations. Responsibly deployed, these interventions can have very beneficial effects on revenue cycle efficiency.

On the other hand, EHRs have come under fire for potentially facilitating systematic "upcoding" for services not medically necessary.[11] While there is certainly potential for abuse, many argue that EHRs have simply allowed providers to more efficiently document and bill for medically necessary services. Similarly, some of the administrative demands of billing on physician time have led to accusations that EHRs are contributing to burnout, though EHRs are more likely just an enabler of administrative complexity.[12]

Executives need to pay attention to the definition of the encounter itself. As with registration, terminology here is imprecise and can be confusing. Some prefer to refer to the billable event as the encounter and the face-to-face meeting with the patient as the visit. But the increasing prevalence of phone, web, and other virtual "visits" makes this topic inherently fluid. Regardless of how you refer to the event, the system must know the rules for the definitions, which are generally determined by the payer and may or may not make sense to the clinician. For example, a 9-month pregnancy may be a single encounter with multiple visits. Similarly, a visit to a doctor's office that results in referral to the emergency room may be combined as a single encounter (the "72-hour rule" or "two-midnight rule"). A visit to different doctors on a single day may be considered a single encounter. The billing system needs to understand these rules. Again, cross-institutional reconciliation may be necessary to ensure complete accuracy in some scenarios.

Managed Care, Value-Based Reimbursement, Coding Rules, and Claims Submission

The most fundamental distinction among practice management systems is support for the various forms of managed care, value-based reimbursement, and the associated coding and reimbursement rules. All this complexity is a significant driver of physician costs.[13] While the traditional fee-for-service model still exists in some form in most markets, some permutation of managed care is the norm in most areas, with various types of value-based incentives layered on top. The critical functionality within modern PMSs is the ability to embed rules engines and workflows to enforce the complex business rules that govern reimbursement. Practices that take on capitation require use of a PMS that is fully capable of tracking expenses and assessing risk. To achieve value-based incentives the system must rigorously track whatever metrics are used to define "value," which may or may not be relevant to the actual clinical encounter (e.g., reminding the doctor to ask about smoking in an otherwise unrelated visit). Because of the diversity of payer rules, the frequency of changes to the rules, and the frequency that patients change payers, the proper setup and maintenance of a PMS is critical for revenue cycle efficiency.

A fundamental aspect of a highly functional PMS is disciplined master-file management. All information systems use a variety of tables and dictionaries to drive the lists and other user interface elements for relevant discrete data capture. In the case of billing systems, there are dozens of relevant master files, such as providers, locations, specialties, payer/plans, procedures, and diagnoses. Some of these dictionaries can be standardized, but some will always be local, and the ability to customize and control these tables is a key vendor differentiator. For large and/or decentralized ambulatory practices, master-file management can be an extremely labor-intensive management effort.

The complexities inherent in managing a provider master-file are instructive. Information technology (IT) managers are vexed by the need to provide users with accurate data without good sources for the data. Even purchased data sets are typically plagued by inaccuracies. This issue is relevant to claims adjudication because many nuances of billing require accurate lookup tables. For example, specialists may need to indicate the license number of a referring physician on the claim or it will be rejected. In the world of managed care, keeping track of who is "in plan" and "out of plan" is a major problem. Many providers who have dropped out of plan will tell you that it may take months or even years for their name to disappear from the payer's list, particularly if they are in a shortage specialty, and provider participation itself may vary by practice location.

Another critical aspect of the sophisticated PMS is a rules engine (and associated task management tools) for evaluating the accuracy and/or validity of billing transactions. Charges must be analyzed for exceptions, discounts, consistency with other claims, the addition of modifiers, or other necessary interventions. The goal of the editing functions is to ensure that every claim that is sent to the payer is a clean claim. Sophisticated PMSs provide native tools (or support third-party rules engine integration) that mimic the adjudication rules used by payers. Coding decision support can sometimes be deployed in real time at the time of charge entry. In addition, claims are often batched and analyzed in bulk, generating exceptions that must be reviewed and edited.

Clean claims mean no rejections, faster payment, and reduced re-processing costs. Not surprisingly, claim editing is another frequent focus of revenue enhancement efforts.

Once through the edit process, a claim is ready to be sent. The vast majority of claims are sent electronically to payers or claims clearinghouses as the intermediary. The ability to print a paper claim remains a requirement of any PMS, if for no other reason than a patient request. In either event, logs of the transactions are essential to avoid disputes over lost claims. Upon receipt, a payer adjudicates the claims, and if a flaw is found, the claim for reimbursement may be denied. Here again, there is an opportunity for efficiency if the payer communicates the denial electronically, using standardized rejection codes. Well-managed practices are continually analyzing denial codes so that practice administrators can track the reasons for rejection over time and correct any systematic problems.

Some proportion of the cost of medical services is often the direct responsibility of the patient. This may be due to co-pays, co-insurance, deductibles, or non-covered services. The PMS must have the capability to generate itemized statements for patients to bill for these "self-pay" balances. Often, this information is extracted from the PMS to specialized statement vendors. Increasingly, progressive ambulatory practices are offering online financial statements and bill pay functions via patient portals. This not only reduces the costs of statement generation and mailing but also helps automate the process of recording the payment against the outstanding balance within the PMS.

Note that pre-adjudication of claims remains a goal to improve efficiency and patient satisfaction by providing costs before a visit or procedure. While there are a few technical challenges to doing this, the primary barrier is that most office charges can only be calculated after the diagnosis is made, the service is rendered, and the complexity is known. Still, this capability will have increasing importance in future PMSs.

Payment Posting and Contract Management

Payments made by payers or patients all must be reconciled or "posted" within the PMS. Payment posting has historically been complex and labor intensive due to a lack of electronic automation. There may be manual effort involved with interpreting paper explanations of benefits (EOBs) and assigning the correct amount of money (via paper checks) to each claim. The procedure can also be error prone, making this whole process a ripe target for automation. Bar coding, optical character recognition, and a variety of other technologies have been applied to try to clean up payment posting, with varied degrees of success.

The use of the HIPAA transaction standard for electronic remittance advice (HIPAA X12N 835 standard) has simplified payment posting by providing an electronic version of the EOB. For ambulatory practices that transact with large, established payers, manual payment posting has largely been replaced by automated processing of electronic remittance advice (ERA). The Accountable Care Act of 2010 mandated the creation of more specific operating rules for electronic funds transfer (EFT). This eliminates the effort of depositing paper checks and simplifies the process of reconciling large payer payments with individual patient balances.

Once posted, there are two more problems the PMS must contend with: overpayment and underpayment. Overpayment most commonly occurs when both the patient and the payer send the provider a payment. This requires a method for refunding which, in many practices, requires a link to a separate accounts payable system. In today's world of managed care conglomerates, underpayment is the more serious problem. Even within one company, claims may be processed by multiple different systems that may not all have the current contract and payment policies loaded. Therefore, inappropriate rejections and underpayments are common and often appear to be idiosyncratic. Further, in many states, there is little accountability by regulators. In a study performed at Weill Cornell and Emory, between 3 and 8 percent of all reimbursements from managed care companies were underpaid compared to contract. While this represents tens of millions of dollars to providers annually, payers are only fined a small fraction of this amount by regulators, leaving enforcement of the contract up to the prowess of the providers' management and information technology.[14]

Contract management systems, integrated or added on to the PMS, are the provider's defense against these errors. If the PMS knows how much the payer is supposed to reimburse for a given procedure, it can alert the provider to underpayments individually or systematically. Underpayments of a few dollars are the most insidious, as the cost of reprocessing the claim will exceed the difference collected. This is why tracking underpayments over time is essential so that underpayments can be addressed in bulk.

Analytics and Business Intelligence

One final critical feature to any PMS is reporting. The biggest payoff to any information system comes from the ability to extract and manipulate data that has been captured during the routine course of business. Cheaper systems come with pre-configured reports and a few tools to manipulate them. More sophisticated systems provide a myriad of options for extracting data and configuring reports. Increasingly, operational reports are embedded directly within the PMS to assist with task management by providing visibility on data quality and staff productivity. Rather than generating a report for a manager to review, the most sophisticated systems create a live task list within the application that staff use to manage their workflow. More complex analytic reports are often executed outside of the PMS to allow for long-term trending of patient access and revenue cycle metrics. These are imperative tools to drive ongoing process improvement efforts.

Ambulatory Clinical Systems

Clinical Systems and Biomedical Devices

There are many types of ambulatory clinical systems. The focus in this chapter will be the core EHR, but the AEHR is often just one piece of a complex system architecture to manage clinical workflow and information storage. The AEHR is often integrated with niche diagnostic and/or procedural systems, such as a lab information system, a radiology information system, and potentially dozens of smaller specialty-based systems. Other highly specialized workflows such as clinical trials management, materials management, and image capture/storage are often addressed via stand-alone systems.

Much of the data generated in the context of routine patient care is via a wide array of biomedical devices. The distinction between clinical systems and biomedical devices is becoming both difficult to make and less important. Traditionally the line between them was apparent. Devices were typically electromechanical, and diagnostic and procedure oriented. From an IT perspective they were data sources. Perhaps the most important distinction was that biomedical devices were regulated by the Food and Drug Administration (FDA). Any changes to their function required recertification. Conversely, information systems were electronic, transaction and documentation oriented, and unregulated in their plasticity.

Some of these distinctions still hold today despite efforts to reduce the arbitrary complexity they impose. Clinically, it is completely natural that the systems a cardiologist or radiologist uses to make a diagnosis should be fully integrated with the systems they use to report their findings. Similarly, from a patient's perspective, the test report is no less a part of their medical chart than the note of the physician who ordered the test or procedure. A few decades ago, the marketplace for these once separate entities appeared to be merging. The leading manufacturers of biomedical devices, like GE and Siemens, have acquired leading vendors of electronic medical records. But the barriers to integration, both technical and regulatory, have prevented true integration from occurring. It is notable that Siemens sold its healthcare software business to a pure-play healthcare software vendor, Cerner, in 2014. Similarly, after acquiring the IDX PMS in 2005, GE recently sold its ambulatory clinical and practice management systems to Veritas Capital.

That said, this chapter will not examine further traditional biomedical devices like electrocardiogram (ECG) and x-ray machines, regardless of how proximal they may have become to clinical systems. One reason for this is that they are still purchased and managed differently in most institutions. But more importantly, biomedical devices do not fit as cleanly into the major thesis of this section. That is, clinical systems are the essential *workflow* managers of ambulatory medicine – or at least they should be.

The reason to emphasize workflow is that it is the key to success when purchasing, implementing, and managing these systems. A brief history of clinical systems shows that this was not always the case. In fact, many, if not most, clinical systems on the market today reveal a *modular* orientation that reflects how their development was funded as much as any well-thought-out technical architecture.

The Ambulatory Electronic Health Record

A Brief History

The first attempts to build electronic medical records were largely in the outpatient arena. Barnett's landmark work in the 1960s with COSTAR[15] emphasized increasing the availability and organization of medical records. Separate modules for registration, scheduling, and the actual clinical encounter form were implemented.

In the 1970s, McDonald at Regenstrief and Stead and Hammond at Duke also developed outpatient medical record systems.[16,17] The Regenstrief system also used encounter form data input similar to COSTAR, but pioneered the emphasis on automated reminders. Stead and Hammond's TMR system actually attempted to go paperless using clerks to enter data.

Throughout the 1970s and 1980s, technology became more affordable and up to the task of building medical records. Computers moved from mainframes to minicomputers in the 1970s and from minicomputers to microcomputers in the 1980s. At this time, most medical centers were organized in a very decentralized manner. Outside the institutions, independent practitioners and small groups were still the norm. Therefore, it is not surprising that the medical record systems that developed reflected this departmental and practice-oriented organization. In the 1990s, when graphical programming and database management tools became ubiquitous, these forces of dis-integration were even more profound. Commercial systems were specialty focused, procedure oriented, and doctor centric.

Large institutions were installing more centralized systems in hospitals, but even there, the industry was moving toward decentralized client-server designs. The sales teams advocated "best of breed" – as much a justification for the way things were as for any nobler architectural reason.

What resulted is a situation many institutions and practices are still in today. Every business unit or clinically distinct entity has (or wants) their own information system that meets its specific needs. There are significant merits to this approach. Many niche systems, in fact, do meet the workflow requirements of a given specialty much better than general purpose systems that are "customized" for their environment. The needs of a cardiology practice offering echocardiography and cardiac graphics are quite distinct from gastroenterologists offering in-office endoscopy, though both are sub-specialties of internal medicine. Venture into radiation oncology, physiatry, ophthalmology, or almost any other common outpatient medical specialty, and you will find radically different functional requirements, workflows, and expectations.

This challenge of sub-specialization exemplifies perhaps the most fundamental strategic IT choice facing an executive managing clinical systems: the choice between an aggregation of interfaced best-of-breed systems and a monolithic system. If each subspecialty can have a better system for themselves if they purchase separately, is the total greater or less than the sum of the parts? Does a unified platform offer economies of scale and degrees of interoperability not feasible with multiple interfaced systems?

This struggle is illustrated in the history of results reporting and order entry systems discussed in the next section. Twenty to thirty years ago, many order entry and results reporting systems were separate. Integration allows loop closure: an order is closed when the result comes back. But in ambulatory practices that order from many different (often external) labs, integration is more complex and costly and might lock such practices in to one laboratory provider.

Recently, the sophistication of large, unified systems and interfacing technology have both improved significantly, so technology itself has not resolved this debate. Large, integrated EHRs are better than ever, and it is also easier than ever to integrate data from sub-specialty systems if they follow the latest standards for data exchange.

Order Entry and Results Reporting

The earliest and most basic clinical systems were result reporting systems that allowed viewing of the output of laboratory and other biomedical devices. Lab data are typically numeric and *relatively* easy to categorize and display. Textual results, such as pathology, microbiology, and radiology results were also fairly analogous to other data routinely managed by early business computers. Graphical results and images arrived later with the more powerful hardware and software required to support these modalities. Radiology results in particular bring in additional complexity, as the non-textual part of the result (the image) is stored and viewed on a picture archiving and communication system (PACS) typically separate from the EHR, requiring additional interface and patient context synchronization needs.

Typically absent from simple result reporting systems is any facility for data *entry*. The user interface characteristics required for data entry and data display are radically different, with the former being far more challenging. Early "monolithic" systems had a relatively modest goal of unifying all the entered data into a single repository, while specialized data entry systems were permitted in departmental silos.[18]

Starting in the 1990s, due to the economics of unrestricted physician orders, many hospitals focused on order entry systems as the centerpiece of their clinical systems efforts.[19, 20] In the ambulatory world, order entry can be a small component of the workflow in some specialties. Further, the economic imperatives are very different in the outpatient world (especially with fee for service), and the ROI from an order entry system may be harder to realize than at a hospital (with prospective payment). That said, ambulatory order entry is still a big business.

Many laboratories and radiology practices will give physicians a result reporting system if they will use their online order entry system. The laboratory gains efficiencies, but they still have to give the physician an incentive to use a potentially less convenient system than paper, especially given the high likelihood that more than one such proprietary system may need to be used. Administrative tasks such as pre-authorization and eligibility checks for ordered procedures further complicate the use of such systems. In large institutions and practices, order entry systems can be very helpful in controlling the flow of referrals. This is achieved through either real-time decision support or through enabling analytics to determine leakage and referral patterns. Order entry systems are all but essential in ambulatory practices under capitation to control utilization.

Evidence suggests that ambulatory computerized provider order entry (CPOE) can be time neutral to physicians, but not all order entry systems are created equal.[21] The minimal systems, some of which are now free, do little more than write prescriptions and support electronic submission to pharmacies. For specialists who prescribe a lot of medications, comprehensive support for refills, including expirations and reminders, can be a major time saver and is frequently the first clinical system installed. Outpatient prescriptions are different from inpatient orders in several respects. The ability to print prescriptions in locally mandated formats is not to be assumed. Inpatient systems also generally have limited formularies, whereas outpatient systems generally need all available drugs. Worse still, in managed care environments, ambulatory systems often have to maintain multiple formularies and distinguish between drugs that are on- and off-plan. A secondary market for vendors that manage pre-authorizations has now emerged, adding yet another layer of system complexity. Due to the variations in cost sharing by outpatient pharmacies, services that either integrate with the outpatient EHR or as independent apps are now available to help reduce the cost burden of medications and would hopefully improve compliance with use.

Inpatient systems tend to be more focused on drips and compound preparations. These exist in the outpatient world as well, such as in oncology infusion centers. Such sites need the full medication administration record (MAR) functionality common to inpatient systems, but they are certainly less common and typically less complex than in the inpatient setting. Conversely, ambulatory centers that dispense drugs often do so without a pharmacist as intermediary. This means that the system must support the functions pharmacists provide. For example, when a sample is given, the system must produce a label with instructions for the patient and log the lot number of the drugs dispensed.

E-prescribing, the transmission of prescriptions electronically, has been expanding rapidly due to recent incentives from the federal government and certain payers. While systems originally did not have bidirectional communication capabilities, more recent versions have added the ability to allow some interaction between pharmacies and practices, such as refill requests and notification of the administration of immunizations in pharmacies. The ability for a medication cancellation notification to be sent to pharmacies has also been widely adopted, which reduces the chances of patients refilling medications that prescribers believe that a patient has stopped. The Centers for Medicare and Medicaid Services (CMS) will require Part D providers support real-time formulary and benefit tools as of January 2021,[22] which many of the leading systems now support. Executives should be aware that the government mandates have created powerful transaction intermediaries who can force contract terms that are harmful to providers and patients.

Similarly, prescription fill information is becoming available electronically from payers. The availability of this information has the potential to alter physicians' ability to monitor patient compliance. Policies around viewing fill-history prior to ordering narcotic medications have been implemented to prevent abuse;[23] however, there is great variability in their execution from state to state. In some cases, failure to comply can lead to fine and loss of licensure. Depending on the requirements, EHR systems can facilitate these workflows by providing point-of-care clinical decision support (CDS) alerts that serve as a reminder to comply with the requirements, and in states that permit it, the system can automate queries to the state's prescription drug monitoring program (PDMP). Lack of a national patient identifier and limited sharing of fill histories between states limits the utility of such efforts. Because ambulatory patients administer their own individual doses and may not submit claims for every prescription filled, the reconciliation of fill data with the original prescription is still imperfect. Further, the mismatch between AEHR and pharmacy master files generates a lot of noise when originating systems cannot match a returning filled prescription. The potential of this capability to improve care is large,[24] but too little has been done to contemplate the workflow impact these data will have on routine visits. Physicians may object to another uncompensated demand on their time. Participation in a well-designed value-based payment contract can help address this concern.

For laboratory orders, key features in an ambulatory environment again differ from the inpatient world. Most hospitals send all their lab specimens to one laboratory. In the outpatient world, this may be desirable, but managed care contracts often mandate the use of a particular lab. The ability to control default routing rules based on contracts is a vital revenue control point for sites that maintain their own laboratory. Routing to the most affordable laboratory for a particular payer is also a key determinant of patient satisfaction.

True integration with multiple laboratories is technically very challenging, but it is also very desirable for many reasons. If the outbound order and the incoming result are linked (loop closure), then there is more potential for features like alerts and reports. For example, a common cause of malpractice claims is the failure to note an abnormal Pap result. Systems with loop closure can alert a physician both to the arrival of an abnormal result and the *failure* of any result to return after a specified time, thereby diminishing the risk of lost data.

The most difficult aspect of linking to multiple labs is reconciling the coding systems for the orders and the results. As of this writing there is no satisfactory coding system for either orders or results, and those that do exist are poorly cross-mapped. CPT is often used when placing orders, but it is too imprecise and incomplete to be used exclusively. Similarly, Logical Observation Identifiers Names and Codes (LOINC) is the dominant standard for coding results but it is also very incomplete and idiosyncratically applied. Certain areas, such as microbiology and transfusion medicine, remain particularly problematic. The National Library of Medicine funded an effort to map CPT and LOINC.[25] While this helped, the fact remains that operations managers faced with multiple laboratories need to commit considerable resources to map procedures and result components. Failure to accurately map the clinical tests can severely compromise the usability of the EHR.

The ability to configure order sets in ambulatory systems is not dissimilar to inpatient order entry systems. Likewise, clinical decision support rules have similar value in both settings. In the outpatient world, there is the additional uncertainty of knowing all medications a patient is taking. This is a topic of considerable conflict in organizations with shared charts. Some specialists object to seeing the full list of medications in their chart, fearing responsibility for drugs they do not prescribe. This is mostly an issue of legal liability and not necessarily medical care. However, it can require system managers to jump configuration hurdles before specialists will buy in to a common EHR.

The Joint Commission made medication reconciliation one of its national patient safety goals in 2005.[26] They require that providers exchange a complete list of the patient's medications at transitions of care. They explicitly include discharge to ambulatory settings. A shared electronic medical record should make this process easier, if not automatic, with the record itself. A seamless handoff between EHRs requires a substantial improvement in state-of-the-art interfacing technologies. The Joint Commission based their recommendation on staffing and process models from the inpatient world[27] and implementing their ideas outside of hospitals has proven difficult. (See Chapter 6.)

Analogous to diagnosis-related group (DRG) reimbursement in inpatient settings, one of the more complex features in ambulatory order entry is "medical necessity" checking. The quotation marks here are to emphasize that the definition of medical necessity is an insurance construct and not a clinical assessment per se. The primary impetus for this requirement comes from Medicare. Through a process called National and Local Coverage Determinations (NCD/LCD; previously called Local Medical Review Policies [LMRP]), Medicare will only reimburse for tests that it deems medically necessary.[28] Because these rules frequently do not meet the needs of individual patients, physicians need to be alerted when they are ordering a test that is not covered. For example, a patient with cancer might need heart tests prior to taking a cardiotoxic drug. It would be clinical malpractice *not* to perform the test, but it may still not be considered "medically necessary" by Medicare in terms of reimbursement.

There are two major reasons to generate NCD/LCD alerts. The first is the intended effect of the regulation: to draw attention to the physician that the test or drug may not be clinically indicated and that an alternative should be sought. The second reason is to alert both patient and provider that charges will go unpaid by the carrier. For providers, particularly laboratory and radiology facilities, this can be a key source of uncollected debt. The ordering provider should give the patient an advanced beneficiary notice (ABN) that alerts the patient how much they are likely to be charged for what the payer may deem unnecessary.

The process for documenting medical necessity is fairly crude. The diagnostic code (typically ICD-10) that the physician associates with the order (typically coded by CPT) either matches or does not match an approved list designed by the NCD/LCD. Practices that are very focused on downstream revenue may seek even more sophisticated alerts to question providers who order tests with codes that they may incorrectly be using as "rule outs" rather than using symptom codes. This is presently at the boundary of commercial system functionality.

The last major category of order entry functionality is referrals. These are similar to inpatient consult orders but are a great deal more complex due to third-party reimbursement rules and geographic variation inherent to outpatient care. In many managed care plans, the ordering provider is supposed to solicit an eligibility and pre-approval code before sending a patient to another specialist. Some systems automate this process to some extent, but the rules and documentation requirements are quite variable, making full automation very difficult. If providers find themselves or their staff spending hours soliciting these approvals, executives would be wise to spend as much time re-negotiating contracts to simplify and standardize these procedures. Otherwise, they might be trying to get the IT staff to automate an unnecessarily chaotic process.

In an ideal patient experience, the referrals can be linked to the scheduling process. This is quite plausible if the order entry system is integrated with the scheduling system and the payer rules allow for such simplification. In reality, this kind of service is most likely to be found only in highly integrated care delivery systems, regardless of their IT infrastructure.

Documentation

While results reporting and order entry remain the core of many electronic medical records, the key to the ambulatory medical record is documentation, particularly physician documentation. This is also the most technically difficult challenge for any medical record system for several reasons. The major challenges in medical informatics generally come together in physician documentation. User interface design, workflow management, structured vocabulary, database performance, and hardware limitations are all major limiting factors to what we can practically deliver to support the most elemental component of medical care: the doctor-patient interaction.

There exists a very fine balance between entering documentation in EHRs via structured versus unstructured documentation. Structured documentation allows the clinician to discretely capture their observations about patients. The most common forms use checkboxes and other tools that limit the clinician's choices to only those that have been previously programmed. This method provides rich reporting and affords the system greater capabilities to know what is contained in a note. Unstructured documentation in an EHR allows for more free-form narrative while still providing legibility, practice standardization, and ubiquitous access. Even though unstructured documentation may involve fewer clicks, it still potentially requires more time for the clinician to enter it into the system than pen and paper.

Many notes are a hybrid between structured and unstructured data. For example, the physical exam may be documented in a structured manner, while the assessment and plan are entered in via free text. The speed at which clinicians can document in the system has become a great concern. In order to reduce the amount of time required, EHR vendors and health systems have developed methods that off-load some of the data entry tasks to others beside the clinician. Patient-entered information can aid clinicians in documenting visits. Some patients log in to web portals, while others may use tablets to interact with EHRs to provide both patient-specific and visit-specific information. For example, a patient may fill out both their past medical history and their review of systems using these tools. The clinician can then review the patient's responses with the patient and choose to accept or reject their inclusion in the documentation.

Dictation can be used to enter non-structured data into electronic medical record systems. Voice recognition software and trained professional transcriptionists are both widely used in practices using electronic medical record systems. As the accuracy of voice recognition software has increased, so has its usage. In order to assist clinicians in entering structured data, some systems use similar software to "read" a provider's documentation and then suggest possible discrete data for the clinician to approve and include in a patient's chart.

Practices using physician extenders or supervising residents and students will have complex co-signature and/or attestation requirements. Another method to speed up documentation is to hire scribes to perform most, if not all, of the documentation tasks in the EHR. The scribe must be present (either physically or remotely via teleconferencing technologies) while the provider interacts with a patient, and they record the information exactly as the clinician describes it. The clinician can then review the documentation and attest that it is an accurate reflection of what occurred during the visit. Scribes can reduce the amount of time that clinicians spend documenting in the EHR, and there is some evidence that the increase in productivity can offset the cost of the services.[29]

Copy and paste functionality in the EHR presents a quandary for many who manage these systems. While the use of copy and paste can dramatically reduce the amount of data entry that a clinician has to do, if the content is not edited properly to reflect what occurred during the patient's visit, it can often prove to be confusing to those who want to know what actually occurred, and it can propagate inaccurate or stale data. In addition to copy and paste, many EHRs have functionality that allows clinicians to import large amount of data into their notes from other areas of the patient record. This phenomenon, often referred to as "note bloat," creates very lengthy notes that can be very difficult to comprehend.[30]

In addition to the above issues, the manner in which a clinician documents visits varies depending upon their specialty. Drawing is a basic element of some physician documentation, such as ophthalmology, that is completely absent in some specialties. Similarly, photography is essential in plastic surgery but optional in most general internal medicine practices. Flowsheets are the primary method of documenting in some specialties, particularly those with repeated visits over a finite period of time such as obstetrics or in practices

focused on a particular disease or procedure, such as diabetes or dialysis. Many "disease management" systems focus on this kind of documentation. Some practices have extensive form completion requirements (e.g., general pediatrics) or practices with heavy managed care oversight (e.g., cognitive psychology). Similarly, specialists who do procedures have very different documentation requirements than those doing evaluation and management.

In academic medical centers, the ability to extract data generated at the point of care into research databases is critical to the research mission over and above immediate clinical needs. The American Society of Clinical Oncology (ASCO)[31] recently released a recommended standard for structured documentation of cancer visits to improve research use of the data as well as interoperability. In 2018 Roche, the global pharmaceutical company, purchased Flatiron Health, which provides an oncology EHR to physicians in return for data that is used for research and drug development.[32] Tech giants such as Google have similar plans.[33] This represents what may be a new era for AEHRs whereby the downstream value of the data drives the payment and usability of the system. It remains too soon to tell if such initiatives will lead to usable systems and gain acceptance despite the ethical conflicts.

Any practice with a wide referral base outside the EHR user base will require a robust inbound and outbound data exchange as well as a scanning system to handle paper brought into the office. Using the Consolidated-Clinical Document Architecture (C-CDA) HL-7 standard, both discrete data such as medications and free-text elements like notes can be sent between systems. Correspondence will migrate towards health information exchange (HIE), as discussed elsewhere in this book, to ensure that an accurate clinical assessment is delivered between clinicians.

Most practices will use a combination of these tools. The challenge for the executive is to differentiate these essential business functions from optional features that may slow down implementation and run up costs. The key to understanding which features provide value and which do not is to examine workflow. This is where systems that deliver functionality in modules reach their limits. All the features in the world can be present in a system, but if they do not hang together for the users in a manner that flows logically within real world use, then the system may cause more harm than good. The unwritten requirement is to select and implement these functions without compromising productivity or provider sanity.

Over the past few decades, inherently modular or interfaced systems have given way to more unified and integrated systems. The market is now dominated by a few large companies that provide more integration out of the box. Recent advances in APIs such as Fast Healthcare Interoperability Resources (FHIR) and other technologies for system interchange have made it attractive to add missing features to integrated EHRs. These can be very attractive individually but present usability challenges in aggregate.

The greatest potential of fully integrated systems comes when they can predict where the user will go next and lead the provider through the visit. This was not possible with older modular systems, and there is a significant danger that contemporary add-ons will further disrupt the workflow to search for different functions.

Fully predictive workflow is beyond the current state of the art in commercial clinical systems. Still, it is where today's executive should be looking when deciding what is needed.[34] Workflow analysis quickly leads to the recognition that system integration is required to make sure data flows in a manner coordinated to the work.

Through the examination of workflow, four additional key functions of clinical systems that go beyond any individual module are revealed as essential to the system architecture: decision support, messaging, interfaces, and patient data entry.

Decision Support

Most modern clinical systems have some form of rules and alerts engine to improve quality, revenue, and compliance. These tools, discussed extensively elsewhere in this book, can improve safety and help narrow the gap between knowledge and practice.[35] Contemporary descriptions of CDS have been more liberal and include tools for providers, patients, and administrators that facilitate decision-making by means of alerts, reminders, flowcharts, guidelines, condition-specific order sets, defaults, and care plans.[36] We confine our discussion to knowledge-based systems integral to an AEHR which have the following cardinal components: (a) data or trigger, (b) knowledge base, (c) rules/inference engine, and (d) user interface/action.

Patient safety alerts such as drug-allergy and drug-drug interaction alerts are examples of simple point-of-care warnings, and they have great potential to help avoid adverse events. The construct is fairly simple: if an ordered medication (trigger) is known to interact with another medication on the patient's record (knowledge base, defining pairs of interacting drugs), it will generate (rules engine) an alert (user interface/action) to warn the ordering provider. The complexity lies in how the knowledge base defines the severity or level of evidence behind the interactions and how well the rules engine can make use of it. "Alert fatigue" may result from misconfiguration of these rules and can be potentially dangerous and counterproductive by overwhelming clinicians with excessive alerts.[37,38,39,40] It is worth pointing out that for this reason, traditional interruptive pop-up alerts are finding less favor when compared to newer approaches such as subtle user interface indicators, nudges, and in-line alerting.[41,42]

Modern systems also allow for real-time alerts that can actively modify how care is delivered. Adoption of best-practice tenets such as Choosing Wisely and prevailing guidelines on disease management or screening are archetypal use cases of decision support, with demonstrated efficacy in literature.[43,44,45,46] Another effort with regulatory underpinnings is a new program to increase the rate of appropriate advanced diagnostic imaging services provided to Medicare beneficiaries, which is described under the Protecting Access to Medicare Act (PAMA) of 2014, section 218(b).[47,48] This appropriate use criteria (AUC) program is set to be fully implemented on January 1, 2023, and requires clinicians ordering imaging studies such as CT, MRI, nuclear medicine, or PET scans to consult a Clinical Decision Support Mechanism (CDSM) to facilitate evidence-based ordering. CDSMs are vendors approved by CMS that implement rules developed, modified, or endorsed by qualified provider-led entities (QPLE), which are typically specialty societies, academic institutions, or institutes comprising practitioners predominantly engaged in direct patient care. The AUC program is to be implemented in ambulatory, emergency department (ED), and inpatient practices; however, some of the requirements may be a bit more demanding in ambulatory practices. Challenges in ambulatory practices (and EDs) pertain to billing requirements, the use of CDSM portals, the use of CDSMs integrated in AEHRs, or the need to account for complex workflows when patients are sent to external imaging centers.

Besides bringing the latest evidence to patient care, CDSMs serve as a means to meet various pay-for-performance measures and quality metrics. Having a structured construct for acting upon and recording these metrics greatly facilitates documentation and reporting. This can have a significant financial impact and can possibly affect physician or hospital repute or ranking.[49]

For example, metrics such as the proportion of patients over the age 65 receiving a pneumococcal vaccine would be meaningless if the vaccine were given at an outside facility and recorded as free text in the clinician's documentation. But an alert triggered by virtue of its absence in the "immunization section" offers the clinician an opportunity to record this fact in a discrete, structured format. Additionally, systems can help clinicians meet the documentation requirements for value-based care programs that often require that problems with certain hierarchical condition category (HCC) values are addressed at least annually. Savings are based upon expected costs, and these conditions are key to predicting expenditures.

From an implementation standpoint, the use of decision support tools requires a great deal of discretion and unremitting evaluation. For ambulatory systems managers, a good starting point is whatever alerts can be purchased in a subscription form so that the knowledge base is easy to maintain. Drug interactions, medical necessity rules, and formulary lists are some examples of commercially available rule sets that are maintained by the vendor. Still, these would need to be configured in order to suit the purposes of one's practice and providers. We recommend two approaches to help with this local configuration: "repeat your history" and "model thy neighbor." Chances are that most new implementations are supplanting an existing EHR, and if the previous EHR utilized a CDS configured to a satisfactory level, then it makes sense to simulate the configuration in the new setup to attain a comparable level of historical alert volume and overrides. By "model thy neighbor" we propose replicating the configuration of clinical practices or organizations that have a close enough constellation of AEHR, knowledge content vendor, clinician culture, and outlook to your setup. EHR vendors often help facilitate identifying "institutions like me," and the shared knowledge can provide a great starting point when deploying CDS. Another sensible strategy is to first introduce alerts of high value (e.g., high-severity drug interaction alerts) and high specificity and gradually dial up the potential alert sensitivity. Establishment of committees with technical and clinical representation to review parameters such as alert volume, alert acceptance, and clinical impact on an ongoing basis can help achieve the ideal configuration.[50,51]

An emerging trend for decision support implementation is the use of APIs to allow the delivery of point-of-care decision support via real-time communication between EHRs and external knowledge engines. Rather than embedding complex and dynamic rule algorithms within EHRs, web services are employed to relay key clinical characteristics or conditions to an external entity at defined workflow trigger points. The decision support content is then transmitted back to the EHR, often in an actionable format. This type of implementation is particularly applicable for programs such as the AUC under the PAMA law described earlier. The AEHR (user interface), the QPLE content (knowledge), and the CDSM (rules engine) in most cases would be provided by separate vendors/corporate entities, and the best method to make these operate in harmony would be achieved through web services–based integrations. In a similar vein, CDS Hooks is a promising Health Level 7 (HL7) specification to allow for more sophisticated decision support integration.[52] CDS Hooks allows for the return of decision support "cards" that can contain not only textual feedback but links to external content as well as customized SMART applications. From a medical liability perspective, it is imperative that the contributions of one or more outside resources be "tagged to permit easy auditing in the event of an adverse outcome related to the content/recommendation provided (See chapter 27 Medical-Legal: Attorney's Perspective).

In summary, the two quintessential challenges for ambulatory managers implementing decision support are knowledge maintenance and improving the relevancy of alerts. For knowledge maintenance, subscribing to third-party CDS content wherever possible, and having a distributed ownership for reviews and updates of guideline content by specialty or department are recommended. To improve relevancy of alerts, constant evaluation and adjustment of AEHR rule configurations is necessary. Rules engines are becoming more sophisticated in their utilization of discrete data elements to improve alert specificity. Machine learning techniques to recognize clinical data patterns hold great potential in making alerts more relevant than traditional knowledge-based systems. Such systems can potentially adapt to alert override patterns and determine which ones hold more relevance for particular specialties, disease states, or patient populations. However, we need to wait until such systems become pragmatic for EHR integration and have proven efficacy and safety.[53] (See Chapter 5.)

Messaging and Communication

Messaging could perhaps be viewed as a module itself. Indeed, if a practice had limited funding, the cheapest and easiest system to implement to increase efficiency might be an instant messaging system. But within a full-featured EHR, clinical messaging can become the central task management tool of a practice. The key difference is the ability to route a message within the context of a patient's chart. This context extends the physician's capacity to utilize support staff, freeing the physician for more productive work. Leading products categorize messages into multiple queues such as new results, orders awaiting co-signature, messages from colleagues, and even personal notes. Messages can go to multiple staff at once to work down a queue and can be rerouted during vacations or for on-call coverage.

Some systems clearly separate messaging from task management. In larger practices, this is probably wise. As the physician workflow progresses along the patient encounter, a variety of tasks queue for the ancillary staff, such as rooming and taking vitals, drawing blood, and processing referrals. How elegantly these processes are integrated with the system will dictate the success of managing the entire practice workflow rather than just isolated pieces of it.

Secure messaging is generally inherent within a given EHR. Meaningful Use (MU) provided the incentive to increase the use of secure messages both between EHRs and with patients themselves. Secure messaging between patient and physician most commonly occurs using a patient portal that is tethered to the EHR. Patients can send messages to their providers seeking medical advice or requesting appointments, refills, and referrals. Providers can actively engage patients regarding diagnostic testing results, health maintenance needs, and patient-specific education. When the patient has a new communication from the practice, they receive a tickler message with minimal or no patient health information (PHI) sent to their designated email address. They then log into the portal for the actual message. While this does create an extra step, it provides the assurance that the message was delivered in a secure manner.

Secure messaging between EHRs is rapidly becoming an industry standard function. For physician-to-physician communication, the Consolidated-Clinical Document Architecture (C-CDA)[54] format was chosen by CMS as part of the MU requirements for Stage 2. The format allows EHRs to exchange discrete data in a manner that foreign systems can digest. Medications, problem lists, immunizations, progress notes, and lab results can be shared between systems, in addition to narrative messages between providers.

As payers increase the demands to encourage patient involvement in their care, new communication methods between patient and practice will be established. This includes the use of text messaging technologies to remind patients about important health-related tasks. The further extension of this will be the delivery of data taken in the patient's home back to the practice's EHR. Glucometers, blood pressure cuffs, and activity monitors are but some of the devices that can securely communicate information back to practices. (See Chapter 16.)

System Integration and Intra-operability

Interfaces are the glue between modules of non-integrated systems and the mechanism for sharing data across entirely dissimilar systems. The richness and complexity of interfaces is more than enough of a topic for a whole book in itself. Some key points to understand about interfaces in ambulatory systems relate to what interfaces can and cannot accomplish and what buzzwords to look out for when evaluating systems.

Early efforts at interfaces were so-called point-to-point custom interfaces that required coding far too extensive for all but the largest ambulatory providers. In 1979 the American National Standards Institute (ANSI) chartered the Accredited Standards Committee (ASC) X12 "to develop uniform standards for inter-industry electronic interchange of business transactions – electronic data interface (EDI)." In the past 40 years, that body has developed more than 320 business-to-business transaction sets.[55] In the late 1980s, healthcare joined the EDI standardization process with the creation of HL7, a set of semantic standards for exchanging data between healthcare information systems. HL7 was accredited by ANSI in 1994.[56]

The HL7 standards define many of the key transactions that are necessary to implement clinical and practice management systems. Anyone attending to practice workflow quickly realizes that more and better interfaces are critical to provider efficiency.[57] Besides the basic insurance transactions, ambulatory systems generally rely on ADT/registration and scheduling interfaces. HL7 includes a wide array of transactions that support clinical processes, including transmission of orders, results, and documents. These HL7 interfaces support common EHR integration with laboratories, radiology systems, transcription providers, pharmacy systems, and a host of specialty niche diagnostic and procedural systems.

While HL7 interfaces continue to be the mainstay of local transactional integration, there are obvious deficiencies and inadequacies. The first problem is the need for multiple interfaces itself. Interfaces are rarely plug and play, and even once implemented they generate error queues and exceptions that require policies, procedures, and staff resources to handle. In a large healthcare system, an interface group may be dedicated to these issues. In a small ambulatory practice this is often impossible, and the errors either go uncorrected or the interface might need to be eliminated.

Ambulatory practices within larger institutions face the related problem of scale. While large IT shops may have the staff to handle implementation and error queues, the priorities of integrating a single obscure medical device may be quite low compared to a new laboratory feed for the whole hospital. But without that device, the single physician or practice cannot do their job. For example, it may be easier for a whole hospital to do without an interface to a spirometer than for an allergist or pulmonologist in their private office.

A second problem rests in the interfaces themselves. As HL7 is primarily a *semantic* standard, it dictates what the message means, not how it is said. There are two problems left unsolved. First, the semantic standards are quite limited. HL7 covers the basics only, and enormous flexibility remains such that two vendor systems can both be "compliant" and not be able to understand one another. Second, HL7 does not standardize how messages are sent. This is called *syntax*. HL7 has integrated a widespread syntactic standard called XML (Extensible Markup Language) into its new standards, which should help ease this problem, though adoption is far from complete.[58]

Though HL7 interfaces have remained an efficient mechanism for transacting between clinical systems, there has been a persistent push for more complete yet simplified interoperability. This initially manifested itself as a debate about the best way to combine semantic and syntactic standards. Those who had wide-ranging systems with rich feature sets favored comprehensive standards to move and reconcile data between systems. Those who had fewer resources or more modest ambitions about data normalization have been willing to settle for far simpler standards.

Competing standards emerged for transmitting electronic patient snapshots at transitions of care. Ultimately, HL7 created C-CDA to harmonize various standards.[59] C-CDA has become the favored standard for transmission of structured patient data between systems. But the inadequacy of all these standards for true interoperability remains.

Improving interoperability between clinical systems has been a focus of the federal government via both certification standards as well as MU incentives. In 2016, with the passage of the 21st Century Cures Act, the government moved beyond incentives and certification toward penalties for the failure to exchange data, or so-called information blocking.[60]

Meanwhile, HL7 itself has undergone a reformation with the FHIR approach.[61] FHIR uses more contemporary internet-based standards like Hypertext Transfer Protocol (HTTP) to communicate and is less proscriptive regarding context than the prior versions of HL7. But it still fails to overcome how clinical data is mapped and used within EHRs, and it can only pull data on one patient at a time. Vendors generally have their own competing proprietary APIs with richer support. Executives evaluating AEHRs certainly need to pay attention to how systems support FHIR and the ambivalence or progressiveness of the vendor's attitude toward this new form of exchange.

Patient Engagement Tools

Evidence suggests that engaging with patients to increase health literacy and to conduct shared decision-making can lead to higher patient satisfaction, increased positive behavioral change, and even improved health outcomes.[62] Personal health records (PHRs) are seen by many as a key technology to assist with patient engagement. PHRs contain an individual patient's health information, including medical history, lab test results or imaging studies, medication and problem lists, and so forth. They are accessible via the internet (sometimes referred to as a patient portal) or a smartphone app, and they are controlled and accessed by patients or their proxies. When a PHR is connected to an EHR, it is sometimes referred to as a "tethered" patient portal. The main advantage of a tethered portal is easier communication between patients and providers, whereas non-tethered PHRs offer patients the ability to aggregate data from multiple unaffiliated providers. Adoption of stand-alone (non-tethered) PHRs has not been widespread, though the recent entry of Apple into the market may change that. EHR-connected portals are increasing in use, especially given the critical role they play in the MU incentive programs.[63]

Functionalities required to meet several of the core objectives of MU and subsequent Promoting Interoperability Programs were either dependent on or benefited from implementation and utilization of a patient portal. Examples include online access to health information, the ability to download health information or transmit it to a third party, secure messaging between patients and their providers, and the provision of tailored educational resources to patients based on their data in the EHR.[64]

Recently, there have been efforts to move beyond using portals to share structured chart data, such as laboratory and test results, to truly opening the medical record and allowing patients to read the narrative notes written by their clinicians. The OpenNotes project (www.myopennotes. org) was initiated in 2010 by a multi-institutional group of research collaborators. Their objective was to promote sharing narrative visit notes with patients as a way to increase transparency and support communication between clinicians and their patients.[65] A survey of patients from the initial pilot sites suggested that providing access to clinical notes could positively impact adherence to medication regimens.[66]

One workflow-optimizing role that the patient portal can play is to facilitate patient data entry (PDE). Through these services, patients can be given questionnaires, consents and authorizations, or even clinical interviews. As vendors begin to integrate these technologies into the full EHR, the power to radically alter physician workflow becomes apparent. If a patient can fill out their complaints, family, social and past medical history, and review of systems online prior to meeting with the physician, several positive consequences will result. Computerized interviews provide more data; allow for asking more sensitive questions; give patients more time; can be adapted for language, hearing impairments, and education level; and when fed into the AEHR, they can lower the amount of time physicians spend documenting.[67] Further, by obtaining structured data before the patient is seen, these systems provide clues the computer needs to present physicians with the most appropriate content and structure for their own workflow.

Some vendors support PDE for more quantitative types of data, such as weight and blood pressure measurements and blood glucose measurements for patients with diabetes. Support is also expanding for device integration to help automate the data entry process for patients. For example, some vendors provide interfaces that will allow data uptake from an array of devices such as glucometers, fitness trackers, scales, and other internet-enabled devices. More and more consumer devices, wearable technologies, and smartphone apps are coming out that collect health-related data. It is reasonable to assume that EHR vendors will continue to expand their capabilities to interface with and digest this patient-generated data. Although these systems are still at the cutting edge of clinical computing today, the very first computer applications for medicine – a half century ago – were patient interviewing tools.[68, 69] The goals of those systems remain compelling today. With the adoption of patient portals rapidly accelerating, these kinds of techniques should become easier. Of course, a challenge that remains is helping physicians understand what exactly to do with all of these new sources of patient-generated data, especially if there are no established, evidence-based guidelines on how they should be interpreted or acted upon.

Virtual care is a growing area for patient engagement. Many systems offer the ability for patients to have encounters provided via video through either their smartphones or computers. Additionally, completely asynchronous encounters for narrowly focused complaints are possible through e-visits. For example, if a woman believes that she a urinary tract infection (UTI), she is able to fill out the information providers need to evaluate and treat a UTI. She fills out the data, and then a provider evaluates it and makes a treatment decision based upon the reported information. As with the new forms of data exchange mentioned earlier, these new types of clinical interactions are likely to increase in popularity as access to high-speed internet and general comfort and experience with tele-presence technologies increases. (See Chapter 2.)

Clinical Reporting and Analytics

As described earlier in this chapter, reporting and analytics are key functionalities of PMSs, but such tools are also becoming a critical functionality in the clinical and clinician-facing parts of ambulatory EHRs. Traditionally, EHR-based reporting functions have been used for operational/financial purposes or to extract clinical data for secondary research use. In the setting of shifting models of care and reimbursement, there is an increased appetite for clinically meaningful and actionable analytics based on the data in EHRs. Both the Accountable Care Organization (ACO) and Patient Centered Medical Home (PCMH) delivery models depend heavily on EHR implementation and analytic capabilities.[70]

At the organizational level, reporting and analytics that are based on clinical data are utilized by a variety of stakeholders, from quality officers and clinic/department heads to care management teams. The transition from paper charts to electronic records with structured data entry enables analytics at the population level to help ensure appropriate preventive screening and chronic disease care. Reporting and business intelligence tools can identify gaps in care in order to focus efforts in areas that will yield the most benefit for an organization's patient population. Beyond finding patients with known care gaps, there is much buzz surrounding "big data" analytic methods and the potential to use data mining techniques to identify at-risk patients and to develop predictive models that reveal opportunities for clinical interventions that have not previously been possible.[71]

At the provider level, clinical analytics will likely play an increasing role as well. One consequence of our work to provide a comprehensive, exchangeable electronic health record that spans time (birth to death) and space (different care settings) is that it becomes challenging for a clinician to thoroughly review even one patient's aggregated data. As difficult as it is to digest all of this individual patient data, an even greater challenge for the clinician arises as we move from a fee-for-service model to incentivizing physicians based on outcomes of the entire patient panel. In that context, clinicians must be concerned with monitoring their panel as a whole and stay vigilant for patients who are outliers in terms of management or outcomes. As value-based reimbursement paradigms have expanded, there has been increasing need for broader and more sophisticated data aggregations. Specifically, patient panel management demands the ability to join clinical data from within a provider's EHR to the administrative claims data held by government and commercial payers.

The concept of a data-driven dashboard is making its way from the business and financial sectors into the healthcare setting as one method to address such information overload challenges. Dashboards generally leverage visualization techniques to summarize complex data in a real-time or near real-time fashion, and they are most effective when linked to workflow tools to enable users to quickly take action. It is common to see dashboards in the acute care setting as a means of quickly summarizing patient data and helping to triage hospital resources (e.g., obstetrics, intensive care units, or EDs).[72,73] In the ambulatory setting, clinical dashboards can help summarize all of the longitudinal data the EHR contains about an individual patient, and they can also give a bird's-eye view of a provider's entire patient panel.[74] When integrated directly into the EHR, dashboards are even more useful, as they are directly actionable within the clinician's primary workflow system.

Infrastructure Considerations

The infrastructure issues for ambulatory systems are similar to inpatient systems but different in emphasis. The scale of ambulatory systems varies from single physician offices to large multistate groups with thousands of providers. Obviously, very different technologies are needed to serve these different constituencies. Regardless of size, the most fundamental questions that need to be answered early are the degree to which one can and wants to support and control the system for customization, integration, and data extraction/reporting.

The answers to these questions will map in part to internal IT capabilities and partly to the functions and design of the software itself. Increasingly, vendors are providing software as a service (SaaS) or hosted offerings as well as traditional, on-premise software. Hosted and traditional solutions are often identical, in that you have your own instance of the software configured and dedicated for you. The difference is that the hosted solution is not in your data center and may or may not be configured by someone else. SaaS (often synonymous with cloud-based) solutions are shared with other clients and usually require less configuration but conversely are less customizable.

If you have a lot of remote rural sites with variable networking infrastructures, then a system that relies on high bandwidth connectivity could prove frustrating. Conversely, if you lack the technical expertise to manage your own system, then a hosted or cloud solution will be attractive. If workstation management presents challenges, then a thin-client or web-based architecture may be appealing. But if your needs are specialized and not supported by the vendor's vision of how you should practice, then a highly configurable system may be your only choice.

Supportability and reliability are key issues that differ in the ambulatory world. Ask yourself about the impact of the loss of a single computer to a busy outpatient center without technical support for 24 or 48 hours. Is that acceptable? Can you afford a shorter time frame? Downtime happens, by accident or design. Does your system provide you with the backup tools to get by for an hour, a day, or a week?

Conversely, diffuse geography may put you at the mercy of an unreliable internet provider or application service provider (ASP). In that case, your workflow may be forced to accommodate the idiosyncratic infrastructure rather than vice versa. Better systems provide static copies of patient records on a local system in case of lost connectivity.

Interoperability with inpatient records varies in importance by practice and specialty. Security and privacy issues similarly may differ according to the interoperability of the workflow both locally (e.g., nurse and doctor charting on the same patient in the same room) and regionally (e.g., sub-specialty referrals across a multi-entity organization).

It is also important to ask if reporting is integrated or separate from the core system. The system that supports day-to-day operations needs to be oriented toward high-speed, single-patient transactions. Reporting systems generally look across patients and do not require sub-second response times. Therefore, these jobs are often separated into different systems. If you need your data for advanced reporting or research above and beyond canned reports provided in the transactional system, then a robust real-time or daily export of your data to a reporting system is required.

A more detailed discussion of infrastructure is beyond the scope of this chapter. One rule of thumb to keep in mind is that while it may seem expensive, infrastructure is rarely a good place to skimp. Hardware is often the cheapest way to hide the inadequacies of software. But this is only true if you focus on the real bottlenecks as opposed to technical fashion or fads. When selecting infrastructure components, it is important to plan for the future but be realistic about the pace of institutional change. Otherwise, one risks wasting money on capacity that will not be used before it becomes obsolete.

Costs and Return on Investment and Meaningful Use

Thanks, in part, to the federal MU incentive payments, most physician practices now have an AEHR.[75] Not surprisingly, PMSs have far greater market penetration than purely clinical systems. As discussed above, PMSs provide a direct impact on revenue and cost control. The value of purely clinical ambulatory systems is often more abstract or delayed. Chismar and colleagues have presented an economic model of EHR adoption that illustrates how larger entities like payers and hospitals gain more quickly from EHRs than small providers.[76] Scrutiny of other models that show benefit from EHRs also reveal the system benefits are greater than those to the individual physician.[77,78] That doesn't mean the value is not present, but given the large startup costs, physicians are poorly incented to adopt systems that benefit others more than themselves – especially if system adoption costs them more than the prime beneficiaries. (See Chapter 11.)

At a high level, the value of the EHR to society is potentially huge.[79] Enhanced quality, better outcomes, an improved patient experience, and lower total costs are all great. But should the individual doctor or practice foot the bill? There are plenty of other barriers to adoption of EHRs, including physician resistance to change, concerns about productivity, the complexity of installation, and conversion of existing paper medical records.[80, 81, 82]

The value equation was altered considerably by federal incentive payments built into the American Recovery and Reinvestment Act of 2009 and the Health Information Technology for Economic and Clinical Health Act (HITECH).[83] HITECH designated billions of federal dollars to incentivize the adoption of health information technology (HIT) via grants for education projects that integrated EHR technology into the clinical education of health professionals, funding for strategic health IT projects, and bonus payments for providers and hospitals to adopt certified HIT.

In order to promote the adoption of the EHR, the federal government designed a CMS bonus payment program (via both Medicare and Medicaid) for both eligible providers and hospitals. The program was initially designed to make incentives available for five years, with early qualification leading to maximum potential monetary bonus. The program's incentives taper and then transition to penalties via withholding of escalating percentages of Medicare/Medicaid reimbursement. In May 2014, CMS proposed revised deadlines.[84]

The EHR incentive program mandated that hospitals and providers use certified EHR technologies in order to qualify for bonuses. EHR certification standards and bodies are described in detail elsewhere in this book, but they continue to evolve via ongoing national committee work and legislation. In addition to installing a certified EHR system, providers and hospitals must demonstrate that they are using the technology in a meaningful fashion. The now ubiquitous term Meaningful Use (MU) refers to these sets of important behaviors. Conceptually, the MU objectives are those behaviors or functions that promote a core set of health outcome priorities delineated by the federal government. Those key priorities include:

■ Improve quality, safety, efficiency, and reduce health disparities
■ Engage patients and families
■ Improve care coordination
■ Improve populations and public health
■ Ensure adequate privacy and security protections for personal health information.

The detailed mechanics of the incentive programs are beyond the scope of this summary. In general terms, the HITECH act mandated that the MU objectives would be defined in stages, with escalating sophistication of objectives and behavioral thresholds. The program evolved through three stages until 2018, at which time the MU program was essentially retired in favor of the Promoting Interoperability components of the CMS Quality Payment Program (QPP).[85]

The Promoting Interoperability Program scoring paradigm is summarized in Table 4.2, excerpted from a CMS fact sheet.[86]

While the federal incentive programs dramatically altered the economics of EHR adoption, it is only temporary. Further, money is only one barrier in a properly considered ROI equation. Doctors also care about quality, time, convenience, regulatory compliance, and a host of other issues that must all be taken into account to truly calculate ROI. This is, of course, not feasible, and the inadequacy of the literature to date reflects that.

For example, some studies show ROI by reducing duplicate orders.[87] Under capitation that is valid, but under fee for service, one's revenue might fall. At our center, we recovered millions of dollars of revenue that was going to outside providers that our EHR very gently pointed back inside. The cost was borne by our doctors and the benefit accrued by our hospital. From a business

Table 4.2 Promoting Interoperability Program Scoring Paradigm

Objectives	Measures	Maximum Points Available
Electronic Prescribing	e-Prescribing	10 points
	Bonus: Query of Prescription Drug Monitoring Program (PDMP)	5 points
	Bonus: Verify Opioid Treatment Agreement	5 points
Health Information Exchange	Support Electronic Referral Loops by Sending Health Information	20 points
	Support Electronic Referral Loops by Receiving and Incorporating Health Information	20 points
Provider to Patient Exchange	Provide Patients Electronic Access to Their Health Information	40 points
Public Health and Clinical Data Exchange	*Choose any two of the following*: Syndromic Surveillance Reporting Immunization Registry Reporting Electronic Case Reporting Public Health Registry Reporting Clinical Data Registry Reporting Electronic Reportable Laboratory Result Reporting	10 points

perspective, this is a big win for the medical center, but it will not show up in academic studies of ROI. From society's perspective, this was just a cost shift and not a real reduction in the total cost of healthcare.

Other studies have shown return from up-coding, and the converse is also touted as a benefit by improving regulatory compliance.[88] Other financial benefits include reduced transcription costs, reduced chart pulls, decreased charge posting costs, pay for performance incentives, and various other efficiencies.

Critics of these studies abound.[89] Costs of implementation are difficult to account for in an accurate manner. Once the EHR is live, there are hidden costs rarely accounted for in any analysis. Dealing with temporary employees is far more complex in an automated environment where training is more involved and less intuitive than in the paper world. Conversely, benefits like integrated access to reference materials or advanced reporting capabilities are extremely difficult to assign value to in a finite period of time. Even the cost of the software itself is hard to standardize and is almost always overemphasized as a cost relative to the much higher intangible costs such as disruption, morale effects, and functional losses from system deficiencies.

For our faculty practice at Weill Cornell, we attempted to address some of these issues by looking at bottom line measures of productivity. We implemented a commercial EHR between 2001 and 2007. We compared monthly visit volume, charges, and work relative value units (wRVUs) before and after each provider's EHR implementation go-live date. We also compared these data to a group of physicians who did not implement, though they had too many confounds to be considered formal controls. Our data matched the anecdotal impression in the industry showing that those practitioners who adopted the EHR had a statistically significant increase in average monthly patient visit volume (nine visits per provider per month), whereas the non-adopter cohort's visit volume was statistically unchanged. Likewise, while both groups had significant increases in average monthly charges, only the adopters showed a statistically significant increase in wRVUs (12 per provider per month).[90]

HIMSS (the publisher of this book) publishes an online tool[91] that highlights scores of individual benefits and provides anecdotes about providers who achieved them. It is primarily inpatient focused, but it is relatively easy to adapt many of the constructs to the ambulatory world. The plural of anecdote is not data.

While these and other data[92] suggest that EHRs do not harm productivity and probably help it, we believe the value of the EHR ultimately needs to be judged like that of an elevator in a skyscraper. It has become an essential tool of the trade.[93, 94] Too few ROI analyses ask what the ROI is of the analysis itself. Like the word processor and the typewriter, email and the fax machine, or cars and the horse, the EHR will come and will transform ambulatory care. Today's executives need to manage the change, not attempt to justify it.

While the ROI of the EHR and its effect on clinical productivity will continue to be scrutinized, there has been increasing attention on the relationship between health information technology and clinician well-being. With physician burnout rates rising, the EHR has been invoked as a primary cause of clinician stress and work dissatisfaction. In fact, there have recently been several high-profile articles in the lay press that highlight physician struggles with their computer systems.[95, 96] Social media has fanned the flames of discontent. A Twitter account dedicated to complaints about one major EHR's usability has attracted over 20,000 followers.[97]

Clinical informaticians are apt to debate whether the EHR is truly the root cause of dissatisfaction or whether the EHR is simply the symptom of a broken healthcare delivery system. Defenders of the EHR will point out that the combination of the rising complexity of healthcare data, ever-increasing regulation, bizarre reimbursement paradigms, and security/privacy barriers all contribute to system usability challenges. End users of the EHRs, though, continue to lament the awkward and inefficient EHR user interface and point to the seemingly faster pace of innovation in other sectors of society.

Whether the cause or the effect, there is mounting evidence that points to the association of HIT with clinician stress and burnout.[98] As such, there is renewed interest in improving EHR usability and identifying best practices for system implementation and optimization. Certainly, technological advances hold promise, especially in the realm of artificial intelligence to support virtual assistance and APIs to create enhanced system user interfaces. However, process improvement, training, and team-based care may ultimately be the most powerful tools to improve clinician well-being. Frequently, simple surveys of clinicians can identify and help address longstanding system misconfigurations and inefficiencies.[99] In forming the ARCH collaborative, KLAS Research convened a group of provider organizations attempting to use survey and benchmarking data to identify drivers of clinician satisfaction with the EHR.[100]

The Future of the Ambulatory EHR

Predicting the future direction of the ambulatory EHR industry is relevant but challenging. Vendors still rapidly come and go, and the technology is evolving quickly. What you buy today will be obsolete soon; expect it, and plan accordingly. Assume your vendor will change by protecting your data and your investment in the knowledge it took to automate your practice. As a rule of thumb, only 20 percent of implementation costs are vendor fees. Not all of the remaining 80 percent is lost if you will need to change vendors. Wise process redesign will deliver value now and in the future, independent of the specific technical platform. The delayed returns from automation will also translate from one system to the next, as they come from the EHR technology itself, not necessarily from any given brand.

Large vendors with full inpatient and outpatient suites offer the hope of increased interoperability. By 2012, only 16 vendors accounted for 75 percent of the market.[101] While pure software companies like Epic and Cerner are currently on top, bigger conglomerates like GE offer both biomedical devices and EHRs in their suites. And yet, interoperability remains elusive. Will these vendors oversimplify and cut the wrong costs? Will their size and oligopoly power destroy innovation? Consider the conflicting incentives facing just one vendor with multiple product lines and seemingly competing interests. Will a vendor that sells MRIs and EHRs support an EHR to help reduce the overutilization of expensive MRIs – a business with far more profit potential than software? Large HIT software vendors are also employers who need to control medical insurance costs. Interoperability with competitors would reduce healthcare expenditures, but it might cause loss of market share. How large HIT vendors balance their own internal conflicts could have as much an impact on the future of the industry as technology itself.

The technology is also hard to predict. The big problems facing clinical informatics for the past 40 years have not fundamentally changed. The nature of the human-machine interface, the physical limits of hardware, and the complexity of medical vocabulary are still problems today. The expansion of the EHR outside academia only adds new problems of scale, configurability, flexibility, complexity, control, and ever-lower fault tolerance.

The next-generation EHR, evolving today, is focused on integration, standards, ubiquity, mobility, reliability, quality, outcomes, and of course, workflow. Dangers to look out for include oversimplification, information overload, alert fatigue, overdependence, and depersonalization. The next generation of ambulatory care is also emerging today full of potential opportunities and dangers. As a key part of that future, the AEHR is surely both an opportunity and a challenge.

About the Authors

Curtis L. Cole, MD, is the Assistant Vice Provost and Chief Information Officer for Weill Cornell Medical College (WCM), where he is also the Frances and John L. Loeb Associate Professor of Libraries and Information Technology and an Associate Professor of Clinical Medicine and Population Health Sciences. After medical school at Cornell and residency at the then New York Hospital, he was a Clinical Investigator in Medical Informatics. He has led the implementation of several EMR systems and WCM's TruData terminology server. As CIO, Dr. Cole is also responsible for the other core information systems that support research, education, and administration at the college. His current work focuses on the secondary use of clinical data for research and education. He is active mentoring students at WCM and CornellTech in the development of new health information technologies.

Adam D. Cheriff, MD, is the Chief Medical Information Officer and Chief of Clinical Operations for the Weill Cornell Physician Organization. In addition to managing the implementation and support of Weill Cornell's shared ambulatory electronic health record and practice management system, Dr. Cheriff is responsible for Weill Cornell's data warehouse, data dictionary, on-line physician directory, and patient portal.

As Chief of Clinical Operations, Dr. Cheriff focuses on process improvement around capacity planning, patient access, and digital engagement. He has maintained an active internal medicine practice while overseeing clinical operations for Weill Cornell Medicine. Dr. Cheriff's interests and expertise include clinical system usability, interoperability standards, provider productivity, and process improvement. His research efforts have centered around measuring the effects of the EHR on provider productivity, medication prescribing accuracy and safety, and reduction of administrative waste in provider-payer interactions.

J. Travis Gossey, MD, MS, MPH, practices Internal Medicine in New York City. He also serves as the Associate Chief Medical Information Office for Weill Cornell Medicine. As part of this role, he advances ambulatory areas of the electronic medical record system; health information exchange and interoperability; telemedicine; and the patient digital experience including the patient portal. He has been active in informatics since 2005.

Sameer Malhotra, MD, MA, is the Senior Director of Clinical Informatics at Regeneron Pharmaceuticals where he leads initiatives on clinical and genomic data integration, and development of analytical platforms for research. Previously, he was the Medical Director of Informatics at Weill Cornell Medicine where for the over 12 years he implemented, optimized, and integrated health IT systems for patient care. He has extensively worked on Clinical Decision Support (CDS) Systems, Radiology IT systems and nurtured the first integration of genomic data into the organizations electronic health record. He continues to maintain a faculty appointment in the Departments of Medicine and Population Health Sciences at Weill Cornell. Dr Malhotra provides patient care as a hospitalist at NewYork–Presbyterian Hospital. He teaches, mentors students and directs courses on Health Informatics in the Masters and Executive MBA programs at WCM.

Daniel M. Stein, MD, PhD, is the Associate Chief Information Officer at Memorial Sloan Kettering Cancer Center. He leads the Tech Incubation team, which aims to transform cancer care through experimentation with new technologies in a variety of breakthrough domains. Dr. Stein has over a decade of research, teaching, and operational experience in Clinical Informatics, primarily working with clinician- and patient-facing systems with a focus on supporting safe, effective and collaborative care. He mentors and teaches graduate students as Adjunct Assistant Professor and "Clinical Innovator in Residence" at Cornell Tech, and as Assistant Professor of Healthcare Policy and Research at Weill Cornell Medicine.

Notes

1. Berwick DM, Hackbarth AD. Eliminating Waste in U.S. Health Care. *JAMA*. 2012;307(14):1513–1516.
2. Cutler D, Wikler E, Basch P. Reducing Administrative Costs and Improving the Health Care System. *New England J Med*. 2012;367(20):1875–1878.
3. Carpenter PC, Chute CG. The Universal Patient Identifier: A Discussion and Proposal. *Proc Ann Sym Comp Appl Med Care*. 1993:49–53.
4. Social Security Numbers. Electronic Privacy Information Center. September 2004. www.epic.org/privacy/ssn. Accessed March 19, 2006.
5. Bittle MJ, Charache P, Wassilchalk DM. Registration-Associated Patient Misidentification in an Academic Medical Center: Causes and Corrections. *Jt Comm J Qual Patient Saf*. 2007;33:25–33.
6. Ritz, D. It's Time for a National Patient Identifier. July 11, 2013. http://www.himss.org/News/News Detail.aspx?ItemNumber=21464. Accessed June 29, 2014.
7. Dooling JA, Durkin S, Fernandes L, et al. Managing the Integrity of Patient Identity in Health Information Exchange (Updated). *J AHIMA*. 2014;85(5):60–65. http://www.ncbi.nlm.nih.gov/pubmed/24938040.

8. Shattuck J. In the Shadow of 1984: National Identification Systems, Computer-Matching, and Privacy in the United States. Hast LJ. 1983. http://heinonlinebackup.com/hol-cgi-bin/get_pdf.cgi?handle= hein.journals/hastlj35&section=46.

9. Physicians at Teaching Hospitals Audits. www.aamc.org/advocacy/library/teachingphys/phys0040. htm. Accessed March 12, 2006.

10. CMS. Transaction & Code Sets Standards. http://www.cms.gov/Regulations-and-Guidance/HIPAA-Administrative-Simplification/TransactionCodeSetsStands/index.html?redirect=/TransactionCode SetsStands/.

11. Abelson and Creswell. U.S. Warning to Hospitals on Medicare Bill Abuses. http://www.nytimes. com/2012/09/25/business/us-warns-hospitals-on-medicare-billing.html?_r=0.

12. Downing NL, Bates DW, Longhurst CA. Physician Burnout in the Electronic Health Record Era: Are We Ignoring the Real Cause? *Ann Intern Med*. 2018;169:50–51. doi:10.7326/M18-0139.

13. Morra D, Nicholson S, Levinson W, Gans DN, Hammons T, Casalino LP. US Physician Practices Versus Canadians: Spending Nearly Four Times as Much Money Interacting with Payers. *Health Affairs*. 2011;30(8):1443–1450.

14. Zall RJ. The Truth About Managed Care: The Silent Provider Discount. *Managed Care Quarterly*. 2004;12(1):11–15.

15. Grossman JH, Barnett GO, Koespell TD. An Automated Medical Record System. *JAMA*. 1973;263: 1114–1120.

16. McDonald CJ, Overhage JM, Tierney WM, et al. The Regenstrief Medical Record System: A Quarter Century Experience. *Int J Med Inf*. 1999;54:225–253.

17. Stead WW, Brame RG, Hammond WE, et al. A Computerized Obstetric Medical Record. *Obstet Gynecol*. 1977;49(4):502–509.

18. Clayton PD, Sideli RV, Sengupta S. Open Architecture and Integrated Information at Columbia-Presbyterian Medical Center. *MD Computing*. 1992;9(5):297–303.

19. Ash JS, Gorman PN, Seshardri V, et al. Computerized Physician Order Entry in US Hospitals: Results of a 2002 Survey. *J Am Med Inform Assoc*. 2004;11:95–99.

20. Cutler DM, Feldman NE, Horwitz JR. US Adoption of Computerized Physician Order Entry Systems. *Health Affairs*. November–December 2005;24(6):1654–1663.

21. Marc Overhage, Susan Perkins, William M Tierney, Clement J McDonald. Controlled Trial of Direct Physician Order Entry: Effects on Physicians' Time Utilization in Ambulatory Primary Care Internal Medicine Practices. *J Am Med Inform Assoc*. 2001;8(4):361–371.

22. https://www.federalregister.gov/documents/2019/05/23/2019-10521/modernizing-part-d-and-medi care-advantage-to-lower-drug-prices-and-reduce-out-of-pocket-expenses. Accessed November 27, 2019.

23. NYS Department of Health. I-STOP/PMP – Internet System for Tracking Over-Prescribing – Prescription Monitoring Program. https://www.health.ny.gov/professionals/narcotic/prescription_ monitoring/. Accessed June 29, 2014.

24. Baehren DF, Marco CA, Droz DE, Sinha S, Callan EM, Akpunonu P. A Statewide Prescription Monitoring Program Affects Emergency Department Prescribing Behaviors. *Ann Emerg Med*. 2010;56(1):19–23.

25. NIH. UMLS: LOINC To CT Mapping. http://www.nlm.nih.gov/research/umls/mapping_projects/ loinc_to_cpt_map.html. Accessed July 17, 2010.

26. The Joint Commission. 2014 National Patient Safety Goals. http://www.jointcommission.org/ PatientSafety/NationalPatientSafetyGoals. Accessed May 14, 2006.

27. Rozich JD. Standardization as a Mechanism to Improve Safety in Health Care. *Joint Commission Journal on Quality and Safety*. 2004;30(1):5–14.

28. CMS. Medicare Coverage Center. http://www.cms.hhs.gov/center/coverage.asp. Accessed March 18, 2006.

29. Bank AJ, Obetz C, Konrardy A, et al. Impact of Scribes on Patient Interaction, Productivity, and Revenue in a Cardiology Clinic: A Prospective Study. *Clinicoecon Outcomes Res*. 2013;5:399–406.

30. Hirschtick RE. A Piece of My Mind. Copy-and-Paste. *JAMA*. 2006;295:2335–2336.

31. https://mcodeinitiative.org/. Accessed November 27, 2019.

32. https://flatiron.com/press/press-release/roche/. Accessed November 27, 2019.

33. https://www.wsj.com/articles/google-s-secret-project-nightingale-gathers-personal-health-data-on-millions-of-americans-11573496790. Accessed November 27, 2019.

34. East TD. The EHR Paradox. *Frontiers of Health Series Management*. 2005;22(2):33–35.

35. Bates DW, Kuperman GJ, Wang S, et al. Ten Commandments for Effective Clinical Decision Support: Making the Practice of Evidence-Based Medicine a Reality. *J Am Med Inform Assoc*. 2003;10(6):523–530.

36. Berlin A, Sorani M, Sim I. A Taxonomic Description of Computer-Based Clinical Decision Support Systems. *J Biomed Inform*. 2006;39(6):656–667.

37. Koppel R, Metlay JP, Cohen A, et al. Role of Computerized Physician Order Entry Systems in Facilitating Medication Errors. *JAMA*. 2005;293(10):1197–1203.

38. Phansalkar S, Van Der Sijs H, Tucker AD, et al. Drug – Drug Interactions That Should Be Non-Interruptive in Order to Reduce Alert Fatigue in Electronic Health Records. *J Am Med Informatics Assoc*. 2012:1–5.

39. Van Der Sijs H, Aarts J, Vulto A, Berg M. Overriding of Drug Safety Alerts in Computerized Physician Order Entry. *J Am Med Informatics Assoc*. 2006;13(2):138–147.

40. Isaac T, Weissman JS, Davis RB, et al. Overrides of Medication Alerts in Ambulatory Care. *Arch Intern Med*. 2009;169(3):1337; author reply 1338. http://www.ncbi.nlm.nih.gov/pubmed/19786683.

41. Blecker S, Pandya R, Stork S, Mann D, Kuperman G, Shelley D, Austrian JS. Interruptive Versus Noninterruptive Clinical Decision Support: Usability Study. *JMIR Hum Factors*. 2019;6(2):e12469. doi: 10.2196/12469. PMID: 30994460; PMCID: PMC6492060.

42. Thaler R, Sunstein CR. *Nudge: Improving Decisions About Health, Wealth, and Happiness*. New York: Penguin Books; 2009.

43. McDonald CJ, Hui SL, Tierney WM. Effects of Computer Reminders for Influenza Vaccination on Morbidity During Influenza Epidemics. *MD Comput*. 9(5):304–312. http://www.ncbi.nlm.nih.gov/pubmed/1522792. Accessed June 27, 2014.

44. Shea S, DuMouchel W, Bahamonde L. A Meta-Analysis of 16 Randomized Controlled Trials to Evaluate Computer-Based Clinical Reminder Systems for Preventive Care in the Ambulatory Setting. *J Am Med Inform Assoc*. 3(6):399–409. http://www.pubmedcentral.nih.gov/articlerender.fcgi?artid=116324&tool=pmcentrez&rendertype=abstract. Accessed June 27, 2014.

45. Rao VM, Levin DC. The Overuse of Diagnostic Imaging and the Choosing Wisely Initiative. *Ann Intern Med*. 2012;157(8):574–576.

46. Johnston ME. Effects of Computer-Based Clinical Decision Support Systems on Clinician Performance and Patient Outcome: A Critical Appraisal of Research. *Ann Intern Med*. 1994;120(2):135.

47. The Protecting Access to Medicare Act (PAMA) of 2014, Section 218(b), amended Section 1834(q) of the Act to establish the AUC program to increase the use of AUC for advanced diagnostic imaging services provided to Medicare patients. https://www.cms.gov/Outreach-and-Education/Medicare-Learning-Network-MLN/MLNProducts/Downloads/AUCDiagnosticImaging-909377.pdf. Accessed December 23, 2019.

48. Hentel KD, Menard A, Mongan J, et al. What Physicians and Health Organizations Should Know About Mandated Imaging Appropriate Use Criteria. *Ann Intern Med*. 2019;170:880–885. https://doi.org/10.7326/M19-0287.

49. Mukamel DB, Mushlin AI. The Impact of Quality Report Cards on Choice of Physicians, Hospitals, and HMOs: A Midcourse Evaluation. http://www.ingentaconnect.com/content/jcaho/jcjqs/2001/00000027/00000001/art00002. Accessed June 29, 2014.

50. Long A-J, Chang P, Li Y-C, Chiu W-T. The Use of a CPOE Log for the Analysis of Physicians' Behavior When Responding to Drug-Duplication Reminders. *Int J Med Inform*. 2008;77(8):499–506.

51. Turning Off Frequently Overridden Drug Alerts: Limited Opportunities for Doing It Safely. 2008; 15(4):439–448. doi:10.1197/jamia.M2311.Introduction.

52. HL7 CDS Hooks. https://cds-hooks.hl7.org/.

53. Abbasi M, Kashiyarndi S. Clinical Decision Support Systems: A Discussion on Different Methodologies Used in Health Care. 2006. http://www.idt.mdh.se/kurser/ct3340/ht10/FinalPapers/15-Abbasi_Kashiyarndi.pdf. Accessed June 29, 2014.

54. HL7 Implementation Guide for CDA® Release 2: IHE Health Story Consolidation, Release 1.1 – US Realm. http://www.hl7.org/implement/standards/product_brief.cfm?product_id=258. Accessed June 8, 2014.

55. http://www.x12.org/about/asc-x12-about.cfm/. Accessed November 28, 2019.

56. Health Level Seven International. www.HL7.org.

57. Walker J, Pan E, Johnston D, et al. The Value of Health Care Information Exchange and Interoperability. *Health Affairs Web Exclusive*, January 19, 2005. http://content.healthaffairs.org/cgi/content/abstract/hlthaff.w5.10. Accessed March 18, 2006.

58. Mead CN. Data Interchange Standards in Healthcare IT – Computable Semantic Interoperability: Now Possible but Still Difficult. Do We Really Need a Better Mousetrap. *J Healthcare Inform Manag.* 2006;20(1):71–78.

59. Health Level Seven International. HL7/ASTM Implementation Guide for CDA® R2 –Continuity of Care Document (CCD®) Release 1. https://www.hl7.org/implement/standards/product_brief.cfm?product_id=6.

60. https://www.healthit.gov/topic/information-blocking. Accessed November 28, 2019.

61. http://hl7.org/fhir/. Accessed November 28, 2019.

62. Coulter, A. Patient Engagement: What Works? *J Ambul Care Manage.* 2012;35:80–89.

63. Turner K, Hong YR, Yadav S, Huo J, Mainous AG. Patient Portal Utilization: Before and After Stage 2 Electronic Health Record Meaningful Use. *J Am Med Inform Assoc.* 2019;26(10):960–967. https://doi.org/10.1093/jamia/ocz030.

64. CMS Meaningful Use EHR Incentive Programs. (n.d.). http://www.cms.gov/Regulations-and-Guidance/Legislation/EHRIncentivePrograms/Meaningful_Use.html. Accessed June 12, 2014.

65. Delbanco T, Walker J, Darer JD, et al. Open Notes: Doctors and Patients Signing On. *Ann Intern Med.* 2010;153(2):121–125.

66. DesRoches C, et al. Patients Managing Medications and Reading Their Visit Notes: A Survey of OpenNotes Participants. *Ann Intern Med.* 2019;171(1):69–71. doi: 10.7326/M18-3197.

67. Bachman JW. The Patient-Computer Interview: A Neglected Tool That Can Aid the Clinician. *Mayo Clin Proc.* 2003; 78(1):67–78.

68. Brodman K, van Woerkom AK, Erdmann AJ, Jr. Goldstein LS. Interpretation of Symptoms with a Data-Processing Machine. *AMA Archives of Internal Medicine.* 1959;103:776–782.

69. Brodman K, Erdmann AJ, Jr., Lorge I, Wolff HG. The Cornell Medical Index; An Adjunct to Medical Interview. *JAMA.* 1949;140:530–534.

70. Bitton A, Flier LA, Jha AK. Health Information Technology in the Era of Care Delivery Reform. *JAMA: The Journal of the American Medical Association.* 2012;307(24):2593–2594.

71. Groves P, Kayyali B, Knott D, Van Kuiken S. The "Big Data" Revolution in Healthcare. *McKinsey Q.* 2013.

72. Stone-Griffith, S., Englebright, J. D., Cheung, D., Korwek, K. M., & Perlin, J. B. Data-driven process and operational improvement in the emergency department: the ED Dashboard and Reporting Application. *J Healthcare Manag/Am College Healthcare Execut.* 2012;57(3):167–80.

73. Egan M. Clinical Dashboards: Impact on Workflow, Care Quality, and Patient Safety. *Crit Care Nurs Q.* 2006;29(4):354–361.

74. Koopman RJ, Kochendorfer KM, Moore JL, et al. A Diabetes Dashboard and Physician Efficiency and Accuracy in Accessing Data Needed for High-Quality Diabetes Care. *Ann Fam Med.* 2011;9(5):398–405.

75. Hsiao C. Office-Based Physicians Are Responding to Incentives and Assistance by Adopting and Using Electronic Health Records. *Health Affairs.* 2013;32(8):1470–1477.

76. Chismar WG, Thomas SM. The Economics of Integrated Electronic Medical Record Systems. *Medinfo.* 2004;11(Pt 1):592–596.

77. Wang SJ, Middleton B, Prosser LA, et al. A Cost-Benefit Analysis of Electronic Medical Records in Primary Care. *Am J Med.* 2003;114:397–403.

78. Miller RH, West C, Brown TM, et al. The Value of Electronic Health Records in Solo or Small Group Practices. *Health Affairs.* 2005;24(5):1127–1137.

79. Hillestad R, et al. Can Electronic Medical Record Systems Transform Health Care? Potential Health Benefits, Savings, and Costs. *Health Affairs*. 2005;24(5):1103–1117.
80. Kaushal R, et al. Imminent Adopters of Electronic Health Records in Ambulatory Care. *Inform Prim Care*. 2009;17:7–15.
81. Gans D, Kralewski J, Hammons T, Dowd B. Medical Groups' Adoption of Electronic Health Records and Information Systems. *Health Affairs*. 2005;24(5):1323–1333.
82. Miller RH, Sim I. Physicians' Use of Electronic Medical Records: Barriers and Solutions. *Health Affairs*. 2004;23(2):116–126.
83. http://www.hhs.gov/ocr/privacy/hipaa/understanding/coveredentities/hitechact.pdf.
84. Press Release: CMS Rule to Help Providers Make Use of Certified EHR Technology. http://www.cms.gov/Newsroom/MediaReleaseDatabase/Press-releases/2014-Press-releases-items/2014-05-20.html. Accessed June 8, 2014.
85. Quality Payment Program. https://qpp.cms.gov/.
86. 2019 Medicare Promoting Interoperability Program Scoring Methodology Fact Sheet. https://www.cms.gov/Regulations-and-Guidance/Legislation/EHRIncentivePrograms/Downloads/ScoringMeth_FactSheet-.pdf.
87. Bates DW, Kuperman GJ, Rittenberg E, et al. A Randomized Trial of a Computer-Based Intervention to Reduce Utilization of Redundant Laboratory Tests. *Am J Med*. 1999;106:144–150.
88. Barlow S, Johnson J, Steck J. The Economic Effect of Implementing and EMR in an Outpatient Clinical Setting. *JHIM*. 2004;18(1):5–8.
89. Walker JM. Electronic Medical Records and Health Care Transformation: EMR Supported Health Care Transformation Is Too Immature for Credible Estimates of Its Costs or Benefits. *Health Affairs*. 2005;24(5):1118–1120.
90. Cheriff AD, et al. Physician Productivity and the Ambulatory EHR in a Large Academic Multi-Specialty Physician Group. *Int J Med Inform*. 2010;79:492–500.
91. HIMSS Realizing the Value of Health IT Value Steps Interactive Tool. http://www.himss.org/ResourceLibrary/ValueSuite.aspx#/steps-app. Accessed June 9, 2014.
92. Buntin MB, et al. The Benefits of Health Information Technology: A Review of the Recent Literature Shows Predominantly Positive Results. *Health Affairs*. 2011;30:464–471.
93. Goodman C. Savings in Electronic Medical Record Systems? Do It for the Quality. *Health Affairs*. 2005;24(5):1124–1126.
94. King J, et al. Clinical Benefits of Electronic Health Record Use: National Findings. *Health Serv Res*. 2014;49;1(II):392–404.
95. Gawande Atul. Why Doctors Hate Their Computers. *New Yorker*. November 12, 2018.
96. Fry E, Schulte F. Death by 1,000 Clicks: Where Electronic Health Records Went Wrong. *Fortune*. March 2019.
97. EPICparodyEMR. https://twitter.com/epicemrparody?lang=en.
98. Gardner RL, Cooper E, Haskell J, Harris DA, Poplau S, Kroth PJ, Linzer M. Physician Stress and Burnout: The Impact of Health Information Technology. *J Am Med Inform Assoc*. 2019;26(2):106–114.
99. Ashton M. Getting Rid of Stupid Stuff. *N Engl J Med*. 2018; 379(19):1789–1791.
100. The ARCH Collaborative. https://klasresearch.com/arch-collaborative.
101. Gold M, et al. Evolving Vendor Market for HITECH-Certified Ambulatory EHR Products. *Am J Manag Care*. http://www.ajmc.com/publications/issue/2013/2013-11-vol19-sp/evolving-vendor-market-for-hitech-certified-ambulatory-ehr-products/1. Accessed June 9, 2014.

Chapter 5

Clinical Decision Support System

Parag Mehta, MD FACP

Contents

> Catch human errors before they occur or block them from causing harm.
>   – The Agency for Healthcare Research and Quality

The Agency for Healthcare Research and Quality promotes a systems approach that aims at the prevention of error. Clinical decision support systems (CDSSs) are at the forefront of this aim.[1] CDS has evolved dramatically over the past 25 years and will likely evolve just as dramatically, or more, so over the next 25 years. Increasingly, the clinical encounter between a clinician and a patient will be supported by a wide variety of cognitive aides to support diagnosis, treatment, care-coordination, surveillance and prevention, and health maintenance or wellness.[2]

What Is Clinical Decision Support (CDS)?

Clinical decision support (CDS) provides clinicians, staff, patients, or other individuals with knowledge and person-specific information, intelligently filtered or presented at appropriate times, to enhance health and health care. CDS encompasses a variety of tools to improve

DOI: 10.4324/9780429423109-5

Table 5.1   CDS Functions

Function	Example
Alert	Highlighting abnormal results
Reminder	Recommend preventive service – e.g., vaccination, mammogram
Critique	Rejecting an electronic order, e.g., duplicate medication
Predict	Calculation of score
Diagnose	Sepsis alert
Assist	Choice of antibiotics based on culture results

decision-making in the clinical workflow (See Table 5.1). CDS includes computerized alerts and reminders to care providers and patients; clinical guidelines; condition-specific order sets; focused patient data reports and summaries; documentation templates; diagnostic support; and contextually relevant reference information. A systematic review of 100 studies found that CDS systems improved practitioner performance in 64% of the studies assessing this outcome, including 4 out of 10 diagnostic systems, 16 of 21 reminder systems, 23 of 37 disease management systems, and 19 of 29 drug dosing or prescribing systems.[3]

Why CDS?

Of all the tasks that clinicians face, medical decision-making is among the most challenging. To make the right diagnosis, a clinician must first actually consider that diagnosis within a list of all possible diagnoses. Second, a clinician must determine which questions, physical exam findings, laboratories, or imaging will best narrow this list as far as possible, while taking into account the costs and risks of the tests as well as the consequences of a missed diagnosis. Third, a clinician must offer the best possible therapy, taking into account national clinical guidelines and local drug formularies. Finally, clinicians must accomplish all of the above tasks without committing gross medical errors, such as drug–drug interactions and life-threatening allergic reactions.[4]

CDS Has Many Vital Benefits

Increased quality of care and enhanced health outcomes
Avoidance of errors and adverse events
Improved efficiency, cost-benefit, and provider and patient satisfaction

CDS requires computable biomedical knowledge, person-specific data, and a reasoning or inferencing mechanism that combines expertise and data to generate and present helpful information to clinicians as care is being delivered. This information must be filtered, organized, and presented in a way that supports the current workflow, allowing the user to make an informed decision quickly and take action. Different types of CDS may be ideal for different processes of care in various settings.

Implementation and Integration

The very first step towards implementing a CDS intervention depends upon what constitutes relevant medical knowledge to be represented. This knowledge may come in the form of national guidelines, the view of domain experts at the hospital, or a hospital policy committee.[4] CDS is not merely an alert. It analyzes an extensive amount of electronic data to provide guidelines in clinical settings and diagnostic and management support. EHRs integrated with clinical decision systems are meant to provide physicians and the health care team with relevant patient information that can improve clinical efficiency, patient safety, and overall health outcomes. The CDS Five Rights concept states that CDS interventions must provide:

1. The right information (evidence-based guidance, response to clinical need)
2. To the right people (entire care team – including the patient)
3. Through the right channels (e.g., EHR, mobile device, patient portal)
4. In the right intervention formats (e.g., order sets, flowsheets, dashboards, patient lists)
5. At the right points in the workflow (for decision-making or action)

Effective CDS must be relevant to those who can act on the information in a way that supports completion of the right action. CDS is intended not to replace clinician judgment, but rather to provide information to assist care team members in managing the complex and expanding volume of biomedical and person-specific data needed to make timely, informed, and higher quality decisions based on current clinical science. CDS tools can be directed toward reduction of errors and adverse events, promotion of best practices for quality and safety, cost profile improvements, rapid response to public health emergencies, and more – such as supporting shared decision-making or tailoring plans of treatment to patient preferences.

Successful CDS Designs

Provide measurable value in addressing a recognized problem area or areas for improvement
Leverage multiple data types to bring the most current and relevant evidence and evidence-based practice recommendations to bear on clinical decisions
Produce actionable insights from the abundant multiple data sources
Deliver information to the user that allows the user to make final practice decisions, rather than being opaque and acting autonomously
Demonstrate good usability principles, including clear displays and rapid action options
Testable in small settings with a clear path to more substantial scalability
Support successful participation in quality and value improvement initiatives
Provide relevant information in real-time, which fits into workflow
Follow–Plan–Do–Study–Act Cycle

The desired outcomes for CDS include (See Table 5.2):

■ Improve efficiency
■ Earlier detection/screening
■ Diagnosis/Treatment protocol

Table 5.2   CDS Is Used to Achieve Many Desired Results

Regulatory	Required signature by an attending	Mandatory pop-up upon opening the chart
Quality	Foley justification	Pop-up to write a justification
Sepsis	When criteria met for sepsis	Notification via a pager system
Financial	Reminder for billing and completion	
Prevention	Health maintenance	Shows what is due, completed
Notification	Rapid response team	Physician get the notification of an occurrence

- Prevent adverse outcome
- Follow-up management
- Cost reductions/convenience

A particular hospital in NY was successful in decreasing sepsis mortality rate by 23% after implementing a computerized surveillance algorithm that alerted providers to new diagnoses of sepsis or worsening vital signs, and also provided reminders about best practices for treating patients with the deadly condition. CDS is also being utilized to implement 'reflex isolation' in patients with EHR showing recent MRSA, VRE, or CRE infections in an attempt to reduce the dissemination of infection.

CDS makes a tremendous contribution to diagnosis and treatment, preventive care, and chronic disease management. In a meta-analysis of randomized controlled trials of physician reminders to improve preventive care, both screening and immunization rates were noted to be higher among physicians exposed to CDS.[4] In a systematic review of clinical alerts to improve safe physician prescribing, 23 studies demonstrated a beneficial effect on prescribing practices, 5 studies demonstrated a positive effect on clinical outcomes, and 4 studies demonstrated no change in prescribing practices.[5]

But, at the same time, the high number of alerts fired becomes overwhelming, which can contribute to physician burnout. EHR contains a vast amount of data, and a physician, along with his health care team, needs that vital piece of relevant information that would contribute to informed decision-making in patient care without creating any cognitive burden. Alert flooding can impede the optimal use of clinical decision support systems and lead to alert fatigue, which can desensitize a physician to clinically relevant information. Alerts prevent adverse events, but it is essential that alerts are funneled down to highlighting only the clinically significant ones. According to an analysis by Kesselheim et al., 'More finely tailored or parsimonious warnings could ease alert fatigue without imparting a high risk of litigation for vendors, purchasers, and users.'[7]

If an alert is chosen as the method of CDS, the alert can be interruptive or non-interruptive.

The modeless alert appears in the background or on the toolbar. It stays on the screen, available for use, but allows other activities and is retrievable when the clinician is ready. An example is an unread lab result indicator on the toolbar. A modal is a pop-up alert, such as a reminder, which requires acknowledgment before continuing.[6]

In coming years, with help of machine learning, artificial intelligence, and standardization of data, we expect that CDS will evolve and fit into the individual provider workflow and improve patient safety. EHR has longitudinal information, and that information can be presented with five rights with help of CDSS. At present it is useful in most cases but also can lead to alert fatigue.

A Use Case

What follows is an example of the number of alerts received over a month at one institution – the number is as high as 1.1 million, of which 20.3%, that is, 140,293 alerts, were overridden. Amongst these 1.1 million alerts, as many as 691,719 alerts were overridable. These alerts include discern, multum, and non-medication alerts.

CDS is an integral part of EHR, and addressing the following may help in tweaking CDS for better utilization of its functions (See Figures 5.1–5.3):

■ The use of tiered alerts, which have been shown to improve acceptance of alerts. Tiered alerts vary in the degree of alert disruptiveness. User options are modified based on the seriousness of the situation prompting the alert. For example, an alert with low risk is

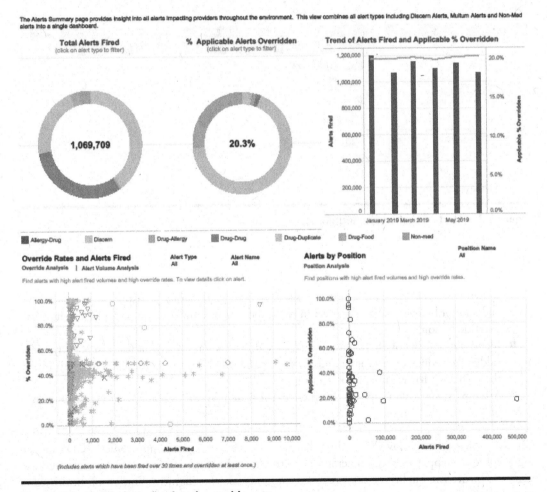

Figure 5.1 Total alerts fired and override rate

The Alerts Fired Page identifies those alerts that are triggering the most within the environment. Using this data may help identify system configuration issues that are causing unneeded alerts.

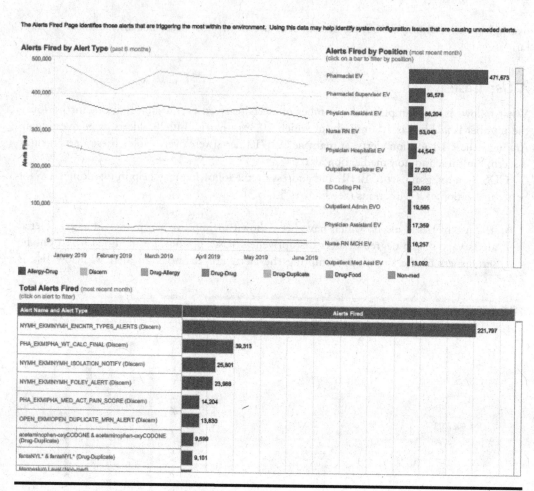

Figure 5.2   Alerts fired by type and position

shown passively, while a life-threatening drug–drug interaction is displayed automatically and cannot be overridden. An alert in the middle may show up automatically but have an override option.[5]

■ Identify categories of alerts that might be good targets for refinement (e.g., frequently over-ridden) to reduce alert fatigue and maximize the number of relevant alerts and minimize those that are irrelevant and distracting.

■ Attempt to make alerts appear elsewhere in the system, in a different way, at a different time, or not at all.

The available evidence shows that while there is significant room for improvement, CDS in the right context – appropriately implemented with the right kind of management – can reduce errors, improve the quality of care, reduce cost, and ease the cognitive burden on health care providers.

The Alerts Overridden page identifies high frequency alerts that are being overridden the most. Using this data may help identify alerts that are not properly impacting provider decision making.

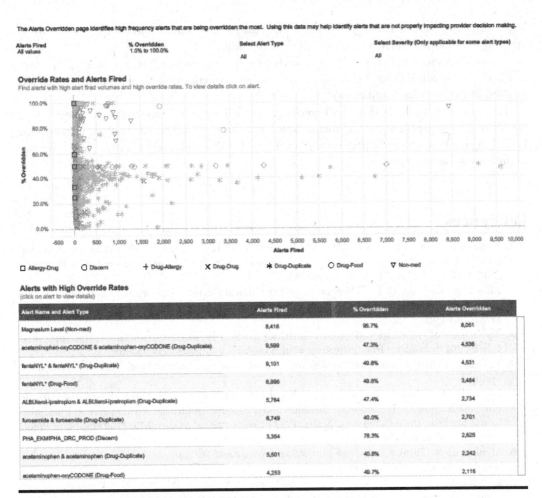

Figure 5.3   Alerts by high override rates

About the Author

Dr. Parag Mehta, MD, FACP, is the Senior Vice Chairman of the Department of Medicine at NewYork–Presbyterian Brooklyn Methodist Hospital. He is also the Chief Medical Information Officer (CMIO) and an associate professor of Clinical Medicine at Weil Medical College.

He is board certified in internal medicine, hospital medicine, and hospice and palliative care medicine. He is also certified in health information technology and artificial intelligence in business. He is board certified in OB-GYN from India.

Dr. Mehta is passionate about teaching and has been awarded the Best Teacher and Best Research Mentor Awards on numerous occasions. He is a strong advocate of resident education, patient safety, and quality improvement. As CMIO, he strives to use technology to improve workflow, reduce the cognitive burden, and improve physician well-being. As a wellness champion from ACP, he believes in bringing back the joy in medicine. He actively participates locally and nationally in advocacy efforts for the patient before paperwork. He led the team to achieve the HIMSS7 level at his organization. He can find simple and creative new solutions to complex problems by applying his clinical acumen and analytical thinking skills.

He is an energetic leader who is active with several organizations like the American College of Physicians, Medical State Society of New York, and American Medical Association. He has received numerous honors and awards.

He has an unquenchable thirst for knowledge, and he is on an endless quest to learn new ideas. With his years of experience as a clinician, administrator, and teacher, he takes the utmost pride in training many young and enthusiastic physicians. He feels privileged to have made a difference in the lives of his many patients.

References

1. Khairat, S., Marc, D., Crosby, W., & Al Sanousi, A. (2018). Reasons for Physicians not Adopting Clinical Decision Support Systems: Critical Analysis. *JMIR Medical Informatics* 6:2, e24. Published 2018 April 18. doi:10.2196/medinform.8912.
2. Middleton, B., Sittig, D. F., & Wright, A. (2016). Clinical Decision Support: A 25 Year Retrospective and a 25 Year Vision. *Yearbook of Medical Informatics, Suppl 1*, S103–116. https://doi.org/10.15265/IYS-2016-s034.
3. The Science of Informatics. Bethesda: American Medical Informatics Association. [Internet, cited July 19, 2019]. Available from https://www.amia.org/about-amia/science-informatics.
4. Finnel, J. (2016). *Clinical Informatics Study Guide*. Springer International Publishing: Imprint: Springer.
5. Olson, D. R., Konty, K. J., Paladini, M., Viboud, C., & Simonsen, L. (2013). Reassessing Google Flu Trends Data for Detection of Seasonal and Pandemic Influenza: A Comparative Epidemiological Study at Three Geographic Scales. *PLOS Computational Biology* 9:10, e1003256. https://doi.org/10.1371/journal.pcbi.1003256.
6. Mankowitz, S. (2018). *Clinical Informatics Board Review and Self Assessment*. Cham: Springer International Publishing: Imprint: Springer.
7. Kesselheim, S., Cresswell, K., Phansalkar, S., Bates, D. W., & Sheikh, A. (2011). Clinical Decision Support Systems Could Be Modified to Reduce 'Alert Fatigue' While Still Minimizing the Risk of Litigation. *Health Affairs* 30:12, 2310–2317.

Chapter 6

Medication Errors

Jitendra Barmecha, MD, Z. Last and A. Zaman

Contents

About Medication Errors

A medication error can be considered either an error of commission (incorrect recording) or an error of omission (missing transaction),[1] anywhere along the prescribing pathway, which begins with a provider placing an order for a medication through to the administration of that medication to the patient, which may or may not cause ultimate patient harm. Alternatively, an adverse drug event (ADE) is clearly defined as an event characterized as harm experienced by a patient resulting from exposure to a medication; this is different from an adverse drug reaction (ADR), where harm is caused by a drug at normal doses during normal use (Figure 6.1). The most common types of medical errors can be attributed to medications. Medication errors and subsequent ADEs can not only harm patients driving up direct healthcare costs but can and often do drive up indirect or associated costs such as productivity and or lost wages.[2,3]

---

[1] https://psnet.ahrq.gov/primer/medication-errors-and-adverse-drug-events.
[2] Journal of Managed Care Pharmacy: JMCP January/February 2003 Vol. 9, No. 1 www.amcp.org.
[3] https://www.amcp.org/about/managed-care-pharmacy-101/concepts-managed-care-pharmacy/medication-errors.

DOI: 10.4324/9780429423109-6

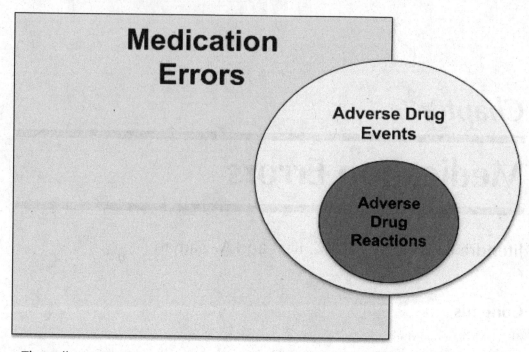

The yellow area represents injuries caused by drug use (adverse drug events). The red area represents harm caused by a drug (adverse drug reactions). The light red area represents harm from appropriate drug use that is generally excluded from studies of adverse drug events. Medication errors are much more common than adverse drug events, but result in harm less than 1% of the time.[1] Conversely, about one quarter of adverse drug events are due to medication errors.[6]

Figure 6.1   Relationship of key terms[4]

The National Coordinating Council for Medication Error Reporting and Prevention (NCC MERP)[5] defines a medication error as follows:

> A medication error is any preventable event that may cause or lead to inappropriate medication use or patient harm while the medication is in the control of the health care professional, patient, or consumer. Such events may be related to professional practice, healthcare products, procedures, and systems, including prescribing, order communication, product labeling, packaging, and nomenclature, compounding, dispensing, distribution, administration, education, monitoring, and use.

---

[4] J. R. Nebeker, P. Barach and M. H. Samore. "Clarifying adverse drug events: A clinician's guide to terminology, documentation, and reporting." *Annals of Internal Medicine*. 2004; 140:795–801.

[5] https://www.nccmerp.org/about-medication-errors.

Category	Category	Description of category
No error	A	Circumstances or events that have the capacity to cause error
Error, no harm	B	An error occurred, but the medication did not reach the patient
Error, no harm	C	An error occurred that reached the patient but did not cause patient harm
Error, no harm	D	An error occurred that resulted in the need for increased patient monitoring but no patient harm
Error, harm	E	An error occurred that resulted in the need for treatment or intervention and caused temporary patient harm
Error, harm	F	An error occurred that resulted in initial or prolonged hospitalization and caused temporary patient harm
Error, harm	G	An error occurred that resulted in permanent patient harm
Error, harm	H	An error occurred that resulted in a near-death event (e.g., anaphylaxis, cardiac arrest)
Error, death	I	An error occurred that resulted in patient death

© 2001 National Coordinating Council for Medication Error Reporting and Prevention. All Rights Reserved.

* Permission is hereby granted to reproduce information contained herein provided that such reproduction shall not modify the text and shall include the copyright notice appearing on the pages from which it was copied.

Figure 6.2   Medication Error Index

Additionally, NCC MERP has adopted a **Medication Error Index**[6] (Figure 6.2) for classifying errors according to the severity of the outcome, utilizing the following definitions:

■ **Harm:** Impairment of the physical, emotional, or psychological function or structure of the body and/or pain resulting therefrom.
■ **Monitoring:** To observe or record relevant physiological or psychological signs.
■ **Intervention:** May include change in therapy or active medical/surgical treatment.
■ **Intervention necessary to sustain life:** Includes cardiovascular and respiratory support (e.g., CPR, defibrillation, intubation, etc.).

As indicated, medication errors can occur anywhere along the prescribing pathway (Figure 6.3) as defined here, with the most common error attributed to the first phase of ordering/prescribing:[7,8]

Typical errors occurring during the prescribing phase can be attributed to the healthcare provider entering the wrong medication or medication formulation, the wrong route of

---

[6] Ibid.
[7] https://psnet.ahrq.gov/primer/medication-errors-and-adverse-drug-events.
[8] Medication Errors: Rayhan A. Tariq; Yevgeniya Scherbak, https://www.ncbi.nlm.nih.gov/books/NBK519065/.

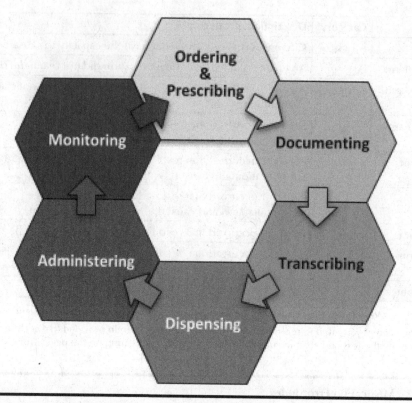

Figure 6.3   Prescribing pathway

administration, the wrong dose, or even the wrong frequency. These types of ordering errors have been shown to account for close to 50% of all medication errors.[9] As pointed out by the NCC MERP, we can now better understand medication errors are an extensive but preventable problem once we break down the root causes to affect meaningful change. As depicted in Figure 6.3, the prescribing pathway follows a circular pattern, whereby the final link in the process, monitoring, leads right back to possible adjustments or re-orders in the ordering and prescribing phase. This feedback loop is a critical design element in mitigating potential adverse drug events and adverse drug reactions.

Impact of Medication Errors

Medication errors are amongst the most common form of medical errors, with harm coming to at least 1.5 million people every year. The extra medical costs of treating drug-related injuries occurring in hospitals alone are at least $3.5 billion a year, and this estimate does not consider lost wages and productivity or additional healthcare costs.[10] Medication error morbidity and mortal-

---

[9] Ibid.
[10] Institute of Medicine. "Committee on identifying and preventing medication errors, preventing medication errors." *National Academies Press.* 2007:124–25; Matthew C. Grissinger et al. "The role of managed care

ity costs are estimated to run $77 billion dollars per year.[11] Preventing medication errors can and will mitigate intrinsic and extrinsic costs. While preventable, medication errors can have a broad range of severity, with the worst-case outcome resulting in serious patient harm and even death. As indicated previously, a medication error resulting in injury or harm would be categorized as an adverse drug event (ADE).

Although most medication errors do not result in patient injury, those that do are more likely to occur at the prescribing (56%) and administering (34%) stages in the hospital setting and are more commonly intercepted at the former stage (48%) than at the latter (0%).[12] With regard to administration errors, there is usually no one between the nurse (or other person administering the drug) and the patient to perceive or foresee the error.

There are many factors that can add to the reason that providers make medication errors. These may include lack of training, insufficient experience and drug knowledge, the unfamiliarity of the patient, and lack of risk perception. External factors leading to medication errors in physicians and nurses may include interruptions, busy workloads, time restraints, high patient census, or a lack of adequate resources. Understanding what causes medication errors will better assist healthcare providers to achieve error reduction.

Reducing Medication Errors – Strategy, Product Design, and Systems

Once the potential causes of medication errors have been identified, strategies can be deployed to minimize and or eliminate the prevalence across the full spectrum of the prescribing pathway. There are many tools and resources being developed to prevent or reduce medication errors. Utilizing available technology geared towards medication safety is crucial to successful mitigation of errors. Examples of such tools include the use of clinical decision support (CDS), automated dispensing machines (ADM), barcode medication administration (BCMA), smart infusion pumps, robotic process automation (RPA), and artificial intelligence (AI).

Starting with prescribing medication errors, computerized physician order entry (CPOE) systems that inherently eliminate potential handwriting errors should leverage medication reconciliation at transitions of care with embedded clinical decision support (CDS) and thus bring awareness of potential interactions and adverse side effects. Clinical decision support (CDS) systems have become a major part of the early detection and warning system of most EMRs. Effective clinical decision support systems are an important step in enhancing the quality of healthcare as well as improving the safety and efficiency of CPOE systems[15] running on top of an Electronic Medical Record (EMR); CDS systems have been the single most effective error prevention strategy to date by providing physicians with dosing suggestions, assisting them with calculations and monitoring,

pharmacy in reducing medication errors." *Journal of Managed Care Pharmacy*. 2003; 9(1): 62–65; Academy of Managed Care Pharmacy. "AMCP's framework for quality drug therapy." http://www.fmcpnet.org/index.cfm?p=132D8447 (accessed February 17, 2010).

[11] Matthew C. Grissinger, et al. "The role of managed care pharmacy in reducing medication errors." *Journal of Managed Care Pharmacy*. 2003; 9(1):62–65.

[12] D. W. Bates and P. Sarah. "Slight. medication errors: What is their impact?" *Mayo Clinic Proceedings*. 2014; 89(8):1027–1029.

and checking for harmful drug–allergy, drug–drug, and drug–disease interactions.[13,14,15] CDS systems help providers process and utilize large amounts of data from multiple sources right at the time of order entry to guide diagnosis and care processes with the presentation of targeted, action-able alerts, and/or evidence-based guidelines. Appropriately implemented, CDS systems can not only improve patient safety, quality of care, and patient outcomes but also reduce workload and cost.[16] However, well-designed CDS systems should not look to replace a provider's analytic skills and critical thinking when assessing a patient, taking care to avoid the potential for alert fatigue, which can become prevalent. A well-implemented CDS system will produce fewer bypassing alerts based upon a provider's normal workflow or scope of practice, looking only to provide those alerts relevant to a medical error or misdiagnosis. CDS systems can be used in many ways, including the reduction of medication errors, monitoring of labs for signs of deterioration, and assisting in the appropriate use of imaging studies. Additionally, CDS systems can and are used to accurately and quickly calculate appropriate evidence-based risk scores and present actionable data in real time. However, it is important to remember that effective CDS systems should be reviewed, tested, and updated regularly to ensure error-free utilization and no increase in alert fatigue.

CPOE with real-time alerts can catch more errors than when orders were written on paper. In conjunction with varying severity of alerts, EMRs can be layered with other safety measures to decrease order entry errors. Such safe practices should first look at distractions providers face during the ordering process. Distractions can and should be minimized by deploying strategically placed, quiet zone, order entry stations. Additional measures to minimize dispensing errors can also focus on policy development and enforcement to eliminate the use of abbreviations; leverage pharmacist oversight embedded into the prescribing pathway; utilize tall man lettering[17] to mini-mize look-alike, sound-alike (LASA) medications; and introduce carefully designed order sets and mandatory hard stops. The implementation and interface of CPOE systems with smart infusion pumps, automated dispensing cabinets, robotics, and surveillance systems along with additional scrutiny to those medications identified as high-risk will help to ensure error reduction along the prescribing pathway. At the time of medication administration, the utilization of scanned bar-codes in the process of bar-coded, knowledge-based medication administration (KBMA) should be the standard to help ensure the five rights of medication administration[18] (the right patient, the right drug, the right dose, the right route, and the right time) to additionally reduce medication errors. Today, nearly all packaging by manufacturers contains a barcode that can be scanned and added to a drug database. The UPC barcodes on medication packaging typically contain a variant of the National Drug Code (NDC) number, which identifies the unique drug, dosage form, and strength of the product. These unique codes help to identify and differentiate drug strength and doses, thus decreasing the chance of errors (See Figure 6.4).

Similarly, in the ambulatory care setting, electronic prescribing is one of the most important safety strategies to reduce medication errors. From a practical standpoint, this also has the added

[13] D. W. Bates and A. A. Gawande. "Patient safety: Improving safety with information technology." *The New England Journal of Medicine.* 2003; 348: 2526–2534.

[14] D. W. Bates, L. L. Leape, D. J. Cullen et al. "Effect of computerized physician order entry and a team interven-tion on prevention of serious medication errors." *JAMA.* 1998; 280: 1311–1316.

[15] S. P. Slight, D. L. Seger, K. C. Nanji et al. "Are we heeding the warning signs? Examining providers' overrides of computerized drug-drug interaction alerts in primary care." *PLoS One.* 2013; 8: e85071.

[16] https://www.fortherecordmag.com/archives/0517p10.shtml.

[17] https://www.ismp.org/sites/default/files/attachments/2017-11/tallmanletters.pdf.

[18] http://www.ihi.org/resources/Pages/ImprovementStories/FiveRightsofMedicationAdministration.aspx.

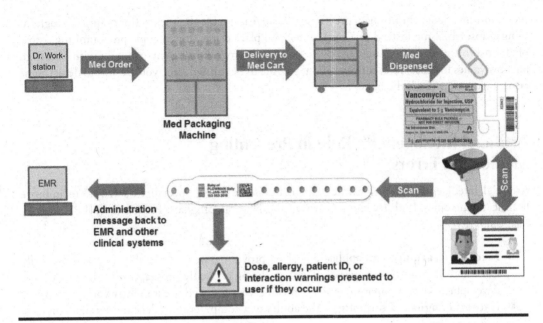

Figure 6.4 Bidirectional interface process flow[19]

Illustration depicts an example of an integrated hospital workflow consisting of computerized physician order entry, ADM vending, barcode medication administration, and corresponding CDS warnings upon scanning.

* Permission is hereby granted to reproduce Bidirectional Interface Process Flow Diagram by Dave Newman at HealthcareITSkills.com.

benefit of increased workflow efficiency, fewer calls to providers to clarify prescriptions due to legibility issues, and possibly increased patient satisfaction from having the prescription ready before heading to the pharmacy for pick up.

Automated medication dispensing systems are now commonly used as a less time-consuming process of dispensing medications. Automated pharmacy dispensing systems are more efficient at performing pharmacists' tasks that require tedious, repetitive motions, high concentration, and reliable record keeping, which can all lead to medication dispensing errors.[20] When used properly, automated dispensing machines (AD's) or automated dispensing cabinets (ADCs) help to reduce medication errors and improve patient safety. Many automated dispensing systems also utilize the bar-coding technology mentioned earlier to safeguard the right drug, dose, and dosage form is used.

Utilization of smart infusion pumps is the safest way to mitigate medication errors involved with administration of IV medications. Smart infusion pumps act as a final check before IV medication administration, and when drips are standardized, it can help to prevent errors resulting from incorrect dose, solution concentration, rate of administration, and human error during pump

[19] Dave Newman. "What Is a Bidirectional Interface?" *Healthcare IT Skills*, 27 January 2019, healthcareitskills.com/bidirectional-interface/.

[20] "Medication Errors." *AMCP.org*, www.amcp.org/about/managed-care-pharmacy-101/concepts-managed-care-pharmacy/medication-errors.

programming. Smart pumps help prevent errors such as double-digit entry (for example, programming a dose of 77 mg instead of 7 mg) or decimal place errors (for example programming a dose of 205 mL/hr instead of 2.5 mL/hr). By appropriately programming smart pumps with max high and low values for dose, rate, concentration, volume to be infused, etc., you are able to detect these errors before they reach the patient.

Artificial Intelligence's Role in Preventing Medication Errors

Artificial intelligence (AI) in healthcare constitutes the use of specialized software to improve healthcare outcomes. Both Machine Learning and Natural Language Processing (NLP) are gaining popularity.[21]

- **Machine Learning** is an application of AI providing systems the ability to automatically learn and improve from experience without being explicitly programmed, focusing on the development of computer programs that can access data and use it to learn for themselves.[22]
- **Natural Language Processing** is the ability of a computer to understand human language as it is spoken.[23]

The use of artificial intelligence can be broken down into several areas.[24] **Improve medication safety** by utilizing screening systems that can generate alerts that may otherwise be missed utilizing conventional CDS systems. Additionally, patterns can be identified in transactions that can be leveraged to produce alerts when outliers to those patterns arise.[25] By utilizing the powerful computing capabilities available, millions of clinical records can be studied to understand and identify "normal" prescribing patterns under very specific situations. Patterns can be identified by location (inpatient, outpatient, unit), provider type, patient type, or any combination to better understand and define what would constitute an outlier. Additionally, AI can **predict health risks and outcomes across large populations** with algorithms that can be used to quickly calculate and predict risk scores, presenting potential interventions for those populations of high-risk patients. Or, AI can **reduce the time and expense** necessary to improve the accuracy of medication dosing with potentially tremendous savings over the management of medication errors.

Robotic Process Automation (RPA)

Through utilization of robotic process automation (RPA), a healthcare facility or clinic may be able to automate many complex tasks that are normally performed by medical professionals or

---

[21] http://www.healthtechzone.com/topics/healthcare/articles/2019/11/14/443751-six-ways-artificial-intelligence-transforming-medication-management.htm.

[22] https://expertsystem.com/machine-learning-definition/.

[23] https://searchbusinessanalytics.techtarget.com/definition/natural-language-processing-NLP.

[24] http://www.healthtechzone.com/topics/healthcare/articles/2019/11/14/443751-six-ways-artificial-intelligence-transforming-medication-management.htm.

[25] https://www.medgadget.com/2018/10/medaware-uses-ai-to-detect-potential-medication-errors-interview-with-dr-gidi-stein-ceo.html.

administrators. RPA can help improve workflow efficiency, quality, and consistency while allowing better allocation of manpower to other important tasks. Robotic medication storage and dispensing units can help automate tasks in both inpatient and outpatient settings. Many high prescription volume outpatient pharmacies utilize robots to store and dispense frequently used medications. These robots effectively free up pharmacy technicians to perform other tasks as the robot will count out the pills, fill, and label prescription bottles. Similarly, robots utilized in the inpatient pharmacy setting can automate the medication dispensing and supply process as well as assist in ordering when there is a low quantity of medications. This can help ensure that medications are readily available, in stock, and picked correctly by pharmacy staff.

Automating the IV compounding workflow using a robot to compound the medication will greatly help free up the pharmacist's time to focus on more valuable and meaningful professional activity while ensuring appropriate compounding procedures were followed. The IV robot can be used to compound IV batches or individual patient specific doses. There are delivery robots in use that will perform tedious tasks such as delivering food, medications, or linens to various areas in the hospital, which frees up staff to perform other, more important tasks. These robots can navigate around the hospital by using lasers to detect their surroundings and avoid obstacles much in the way that self-driving cars operate.

By 2025, global medical robot expenditures will increase by approximately 20% to $24.6 billion.[26] While the upfront expense of purchasing and setting up robotic processes can be high, there is value, time, and cost savings added when projecting out long term. A robot does not suffer from fatigue or exhaustion as humans do, so they can work longer and with more consistency. These robots are programmed with safeguards in place to help ensure safety, security, and accuracy.

Innovations in Medicine

As technology continues to advance at unprecedented rates, it offers new options for expanding care and safety in medicine. There are many examples of technology being used to increase medication compliance, increase treatment efficacy, and decrease medication errors. Take, for instance, medication pill trays – normally you would think of a plastic container labeled morning and evening for Sunday through Saturday. In the market currently, you will find a wide range of "smart" pill organizers, or "smart packs," which are electronic pill trays that can perform a wide range of tasks. Many of these pill trays can be paired with an app on your smartphone; depending on which type of smart pack you have, they can sound alarms during administration time, send notifications to you via text or email if a dose was missed, record whenever a medication was taken out, and give a reminder to the patient when the next dose is due or refill is required. Use of devices such as these can increase medication adherence rates and decrease omission.

Smart inhalers can be of use to reduce medication errors in asthma and COPD treatment. These smart inhalers use built-in Bluetooth to pair to an app on your phone, which can do various things such as keeping track of your inhaler compliance, notify you if you are using your inhaler incorrectly, or even letting you know if you are traveling in a high pollen area (so you can decide if

[26] Zion Market Research. "Medical Robots Market by Product Type (Robotic Systems and Accessories and Instruments), by Application (Orthopedic, Neurology, Laparoscopic, Cardiology, and Others), and by End-User (Clinics, Ambulatory Surgical Centers, and Hospitals): Global Industry Perspective, Comprehensive Analysis, and Forecast, 2018–2025." *Global Medical Robot Market Size 2018: By Type, Applications, Industry Share, Trends, Growth, Analysis and Forecast, 2025*, www.zionmarketresearch.com/report/medical-robot-market.

you want to steer clear or not). Using this can help improve patient compliance and reduce errors from improper inhaler use.

Another such example of this is the advent of precision medicine. According to the Precision Medicine Initiative, precision medicine is "an emerging approach for disease treatment and prevention that takes into account individual variability in genes, environment, and lifestyle for each person."[27] Precision medicine will allow practitioners and researchers to predict with greater accuracy which treatment options and prevention strategies for a particular disease will work better in which groups of people. This is different from the traditional "one-size-fits-all" method, where disease treatment and prevention was developed with the average person as the target population, which really didn't consider the differences between individuals. Tailoring medication options may limit the number of treatment options to those that are most efficacious with a decreased likelihood of an adverse drug reaction or prescribing error.

Delving further into personalized medicine, you will find other advancements in medicine such as 3D-printed drugs. Known as additive manufacturing, 3D printing starts with a computer-aided design of a digital model of the product. The design is then sliced into thousands of horizontal layers that will form the digital file for feeding into a 3D printer. It will then use different materials to print the product layer by layer, transforming two-dimensional layers into a 3D product.[28] The application of this is wide-ranging from being able to create personalized pills that come in different shapes, sizes, textures, solubility, and rate of delivery than what is commercially available. You can even "print" polypills, which contain multiple drugs, into one pill to make adherence easier. This can be useful for patients who are young, elderly, unable to swallow, or unable to follow complex treatment plans. When this becomes readily available, there are many ways that it will be able to help reduce errors.

Reporting Medication Errors

An important and not to be overlooked component of any effective program to reduce medication errors must include the adoption of an effective reporting system. Identification of medication errors is the first and most important step towards making meaningful changes to workflows and systems to prevent similar errors from reoccurring. Even those errors as indicted by NCC MERP as category A (no error) and B (did not reach the patient) must be reported, reviewed, and acted upon. The organization should have a policy to encourage the reporting of any adverse event without the risk of repercussions. Additional reporting options outside of the organization include:

- ISMP Medication Errors Reporting Program (MERP) (link is external)[29] 1-800-233-7767
- U.S. Food and Drug Administration's MedWatch Reporting Program (link is external)[30] 1–800-FDA-1088

---

[27] "What is precision medicine? – Genetics home reference – NIH." *U.S. National Library of Medicine*, National Institutes of Health, ghr.nlm.nih.gov/primer/precisionmedicine/definition.

[28] Stephen Huang and James Huang. "3D printing drugs: More precise, more personalised." *PharmaTimes*, PharmaTimes Media Limited, 19 January 2018, www.pharmatimes.com/magazine/2018/janfeb/3d_printing_drugs_more_precise,_more_personalised.

[29] https://www.ismp.org/report-medication-error.

[30] https://www.fda.gov/safety/medwatch-fda-safety-information-and-adverse-event-reporting-program.

About the Authors

Jitendra Barmecha, MD, MPH, SFHM, FACP, is Chief Information Officer and Senior Vice President of Information Technology and Clinical Engineering for St. Barnabas Health System (SBH). He leads IT and analytics strategy for population health management for SBH, which is a leading DSRIP Performing Provider System in the Bronx. His team is responsible for managing and upgrading the technical infrastructure, ensuring clinical IT systems, and patient monitoring devices are well integrated in the EHR.

As a senior executive team member of SBH's COVID-19 pandemic command center, Dr. Barmecha has been instrumental in providing technology, telecommunication, biomedical engineering, clinical, and public health knowledge and resources to the emergency response effort. As telehealth became a necessity during the pandemic, he contributed to the publication of telehealth manuals for both the American Medical Association and the American College of Physicians.

Dr. Barmecha holds numerous board and committee leadership positions, including serving as chair of the Digital and Telehealth Advisory Board of the American College of Physicians and an executive member of the New York eHealth Collaborative's Physician Advisory Group. He is a fellow of the American College of Physicians and a governor of the New York State chapter, as well as a senior fellow of the Society of Hospital Medicine.

In addition to IT leadership, Dr. Barmecha continues his passion for bedside patient care as a hospitalist. He enjoys teaching clinical staff and medical students, and he routinely lectures on healthcare management, technology, digital medicine, innovation, and health policy.

Chapter 7

Racing against the Clock, Winning Back Time Spent in EHR

Parag Mehta, MD FACP

Contents

The introduction of a new structured and standardized EHR has led to a higher documentation burden and less time for dedicated patient care.[1] Because of changes in how insurance companies and the government pay for medical care, physicians now need to meticulously document their care on the computer, causing many physicians to spend more time with their desktops than with their patients.[14] In fact, physicians are spending around 35% of their time recording patient data in Electronic Health Records (EHR).[1] EHRs that were meant to improve quality, safety, and efficiency in clinical settings are instead making physicians feel disconnected from their patients. Therefore, it is no surprise that EHR is one of the top reasons for physician burnout.

Despite these drawbacks, EHRs are here to stay and can serve as powerful tools to revolutionize the art of medicine – it is up to the providers to make a bad system better or a good one great. EHRs have tremendous potential to improve efficiency and increase positive patient outcomes and population health. Potential improvements in population health result from EHRs' ability to organize and analyze a large amount of patient information, monitor patterns of infectious diseases, manage patients with chronic diseases, and identify populations with higher risk factors. For example, the presence of EHR made it possible to detect the increase of unsafe lead levels in children in Flint, Michigan, after the city changed its water supply.

To achieve the maximum potential of EHR, it is essential to look into its current state of use and improve its design to better fit physician workflow and remove redundancies while also reevaluating its current emphasis on regulatory and administrative requirements.

DOI: 10.4324/9780429423109-7

Where is the time spent in EHR? It is divided into the following categories.

Actual active time was calculated by the system based on mouse mile (movement of mouse), keyboard strokes, and clicks.

- Reviewing
- Documenting
- Ordering
- Billing and coding
- Managing inbox
- Managing alerts

There is significant variation among users pertaining to the time spent in EHR. It varies depending on the position, resident years in training, and the attending physician, specialty, training on EHR use, and the institution.

Data on time spent by national health system leaders shows that the average time spent in EHR per patient is 13:15 minutes (See Table 7.1). This data is over one year, consisting of more than a million encounters.

Comparison of data from one institution showed an average time of 14:44 minutes for an outpatient setting, which is similar to multiple organizations. This data is over one year, consisting of more than a million encounters. See Figure 7.1. Inpatient time spent in EHR. See Figure 7.2.

Table 7.1   Time Spent on EHR in Different Settings

Settings	Leaders
Ambulatory	0:06:39
Inpatient	0:13:04
ED	0:15:04
Average of all	0:13:15

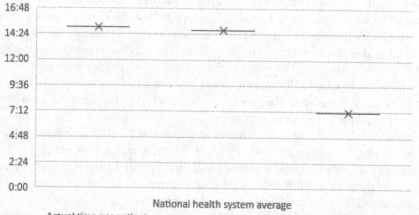

Figure 7.1   Outpatient time spent in EHR

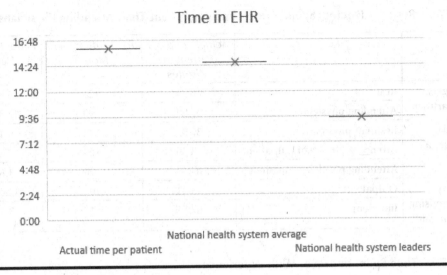

Figure 7.2   Inpatient time spent in EHR

Table 7.2   Time Spent on Each Component Based on Specialty

Inpatient	Medicine	Surgery	OB/GYN
Review	0:03:28	0:04:33	0:02:52
Order	0:01:17	0:03:41	0:00:53
Documentation	0:03:51	0:04:15	0:03:25

Looking further into the data for one teaching institution, the average time spent among all users with more than a million encounters per year is 13:28 minutes. Most time across different specialties is spent in the review and documentation of the chart (See Table 7.2). Time spent in EHR by residents is more comparable to the attending physicians. The least amount of time is spent by the supervising physician (See Table 7.3).

There is a wide variation in time spent per patient based on the position (resident vs. attending physician), as seen from the use case, which happens to be a teaching hospital. Most users, however, have a duration of 9:35 minutes per patient. Time spent by residents improves with training in EHR (See Table 7.4). Time spent is 40 minutes per patient in July compared to May, which is 29 minutes.[3]

An EPRE was defined as the total amount of time spent per patient record on a single day. Time spent was rounded to the nearest hour or minute. Total time spent was total hours spent on the electronic health record in a month per physician. The EPRE per physician was the average number of EPREs per physician per month. Time per EPRE was the average minutes spent per EPRE. It should be noted that data from May represent the previous class of interns for comparison purposes. July is compared to May, which is 4 minutes.

Reasons for the time spent in EHR

■ Poor workflow
■ Interface design and cluttered screen

Table 7.3   Resident Doctors Spend More Time per Patient Than Attending Physicians

	Per User	Actual Time per Patient in Minutes	Total Patients per Month	Patients per Day
Emergency Department	Resident	46:31	107	5.09
	Attending physician	30:24	90	12.8
Internal medicine	Resident physician	30:32	142	6.17
	Attending physician outpatient	13:30	105	7
	Attending physician inpatient	07:39	20	1.6
Surgery (supervising physician)	Outpatient	3:31	101	12.06
	Inpatient	02:51	17	3.4

Table 7.4   Time Spent Improves With Experience

	Interns (N = 41)			
	May	July	October	January
Total EPRE	8815	8099	9072	8806
Time spent per month, h	104	132	121	110
EPRE per intern	215	198	227	220
Time per EPRE, min	29	40	32	30

- Inadequate training
- The administrative and regulatory requirement
- Inbox management
- Overwhelming alerts

What Can Be Done to Address This Issue?

1. **Customize the EHR interface to workflow and specialty to reduce the appearance of the cluttered screen human–computer interaction.** The out-of-the-box desktop view from the EHR vendor may not have the information organized in a way that helps a physician find what he or she needs, and there are often tabs or other information they do not need. Customize the view for each physician in a way that suits them best. It is necessary to assess and analyze the current workflow in order to re-engineer it for better outcomes. The elements displayed can be customized to meet workflow preferences, e.g., writing an order for Coumadin will show indication, previous dose, order for PT/INR, and any other medication that has drug interactions, all seen on one page. There are a few rules worth understanding to improve workflow:

   a. **Hick-Hyman Law.** This expresses user response time as a function of a number of possible responses (n) – predicts user response to hierarchical menus, response to finding correct an option among an unfamiliar list (like a non-QWERTY keyboard). Law predicts: Response Time $RT = a + b*log2(n)$.

b. **Keystroke-Level Model (KLM).** Time to task completion is the sum of the time spent key-stroking, pointing, homing, drawing, mental operator (thinking), system response operator (waiting). It can help to anticipate which functions are most amenable to short-cuts and "hotkeys."

2. **Single sign-on and improvement in the password process.** Physicians should not spend any time typing passwords into workstations in practice. Instead, provide a proximity password device or other technology solution that does not require the physician to enter a password on a keyboard each time they enter a new room.

3. **Preparation of chart before visit and information exchange among different EHRs.** It takes significant time to obtain information from outside records. Labs, imaging, medications, past history, family history, social history, immunization records, health care proxy, and advance directives remain unchanged and should be easily imported in a meaningful way and reconciled.

4. **Teamwork and delegation.** There are certain aspects of EHR that lead to increased time spent on EHR, including pajama time (family physicians spend 86 minutes doing administrative work after hours or at home),[5] rather than in patient interaction significantly contributing to work–life imbalance and ultimately physician burnout. Several parts of the EHR can be filled by the patient before the visit: health maintenance, chief complaints, and ROS can be capture by appropriately trained staff before the visit and before the physician enters the exam room. Several activities and education can also be completed by physician extenders, including but not limited to patient education and follow-up appointment. Sharing clerical tasks can result in each team member working at the top of his or her skill set.[6]

5. **Training optimal, individualized, and retraining to stay current with software upgrades to take advantage of new features.** Interns spend at least five hours a day on the EHR caring for a maximum of ten patients.[3] Increased familiarity reduced time spent on clinical documentation, but a significant portion of an intern's day was still consumed by clinical computer work, which took time away from education, patient care, and, more importantly, motivation to provide high-quality care.[3] There is a high correlation between using personalization settings and physician satisfaction. EHR systems often have features that allow rapid access to data or customization options that physicians do not even know about, so investing time in training can pay off in long-term time savings and frustration reduction. When training is complete, physicians can create filters and preference lists and know how to find the data they need to deliver quality care.

6. **Time management and reduction in waste.** Most EHRs have charts that can show precisely where physician time is being spent on the software. Compare these results and efficiency among multiple physicians in practice. Share best practices to improve everyone's efficiency.

7. **Inbox management.** The study of physicians in a multispecialty practice found that in-basket messages generated by the EHR itself accounted for nearly half the 243 weekly in-basket messages received per physician, on average – 114 of them, far more than the 53 notes received from colleagues and 30 from patients.[7] More than one in three physicians reported experiencing burnout symptoms, and 29% said they plan to cut back clinical work time in the upcoming year. "Receiving more than the average number of system-generated in-basket messages was associated with a 40% higher probability of burnout and 38% higher probability of intending to reduce clinical work time," according to the report.[7] The challenge lies in how the messages are generated – nearly half of those in the study came from EHR algorithms. Family physicians and internists received more than 2.5 times as many

system-generated messages as surgeons did and five times as many as nonsurgical procedur-alists.[7] Physicians often waste too much time reviewing or approving items that could have been handled by someone else with a lower licensure level. Create a system where a member of the staff reviews all "in-basket" items before sending them to a physician. Items that do not require physician input can be rerouted to the appropriate person. Only appropriate messages to be sent to the right person. Define the importance and appropriate header to identify the reason for the message.

8. **Find the time-saving documentation method that works best for each physician.** Mul-tiple studies show similar findings. In one study of family physicians in a teaching hospital, the average visit length was 35.8 minutes, including 2.9 minutes working in the EHR before the physician entering the room, two minutes working in the EHR while in the room, and 6.9 minutes on EHR work outside of typical clinic hours. The average visit included 7.5 min-utes of non-face-to-face time, much of which was spent with the EHR. The average patient visit comprised 16.5 minutes of face-to-face time with the patient. First-year residents, or interns, spend nearly 90% of their work time away from patients, half of which is spent interacting with electronic health records and documentation. Most of that time, 10.3 hours, was spent on interacting with EHRs.[8] Use voice recognition, dictation, scribes (the scribe can also order labs and x-rays as requested by the physician; a physician can focus on the patient and does not need to navigate the EHR or worry about inputting data at all), templates, remote scribes, or some combination of these. The critical point is that every physician works differently, and it is essential to find the way with which each physician is most comfortable and make it available. This will improve facetime with the patient and lessen screen time.

9. **Create a centralized prescription refill plan.** Where possible and allowed by law, staff RNs or other licensed clinicians may handle mundane prescription refills.

10. **Install a printer in each exam room.** If physicians are spending time walking back and forth, printing out information from the EHR, consider installing a printer in each exam room. The cost of a printer is far less than the doctor's time.

11. **Encourage use of the patient portal.** In the future, patients are expected to be able to view EHRs through a patient portal from their own devices, enabling the population to stay bet-ter informed about their health. By logging into a patient portal, patients would be able to see the results of a recent lab test, for example, or find out when they last had a tetanus shot, awarding the patient with the agency to make informed decisions about their care.[9] Encour-aging patients to access their portal also adds to efficiency, in particular where a caregiver is responsible for multiple patients.[9]

12. **Minimizing downtime** and maintaining an adequate speed of hardware and network, the size of the screen, and the dual monitor does make a difference.

13. **Reducing a click burden.** According to an *American Journal of Emergency Medicine* study, an ER doctor makes around 4,000 computer clicks throughout a single shift. Based on a 2017 review in the *Annals of Family Medicine*, on average, doctors spend 5.9 hours out of an 11.4-hour workday on EHRs, compared with 5.1 hours spent with patients.[10] "One less click at a time" by Guo et al. (Figure 7.3) describes several initiatives – creating smart templates, auto text, text macros, use of the handheld device – making it easier to combine multiple clicks into one action item. Physician-driven changes to EHR systems – including a mobile documentation application; abnormal test results auto-populated into an EHR patient sum-mary; physician alerts to reduce inappropriate test ordering; and a network of safety alerts on a dashboard – led to decreased click burden and allowed physicians to spend less time on the computer and more time with patients.

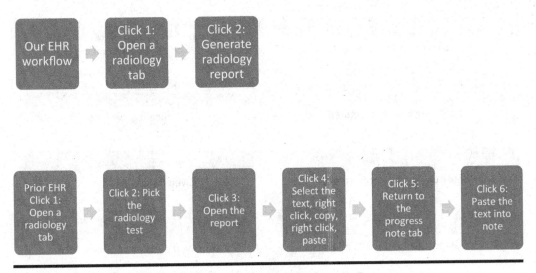

Figure 7.3   Reducing click burden by combining multiple tasks into one

14. **Reevaluate alerts.** The use of tiered alerts is feasible to counteract an overwhelming number of alerts. Tiered alerts have been shown to improve the acceptance of alerts. Tiered alerts vary in the degree of alert disruptiveness. User options are modified based on the seriousness of the situation prompting the alert. For example, an alert with low risk is shown passively, while a life-threatening drug–drug interaction is displayed automatically and cannot be overcome. An alert in the middle may show up automatically but have an overridden option.[11] Identifying categories of alerts might be good targets for refinement (e.g., frequently overridden) to reduce alert fatigue and maximize the number of relevant alerts and minimize those that are irrelevant and distracting.

Despite all the obstacles encountered with the use of EHR, doctors, hospitals, and labs can share a mutual patient's health information – digitally, in real time – so that they can work more effectively as a team. This digital platform makes it convenient for a provider to stay in the loop on illnesses, treatments, and surgeries, thus mitigating errors and improving the quality of care.[9] Medical advancement is mainly dependent on research.[9] Digital records – as opposed to handwritten – inherently lead to increased legibility and comprehensiveness, which makes it easier for researchers to access information, identify subjects, track the quality of care, and conduct essential research.[9] EHR use is at the core of the Quality Payment Program, with both MIPS (Merit-based Incentive Payment System) and APMs (Alternative Payment Models) requiring the use of certified EHR technology to qualify for positive Medicare payment adjustments. These measures reflect the potential to improve patient-centered care and the quality of care delivered to patients. More specifically, they foster both the inclusion of persons and family members as active members of the health care team and the creation of partnerships with health care providers. These measures can also include patient-reported experiences and outcomes that reflect greater involvement of patients and families in decision making, self-care, activation, and understanding of their health condition and its effective management."

Users and developers are joining technology, such as machine learning and AI, with organizations and ONC, creating hope of finding a balance between technology and medicine, art and science. The steps to convert data to wisdom which assists in decision-making is seen in Figure 7.4.

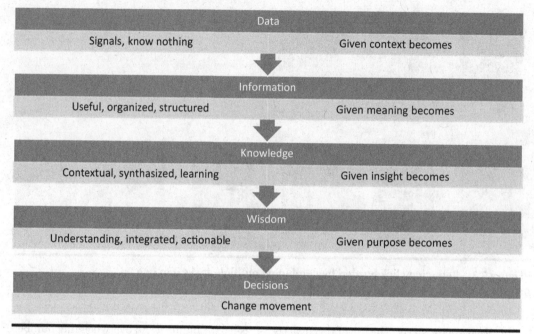

Figure 7.4 Data to decision

About the Author

Dr. Parag Mehta, MD FACP, is the Senior Vice Chairman of the Department of Medicine at NewYork–Presbyterian Brooklyn Methodist Hospital. He is also the Chief Medical Information Officer (CMIO) and an associate professor of Clinical Medicine at Weil Medical College.

He is board certified in internal medicine, hospital medicine, and hospice and palliative care medicine. He is also certified in health information technology and artificial intelligence in business. He is board certified in OB-GYN from India.

Dr. Mehta is passionate about teaching and has been awarded the Best Teacher and Best Research Mentor Awards on numerous occasions. He is a strong advocate of resident education, patient safety, and quality improvement. As CMIO, he strives to use technology to improve workflow, reduce the cognitive burden, and improve physician well-being. As a wellness champion from ACP, he believes in bringing back the joy in medicine. He actively participates locally and nationally in advocacy efforts for the patient before paperwork. He led the team to achieve the HIMSS7 level at his organization. He can find simple and creative new solutions to complex problems by applying his clinical acumen and analytical thinking skills.

He is an energetic leader who is active with several organizations like the American College of Physicians, Medical State Society of New York, and American Medical Association. He has received numerous honors and awards.

He has an unquenchable thirst for knowledge, and he is on an endless quest to learn new ideas. With his years of experience as a clinician, administrator, and teacher, he takes the utmost pride in training many young and enthusiastic physicians. He feels privileged to have made a difference in the lives of his many patients.

References

1. Joukes, E., Abu-Hanna, A., Cornet, R., & de Keizer, N. F. (2018). Time spent on dedicated patient care and documentation tasks before and after the introduction of a structured and standardized electronic health record. *Applied Clinical Informatics*, 9(1), 46–53. doi:10.1055/s-0037-1615747.
2. Your Doctor May Spend More Time with a Computer Than with You. (n.d.). Retrieved from https://www.forbes.com/sites/peterubel/2017/11/24/your-doctor-may-spend-more-time with a computer than with you.
3. Chen, L., Guo, U., Illipparambil, L. C., Netherton, M. D., Sheshadri, B., Karu, E., Mehta, P. H. (2016). Racing against the clock: Internal medicine residents' time spent on electronic health records. *Journal of Graduate Medical Education*, 8(1), 39–44. doi:10.4300/JGME-D-15-00240.1.
4. Young, R. A., Burge, S. K., Kumar, K. A., Wilson, J. M., & Ortiz, D. F. (2018). A time-motion study of primary care physicians' work in the electronic health record era. *Family Medicine*, 50(2), 91–99. https://doi.org/10.22454/FamMed.2018.184803.
5. Berg, S. (2017, September 11). Family doctors spend 86 minutes of "pajama time" with EHRs nightly. Retrieved from https://www.ama-assn.org/practice-management/digital/family-doctors-spend-86-minutes-pajama-time-ehrs-nightly.
6. Solutions to Reduce EHR Burdens and Decrease Physician Burnout. (n.d.). Retrieved from https://www.norcal-group.com/wellness/solutions-to-reduce-ehr-burdens-and-decrease physician burnout.
7. Milliard, M. (2019, July 3). EHR messaging improvements could be key to reducing physician burnout. Retrieved from https://www.healthcareitnews.com/news/ehr-messaging-improvements-could-be-key-reducing-physician-burnout.
8. Chaiyachati, K. H., Shea, J. A., Asch, D. A., et al. (2019, April 15). Assessment of inpatient time allocation among first-year internal medicine residents using time-motion observations. *JAMA Internal Medicine*, 179(6), 760–767. doi:10.1001/jamainternmed.2019.0095.
9. Electronic Health Records: A Blessing or Burden? (2017). Retrieved from https://jordansc.com/electronic-health-records-blessing-burden/.
10. Sentinel Event Newsletter – Maine.gov. (n.d.). Retrieved from https://www.maine.gov/dhhs/mecdc/public-health-systems/rhpc/documents/SENewsletter0619.pdf.
11. Mankowitz, S. (2018). *Clinical Informatics Board Review and Self Assessment*. Cham: Springer International Publishing: Imprint: Springer.
12. Arndt, B. G., Beasley, J. W., Watkinson, M. D., Temte, J. L., Tuan, W. J., Sinsky, C. A., & Gilchrist, V. J. (2017). Tethered to the EHR: Primary care physician workload assessment using EHR event log data and time-motion observations. *Annals of Family Medicine*, 15(5), 419–426. doi:10.1370/afm.2121.
13. Kroth, P. J., Morioka-Douglas, N., Veres, S., Pollock, K., Babbott, S., Poplau, S., Corrigan, K., & Linzer, M. (2018, July). The electronic elephant in the room: Physicians and the electronic health record. *JAMIA Open*, 1(1), 49–56. https://doi-org.eres.qnl.qa/10.1093/jamiaopen/ooy016.
14. Read-Brown, S., Hribar, M. R., Reznick, L. G., et al. (2017). Time requirements for electronic health record use in an academic ophthalmology center. *JAMA Ophthalmology*, 135(11), 1250–1257. doi:10.1001/jamaophthalmol.2017.4187.
15. Guo, U., Chen, L., & Mehta, P. H. (2017). Electronic health record innovations: Helping physicians – One less click at a time. *Health Information Management Journal*, 46(3), 140–144. https://doi.org/10.1177/1833358316689481.
16. Shryock, T. (2018, March 9). 8 ways to reduce physician frustration with the EHR. Retrieved from https://www.medicaleconomics.com/health-law-and-policy/8-ways-reduce-physician-frustration-ehr.
17. Goldstein, I. H., Hribar, M. R., Reznick, L. G., & Chiang, M. F. (2018). Analysis of total time requirements of electronic health record use by ophthalmologists using secondary EHR data. *AMIA . . . Annual Symposium Proceedings. AMIA Symposium*, 2018, 490–497.
18. Mearian, L. (2019, May 22). Poorly designed systems make doctors a slave to their HER. Retrieved from https://www.computerworld.com/article/3397039/poorly-designed-systems-make-doctors-a-slave-to-their-ehr.html.

19. Born, E. (2019, January 24). The EHR and physician burnout. Retrieved from https://alidadegroup.com/ehr-physician-burnout/.

20. Gold, M., & McLaughlin, C. (2016). Assessing HITECH implementation and lessons: 5 years later. *The Milbank Quarterly, 94*(3), 654–687.2. Lakbala, P., & Vindaloo, K. (2014). Physicians' perception and attitude toward the electronic medical record. *Springerplus*, 3:63-1801-3-63. collection 2014. doi:10.1186/2193-1801-3-63.

21. Collier, R. (2017). Electronic health records contributing to physician burnout. *CMAJ: Canadian Medical Association Journal = Journal de l'Association Medical Canadienne, 189*(45), E1405–E1406. doi:10.1503/cmaj.109-5522.

22. Kelly, Y. (2016, September 6). Half of physician time spent on EHRs and paperwork. Retrieved from https://www.jwatch.org/fw111995/2016/09/06/half-physician-time-spent-ehrs-and-paperwork.

23. Rajagopoal, R. (2018). What can physicians do to stop spending too much time on their EHR? Retrieved from https://www.medicaltranscriptionservicecompany.com/blog/physicians-do-to-stop-spending-too-much-time-on-ehr/.

Chapter 8

Hospital Systems
History and Rationale for Hospital Health IT

Virginia Lorenzi, MS, CPHIMS

Contents

DOI: 10.4324/9780429423109-8

A History of Health IT

The typical modern-day hospital relies heavily on technology to support its clinical and administrative functions. This was not always the case. The advancement of computer technology, the sophistication of regulations surrounding payment, and the Electronic Health Records (EHR) Incentive program have all played a part in these changes. In the last decade, hospitals have exchanged paper processes for computer-reliant processes, especially with regard to the medical record.

Technology has changed significantly over the years – these changes have enabled and transformed health IT solutions used in clinical and administrative workflow. In the 1960s, hospitals with computers had a mainframe computer and a monolithic system referred to as the hospital information system (HIS).[1]

Over time, some of these systems expanded to include functionality to support ancillary departments, and some even supported clinical functions such as order entry (orders were typically entered by clerks). In the 1970s, the availability of minicomputers made it possible for departments of large hospitals to have their own niche systems.[2] For example, the laboratory would have its own laboratory information system (LIS), and the radiology department would have its own radiology information system (RIS). Many departments liked the flexibility of selecting systems uniquely specialized in their domain. This concept of having multiple systems to support different functional areas is often referred to as a "best of breed" architecture. The advent of the minicomputer also provided an opportunity for computerization in smaller hospitals. Smaller hospitals could have an HIS on a minicomputer. Microprocessors became available in 1975, and IBM introduced the IBM Personal Computer (PC) in 1981. Personal computers presented many more opportunities because of their affordability for niche systems and distributed architectures. Around the same time, local area networks (LANs), and the Internet were beginning to gain traction. Connectivity between systems was possible, providing further support for a more distributed "best of breed" approach to health IT versus the single HIS approach of the 1960s.[2] Opportunities to improve display of clinical and operational data were further advanced with the development of more advanced display technology and the concept of a graphical user interface. The first health IT systems were developed in the 1960s and 1970s, and surrounding that development, the field of health informatics emerged. A few examples of early systems:

- A laboratory information system and later a Medical Information System (MIS) named COSTAR at the Massachusetts General Hospital (MGH)
- Health Evaluation through Logical Processing (HELP) system at LDS Hospital and the University of Utah
- PRoblem Oriented Medical Information System (PROMIS) at the University of Vermont, which implemented Larry Weed's Problem Oriented Medical Record concept
- Veterans Health Information System and Technology Architecture (VISTA), an electronic health record for the Veteran's Administration

In 1979, both Cerner Corporation and Epic Systems Corporation were founded – these two companies currently dominate the EHR market.[3]

Yet, as of the early 1990s, health IT was still not prevalent and was primarily limited to large sites and academic medical centers. Electronic order entry was primarily done by clerks, and the patient record – or at least many parts of it – remained on paper at many hospitals. In 1991, the Institute of Medicine published a report, "The Computer-Based Patient Record: An Essential Technology for Health Care," which identified this issue:

In spite of more than 30 years of exploratory work and millions of dollars in research and implementation of computer systems in health care provider institutions, patient records today are still predominantly paper records. This evident lack of diffusion of information management technologies in the health care sector has limited the tools available for effective decision making from the bedside all the way to the formulation of national health care policy.

The report also set a vision for the future: "We envision the day when the physician's computer workstation is an integral part of the normal practice environment" so physicians can "obtain patient information when they need it, where they need it."[4]

Financial pressure and payment reform have traditionally been the central driving force for health IT in hospitals. Prior to the 1970s, hospitals charged the costs they incurred in care delivery to insurance companies. In the late 1960s, after the creation of Medicare and Medicaid, U.S. healthcare spending increased at an exponential rate.[5] To address this problem, CMS adopted the Diagnostic Related Group model for hospital reimbursement:

> Inexorably rising medical inflation and deep economic deterioration forced policy-makers in the late 1970s to pursue radical reform of Medicare to keep the program from insolvency. Congress and the Reagan administration eventually turned to the one alternative reimbursement system that analysts and academics had studied more than any other and had even tested with apparent success in New Jersey: prospective payment with diagnosis-related groups (DRGs). Rather than simply reimbursing hospitals whatever costs they charged to treat Medicare patients, the new model paid hospitals a predetermined, set rate based on the patient's diagnosis.[6]

The idea of limiting payment to only what seemed fair for a diagnosis meant that hospitals had to develop tighter controls on operations to ensure they were able to provide efficient care. More efficient protocols were developed over time with the advent of managed care and the beginnings of a shift towards pay-for-performance over pay-for-service. Computer systems to manage financial, clinical, and operational aspects of the hospital were helpful in meeting these new requirements.

In the 1990s, some hospitals were not able to remain viable as payment structures changed, and it was a common occurrence to read news about hospitals going out of business or merging. As hospitals merged or affiliated with other delivery organizations across the continuum, the architecture of health IT within these organizations also changed. Health IT services commonly became centralized and standardized so that the same health IT was deployed at multiple sites in the network.

In addition, there has been a longstanding problem with hospital staffing, especially nurse shortages. Computers were seen as a solution to help reduce the problems with staffing by providing automated support of workflows of key hospital workers.[7]

Probably the most important catalyst to the modern day EHR was the "To Err is Human" report published in 1999 by the Institute of Medicine. This report noted that:

> Health care in the United States is not as safe as it should be – and can be. At least 44,000 people, and perhaps as many as 98,000 people, die in hospitals each year as a result of medical errors that could have been prevented.[8]

In addition, that:

> Among the problems that commonly occur during the course of providing health care are adverse drug events and improper transfusions, surgical injuries and wrong-site surgery, suicides, restraint-related injuries or death, falls, burns, pressure ulcers, and mistaken patient identities. High error rates with serious consequences are most likely to occur in intensive care units, operating rooms, and emergency departments.[8]

The report goes on to explain that these errors are not usually the cause of any one person but instead are a systemic problem that included many missed communication opportunities. A hospital, a place of healing, was now considered downright dangerous. A handbook was even published entitled *You, the Patient*, which described how to take charge of your health and included a chapter on surviving a hospital stay. It opens with the quote:

> Only $2,900 a Night and Free Sponge Baths – What a Deal!
> Just Make Sure You Check Out.[9]

A follow-up Institute of Medicine report, *Crossing the Quality Chasm*, emphasized that "IT has enormous potential to improve the quality of health care" and recommended the development of a "National Health Information Infrastructure."[10] Health IT was seen as an essential tool in the improvement of the quality of care. As hospitals became more automated, health IT was used for automated clinical decision support aimed at improving quality, and for the measurement and reporting of quality information so that benchmarking and comparisons could be made and compliance could be assessed. Payment reform used quality indicators in determining payment. For example, if a patient has a "HAC" (hospital acquired condition) during their stay, the hospital is not allowed to bill CMS.

A landmark event in U.S. health IT history was the 2004 creation of the Office of the National Coordinator of Health Information Technology (ONC). This creation marked the beginning of a concerted effort by the federal government to encourage hospitals to adopt EHR technology. Since the functionality of EHRs widely varied, the standards development organization called Health Level Seven (HL7) was tasked with creating a standard functional model of an EHR system. The EHR system functional model could be used to establish criteria for the certification of EHR functionality. The ONC commissioned a private, not-for-profit organization called the Certification Commission for Healthcare Information Technology (CCHIT) to create a voluntary EHR certification program. However, not many EHRs became certified due to the complicated requirements for EHRs set by CCHIT, the lack of perceived value for the vendor, its voluntary nature, and its lack of incentives. In addition, even if an EHR were certified, a hospital was free to choose which features of the EHR to implement in clinician workflow. As a result, many of the benefits of the EHR were not realized when implemented at provider sites.

The rising cost of healthcare in the U.S. continued to be a major concern, and more reform was needed. While the direction of reform was not clear, the concept of value-based care was generally agreed on as well as the possibility that health IT could be useful in improving efficiencies in the system and reducing cost. A bill aimed at expanding health IT across the country, called the HITECH bill, was circulated in Congress, but it required funding.

Built on this initial work, the American Recovery and Reinvestment Act of 2009, a funding bill designed to stimulate the economy, included HITECH as a section. HITECH introduced the concept of an EHR Incentive program in which hospital providers who had Medicare or

Medicaid would need to adopt certified health information technology and then meaningfully use it. It also provided for incentives, support, and education for health IT adoption and the promise of eventual penalties. Subsequent regulations that implemented the law included rules for EHR vendors and rules for providers. These rules established a staged approach to ensure adoption of EHR technology across the United States. With the EHR Incentive program, a dramatic update in EHRs began to occur. Now hospitals were incentivized to buy and use the functionality of certified EHRs, and vendors were encouraged to build and certify applications that provided more robust functionality. The impact of the program was transformative for the industry. Hospital EHR adoption climbed from 9% in 2009 to over 95% in 2017.[11]

This was followed by additional laws aimed at increasing the functionality and use of health IT, especially with respect to patient engagement and interoperability – the MACRA law and the 21st Century Cures law. There was a strong emphasis on the importance of connecting all of the technology together in an interoperable ecosystem so that information would flow where it was needed to support patient care, to engage patients in their care, and to manage the health of the public.

Summary of Health Information Technology in the Hospital

Health IT in the hospital consists of systems in these broad categories:

1. Technology related to patient care provision (EHR)
2. Systems supporting the administration of the hospital
3. Departmental systems supporting care provision
4. Integration technology
5. Analytics systems
6. Information services support and infrastructure

Care Provision Systems – EHR Technology

The EHR in the Inpatient Setting

Inpatient and outpatient settings have similarities, but a key difference is that the inpatient EHR is encounter specific, concerned about a single multi-day encounter for the patient and not as much about his or her record over the continuum of care. This differs from ambulatory primary care, the focus of which is care across the continuum. A hospital stay is a major event requiring an acute level of care. *Acute care* is defined as "the health system components, or care delivery platforms, used to treat sudden, often unexpected, urgent or emergent episodes of injury and illness that can lead to death or disability without rapid intervention."[12] That care requires a specialized 24/7 environment; a wide range of clinical and support staff; and a lot of clinical interventions, testing, and technology in a short time period. The amount of data collected related to patients during their stay will be substantial – medication administration records, x-rays, lab tests, cardiology interventions, therapy and specialty consults, nursing interventions, vital signs, and more. EHR systems are designed to support the workflows of numerous clinicians – doctors, nurses, assistants, and allied health workers. As noted earlier, the functionality of an EHR ranges from a comprehensive system that includes administrative and ancillary functions to one that is focused on the main clinical processes on a nursing unit.

Physicians use the EHR to review results and data collected by other care workers, to write their notes, and to write their orders. Orders entered into the EHR initiate workflows that involve ancillary departments and other care team members. For example, a medication order would trigger a message to the pharmacist, who would review the order and determine how to fill and dispense the medication. The medication order would also trigger a message to nursing for medication administration. The nurses chart medications in the Medication Administration Record (MAR).

The EHR Incentive program encouraged adoption of basic EHR functionality with Stage 1 and then additional functionality in each subsequent phase. For example, an important function in Stage 1 was to ensure that hospitals could meet a low threshold showing that a percentage of medication orders were entered into the EHR electronically – the computerized provider order entry (CPOE). In Stage 2, this threshold was increased, and laboratory and radiology orders were included. Stage 2 also introduced the concept of electronically assisted medical administration (EMAR). Both CPOE and EMAR are seen as beneficial to patient safety, because the computer assists in safe medication ordering, including checking for drug–drug interactions and allergies, as well as safe medication administration – ensuring that the right patient is getting the right medication.[13] CPOE, when integrated with ancillary systems, can also improve efficiency, because the ancillary staff receives and responds to an order electronically instead of paper communication and double entry. The EHR functionality required for the EHR Incentive program is obtained from Certified EHR Technology (CEHRT); however, that technology does not have to be provided using a single comprehensive EHR. Instead, multiple CEHRTs could be used that each provide some of the needed functions, which allows the provider to mix and match to reach 100% functionality. One example would be for a provider to use a different patient portal than the portal its main EHR vendor provides. The requirements for certification of EHRs are well documented at www.healthit.gov and in other parts of this text. However, it is important to note that the functionality required for the EHR Incentive Program does not represent all functionality that has been recommended for EHRs; it is a prioritized subset. Also, the regulations allowed a hospital to obtain the required functionality as a set of certified components. Therefore, while one possibility was to obtain all of the required functionality from a single vendor, it was also possible to obtain functionality from multiple vendors. An example would be to use a separate vendor for the patient portal functionality.

In most large hospitals, there are numerous systems that together make up the health IT functionality of the organization. These are connected to ensure the flow of information to support workflow of the hospital via a special kind of middleware referred to as an interface engine. For example, a hospital might have patient administration or one or more ancillary systems or supporting systems that are separate from the EHR and interfaced. Some smaller hospitals still utilize a model similar to the HIS model of the 1960s, but one that uses modern technology and functionality. When organizations consolidate, there may be a multitude of competing health IT systems and the need for interfaces between systems of double data entry. Networks of hospitals and healthcare services can benefit by streamlining and standardizing health IT. If an enterprise utilizes the same health IT vendors or a unified system across entities in its network, care coordination across an enterprise is improved.

The HL7 Functional Model[14] covers EHR functionality in a more comprehensive manner than the EHR Incentive program. It provides details on function points that an EHR *shall*, *should*, or *may* have in the categories of care provision, care provision support, administration support, and population health support. All of these are important functionality that hospitals automate today using health IT either in a monolithic EHR solution or through a set of collaborative health

IT technologies. Central to patient care are the care provision functions of the EHR Functional Model. These are as follows:

1. Manage clinical history
2. Render externally sourced information
3. Manage clinical documentation
4. Manage orders
5. Manage results
6. Manage medication, immunization, and treatment administration
7. Manage future care
8. Manage patient education and communication
9. Manage care coordination and reporting

HIMSS takes another approach by summarizing EHR functionality at a high level and providing a measurement of adoption using the HIMSS Analytics EMR Adoption Model (EMRAM). The model has eight stages, starting with Stage 0, with each stage building on the one before. Hospitals are assessed based on this model to determine what stage they have achieved. Figure 8.1 shows

EMR Adoption Model

Stage	Cumulative Capabilities	% of Hospitals
Stage 7	Medical record fully electronic; CDO able to contribute to ICEHR as byproduct of SEHR	0.0%
Stage 6	Physician documentation (structured templates), full CDSS (variance & compliance), full PACS	0.1%
Stage 5	Closed loop medication administration	0.5%
Stage 4	CPOE, CDSS (clinical protocols)	3.0%
Stage 3	Clinical documentation (flow sheets), CDSS (error checking), PACS available outside Radiology	18.0%
Stage 2	CDR, CMV, CDSS inference engine, may have Document Imaging	38.8%
Stage 1	Ancillaries – Lab, Rad, Pharmacy	18.9%
Stage 0	All three Ancillaries not installed	20.7%

December 31, 2006

Figure 8.1   EMR Adoption Model, 2006[15]

US EMR Adoption Model[SM]

Stage	Cumulative Capabilities	2014 Q1	2014 Q2
Stage 7	Complete EMR; CCD transactions to share data; Data warehousing; Data continuity with ED, ambulatory, OP	3.1%	3.2%
Stage 6	Physician documentation (structured templates), full CDSS (variance & compliance), full R-PACS	13.3%	15.0%
Stage 5	Closed loop medication administration	24.2%	27.5%
Stage 4	CPOE, Clinical Decision Support (clinical protocols)	15.7%	15.3%
Stage 3	Nursing/clinical documentation (flow sheets), CDSS (error checking), PACS available outside Radiology	27.7%	25.4%
Stage 2	CDR, Controlled Medical Vocabulary, CDS, may have Document Imaging; HIE capable	7.2%	5.9%
Stage 1	Ancillaries - Lab, Rad, Pharmacy - All Installed	3.2%	2.8%
Stage 0	All Three Ancillaries Not Installed	5.6%	4.9%

Data from HIMSS Analytics[TM] Database © 2014   N = 5,449   N = 5,447

Figure 8.2   EMR Adoption Model, 2014[15]

the EMR Adoption Model and the rate of U.S. EMR adoption as of 2006. Figure 8.2 is the 2014 version of the model. A comparison of these models shows how much HITECH has served as a catalyst for EHR adoption and robustness.[15]

The success of EHR adoption and sophistication of available technology led to HIMSS revising their EMR Adoption Model in 2018.[16] Figure 8.3 shows the current adoption model – by comparing to the prior models, one can see how the model has evolved to reflect the sophistication of the field.

Patient Care Devices and the Smart Health Care Setting

The EHR itself can have many appendages. There are numerous small devices and technologies that interact with the EHR in a patient's care. Vital signs equipment measures pulse, oxygen level, and blood pressure. Other equipment includes spirometers, fetal monitors, ventilators, and infusion pumps. There are point-of-care (POC) testing devices such as glucometers, portable x-rays, and portable EKG machines. Identification technology such as RTLS (real-time locating system) and RFID (radio frequency ID), barcodes, and biometrics as well as signature pads can be used to identify patients, clinicians, and equipment. Data input technology such as smart phones, tablets, kiosks, and dictation systems are also used. Workstations on wheels (WOW), high-resolution viewing stations, and mobile devices like wireless tablets allow clinicians to interact

STAGE	**HiMSS** *Analytics* **EMRAM** EMR Adoption Model Cumulative Capabilities
7	Complete EMR; External HIE; Data Analytics, Governance, Disaster Recovery, Privacy and Security
6	Technology Enabled Medication, Blood Products, and Human Milk Administration; Risk Reporting; Full CDS
5	Physician documentation using structured templates; Intrusion/Device Protection
4	CPOE with CDS; Nursing and Allied Health Documentation; Basic Business Continuity
3	Nursing and Allied Health Documentation; eMAR; Role-Based Security
2	CDR; Internal Interoperability; Basic Security
1	Ancillaries - Laboratory, Pharmacy, and Radiology/Cardiology information systems; PACS; Digital non-DICOM image management
0	All three ancillaries not installed

Figure 8.3 EMR Adoption Model enhanced requirements 2018+[16]

more efficiently with the EHR in the workplace. Telemedicine technology has also become commonplace in the hospital setting. A primary use case for telemedicine is to provide the ability for specialists to consult remotely – this is useful for in demand specialists such as radiologists and psychiatrists. It is also especially useful for the rural hospital where specialists are scarcer. Technology in a hospital room could include floors that detect a patient falling, beds that can monitor a patient's vital signs, and technologies that listen and respond to patient and clinician commands.

Administration

One of the oldest areas of automation in the hospital is administration. Patient administration is the identification of patients and the management of their hospital encounters, including scheduling, census management, admissions, transfers, and discharges. Insurance information is collected and automatically checked for authorization with insurance companies. Medical records systems ensure that all of the documentation for the patient is complete and that encounters are coded accurately. Patient accounts and revenue cycle management are closely integrated with patient administration as well. A quality system can support the reporting of quality measures to regulatory bodies. There are also general hospital management functions that are supported by computer systems – human resources, nurse scheduling, time tracking, general accounting, learning management system, and materials management are all examples.

Provider-Facing Applications and EHR Add-Ons

It is also more common for providers to have applications on their smart phones or portable devices to help them with care. An application might be used for secure texting or to help with patient handoff and change of shift. Applications can also be integrated into the EHR using SMART-on-FHIR technology. The SMART Health IT[17] (substitutable medical apps, reusable technology) concept was originally developed at Boston Children's Hospital.

> SMART Health IT is an open, standards based technology platform that enables innovators to create apps that seamlessly and securely run across the healthcare system. Using an electronic health record (EHR) system or data warehouse that supports the SMART standard, patients, doctors, and healthcare practitioners can draw on this library of apps to improve clinical care, research, and public health.
> (https://smarthealthit.org/an-app-platform-for-healthcare/about/)

These SMART Health IT applications security communicate and exchange information with EHRs and other health IT systems using internet RESTful APIs that conform to the HL7 FHIR standard. Starting in 2019, most of the major EHR vendors implemented SMART-on-FHIR conformant APIs, allowing both patient and provider applications to connect to the EHRs. Examples of applications include workflow-specific risk calculators or an app that facilitates care coordination with social services.

Departmental Systems

Larger hospitals often have several health IT systems within a department to support its operations. The next three sections cover three of the main ancillaries at a hospital: laboratory, pharmacy, and radiology. The fourth section lists other kinds of departments that potentially have automation. Recall that the number of systems depends on how much vendor consolidation exists at the hospital – however, even where there is a centralized architecture, each department uses their own modules of the central system and may also have additional departmental systems to carry our operations of the department.

Health IT in the Laboratory

In a highly automated laboratory, there might be a laboratory information system (LIS), a specimen tracking system, a robotics system controlling specimen flow, a dashboard showing the current state of high-priority tests, and many different automated laboratory devices. The most common tasks relate to testing blood specimens. If the LIS is separate from the EHR, the LIS learns about a new lab order via an inbound HL7 interface. In a highly automated environment, phlebotomists and nurses use mobile devices to identify patients by barcode and print specimen labels with patient and order identification via wireless mobile printers. The labels are placed on the blood collection test tubes. Drawn specimens arrive at the lab in tubes and then are placed in robotics equipment, which divides the sample into smaller samples for specific tests (aliquoting). Each sample is automatically routed to the appropriate testing device. Once the testing is done, the result is uploaded to the LIS and validated against past results. Verified results are sent back to the EHR via an HL7 results interface.

Hospital laboratories may also interact with other EHRs and LISes since they may process tests sent to them from ambulatory clinics or outside doctors or labs and may send out some of their testing work to outside labs.

There are also specialized lab systems or functions such as pathology and blood bank. Pathology workflow is different, often involving specialized specimen preparation and review by a clinical pathologist. Blood bank systems might support blood typing, as well as the management of blood products. There are also computerized storage and dispensing cabinets for blood products in some operating rooms.

Health IT in the Pharmacy

In a hospital, medications are ordered by clinicians, dispensed by the pharmacy, and administered by nursing. In a fully automated environment, the clinician enters the order in the EHR and drug–drug and drug–allergy checking is performed, as well as other clinical decision support. If the pharmacy system is separate from the EHR, the order is sent to the pharmacy information system (PHIS) via an HL7 interface. The received order is verified by a pharmacist, who may then specify compounding, mixing, and dispensing information. Complex medications such as multi-ingredient IVs (intravenous) must be mixed. There is specialized robotic equipment in hospital pharmacies that can help with the counting and filling of pills, as well as the mixing of IVs. When the medication is ready to be dispensed, it might be placed in an automatic dispensing system. Automated dispensing systems are located near where medications are dispensed (such as on the nursing unit) and allow for careful control of medication inventory and appropriate dose dispensing. Electronic medication administration technology allows the nurse to scan the barcode on the medication and on the patient's wristband to be sure that the medication and the patient match before administration.

Health IT in Radiology

The process of radiology begins with the ordering of an imaging exam by the clinician. In an automated environment, the order would be entered into the EHR, and if the RIS is a separate system, it is sent to the RIS via an HL7 interface. An important function of the RIS is scheduling the patient for the procedure – numerous resources must be booked on behalf of the patient – radiology staff, room, and equipment. There are many kinds of exams – examples include x-rays, computed tomography (CT) scans, magnetic resonance imaging, ultrasounds, and positron emission tomography-CT scans. Advanced imaging could include 3D and/or holographic radiology images. Radiological images are represented using the DICOM (Digital Imaging and Communications in Medicine) standard. The images can be quite large and are usually stored on a picture archiving and communication system (PACS). Once the imaging is complete, the next step is that a radiologist reviews the image and reports the findings. The viewing station that the radiologist uses is important and often a high-resolution workstation. Radiologists sometimes use dictation systems to capture their findings. Sometimes, images are reviewed remotely (teleradiology). The text reports are sent to the EHR via an HL7 interface, and the ability to see the image is provided in some way to the EHR. For example, a link to the PACS could be provided. It is now possible for clinicians to access images from mobile devices, as well. Advanced technology such as 3D printers in radiology can help with training and guiding surgery. Artificial intelligence is also an emerging technology with radiology. Using machine learning (a type of artificial intelligence), machines "trained" on large datasets of images can help guide a radiologist in their decisions.

Health IT in Other Departments

The number of health IT systems is as diverse as the number of departments and functions in a hospital. In cardiology, there are systems for EKGs, cardiac catheterization, echocardiology, nuclear medicine, general cardiology, and more. Numerous technologies support the surgery suite, including anesthesiology systems, perfusion systems, automated dispensing cabinets, and RFID technology for surgical supplies and implantable devices, as well as the surgery information system. Transplant information systems manage the receipt and supply of organs for transplant purposes.

There are also systems to support registries – examples include immunization, cancer, and biobank (genetic samples).

Additional departmental systems include systems to support the operations of the dietary department, patient transport, bed tracking and cleaning, patient entertainment, the emergency department, endoscopy, pulmonology, employee health, epidemiology, radiation oncology, credentialing, etc.

Health IT Middleware and Edgeware

Interface Engines

For hospitals that have numerous interconnected systems, an interface engine is an essential tool. Imagine the following scenario:

Once a patient is admitted, the patient's information is recorded on the patient administration system. This triggers the generation of a message containing demographic information about the patient, as well as information about his or her visit to be generated and sent to downstream systems that are interested in the information. Imagine that the hospital also has a pharmacy information system. If the pharmacy system is able to receive this patient administration message, then it can automatically create a record of the patient visit so that any subsequent orders for medications for the patient can be attached to the visit. In a similar way, if the message is sent to the EHR, this message will automatically create the encounter on the EHR, which alleviates the need for a clinician to create the visit and enter in the information.

This has two benefits:

1. Convenience and efficiency for the user of the downstream system
2. Safety for the patient, because when data are hand entered a second time, errors or discrepancies might be introduced

However, as the needs for interfacing increase (imagine interfaces between 50 systems), two problems occur:

1. Each time another system wants an interface, it has to be built on both the sending and receiving system. Eventually an unwieldy number of point-to-point interfaces exist that need to be maintained.
2. Each time an interface is needed, design, negotiation, and detailed mapping are needed to translate from the sender's interface logic to the receiver's interface logic.

Using an interface engine reduces this complexity. An interface engine sits in the middle of all interfacing – taking in all inbound feeds and then filtering, translating, and routing to the destination system. This streamlines the process and reduces the need for as many point-to-point interfaces. Most interfaces used to communication between systems within a hospital use HL7 Version 2 messaging. Common interfaces include:

1. **Patient Administration Interface.** This interface receives messages from the patient administration system about all patient admissions, updates, transfers, and discharges. This information flow is often referred to as the ADT feed. ADT stands for admission, discharge, and transfer.
2. **Billing Interface.** This interface sends out charge information for services provided.
3. **Orders Interface.** The EHR and other clinician-oriented systems that include CPOE would include an outbound interface to send orders to the ancillaries that could fulfill them. In turn, ancillary systems that fulfill clinician orders would have an inbound orders interface.
4. **Results/Documents Interface.** Systems that generate clinical results or documents will send these out to other systems. In turn, the EHR as well as other interested systems (clinical data warehouse, epidemiology, etc.) would receive clinical results and documentation via an inbound interface.

Enterprise Master Patient Index

Complex organizations that involve multiple sites and affiliations often have several assigning authorities of identifiers for patients. For example, a hospital could potentially have two medical records departments, each independently assigning medical record numbers. An Enterprise Master Patient Index owns and manages patient identification across an enterprise with multiple assigning authorities.[18] The EMPI number can become the index or linkage in shared systems and is useful in in cross-network query. The EMPI system manages demographics for the patient across the enterprise, provides an enterprise-unique patient identity (EMPI), and maintains linkages to local identifiers (e.g., MRNs) for the patient. An EMPI also often provides support for quality improvement of the index, suggesting potential duplicates and ID errors. Patient administration systems interface with the EMPI during patient search and new patient creation, making sure that the EMPI has the master copy of demographics and is able to link the enterprise identifier with local identifiers. The interface engine can add the EMPI into interfaces to systems that use the EMPI as an identifier. Enterprise systems use the EMPI to link patient records across the enterprise.

Terminology Services

As hospitals store more and more structured information on computers, the need for terminology management becomes critical. A terminology server manages concepts and their relationships to each other; it also provides mappings between current and historical local terminologies and mappings to standard terminologies. For example, the terminology server might keep track of the concept of a glucose laboratory test as represented in two different laboratory systems managed by the hospital. It might also keep a mapping to the code used to represent glucose in a system no longer used by the hospital. It could also map the local lab codes to the standard terminology LOINC© (Logical Observation Identifiers Names and Codes). Finally, it might map related concepts together – diabetes and A1C tests might both be related to the glucose test. A terminology server is able to provide a multitude of translational services as well as an intelligent repository of hospital metadata. NewYork–Presbyterian Hospital uses the Medical Entities Dictionary, which maintains over 100,000 interconnected concepts.[19] HL7© has published specifications for standard interactions with terminology servers using the HL7© FHIR© standard.

Technology to Support Interorganizational Interoperability

Communication with outside organizations has become more common as we work toward interorganizational healthcare interoperability. Hospitals may be a part of regional Health Information Exchanges (HIEs). If the HIE uses a federated model,[20] it will need to access patient data at the hospital site. In that case, the hospital would have an *edge server*. An edge server contains patient information accessible to other organizations. It provides a secure window into the hospital's patient data for the purposes of HIE. Hospitals will sometimes have their own internal HIEs between affiliated hospitals or sites and their own HIE software. HIE software includes interface management, patient identification services, and patient resource locator services. The initial concept of HIEs was to build regional exchanges between providers. The regional exchanges connected to each other and to a state level HIE, and state HIEs connect together, ultimately resulting in a national interoperability infrastructure. Other interoperability networks have emerged that connect EHR to EHR – such as CareQuality and Commonwell. Hospitals connected to these networks would need to manage those connections. The future direction in the U.S. is to connect all hospitals via a national network of networks referred to as the Trusted Exchange Framework by the Office of the National Coordinator of Health IT.

Analytics

One of the fastest growing areas in health IT is in the area of analytics. In order to manage patients' care better and to improve efficiency, it is extremely important to study datasets collected from the EHR and other systems at the hospital. These data are also useful for research, quality, regulatory reporting, and population health management. Both clinical and business data can be collected and studied and sometimes combined for additional insight. Based on the data, one can determine trends and nuances and begin to support decisions by making predictions using the data. There could be numerous systems involved in the collection of data from many sources, preprocessing ("cleaning") of the data, and storage in specialized database systems optimized for queries that are more population based. The systems supporting analytics include clinical and business data warehouses, business intelligence tools that are able to prepare the data in formats ready for analytics, and analytics tools that allow for patterns to be discovered and displayed. Visualization tools include report writers, portals, dashboards, and others. The insights determined using analytics technology sometimes automatically feed back into the operations of care provision systems to improve care.

Robotics

The use of robots is becoming more common in hospitals. Routine processes in the laboratory and pharmacy can be automated by robots. Robotic process automation can be used to reduce repetitive tasks, allowing administrators to optimize their work efforts. Robots can even clean floors and deliver supplies and food trays.

IT Infrastructure

Finally, there are systems that support the IT service. Security and confidentiality of healthcare information is paramount, and numerous IT systems may be utilized. This might include systems to manage, control, and track access to systems as well as systems that detect potential intrusions. A fast and reliable network is assumed, and there are monitoring tools to keep track of performance and reliability. There are systems to manage service requests and planned changes to the production IT environment, as well as to manage unplanned incidents (service desk calls). Health IT systems are usually hosted on one or more servers housed in off-site data centers or in the cloud. Backup servers and storage are also required in the event of failure.

Conclusion

Hospital stays are intensive and expensive. Patients in hospitals are very sick, and many individuals are involved in their care. Statistics have been reported on the dangers of hospitals to patients due to preventable errors. It is imperative that hospitals serve as safe places of healing, not risky adventures fraught with medical error. Computers hold the promise of organizing data, presenting critical information to users, and improving communication between individuals. With continued rising costs of healthcare and the advent of healthcare reform, health IT in hospitals is more important than ever. ACOs will rely on substantial technology to ensure that information flows seamlessly across the ACO and that information is available to analyze and inform strategy to ensure ACO success.

Health IT is critical for the success of the modern-day hospital. Larger organizations could have over 100 health IT systems and thousands of intelligent devices, with many interconnections. Health IT supports the myriad of administrative and clinical workflows within hospital operations. Each year at HIMSS, attendees witness the power of the health IT role in hospitals. However, in 2020, the international HIMSS Annual Conference Exhibition was canceled as the world was devastated by the COVID-19 pandemic. Yet, the value of Health IT was evident in hospitals fighting the disease. Telemedicine scaled and expanded to levels never seen before, allowing patients and providers to convene virtually. Providers were able to screen patients through specialized EHR workflows and safely send patients home with remote monitoring devices. Health IT made real-time, data-driven lifesaving decisions possible in a quickly changing environment as the demand for beds surged to overflow beds and converted ICUs, testing was developed and rolled out, and new treatments emerged. As dependent as hospitals are on frontline staff, the cleaning staff, and electricity, health IT has become an essential part of healthcare delivery.

About the Author

Virginia Lorenzi, MS, CPHIMS, has been working in health IT for over 30 years with vendor, consulting, provider, and faculty experience. She is currently a Senior Technical Architect at NewYork–Presbyterian Hospital, where she advises on regulatory programs and interoperability and is on the faculty at Columbia University where she helps with workforce and FHIR efforts and serves as Program Director for the Certification of Professional Achievement in Health IT. She has deep experience in interoperability and standards, including over 26 years of active involvement in HL7. She is active in New York HIMSS and enjoys the community it offers to her as well as to students and early careerists in the field.

References

1. Shortliffe EH, Cimino JJ, eds. *Biomedical Informatics: Computer Applications in Health Care and Biomedicine,* 3rd ed. Springer Science and Business Media; 2006.
2. Spronk R. The Early History of HL7, Part 1. *HL7 News.* January 2014.
3. Drees J. KLAS: Epic, Cerner Dominate EMR Market Share. *Becker Hospital Review.* April 30, 2019.
4. Ball MJ, Collen MF, eds. *Aspects of the Computer-Based Patient Record.* New York: Springer-Verlag; 1992.
5. Mayes R. The Origins, Development, and Passage of Medicare's Revolutionary Prospective Payment System. *Journal of the History of Medicine and Allied Sciences.* 2007;62(1):21–55.
6. Goodridge E, Arnquist S. A History of Overhauling Health Care – Nearly 100 Years of Legislative Milestones and Defeats. *The New York Times.* March 2010.
7. Welton JM. Mandatory Hospital Nurse to Patient Staffing Ratios: Time to Take a Different Approach. *The Online Journal of Issues in Nursing.* Accessed September 30, 2007.
8. Institute of Medicine. To Err is Human: Building a Safer Healthcare System. 1999.
9. Roizen MF, Oz MC. *You, The Smart Patient – An Insider's Handbook for Getting the Best Treatment. The Joint Commission.* New York: Free Press; 2006.
10. Crossing the Quality Chasm: A New Health System for the 21st Century is a report on health care quality in the United States. National Institute of Medicine; National Academy Press, March 1, 2001.
11. Percentage of Hospitals, By Type, That Possess Certified Health IT. www.healthit.gov 2017.
12. Hirshon JM, Risko N, Calvello EJB, et al. Health Systems and Services: The Role of Acute Care. *Bulletin of the World Health Organization.* 2013;91:386–388. http://dx.doi.org/10.2471/BLT.12.112664.
13. Enabling Medication Management Through Health Information Technology; Contract HHSA 290–2007–10060-I). AHRQ Publication No. 11-E008-EF. Rockville MD: Agency for Healthcare Research and Quality. April 2011.
14. HL7 EHR System Functional Model, April 14, 2014.
15. HIMSS Analytics. EMR Adoption Models. www.himss.org. 2006 and 2014.
16. HIMSS Analytics. EMR Adoption Model www.himss.org 2020.
17. SMART Health IT. www.smarthealthit.org.
18. Lorenzi V, DaSilva G, Saini S, et al. Who Are You? The NewYork–Presbyterian EMPI Experience. Knowledge. www.amia.org. Accessed January 2015.
19. The Medical Entities Dictionary. http://med.dmi.columbia.edu/. Accessed January 2015.
20. Technical Architecture of ONC-Approved Plans for Statewide Health Information Exchange. *AMIA Annu Symp Proc.* 2011.

Chapter 9

Artificial Intelligence and Hospital Automation

Daniel J. Barchi, MEM

Contents

Any decision a human can make in less than one second can be done by artificial intelligence (AI), according to Andrew Ng, founder of Google Brain and chief scientist of Baidu. In a slightly different approach, renowned computer scientist Donald Knuth has suggested that AI can do essentially everything that requires thinking but fails to do most of what people and animals do without thinking. For example, though people consider differential equations difficult, a computer has no problem solving them with complete accuracy. On the other hand, while humans think catching

DOI: 10.4324/9780429423109-9

a ball is easy, such nearly reflexive action is currently beyond the capability of most machines and robots. A popular internet meme called *Chihuahua or muffin* juxtaposes photographs of Chihuahuas and blueberry muffins. Humans easily recognize the difference between the two, but machines lack the same reliability when tasked with distinguishing between the eyes and nose of a small dog and a muffin containing three blueberries.

AI can be thought of as two broad categories. The first – methods – includes expert systems, machine learning, and neural networks. Learning or smart systems that get smarter as they are exposed to more data fall into this methods category of AI. The second – applications – includes all of the ways we convert intelligence into outcomes. These encompass natural language processing, speech recognition, robotics, and predictive analytics. While the field of AI is broad and becoming more so daily, this chapter is focused specifically on the AI applications we can expect to impact healthcare in the next decade.

AI is developing rapidly, and the better we understand where it is going, the better we will be able to use it today. We are now in an age of Artificial Narrow Intelligence (ANI), where algorithms excel at very specific tasks. The AI algorithms of Pandora, for instance, "know" that if you like Jay-Z, you are likely to be happy if a Drake song queues up next on your playlist. Similarly, if you ask Alexa if you should carry an umbrella today, it knows enough to make appropriate recommendations. At some point in the next 20 years, however, computers will move from this limited-capacity ANI to broader Artificial General Intelligence (AGI), in which a reasonably sized computer will be able to make decisions comparable to those that a human might make. Twenty years beyond AGI in, say, 2060, we may reach the even more capable Artificial Super Intelligence (ASI). It is when we cross the ASI tripwire that we may entirely lose our ability as humans to control machine development. The seemingly benign benefit of ASI could quickly become scary if super-intelligent machines move beyond solving thorny problems and curing cancer to decide that instead of improving the health of humans, perhaps humans are an unnecessary part of life on Earth. This idea of a moment when exponential technology growth profoundly impacts civilization is commonly known as *The Singularity*. While the possible threats of ASI deserve consideration, this potential outcome exists on a distant future horizon. In a 2015 interview with *Wired* magazine, President Obama brought perspective to this concern by stating, "Most people aren't spending a lot of time right now worrying about singularity – they are worrying about, 'Well, is my job going to be replaced by a machine?'"

Shooting for the Moon

Whether we are thinking in the short or long term, it is worth considering the implications of AI for the workforce and on business processes. An early idea was that AI would profoundly influence all areas of service delivery. MD Anderson Cancer Center launched a partnership with IBM's Watson AI platform in 2013, which focused on using cognitive computing to eradicate cancer. MD Anderson labeled its innovative programs as *moon shots*, and the IBM initiative promised to harness MD Anderson's medical records and a big data approach to recommend innovative treatments for patients. A January–February 2018 *Harvard Business Review* article outlined the failure of MD Anderson's AI moon shot and its decision to shutter the program in 2017, after a $62 million investment yielded no significant clinical outcomes. The article pointed out that the cancer center is still experimenting with artificial intelligence; however, its focus is now far narrower. MD Anderson patients can at present use AI for hotel reservations and restaurant recommendations (Davenport & Ronanki, 2018).

MD Anderson's recognition that the value of AI exists not in complex, high-value tasks but rather in simple, commodity processes is reminiscent of the economic lessons learned from the California Gold Rush of 1849. While some early miners dug their way to riches, the first person who became a millionaire from the Gold Rush was newspaperman Sam Brannan, who sold picks, shovels, food, and services to miners. The names we recognize today from that period are not those of the miners but those of merchants who serviced them, including Leland Stanford of Stanford University and Levi Strauss of Levi's eponymous riveted blue jeans.

Finding Solid Footing on Earth

Similarly, the best use of AI in the current business environment may be not in the most visible, customer-facing applications but rather in the routine, repetitive, high-volume, back-office processes common to most industries. In healthcare, for instance, Robotic Process Automation (RPA) offers the opportunity to make finance and administrative requirements more efficient, while freeing our human workforce to focus on higher-value work and patient-focused clinical care.

In their paper published by *The National Academy of Medicine*, Matheny et al. (2019) suggest that AI has the power to reduce costs and improve efficiencies by prioritizing human labor for complex tasks and applying AI to workflow optimization, fraud prevention, waste reduction, and repetitive processes. For all its potential and promise, however, implementation of AI requires human guidance to ensure that the power of this technology aligns with the preferences of its users and the goals of the organization. Human management of AI is also critical to protect against unintended and potentially adverse consequences. This human component is crucial, if we are to maximize the potential of AI and protect against its risks.

Part of the misconception of AI stems from the tendency to use AI as a blanket term for all computer automation. Just as AI should be judiciously and precisely applied to the appropriate well-defined organizational goal, choosing the proper type of AI for the task is critical.

Darrell West and John Allen (2018) argue in their paper that intentionality, intelligence, and adaptability are the essence of AI. They quote the assertion of Shukla Shubhendu and J. Frank Vijay that AI is generally thought to be "machines that respond to stimulation consistent with traditional responses from humans, given the human capacity for contemplation, judgment, and intention [to] make decisions which normally require [a] human level of expertise."

RPA is a separate concept. RPA employs software that automates and standardizes routine and repetitive workflow processes. This software robot performs the same task identically at every attempt. It is not designed to learn or improvise or design improved systems. Where AI has the potential to make systems better, RPA simply does the work it is programmed to complete. RPA is a predictable, precise workhorse that does not make mistakes, grow bored, or lose efficiency but has the power to liberate thinking human employees from rote tasks and better deploy their talents to areas that require the nuance of human judgment.

In technology and those industries most affected by its advances, too much devotion to the cutting edge can undermine the adoption of new tools. Pursuit of the next bright, shiny object should be tempered with restraint and an eye to smooth integration and user experience. The first step to incorporating the next AI opportunity is framing. I work in healthcare and very much believe that people practice the art of medicine for their patients. The human aspect is inseparable. I have yet to meet anyone who desires healthcare delivered by machine, but our hospital system reports high levels of satisfaction from patients who receive care from humans *facilitated by* machine. And this is where the framing of new AI tools is important. Patients and users must feel confident that AI augments, not replaces, doctor care. We believe that the best AI tools support physicians and staff by freeing them of the rote aspects of care, such as making sure that proper tests are ordered and reported, filing insurance claims, monitoring drug interaction, and scheduling appointments so that they can "work at the top of their licensure," allowing them to deliver the best possible care for their patients (Matheny et al., 2019). In other words, we see a future where AI relieves caregivers of low-level tasks so that they can practice the best possible medicine unencumbered. Additionally, AI implementers can develop trust by providing humans the ability to override AI when necessary. This aspect is critically important because of the "understandably low tolerance for machine error" and the circumstances in which AI tools are being implemented in "an environment of inadequate regulation and legislation" (Matheny et al., 2019). Matheny et al. (2019) report what we, too, find in our hospital system that in the near term, we are better to use AI to augment care rather than to fully automate it. When patients and users feel secure in this arrangement, AI actually makes medicine more, not less, human.

Keeping an Eye on What Works

Another important factor in successfully integrating AI is in choosing its area of use. In our current capacity, AI is a more natural fit with certain clinical applications than others. A particularly good match for AI is the detection of diabetic retinopathy, the most common cause of vision impairment and blindness in adults who suffer from diabetes. Diabetic retinopathy occurs when high blood sugar levels damage blood vessels in light-sensitive retinal tissue in the back of the eye. Early detection is critical for managing this condition, but since half of diabetic patients do not see an eye doctor annually, many are not properly screened for diabetic retinopathy, according to Malvina Eydelman, MD, of the FDA Center for Devices and Radiological Health.

In April 2018, the U.S. Food and Drug Administration allowed marketing of the AI device to detect diabetic retinopathy in adults (FDA.gov). The IDx-DR software program analyzes camera images of the eye via an AI algorithm and provides screening decisions without requiring clinician interpretation of the images or results. What this achieves is better, more accurate, specialized care in the familiarity of the primary care setting. In trials, the IDx-DR correctly identified the presence of more than mild diabetic retinopathy with 87.4 percent accuracy and identified the absence of more than mild diabetic retinopathy with 89.5 percent accuracy. An April 2019 study published in *Ophthalmology* found that physicians and AI systems working together are more effective in diagnosing diabetic retinopathy than physicians or AI alone. Once again, AI supports, and even augments, the capability of the physician, and, in this instance, the patient receives the benefit of specialized care in the comfortable presence of a primary care physician.

While experienced specialists may be expert in recognizing risk patterns in retinal images, it is impossible for an individual physician to view the number of images in a lifetime that AI can compare in minutes. In a separate but related topic, deep learning AI was able to predict cardiovascular risk factors from retinal fundus (interior lining of the eyeball) images after training on data from 284,335 patients not previously thought to be present or quantifiable in retinal images (Poplin et al., 2018).

Diagnostic Imaging

The health research unit at Google has recently developed an AI application that can match and even outperform radiologists in the detection of breast cancer. According to the American Cancer

Society, one in eight women will develop breast cancer. Second only to lung cancer, breast cancer kills more than 41,000 women each year. Early detection saves lives, but many cases are missed, allowing tumors to spread, or misdiagnosed, causing unnecessary worry and treatment.

The international team of researchers who developed Google's AI model supplied the algorithm with anonymized mammograms and identified those with confirmed cases of breast cancer. While human radiologists identified cancers that the AI system missed, the AI system caught cancers that the radiologists missed. After trials on mammograms of more than 28,000 women, the AI system reduced missed cases of cancer by 9.4 percent (United States) and 2.7 percent (United Kingdom) and reduced false positive cancer diagnoses by 5.7 percent (United States) and 1.2 percent (United Kingdom) when compared to the original diagnoses made by radiologists. Additionally, radiologists in the United Kingdom indicate that the AI model has the potential to reduce their workload by 88 percent. And that workload reduction can mean more time devoted to their patients – yet another example of AI making medicine more, not less, human.

Operational Recommendations

In addition to improving diagnostics, AI can support operational processes as well. The hospital system where I work, NewYork–Presbyterian (NYP), introduced AI to our clinical areas as a supportive, operational tool. Length of stay is a measure we use to ensure that patients get the care they need and then return home in a timely manner. A patient who comes in for a hip replacement, for instance, should need about two days of care and follow-up tests post-operatively before discharge. If a patient stays longer, the risks of complications, hospital-acquired infections, and higher costs increase. To help prevent these potential concerns, we worked with a small company to use AI to review past hospital processes to predict delays for our current patients. By looking at past encounters, the system identified the scheduling of a physical therapy consult as an obstacle to the timely discharge of orthopedic patients. Now, if a patient is within a day of expected discharge and an order for physical therapy has not occurred yet, the AI system will send a "nudge" to the physical therapy department to prioritize a consult for the patient that same day. Additionally, if the system "sees" that a long queue for an MRI might delay a patient's return home, a nudge is sent to both the physician and MRI teams to determine whether that imaging study can be expedited for discharge or, alternatively, cancelled to be rescheduled as an outpatient appointment. Again, AI is not replacing or overriding clinical care but merely organizing the resources of our entire system to the benefit of both patient and the team of clinicians working to get that patient well and home.

Patients increasingly have access to their doctors and records online. Their prescriptions are sent to pharmacies electronically, where pharmacy reconciliation happens automatically. EMRs have become requirements for reimbursement and offer a level of patient safety far beyond handwritten notes in a paper file that may or may not be in close proximity to the patient.

Medicine is no longer a question of human or machine but rather how the two can deliver the best possible care in concert. One is not necessarily better than the other. We need to keep our attitudes and expectations in the right place – do not blindly trust AI nor fear that a human clinician can be replaced by AI. (Recall the mammography study where AI found cancers humans did not, and humans spotted cancers AI did not.) We can use AI for the same reason that it is standard practice for two radiologists to read images – it is safer that way, and the end result is just too important for mistakes.

I recall a conversation with our daughter about the pride we take in our safety numbers and low morbidity rate. Her response was that, while our numbers may be impressive, they are not exactly the kind of data we can use to market our health system. And while her assessment is correct, keeping people alive and helping them get well is our goal, and why would we not use AI, if it can help us toward that goal by reducing the chance of mistakes?

Triage

When patients have cause to visit emergency departments, their first interaction is often triage. Accurate triage is essential because it quickly establishes the basics of patient condition and assigns a level of urgency to the timeline of care for that individual. Getting triage right means that the resources of an emergency department are appropriately meted to each patient in the proper order. At NYP, we have found that offering low-risk patients the option of telemedicine can be beneficial both in quicker care and discharge for those who choose it and in keeping our exam rooms open for the most urgent cases, where telemedicine would not be appropriate. I mention telemedicine, not because it is an example of AI, but because it is an example of technology improving patient experience by enhancing the ability of physicians to efficiently care for patients.

Albert Rizzo is a psychologist and the director of medical virtual reality at the University of Southern California Institute for Creative Technologies (ICT). He and his research team are working to develop virtual AI robots capable of reading, processing, and responding to human emotions. Dr. Rizzo says, "Our mission isn't to replace human beings where only human beings can do the job." He and his team have designed a virtual reality character named Ellie to help identify veterans who might need therapy when they return home from deployment. Ellie makes eye contact and nods and gestures much like a human therapist would. Ellie even pauses after short answers in an attempt to elicit more information from the veterans served.

Cheyenne Quilter, a West Point cadet who is helping test the program, said of her experience with Ellie, "After the first or second question, you kind of forget that it's a robot." AI Ellie does not diagnose or treat veterans but instead provides data for human therapists to determine the needs of each veteran. "This is not AI trying to be your therapist," said researcher Gale Lucas. "This is AI trying to predict who is most likely to be suffering."

One unsaid advantage to an AI tool like Ellie is the privacy it offers patients. Those who may be intimidated by or resistant to therapy may be more open to Ellie than a human therapist. Ellie could even serve to bridge the gap between avoiding therapy and fully engaging in it.

Balancing Access With Accuracy

Babylon Health is a private company that provides remote healthcare services by way of its text and video application. Through its GP at hand, Babylon Health offers participants in the United Kingdom video appointments 24 hours a day within 2 hours. This access is considered a vast improvement, given that patients typically wait weeks to see to a clinician in the NHS. According to its website, Babylon has harnessed AI "around a doctor's brain" and uses natural language processing to allow computers to "interpret, understand, and then use everyday human language and language patterns" in its communication with patients to provide information, *not* clinical care. The website directly states that the information its application provides is not to be used as a diagnosis.

The problem with this model is easy to identify. GP at hand's close association with the NHS lends it enough credibility that users may choose to ignore the information-only disclaimer and rely on it for diagnoses, especially when regular NHS appointments must be scheduled so far in advance. GP at hand does offer face-to-face appointments in their clinics, but, unlike the application, those hours are limited and require the patient to present at the clinic. It is not difficult to see how a harried parent with a sick child in the middle of the night or someone feverish in bed would not gratefully accept the information provided by GP at hand as a diagnosis.

So, if the information provided is correct, is a diagnosis even necessary for most everyday ailments? Perhaps, not, but accuracy is absolutely necessary, and GP at hand has not reached the threshold of "safe advice 100% of the time," as stated on its website before an advertising regulator requested that the claim be removed in April 2018 (Olson, 2018). Even Babylon doctors questioned the accuracy of the mobile AI health service. When they performed their own audit of the application, they discovered that 10–15 percent of the most commonly suggested outcomes were incorrect or failed to identify signs of serious conditions such as cancer or sepsis (Olson, 2018).

For perspective, *The Journal of the American Medical Association* reports that, on their own, doctors make incorrect diagnoses 15 percent of the time (Livingston, 2016). According to the *JAMA* report, physicians correctly diagnosed cases with greater than 72 percent accuracy, while their AI counterparts were correct 34 percent of the time. Accuracy improved for both groups when naming their three most common diagnoses to better than 84 percent for human doctors and 51 percent for AI applications (Livingston, 2016).

While Babylon clearly states on its GP at hand website that its AI services are not diagnostic nor a substitute for a doctor, Dr. Ateev Mehrotra, author of the *JAMA* study and associate professor at Harvard Medical School, said that he was not surprised that doctors would perform better but also that he could foresee the development of AI programs capable of meeting human accuracy within the next decade. He also went on to say that it would be worthwhile to study how computers could improve the diagnostic accuracy of physicians (Livingston, 2016).

Enhancing Skills

Cardiologists use sonography to capture the image of a patient's heart. They can use this tool to measure the ejection fraction of the left ventricle or the percentage of blood that leaves the heart with each contraction. Cardiologists train for years and often serve two-year fellowships in cardiac imaging to become proficient in delivering this type of care. A company called Caption Health (formerly known as Bay Labs) is testing its EchoGPS cardiac ultrasound guidance software, which uses AI to guide certified medical assistants who have no prior scanning experience to capture echocardiograms.

You could be forgiven for preferring that a cardiologist perform your echocardiogram, but consider for a moment the problem of access to this critical diagnostic tool. Radiologists rarely perform x-rays to diagnose broken limbs; they read x-rays performed by other medical staff. It is a best use of resources solution to have one or two radiologists read the images collected by several medical staff members.

Patrick M. McCarthy, MD, chief of cardiac surgery at Northwestern Memorial Hospital and principal investigator on testing EchoGPS, explains, "Deep learning will have a profound impact on cardiac imaging in the future, and the ability to simplify acquisition will be a tremendous advance to bring echocardiograms to the point-of-care in primary care offices." In this model, patients are served and receive care more efficiently. We do not require pilots to schedule our flights, but we certainly want them flying the plane.

So, we find ourselves at a place where AI can improve access to medical care but not with the same diagnostic accuracy of physicians, as in the case of GP at hand; pick up on certain radiological images that doctors miss, as in mammography studies; perform aspects of triage to determine if further psychological assessment is needed, as in Ellie for veterans returning from war; and capture echocardiograms for referral to cardiologists in primary care settings. Used with care and awareness of its current limitations, AI appears to have greater promise for good than for harm.

Supporting Care Delivery in the Back Office

AI has back-office applications that have the potential to streamline all steps in the delivery of care so that hospital systems may devote more of their resources directly to patients.

Finance

At NYP, we began using RPA to solve the seemingly complex problem of spending thousands of staff hours to manage the procedure of completing, signing, and filing forms to document exceptions to our normal employee timekeeping process. Our goal was to centralize the process and make it more efficient, but doing so would have required creating a new staff of more than 30 employees dedicated full-time to this administrative work. Instead, we collaborated with a small company to automate the entire process through AI and an automated email push/approval process. Though the work to create and enact the process was significant, and the change management process for our users was material, the investment produced immediate cost avoidance and time savings for our frontline staff, now freed to focus more on clinical care.

Claims Follow Up

Like most hospitals, NYP financial staff must process follow-up insurance claims. For each claim, a staff member spends ten minutes to look up the patient's name, date of birth, and date of the clinical encounter and then goes to the insurance company website, enters the data, and looks up and documents the status of the claim for the next step in the follow-up process. RPA teaches a computer-based bot to do the same thing with software. RPA learns the workflow and then repeats it efficiently. What required the financial staff member ten minutes to do, RPA accomplishes in one minute, and RPA can process claims 24 hours a day without interruption.

Claims Appeal

When a hospital learns the reason why a payment from an insurance company has been held or denied, the hospital begins the claims appeal process. Nurses with clinical experience manage the claims and follow-up directly with the insurance companies. For years, the process was to hand each claims nurse a stack of follow-ups and allow him or her to go about the process using experience and skill. Some claims nurses were experts in workman's compensation cases, others in congestive heart failure, and still others in working with a specific insurance company. When we applied AI to this process and assigned nurses to cases that best matched their success profile, we improved our overall success rate. Our 43 percent success rate on claims follow-up with random assignment climbed to 57 percent when cases were matched to nurses who had demonstrated past expertise. In this instance, AI did not do the work itself, but it assigned the best people to do the work.

Challenges of Developing AI for Medicine

AI faces many challenges. If the foundation of AI is data, AI algorithms must be developed with data that reflects and is representative of the populations it serves. The National Academy of Medicine report warns that scaling AI trained on data containing existent inequities and biases will only intensify those inequitable outcomes that we currently work to eliminate. The National Academy of Medicine reports that the subjects of social science research tend to be disproportionately Western and, therefore, not applicable to the greater population. The volume of data AI can analyze helps mitigate this potential bias and provides information that is more applicable to a wider population.

Ethical considerations are at the heart of almost every medical decision. We will need to determine an ethical path forward with regard to data, patient privacy, dignity, and quality of care. Informing patients when AI is used seems to be an important consideration, too.

Considering AI as a Medical Device

As we face these considerations, it may be helpful to classify AI in some way. Is AI a medical device? If so, medical devices are used by medical professionals, and this categorization would require that AI be used by, and not instead of, medical professionals. Such classification would also place AI under FDA regulations. The current statement from the FDA regarding AI is a plan to "reimagine" a regulatory path, since the adaptive nature of AI does not fit the typical steps of pre-market testing and approval. AI is not static; therefore, its oversight must, likewise, be dynamic.

Every day, the delivery of healthcare generates an untold volume of data, and this data has the potential to improve population health by recognizing patterns and making comparisons never before possible. The data we have amassed by using EMRs can potentially be used to draw conclusions and find correlations that would be otherwise impossible for ethical concerns and experimental limitations. EMRs capture real data in real time from real patients outside of laboratories. The sheer number of cases to be compared and analyzed would be outside the realm of human possibility, but AI can crunch this humanly impossible amount of data for very human use on very real humans.

Incorporating AI Into the Clinical Environment

Imagine that you are an oncologist who has spent a career caring for patients with Non-Hodgkin Lymphoma and conducting research on advanced treatments. Part of your research shows that for a specific cohort of patients, immunotherapy is particularly efficacious. Imagine, though, that a new AI-driven oncology system recommends chemotherapy for one of those patients. Your research and experience tell you that one course of treatment is best, but the AI system recommends a different one. What do you do, and what do you tell patients when they ask why? This is the black box problem – the AI system has a high AUC, but we do not understand how the system comes to this decision. While some black box predictions have low risk, such as the ability for AI to predict a patient's gender with 97 percent accuracy based solely on a retinal image, others are riskier. Our ability as a health industry to grow comfortable with accepting AI guidance, even when we do not understand why, and refusing AI guidance when our experience refutes it, will define our ability to use technologies in advanced ways.

Looking Ahead

AI has an undeniable workforce impact. Leaders of healthcare must consider how AI changes jobs and adapt training so that employees learn alongside AI. Accepting the changing nature of AI will keep our workforce nimble and hopefully allow us to avoid the obsolescence of skillsets as employees evolve with AI.

In these ways, we are not substituting AI for human care but are rather using AI to make the administrative process of delivering care and running a hospital more efficient. Today, AI is not ready to make diagnoses or perform surgeries on its own. We can, however, harness AI to improve our decisions, enhance patient safety, and free our providers of time-consuming, routine tasks so that they can deliver the best possible hands-on care to our patients. Elevating the work and minds of the talented people who make up our health system can only enhance our ability to provide the highest quality care to our patients.

I describe information technology as 80 percent people, 15 percent process, and 5 percent technology. People are responsible for determining the use and application of powerful technologies. People must also determine how to best deploy these tools. AI shines for its ability to compare and analyze infinite data sets and potential outcomes, but, no matter how many human-like touches we program and AI learns, there will always be a part of AI that is insufficient for its lack of human touch.

No machine or AI application could have helped my wife in the birth of our two children better than the caring hands of the people who had learned from their experiences of bringing tiny new lives into the world. Yet, AI too has a learning component. The warmth of a nurse's comforting hand during an outpatient procedure cannot be accomplished by way of AI, but the procedure and the nurse's training may be vastly improved for it.

Do we want to remove human doctors from the medical care of humans? I think the answer is definitively no, but AI holds the promise of helping humans care for each other in ways that were once impossible.

About the Author

Daniel J. Barchi, MEM, is Senior Vice President and Chief Information Officer of NewYork–Presbyterian, one of the largest healthcare providers in the United States and the university hospitals of Columbia and Cornell. He leads 2,000 technology, pharmacy, informatics, artificial intelligence, and telemedicine specialists who deliver the tools, data, and medicine that physicians and nurses use to deliver acute care and manage population health.

Daniel previously led healthcare technology as CIO at Yale and earlier as CIO of the Carilion Health System. He was president of the Carilion Biomedical Institute and Director of Technology for MCI WorldCom. Daniel graduated from Annapolis, began his career as a US Naval officer at sea, and was awarded the Navy Commendation Medal for leadership and the Southeast Asia Service Medal for Iraq operations in the Red Sea.

References

Abbott, Brianna. (2020). "Google AI Beats Doctors at Breast Cancer Detection – Sometimes." *The Wall Street Journal*, January 2.

Davenport, Thomas H. and Rajeev Ronanki, Rajeev. (2018). "Artificial Intelligence for the Real World." *Harvard Business Review*, January–February 2018.

Livingston, Shelby. (2016). "Physicians Beat Symptom Checkers in Test of Diagnostic Accuracy." *Modern Healthcare*, December 10, 2016.

Matheny, M., Israni, T. S., Ahmed, M. and Whicher, D. Editors. (2019). "Artificial Intelligence in Health Care: The Hope, the Hype, the Promise, the Peril." *NAM Special Publication*. Washington, DC: National Academy of Medicine.

Mistry, Priyansha. (2016). "AI Therapist Developed for PTSD Counselling." *Technowize Magazine*, April 6.

Mukamal, Reena. (2019). Reviewed by Robert T. Chang, MD and Ravi D. Goel, MD. "Artificial Intelligence Can Support Ophthalmologists, Not Replace Them." *Ophthalmology*, May.

Murphy, Tom. (2019). "Paging Dr. Robot: Artificial Intelligence Makes Way into Health Care." *The Daily Herald*, November 30.

Olson, Parmy. (2018). "This Health Startup Won Big Government Deals – But Inside, Doctors Flagged Problems." *Forbes Daily Cover*, December 17, 2018.

Poplin, R., Varadarajan, A. V., Blumer, K., et al. (2018). "Prediction of Cardiovascular Risk Factors from Retinal Fundus Photographs via Deep Learning." *Nature Biomedical Engineering*, 2, 158–164. doi:10.1038/s41551-018-0195-0.

West, Darrell M. (2018). "What Is Artificial Intelligence?" *Brookings.edu*, October 4, 2018.

Chapter 10

Clinical and Business Intelligence

Ray Hess, FHIMSS, RRT, MSA

Contents

What Is Business Intelligence?

Business intelligence (BI) is a term that is used regularly in the healthcare industry. Most pundits assert that it is vital for effectively managing today's complex healthcare environment. However, many people have a hard time defining what BI is and certainly cannot recall its key elements. This chapter will present a simple overview of BI, starting with defining the term and moving on

DOI: 10.4324/9780429423109-10

to reviewing key elements and a simple strategy for using BI. Once the reader has a basic framework for understanding this key element, the chapter will delve into the merging of clinical data into BI. Finally, we discuss some advanced topics on BI. Know that this chapter only skims the surface of the topic; there are multiple referenced resources the reader should review if a deeper understanding is desired.

Here are several definitions of BI:

Business intelligence is a set of theories, methodologies, architectures, and technologies that transform raw data into meaningful and useful information for business purposes. BI can handle enormous amounts of unstructured data to help identify, develop, and otherwise create new opportunities. BI, in simple words, makes interpreting voluminous data friendly. Making use of new opportunities and implementing an effective strategy can provide a competitive market advantage and long-term stability.[1]

Business intelligence is an umbrella term that includes the applications, infrastructure and tools, and best practices that enable access to and analysis of information to improve and optimize decisions and performance.[2]

Business intelligence software (BI software) is software that turns raw data into information that businesses can use to create growth. BI software helps users to understand the strengths and weaknesses in their organizations by showing them the implications and meanings in their data. This information can be used to improve every aspect of a businsess.[3]

At first glance, these definitions might not appear to answer the question, what is business intelligence? However, there are several key concepts to be found in these definitions.

■ BI is a set of processes, software, or techniques
■ BI takes data and seeks to turn it into information that results in intelligence
■ BI seeks to give understanding to the user
■ BI exists to help manage and improve the functioning of the business
■ BI can show the user opportunities that otherwise may have been missed

Healthcare BI is the tool that allows the user to know about the operations of the healthcare system. It is analogous to a patient's vital signs and test results. They tell the doctor about the patient and provide direction toward the proper treatment. Healthcare BI tells the administrator about the healthcare system and provides direction for how to manage the organization.

Why Is Business Intelligence Important?

This book is filled with chapters showing the complexity of today's healthcare environment. Each chapter presents another in an ongoing list of challenges that faces the current day administrator. BI is the tool that allows leaders to know as accurately as possible how things are going, the performance of their system, the issues that need to be addressed, and opportunities that exist. Without BI, the executive is literally flying blind.

BI provides key and timely information needed to make wise decisions. Despite the importance of BI, why is there confusion and at times a lack of consistency in implementing BI in the healthcare environment? The answer lies in the complexity of creating a solid and effective BI infrastructure. BI has many components, each of which must be understood, implemented, and managed. Getting good BI takes work, time, and resources. There is a commitment that needs to be made to achieve successful results.

Key Elements of Business Intelligence

Here is a list of elements that make up BI. The reader will see that these elements often build or depend on one another. This list is not exhaustive, but it will present some of the core items needed to understand BI and to create a strong BI system.

Data Collection

Data collection is at the foundation of any and every BI process. It is the most basic element of BI, and the effectiveness of any BI program rests on the quality of the data involved. Data represent each element saved in the computer systems from every activity that occurs. It can be data about the patient, such as test result values. It can represent demographics about the patient or the clinicians providing care to the patient, such as address or age. It can be charges, costs, or time values. Data can be anything, and data are everything that is captured by the systems.

Many important pieces of data historically were not captured in systems. A key to BI is understanding what data exist electronically and what data need to be captured and put into systems for future use. Without data, there can be no knowledge of what is going on in a health system. Without the data first being collected into a system, there cannot be any meaningful evaluation or reporting. The first challenge in any BI effort is discovering the state of the healthcare institution's data. BI professionals cannot stop with knowing what data exists but must discover what data are needed to effectively monitor and report on the healthcare system. Over time, BI success depends on collecting key data into a system where it can be used.

Data Governance

Because data are the foundation for producing information, there must be a structure in place to evaluate and manage data. That structure is called data governance. The Data Governance Institute defines data governance this way:

> Data Governance is a system of decision rights and accountabilities for information-related processes, executed according to agreed-upon models which describe who can take what actions with what information, and when, under what circumstances, using what methods.[4]

Data governance represents the rules and definitions that let everyone know how to interact with data. There are many aspects of data governance that are beyond the scope of this chapter. These include data definitions, data quality, data integrity, data completeness, how the data can be used, and by whom. Readers are encouraged to go to the Data Governance Institute website to obtain further information on data governance.

For the purposes of this discussion, key data governance issues revolve around making sure that vital pieces of data are consistently captured using the same definition or process. A simple example is the collection of a patient's pain level. Free text inputs like "moderate" or "slight" are much harder to work with and evaluate than a set numeric pain scale of "1" to "10" with definitions of when to use each number. Having a number over the free text entry allows for a greater ability to collate and track the effectiveness of pain interventions. This is just one simple example of how data governance sets the rules and patterns for capturing usable data. Data governance is an important function that must receive regular attention for BI output to be trustworthy.

Creating a Data Warehouse

Data are created and stored in operational systems throughout the healthcare environment. Most of these systems are designed to optimize the function for which they were designed (an EMR or a cardiology system) and are not designed to provide data for analysis and reporting. A data warehouse is a database system that is designed specifically to hold and manage data for use in BI activities. The data are harvested from the source systems using a process called ETL: extract, transform, and load. Once in the data warehouse, the data can be validated, standardized, and collated for use. There are many resources on data warehousing on the web. The Data Warehouse Institute[5] is one such resource that can provide more information on data warehousing.

Reporting

The creation of reports is one of the oldest and most common BI activities. Data need to be consolidated, filtered, and placed into an easily readable format before they can be used. Reports do just that. The report writer creates a query to pull the appropriate data and then places those data in a report shell to make it easy for people to read and understand. There are many types of reports, but the most basic ones show tabular or graphic representations of summarized data.

Figure 10.1 shows a basic report of inpatient activity for a given month. The report shows the patients summarized by the diagnosis-related group (DRG) based diagnosis and gives details

American Hospital
Inpatient Volume by DRG
For the Month of: May 2014

DRG	Description	Volume	Days	Length	Mortality
795	Normal newborn	144	291	2.0	0
775	Vaginal delivery w/o complicating diagnoses	119	238	2.0	0
871	Septicemia or severe sepsis w/o MV 96+ hours w MCC	83	450	5.4	4
872	Septicemia or severe sepsis w/o MV 96+ hours w/o MCC	39	185	4.7	2
392	Esophagitis, gastroent & misc digest disorders w/o MCC	32	132	4.1	1
603	Cellulitis w/o MCC	31	103	3.3	0
794	Neonate w other significant problems	31	304	9.8	0
774	Vaginal delivery w complicating diagnoses	31	75	2.4	0
470	Major joint replacement or reattachment of lower extremity w/o	26	75	2.9	0
765	Cesarean section w CC/MCC	25	73	2.9	0
766	Cesarean section w/o CC/MCC	24	58	2.4	0
793	Full term neonate w major problems	17	67	3.9	0
291	Heart failure & shock w MCC	15	72	4.8	2
683	Renal failure w CC	15	68	4.5	1
189	Pulmonary edema & respiratory failure	13	47	3.6	1
292	Heart failure & shock w CC	12	55	4.6	1
308	Cardiac arrhythmia & conduction disorders w MCC	12	41	3.4	1
310	Cardiac arrhythmia & conduction disorders w/o CC/MCC	12	32	2.7	0
309	Cardiac arrhythmia & conduction disorders w CC	11	37	3.4	0
690	Kidney & urinary tract infections w/o MCC	11	35	3.2	0
287	Circulatory disorders except AMI, w card cath w/o MCC	10	43	4.3	0
682	Renal failure w MCC	10	42	4.2	1
419	Laparoscopic cholecystectomy w/o c.d.e. w/o CC/MCC	9	13	1.4	0
331	Major small & large bowel procedures w/o CC/MCC	9	39	4.3	0
343	Appendectomy w/o complicated principal diag w/o CC/MCC	9	21	2.3	0
247	Perc cardiovasc proc w drug-eluting stent w/o MCC	9	22	2.4	0
792	Prematurity w/o major problems	9	78	8.7	0
176	Pulmonary embolism w/o MCC	9	37	4.1	0
378	G.I. hemorrhage w CC	8	35	4.4	1

Figure 10.1   Basic DRG Report

like volume of patients, length of stay, and mortality. Depending on the reason for the report, it can be enhanced by adding charges, cost, and reimbursement. If DRGs are too granular, the report (See Figure 10.2) can be changed to show DRG groupings by services such as cardiology, surgery, etc. These data are displayed in a summary report that explodes into DRG detail for each service line. If more detail is needed, a report can be created (Figure 10.3) showing detail at a patient level.

American Hospital
Inpatient Volume by Service Line
For the Month of: May 2019

Service Line	DRG	Description	Volume	Days	Length of Stay	Mortality
CARDIAC SURGERY			15	67	4.5	1
DERMATOLOGY			36	81	2.3	0
ENDOCRINOLOGY			23	89	3.9	1
GASTROENTEROLOGY			91	372	4.1	2
GENERAL MEDICINE			145	599	4.1	4
GENERAL SURGERY			24	68	2.8	0
GI SURGERY			59	183	3.1	0
GYNECOLOGY			6	23	3.8	0
HEMATOLOGY			10	48	4.8	1
INTERVENTIONAL CARDIOLOGY			32	79	2.5	1
MEDICAL CARDIOLOGY			103	483	4.7	3
NEONATOLOGY			67	532	7.9	2
NEPHROLOGY/UROLOGY			63	244	3.9	1
NEUROLOGY			46	135	2.9	0
NEUROSURGERY			7	45	6.4	0
NORMAL NEWBORN			144	293	2.0	0
OBSTETRICS-DEL			204	408	2.0	0
OBSTETRICS-NO DEL			13	39	3.0	0
ONCOLOGY MEDICAL			12	68	5.7	2
ONCOLOGY SURGICAL			4	21	5.3	0
OPHTHALMOLOGY			0	0	0.0	0
ORTHO MEDICAL			13	38	2.9	0
ORTHO SURGICAL			63	234	3.7	0
OTHER			9	39	4.3	0
OTOLARYNGOLOGY			13	38	2.9	0
PLASTIC SURGERY			7	16	2.3	0
PSYCHIATRY			2	8	4.0	0
PULMONARY MEDICINE			71	352	5.0	4
SPINE			5	29	5.8	0
SUBSTANCE ABUSE			1	8	8.0	0
THORACIC SURGERY			7	37	5.3	1
TRACHEOSTOMY			3	15	5.0	1
TRAUMA/INJURIES			2	34	17.0	1
Unclassified			3	14	4.7	0
VASCULAR SURGERY			6	28	4.7	0

Figure 10.2   Service Line Report

American Hospital
Inpatient Discharge Detail
For the Month of: May 2019

Name	Gender	Age	MsDrg	MsDrg Desc	Admit Date	Dsch Date	Length of Stay	Adm Src Desc	Dsch Disp	Dsch Disp Desc
Jane Doe	F	44	603	Cellulitis w/o MCC	4/28/2019	5/2/2019	4	EMERGENCY FROM HOME	AHR	Routine discharge
Mary Smith	F	76	470	Major joint replacement or reattachment of lower extremity w/o MCC	4/29/2019	5/2/2019	3	FAMILY PHYSICIAN REFERRAL	ATE	Trans/disch to extended skilled nursing
John Doe	M	0	795	Normal newborn	4/28/2019	4/30/2019	2	Born inside this hospital	AHR	Routine discharge
Nancy Jones	F	34	775	Vaginal delivery w/o complicating diagnoses	4/30/2019	5/2/2019	2	FAMILY PHYSICIAN REFERRAL	AHR	Routine discharge
Tom Jones	M	61	863	Postoperative & post-traumatic infections w/o MCC	4/29/2019	5/2/2019	3	FAMILY PHYSICIAN REFERRAL	AHR	Routine discharge
Baby Boy Warren	M	0	795	Normal newborn	4/30/2019	5/2/2019	2	Born inside this hospital	AHR	Routine discharge
Tammy Warren	F	37	775	Vaginal delivery w/o complicating diagnoses	4/30/2019	5/2/2019	2	FAMILY PHYSICIAN REFERRAL	AHR	Routine discharge
Roy Dupont	M	78	853	Infectious & parasitic diseases w O.R. procedure w MCC	4/23/2019	5/3/2019	10	EMERGENCY FROM HOME	ATW	TRANS. HHA CARE RELATED TO ADM
Cheryl Hart	F	22	951	Other factors influencing health status	4/30/2019	5/2/2019	2	FAMILY PHYSICIAN REFERRAL	AHR	Routine discharge
Baby Girl Walker	F	0	795	Normal newborn	4/30/2019	5/2/2019	2	Born inside this hospital	AHR	Routine discharge
Grandma Wise	F	72	220	Cardiac valve & oth maj cardiothoracic proc w/o card cath w CC	4/25/2019	5/3/2019	8	FAMILY PHYSICIAN REFERRAL	ATW	TRANS. HHA CARE RELATED TO ADM
Peter Parker	M	56	101	Seizures w/o MCC	4/29/2019	5/3/2019	4	EMERGENCY FROM HOME	AHR	Routine discharge

Figure 10.3   Patient Detail Report

Reports are powerful tools if they are created properly and if the underlying data are solid. They are the basis for most BI activity. Reports are used in all aspects of management. In some places, BI is only reporting. While reporting always needs to be a part of any functional BI structure, it should not be the only tool available to the executive.

Dashboards

Many busy leaders do not have time to wade through complex reports trying to understand what is happening in their institution. They want something that quickly provides them with the information they need to know. They desire information that tells them where to focus their attention. Dashboards are the tool that provides this requirement. A dashboard should be just like the dashboard on a car. It needs to be something that the viewer can glance at quickly to see the status of things. Dashboards are graphic in nature and usually only provide very high-level information. Some advanced dashboards link into drilldown reports and or have alerts that can be set to notify the user if a certain set of conditions occur.

Figure 10.4 shows a basic dashboard for operational activity. It presents the activity by various departments for a given month and year to date. The dashboard, if seen in color, has various items highlighted as red, yellow, or green. This lets the observer know instantly how the metric is doing. The reader should note that the dashboard also contains budget numbers. Budgets are necessary to provide a context for how a function or metric is doing. Without them, a number has no reference and does not provide necessary information needed to determine if everything is okay or not. The role of the dashboard is to give the leader quick understandable information at a glance. The dashboard tells the executive the status of things: either the indicators are okay or there is an issue. Reports and analytics will be used to identify the causes of an issue, not a dashboard. The dashboard only raises the flag that something is off target.

American Hospital
Operational Dashboard: Overall Hospital Indicators For May 2019

Indicators		May 2014	Budget	Variance #	Variance %		Prior Year	Change #	Change %		May 2014	Budget	Variance #	Variance %		Prior Year	Change #
Total IP Discharges, Observation and Extended Stay		1,581	1,501	80	5.4%	●	1,522	59	3.9%	●	17,432	16,663	769	4.6%	●	16,596	836
Inpatient Discharges		1,309	1,276	33	2.6%	●	1,273	36	2.8%	●	13,668	14,224	-556	-3.9%	◐	14,153	-485
Observation Patients		202	225	-23	-10.1%	●	249	-47	-18.9%	●	2,674	2,439	235	9.6%	●	2,443	231
Medical Observation Patients		186	144	42	29.2%	◐	154	32	20.8%	◐	1,837	1,564	273	17.5%	◐	1,555	282
Surgical Observation Patients		16	81	-65	-80.1%	●	95	-79	-83.2%	●	837	875	-38	-4.3%	●	888	-51
Extended Stay		70				●	0	70		●	230				●	0	230
Operational Avg LOS		3.79	3.87	-0.08	-2.0%	●	3.69	0.11	2.9%	●	3.78	3.87	0	-2.5%	●	3.88	-0.10
Emergency Department																	
ED Total		3,902	3,569	333	9.3%	●	3,583	319	8.9%	●	39,504	38,771	733	1.9%	●	38,365	1,139
Total ED Admissions and Observation		950	920	30	3.3%	●	885	65	7.3%	●	9,718	9,994	-276	-2.8%	◐	9,939	-221
ED Admissions		754	776	-22	-2.8%	◐	734	20	2.7%	●	7,814	8,426	-612	-7.3%	●	8,396	-582
ED Observation		196	144	52	35.8%	◐	151	45	29.8%	●	1,904	1,568	336	21.4%	●	1,543	361
ED Discharges		2,952	2,649	303	11.4%	●	2,698	254	9.4%	●	29,786	28,777	1,009	3.5%	●	28,426	1,360
Outpatient Registrations		21,072	21,072	0	0.0%	○	21,575	-503	-2.3%	●	222,702	228,908	-6,206	-2.7%	◐	227,056	-4,354

Figure 10.4   Hospital Dashboard

Analytics

Analytics is a term that can mean many things, and it is being used more and more commonly in the healthcare arena. For this discussion, it represents the process that an analyst uses to understand what the data are showing (See Figure 10.1). Using the previous examples, suppose the dashboard shows that admissions are down; specifically, the report shows that it is cardiology admissions that are lower than expected. In this scenario, analytics would be used to determine what is causing the cardiology patient volumes to have fallen. The analyst would run various reports and use tools to look for the reason for the decrease. Analytics represent the processes that glean information from the data. The information is then used to determine why something is not as expected. Analytics can also be used to look for positive trends and opportunities for growth and development. Analytics represents the process of using data to create information that can provide intelligence for intervention, action, or change.

Benchmarking

The final core element of BI that will be discussed is benchmarking. Benchmarking is the process of getting other institutions' data or external target numbers for the metrics being tracked. Is a length of stay of five days for a given DRG good or bad? How are other hospitals of a similar size and makeup doing with their readmission rates? How much should a knee replacement cost? These are all questions that benchmarking data can help answer.

For benchmarking to work, every participant must use the same definitions and counting methodology. This is external data governance, which represents a key requirement for benchmarking to work. The benchmark requirement must be clear for the benchmark data to be valid and valuable. A good example of this is readmissions. Different payers use different definitions for readmissions. Before one institution can compare itself with other institutions, all must agree on which readmission definition to follow. While this may sound easy, it can often be challenging.

Without agreement, the comparisons are weak at best, useless or dangerous at worst. Properly applied benchmarking data give the leaders fixed external points of reference that allow them to gauge how they are doing or to set realistic targets.

A Solid Business Intelligence Strategy

The seven elements previously mentioned are not an exhaustive list of BI components, but they do represent a good starting point for understanding what needs to be included in a solid BI strategy. This strategy should grow out of the organization's strategic plans. The senior team needs to define the priorities for the institution. Once these are set, the BI team can start to formulate its strategy to support these strategic initiatives. BI support starts with ensuring that the data needed to track and evaluate the strategic initiatives are captured in a consistent and appropriate manner in the data warehouse. The team then creates reports and dashboards to track the metrics around the strategic initiatives. The key priorities for the institution should always drive the BI work plan.

In addition to the strategic plan, the BI strategy must include methods to support regulatory requirements and key clinical and business functions. The BI strategy should never be created in a vacuum; rather, it should be a collaborative and inclusive effort in which all the stakeholders have an opportunity to provide input and express their needs. The BI team will take this information and create a framework for delivering the required information. The plan should be considered the guide for BI development activity, but this cannot be too rigid. Healthcare requirements are constantly evolving, and the BI plan needs to be able to flex as changes occur or new needs arise.

The strategy, once developed, should be presented to the senior team and approved. A strategy will only be effective if it has the support of administration and only if it is known and under-stood by the management team generally. Therefore, the strategy should be presented to the entire management team once it is approved. Many of the managers in the institution will be involved in data governance activities and/or are consumers of the output of the BI efforts. Over time, the BI team will develop a comprehensive set of reports, dashboards, and other tools that give managers the information they need to effectively run their part of the business.

Clinical and Business Intelligence

The title of this chapter is "Clinical and Business Intelligence," but up to this point only BI has been discussed. Until recently, clinical intelligence referred only to data that was used in treating the patient. This book includes a full chapter on clinical decision support (CDS). CDS targets clinicians and helps ensure they are alerted to key elements regarding a patient's care. Over the last several years, there has been a rapidly increasing adoption of EMR technology, resulting in rich databases of clinical data. This clinical data, once used only for patient care and CDS, is now being incorporated into reporting data warehouses and used to provide richer information and intelligence.

In the healthcare environment, clinical data are often a key requirement to making good busi-ness decisions. After all, the business of healthcare and clinical care is what healthcare is about. This merger of the two data sets is important if an institution hopes to survive and thrive in the changing healthcare environment. VTE (venous thromboembolism) is a good example of this concept. VTE is a high-risk condition that is often preventable with proper intervention. It is also the focus of many quality measures and a subject of pay-for-performance payer contracts. CDS will evaluate a patient, recognize the need for prophylactic anticoagulant therapy or other VTE measures, and alert the clinician. The alert is focused on an individual and the care that he or she needs to receive. Clinical and business intelligence (C&BI) aggregates the individual data and tracks trends and compliance. If the VTE prophylaxis rate is unacceptable, C&BI will provide drilldowns to look at the compliance of doctors to the CDS alerts or other factors that may be affecting the success of the VTE measure. By merging the clinical data into the BI warehouse, the system is now able to track a key performance metric that has direct reimbursement implications.

EMR systems are not designed to report data in a grouped fashion. They are optimized for transactional activity focused around one patient. Therefore, the EMR data need to be pulled into a data warehouse where it can be combined with business data in a relational format. This makes it much easier to look at the profitability of patient care, the effectiveness of various treatment regimes, and the performance of clinical programs from an efficiency or outcomes perspective. Understanding data makes the merger of clinical and business data sets a natural extension of historic BI activities. Clinical and business data combined into one large data warehouse is a very powerful source of intelligence for today's leaders. It is a necessary step forward that must be taken in today's healthcare environment.

Advanced Business Intelligence

A discussion of BI would not be complete without reviewing some the new and exciting tools that are currently being developed and used by BI professionals. This section will review four areas that are being integrated into healthcare BI. Many of these tools have been used for years in other industries but only recently in healthcare. These tools allow the BI profession to provide even greater value to the healthcare management team.

Data Mining

Data mining uses artificial intelligence techniques, neural networks, and advanced statistical tools (such as cluster analysis) to reveal trends, patterns, and relationships that might otherwise have remained undetected.[6] There is so much clinical and business data and so many variables to be examined that a computer program is often needed to effectively find patterns in the data. Data mining is the software process that performs these automated searches. The technique has been used for many years in other industries, but it could not handle the complexity of healthcare data until recently. Part of the challenge is that healthcare data is frequently inconsistent from patient to patient. An even bigger problem has been the large volume of unstructured data that exists in healthcare. As data mining software has advanced, it can now start to be applied to healthcare to handle these inherent challenges.

In data mining, the analyst asks a question, creates a profile for the mining tool based on that question, and then the software digs through the data looking for patterns that might provide clues to answer the question. Here is an example of how data mining might be applied in a healthcare setting. Consider a scenario in which there is a certain disease condition with divergent outcomes. One group of patients responds to treatment and recovers while another group seems to languish and not improve. Data mining could be used to profile the two sets of patients and find commonalities in the treatment regime, test results, patient history, genetics, or other elements that may represent hidden factors causing the difference in outcomes. If the sampling size is big enough, this technology can look at treatment sequencing and when interventions during the patient's course of care are most effective.

Data mining is becoming a necessary tool for the BI professional as data sets grow and become more complex. There is too much data to manually process, evaluate, and review. The key to effective data mining is knowing when and where data mining can be applied safely and appropriately to answer complex questions. As healthcare database sizes continue to grow, the use of data mining will become more prominent. It will become a foundational component of a solid BI toolkit.

Modeling and Simulation

Another area of advanced BI is the use of modeling and simulation software. This software allows the user to create a model of a working process or function. The model can be of a clinical unit such as the emergency department or operating suite. It can also be of a process such as registration or the flow for a testing procedure.

Developing the model can be challenging. The user follows strict parameters and often uses statistical representations of actual observed activity that is collected via time and motion studies. Models of physical locations may use a computer-aided design (CAD) drawing to set up a realistic scale rendering of the unit. Models use probability and statistics to randomly determine how the modeled item will function on a given day. The model is then run hundreds or thousands of times, each representing a day, and the output is compared with the actual recorded activity of the unit or function. The model is tweaked until it provides a statistically accurate simulation of the observed values of the targeted unit or process.

Once the baseline model is completed and the iterations have shown it to be statistically sound, the analyst is then able to change one or more factors in the model. Each change represents a potential process change. The model is rerun several hundred or thousand times and the new results are captured. If done correctly, the model will produce a statistically valid representation of how a possible change will alter the overall process being studied. Changes to a working process often have a big impact on time, cost, and cause functional disruption. Simulation software is used to help ensure that the actions being considered will have the desired outcome and ultimately be successful. A model can statistically predict how an alteration will impact the process. It can protect the process from ineffective and costly failures.

In one non-healthcare setting, the weather service uses and presents models regularly. Anytime there is a hurricane, the various models build on the accumulated data and science of meteorology to project the path of the storm. There are often multiple models, and the average drawn from the models is shown by the weather station. The same type of science is being applied in healthcare modeling. Obviously, the storm tracker is not 100 percent accurate; however, it is usually good at determining the general area and time frame for a storm to make land. Healthcare modeling software is evolving just like meteorological storm models did over the years. One difference between the weather service and healthcare modeling, however, is that in healthcare, the model is set to mimic actual processes and then altered to see the effect. As experience is gained, healthcare modeling is becoming stronger and more reliable in predicting the effects of process changes. With many of these advanced concepts, it is often prudent to get expert support when first starting to use these tools.

Forecasting and Predictive Analytics

Forecasting and predictive analytics are similar to modeling and simulation. Using the previous weather analogy, the forecast is not a model of a storm but a scientifically based prediction of rain, the daily temperature, etc. Forecasting is similar in healthcare. The BI analyst uses scientific processes to predict the future. This is seen regularly in healthcare today. There are forecasts of decreased inpatient admissions due to increasing use of observation status or the "two midnight" rule established by the Centers for Medicare and Medicaid Services (CMS). Other forecasts include the actuarial projections of increases in healthcare utilization as the baby boomers move into their senior years. These techniques have been used for population health analysis for many years.

At an individual healthcare institution level, there are also many types of forecasting that can be done. Properly performed, this process can alert the management team to future trends or direct them to the most appropriate choices. Forecasting software can predict how bringing an additional orthopedic surgeon on staff might increase operating room volumes. It can project bed utilization, staffing requirements, or changes in profitability based on proposed alterations in an insurer contract. Forecasting can be a powerful tool, but it must be completely understood and used wisely. Otherwise, the predictions lose their credibility and following them could be dangerous.

Big Data

There are many aspects to big data and many complex definitions. Here is a simple one: data sets, typically consisting of billions or trillions of records, that are so vast and complex that they require new and powerful computational resources to process.[7] *Big data* is a term used to describe the incredible amounts of data stored in computers today and refers to the tools and/or techniques needed to manage and work with those data. Big data in healthcare often refers to vast amounts of clinical data from across the continuum of care, genomics data, and other types of input such as data from devices that continually monitor the patient. All these data are too much for many traditional data warehouse products to manage. New big-data methodologies and systems are being created to work with this vast ocean of data.

As healthcare moves toward population health management and personalized healthcare, the management of these massive data sets will be a key to success. Big data has come to encompass efforts to harness and manage these data, using it to discover and direct care. The sheer volume is causing the industry to develop and use new tools and techniques. However, at the core of this new and exciting element of BI is still the same foundational reality. Data governance, a solid warehouse structure, good querying and reporting tools, and solid analytics are the pillars of big data just as they are for all BI. Layered on top of these pillars are the new tools that take this massive amount of data and turn it into useful information, which then provides intelligence to the manager.

Summary

Business intelligence is a vital part of healthcare management today. It is used to transform data into information and information into intelligence. It is a key factor in assuring the success of a healthcare institution. Good clinical care requires a functioning and financially stable business framework within to operate. BI provides today's leaders with the knowledge they need to manage effectively. Without it, they would be managing blind. The addition of clinical data into the data warehouse allows leaders to gain deeper insight into how their clinical processes are functioning. The merger of clinical and BI allows managers to have a complete view of how the healthcare operation is performing.

This chapter only skimmed the surface of C&BI. Hopefully it has provided the reader with a functional understanding of the basic tenets of the subject. If the reader is interested in additional information on the topic, a reference to a more in-depth review of BI can be found in the notes.[8]

About the Author

Ray Hess, FHIMSS, RRT, MSA, is Director of Data Analytics for Penn Medicine, the University of Pennsylvania Health System, in Philadelphia. Ray has over 40 years of healthcare experience. His information management and process improvement experience includes having overseen business intelligence for 18 years, health information management for 6 years, and workflow automation/clinical decision support efforts for 10 years. He is a Six Sigma Green Belt. His clinical experience includes 10 years in patient care and rehabilitation, and he has administrative experience from managing cardiology services for 4 years. He holds a master's degree in healthcare administration from West Chester University. Hess has addressed audiences throughout the United States and internationally and has published multiple articles and book chapters. Hess is a fellow of HIMSS and is involved in multiple HIMSS communities and projects. He currently oversees data analytics and healthcare information exchange for Penn Medicine.

References

1. Rud O. *Business Intelligence Success Factors: Tools for Aligning Your Business in the Global Economy.* Hoboken, NJ: Wiley & Sons; 2009. ISBN 978-0-470-39240-9.
2. http://www.gartner.com/it-glossary/business-intelligence-bi/. Accessed November 17, 2014.
3. http://businessintelligence.com/dictionary/business-intelligence-software/. Accessed November 17, 2014.
4. http://datagovernance.com/adg_data_governance_definition/. Accessed November 17, 2014.
5. http://tdwi.org/Home.aspx. Accessed November 17, 2014.
6. http://www.businessdictionary.com/definition/data-mining.html. Accessed November 17, 2014.
7. McKinney C, Hess R, Whitecar M, eds. *Implementing Business Intelligence in your Healthcare Organization.* Chicago, IL: HIMSS; 2012. ISBN 978-0-9844577-5-5.
8. http://www.simulation-modeling.com/project_detail.asp?pcid=1&pid=16. Accessed November 17, 2014.

Chapter 11

Promoting Interoperability and Quality Payment Programs
The Evolving Paths of Meaningful Use

Anantachai (Tony) Panjamapirom, PhD,
Naomi Levinthal, MS and Ye Hoffman, MSc

Contents

DOI: 10.4324/9780429423109-11

Introduction

The US health care industry has undergone a number of transformations over the past several decades. In efforts to curb the growing cost of health care services and improve care quality, the federal government has employed different mechanisms, including various types of payment reform. However, many of these efforts did not achieve their intended goals and inadvertently furthered health care system fragmentation.[1–3] Since the turn of the decade, the government has undertaken another round of transformation with an eager focus to shift both providers and payers from largely fee-for-service, volume-based health care delivery to value-based, patient-centered payment models. As the largest payer of health care services, the Centers for Medicare and Medicaid Services (CMS) has launched many new payment models that base providers' payments on quality, efficiency, and effectiveness of care rendered to patients. These payment models often share a common strategy that requires the use of health information technology (HIT) to support care delivery processes. This is because HIT is an essential tool for providers and health systems to improve quality of care, increase efficiency, and promote patient engagement.

The American Recovery and Reinvestment Act of 2009 (ARRA), signed into law to help the country recover from an economic downturn, was also one of the most influential legislations that has shifted the health care industry into the digital era. Incorporated within ARRA, the Health Information Technology for Economic and Clinical Health (HITECH) Act established the Office of the National Coordinator for health IT (ONC) and the CMS Electronic Health Record (EHR) Incentive Programs, also known as meaningful use (MU). Through these initiatives, the HITECH Act mandated Medicare and Medicaid incentive payments for hospitals and clinicians (herein referred to jointly as providers) that were able to demonstrate adoption and "meaningful use" of certified EHR technology (CEHRT).

It is undeniable that the MU program has led to a significant increase in EHR adoption rates. From 2008 to 2017, the EHR adoption rate among office-based physicians more than doubled, increasing from 42% to 86%.[4] Similarly, hospitals have shown a noteworthy EHR adoption rate. As of 2017, 96% of all non-federal acute care hospitals have implemented CEHRT.[5]

While the MU program has made a notable impact on EHR adoption, the complex requirements have also created a number of challenges for providers. Over the years, CMS has aimed to reduce burden, including modifications to the program that postponed certain key requirements to support provider and vendor readiness. At times, CMS has also implemented large-scale changes to completely overhaul the program's requirements and goals. Effective April 2018, the

EHR Incentive Programs was renamed to the Promoting Interoperability (PI) Programs. This chapter focuses on the evolution of PI for two sets of stakeholders: 1) Medicare hospitals and Medicaid hospitals and providers that participate in PI as a standalone program; and 2) Medicare providers that must report PI through the new CMS Quality Payment Program (QPP). This chapter also explains the QPP program, as it reflects the newest set of PI-related reporting requirements.

Promoting Interoperability

The Evolution of PI

At a basic level, the HITECH ACT provides financial incentives to certain eligible providers if they adopt CEHRT and meet all PI program requirements. The first opportunity for providers to collect a payment was 2011. Incentives continued through 2016 for Medicare providers and through 2021 for Medicaid providers, depending on the year the provider began PI participation. While CMS deems the program voluntary, providers are in fact mandated to successfully participate in the program after a certain period to avoid a Medicare financial penalty that started in 2015.

Since the start of the program, CMS has made annual regulatory updates to PI program structure and requirements. Table 11.1 highlights the modifications made effective by each corresponding rule.

The HITECH Act did not specify an end date to the Medicare PI program, unless otherwise required per subsequent statute (e.g., MACRA for the Medicare EP PI program). Additionally, the Act originally mandated that PI became increasingly stringent over time. Even though the Bipartisan Budget Act of 2018[24] removed such statutory requirement, it does not eliminate the PI program. CMS may still choose to increase performance thresholds and evolve PI over time.

Table 11.1   Summary of the PI Evolution and the Corresponding Regulation

Agency	Regulation	Publication Date	Highlights
CMS and ONC	Stage 1[6] and 2011 Edition CEHRT[7]	July 28, 2010	Defined 2011 Edition EHR certification criteria, MU measures, and clinical quality measures (CQMs) to report for Stage 1
CMS and ONC	Stage 2[8] and 2014 Edition CEHRT[9]	September 4, 2012	Defined 2014 Edition EHR certification criteria, MU measures, and CQMs to report for Stage 2; and revised objectives for Stage 1
CMS	2014 Alternate Reporting Options[10]	September 4, 2014	Allowed certain providers to meet a different set of MU objectives and measures than the set they were scheduled to report due to delays with available CEHRT upgrades

(Continued)

Table 11.1 (Continued)

Agency	Regulation	Publication Date	Highlights
ONC	2014 Edition Release 2 Final Rule[11]	September 11, 2014	Revised 2014 Edition EHR certification criteria
CMS and ONC	Modified Stage 2 and Stage 3[12]; and 2015 Edition CEHRT[13]	October 16, 2015	Revised Stage 2 objectives and measures (i.e., Modified Stage 2); finalized Stage 3 requirements (but allowed for public comment); and defined 2015 Edition certification criteria
CMS	2017 MIPS and APM Final Rule[14]	November 4, 2016	Sunset the Medicare MU program for EPs and established the Quality Payment Program (QPP) under MACRA[15]
CMS	2017 OPPS Final Rule[16]	November 14, 2016	Shortened the 2016 and 2017 MU reporting period and eliminated objectives and reduced measure thresholds for Medicare hospitals in 2017 and 2018
CMS	2018 IPPS Final Rule[17]	August 14, 2017	Shortened the 2018 reporting period, and reduced hospital electronic CQM reporting requirements in 2017 and 2018
CMS	2019 IPPS Final Rule[18]	August 17, 2018	Changed the name of MU to PI and overhauled the Medicare hospital requirements with a new scoring methodology and fewer measures
CMS	2019 MPFS Final Rule[19]	November 23, 2018	Updated 2019 QPP policies for Medicare ECs, including a MIPS PI overhaul, and maintained Stage 3 PI requirements for Medicaid EPs with adjustments to some measure thresholds
CMS	2020 IPPS Final Rule[20]	August 16, 2019	Continued most 2019 PI reporting requirements affording program stability to hospitals for the first time in many years
CMS	2020 MPFS Final Rule[21]	November 1, 2019	Updated 2020 QPP policies, maintained required MIPS PI measure requirements, simplified or eliminated bonus opioid measures
CMS	2021 IPPS Final Rule[22]	September 18, 2020	Maintained PI objectives and measures and increased hospital electronic CQM reporting requirements for 2021 and beyond
CMS	2021 MPFS Final Rule[23]	December 28, 2020	Updated 2021 QPP policies, maintained required MIPS PI measure requirements and added an optional alternative bi-directional health information exchange measure

Eligibility, Incentive Payments, Penalties, and Hardship Exception

While CMS has revised a number of program requirements, many components of the program remain constant, such as eligibility, incentive payments, penalties, and hardship exceptions.

Eligibility

Not every hospital or physician is eligible to participate in PI. There are specific eligibility requirements depending on the provider's participation in Medicare and/or Medicaid (i.e., provide medical services to Medicare and/or Medicaid patients and receive Medicare and/or Medicaid reimbursement).

Eligible Hospital (EH)

Hospitals eligible to participate in the Medicare PI program include: "Subsection (d) hospitals,"[25] paid under the Inpatient Prospective Payment Systems (IPPS); critical access hospitals (CAH); and Medicare Advantage hospitals. EHs may also choose to participate and earn incentive in the Medicaid PI program if they have an average length of stay of 25 days or fewer and at least 10% Medicaid patient volumes. Children's hospitals are eligible for only Medicaid incentives and require no minimum Medicaid patient volumes.

In their first year of Medicaid PI participation, EHs can choose to adopt, implement, or upgrade (AIU) CEHRT to earn an incentive. In their second and subsequent participation years, EHs must satisfy PI objectives and measures. To reduce reporting burdens, CMS allows a dually eligible EH (i.e., eligible for both the Medicare and Medicaid PI programs) to attest in either the Medicare or Medicaid PI program in order to be deemed successful in both programs.

Eligible Provider (EP)

Unlike EHs that may be eligible for both Medicare and Medicaid PI incentives by attesting in either program, a dually eligible EP must decide in which program to participate. Once the decision was made, CMS allowed an EP to make a one-time switch between Medicare and Medicaid programs before 2015, after which the EP will remain in the program they participated in in 2014 for future years of the PI program.

An EP must be a doctor of medicine or osteopathy, a doctor of dental surgery or dental medicine, a doctor of podiatric medicine, a doctor of optometry, or a chiropractor. To be eligible for the Medicare PI program, the EP must have at least 50% of all patient encounters in a location that uses CEHRT and cannot be hospital-based. An EP is considered hospital-based if 90% or more of their services are performed in an inpatient setting or emergency department (i.e., place of service [POS] 21 and 23). Starting 2017, CMS sunset the PI program for Medicare EPs. Future Medicare eligible clinician (EC) payments will be based on the QPP established by MACRA (See further details in the Quality Payment Program section).

However, Medicaid EPs may continue to participate in the Medicaid PI program. Medicaid EP eligibility is determined by one of the following three criteria: 1) a minimum of 30% Medicaid patient volume; 2) a minimum 20% Medicaid patient volume and the EP is a pediatrician; or 3) the EP practices in a Federally Qualified Health Center (FQHC) or Rural Health Clinic (RHC) and has a minimum 30% patient volume attributable to "needy individuals." Medicaid EPs include other types of medical professionals beyond medical doctors, such as nurse practitioners and physician assistants. In their first year of participation, Medicaid EPs can demonstrate AIU to earn an incentive, and in subsequent participation years, EPs must satisfy PI objectives and measures.

Other Settings

Some types of care settings are ineligible to participate in PI. Eligibility criteria established within HITECH exclude behavioral health and long-term post-acute care (LTPAC) providers from PI. Legislative efforts to expand the eligibility criteria for benefit of other provider types have not been successful. However, EPs that practice at these settings may report PI if they otherwise meet the eligibility criteria.

Incentive Payments

Providers that successfully meet all program requirements within a program year are eligible for an incentive payment.

Eligible Hospital

EHs could begin participation to receive Medicare incentives in any year from 2011 to 2015, and 2016 was the last year in which the incentives were paid. Any EH that began Medicare PI participation in 2016 or subsequent years is not eligible for an incentive payment. EHs may receive incentives from Medicare for a maximum of four years. Payments to EHs are determined by several factors: discharge volume, Medicare charges, and a transition factor, which phases down the incentive payments over the four-year period. Medicare PI incentives are paid out in a consecutive manner. In other words, once an EH starts receiving a Medicare incentive payment, it must continue to do so until it exhausts all of the remaining incentives. Or else, if the hospital fails to successfully attest for a particular year, it automatically forfeits the associated incentive payment for that year. The hospital may make a comeback and still collect the remaining incentives after a "skip" year.

Hospital discharge volumes, Medicaid charges, and a state-based disbursement calculation determine Medicaid incentive payments, which can be distributed from three to six years in length, depending upon the state. Unlike the Medicare incentive payments, Medicaid EH incentive payments can be paid in non-consecutive years (i.e., an EH could "skip years" and still earn the maximum Medicaid incentive payments). However, starting CY 2017, EHs must receive an incentive payment in the previous year in order to continue to receive any remaining incentives, and 2021 is the final year EHs can earn any remaining Medicaid incentives.

Eligible Provider

Each Medicare EP is eligible for up to five incentive payments of about $43,000 in total, if they began in 2011 or 2012. As required by law, a 2% sequestration cut applies to all Medicare EHR incentive payments for a reporting period that ended on or after April 1, 2013. As a result, the total maximum incentive payments are less than the original value of $44,000. The sequestration cut does not apply to Medicaid EHR incentive payments.

Medicare incentivized EPs to begin PI early, as those who started in 2013 or 2014 receive substantially fewer incentives than those who began participation earlier. Any EP who began Medicare PI participation in 2015 or subsequent years is not eligible for an incentive payment.

Akin to their hospital counterparts, an EP must continue to collect Medicare incentive payments in a consecutive manner.

However, an EP may "skip years" in the Medicaid program and can receive incentives for up to six years. EPs may receive up to $63,750 in total (i.e., $21,250 for their first year of participation and $8,500 for each subsequent year). However, 2016 is the last year an EP can begin participation in the Medicaid PI program, and 2021 is the final year any remaining incentives will be paid.

Penalties or Payment Adjustments

EHs that fail to successfully meet all PI program requirements are subject to penalties, which are levied as a reduction in the hospital's Medicare reimbursement. EPs who fail to meet PI requirements are also subject to payment adjustments. However, from 2015 to 2018 they were applied as a PI-specific adjustment. Starting 2019 onward, the Medicare payment adjustment for EPs is based on their participation in the QPP program that began in 2017. There is no payment adjustment in the Medicaid PI Program.

Eligible Hospital

The first EH PI penalties started in payment year 2015 (i.e., October 1, 2014, based on the federal fiscal year). Adjustments are assessed in the payment year that occurs two years after the program year in which the EH fails to demonstrate PI. The adjustment is applied as a percentage reduction to the annual market basket update. Importantly, the adjustment is not cumulative and applies only in the payment year associated with the year that a hospital fails to demonstrate PI. Table 11.2 shows the percentage reduction associated with a payment year. For EHs, there is a financial imperative to meet PI each year because that reduction to the annual market basket update can equate to millions of dollars. This is because the reduction is taken out of all reimbursements received throughout the year that the hospital is subject to the penalty.

Eligible Provider

A Medicare PI penalty for an EP was applied as a percentage reduction in the Medicare Part B physician fee schedule (PFS) amount for covered professional services starting 2015 and future years (See Table 11.3). Payment adjustments are assessed two years after each year the EP fails

Table 11.2 Medicare EH Payment Adjustments

Payment Year	2015	2016	2017+
Percentage reduction in the annual market basket update	25%	50%	75%

Table 11.3 Medicare EP Payment Adjustments

Percent Adjustment of MPFS Amount	2015	2016	2017	2018
EP is not subject to the payment adjustment for the CMS Electronic Prescribing Incentive Program in 2014	99%	98%	97%	97%
EP is subject to the payment adjustment for the CMS Electronic Prescribing Incentive Program in 2014	98%	98%	97%	97%

to demonstrate PI. An EP eligible for both Medicare and Medicaid PI programs who chooses to participate in the Medicaid program is still subject to Medicare payment adjustment if they do not continue to demonstrate PI. The adjustment starts at 1% in 2015 and increases in the following years until 2018.

Starting in the 2019 payment year (tied to the 2017 performance year), the QPP imposes different rules to determine financial penalties for non-reporters and low performers in the MIPS payment track. Similar to EHs, Medicaid does not impose payment adjustments for EPs, and dually eligible EPs who choose to participate in the Medicaid PI program can avoid Medicare payment adjustment.

Hardship Exception

CMS uses a mechanism called a Hardship Exception application to allow providers with significant hardship to avoid the Medicare PI payment adjustment. If a Medicare-eligible provider (i.e., EH or EP) is unable to successfully demonstrate PI in any given year, the provider can file a hardship application with CMS to avoid the associated payment adjustment. If CMS grants the hardship exception, the penalty is waived for that payment year. If CMS denies the application, the penalty will be applied.

Hardships can be established for several reasons. For example, a provider that experienced a change in ownership for the organization can explain why they were unable to demonstrate PI under that circumstance. New hardship categories may be added through rulemaking and/or statute. For example, the 21st Century Cures Act introduced hardship exception categories for providers unable to meet PI due to CEHRT decertification, or providers that practice predominantly in Ambulatory Surgical Centers. Providers may only receive up to five total exceptions throughout the PI program. CMS publishes associated year-specific hardship exception forms and instructions on its program websites.

The Three Tenets of PI – Reporting Requirements

A successful attestation to PI means providers must satisfy three key tenets of the program: 1) use CEHRT; 2) meet all PI objectives/measures; and 3) report clinical quality measures (CQMs). Providers must attest to these requirements in each year of participation and comply with the specified reporting period and attestation deadline. Each tenet is further discussed next.

Use CEHRT

ONC issues regulations that identify the set of technical standards, implementation specifications, and certification criteria to which EHRs used for PI must be certified. Providers can license CEHRT as separate EHR modules for technologies certified to less than all certification criteria, or as bundled all together from a single module. Providers must select one or more CEHRT products listed in the Certified Health IT Product List (CHPL) website[26] to generate a certification ID for each year they attest to PI. While the website will create a certification ID once the selected products meet 100% base certification criteria, providers must ensure that they include other products needed to meet all required PI measures and reporting requirements. Moreover, it is important that providers confirm with their vendor(s) which exact products they possess because if the providers receive a PI audit, they will need to provide documentation to prove they used those specific systems during their reporting periods.

Meet PI Objectives and Measures

Through program year 2018, PI had three defined stages, with objectives that have one or more performance measures a provider must satisfy. From 2011 to 2014, there was a required set of objectives called Core objectives, and another set from which a provider could choose which objectives were best suited to their scope of practice and capabilities, called Menu objectives. Effective 2015 through 2018, CMS made all objectives required (with some limited year-by-year exceptions that allowed providers to incrementally satisfy requirements in a phased approach). Certain per-measure exclusions are available, for example, when a measure does not pertain to a provider's scope of practice.

The number of objectives an EH versus an EP must meet has traditionally varied over the years (See Table 11.4). Some measures are percentage-based with a required performance threshold, and others require that a task was performed or functionality enabled over a reporting period. All providers in their first year of PI can choose any consecutive 90-day time frame within their program year, and in other years the reporting periods vary between a program year, or program year-quarter, or 90-day period. Reporting period requirements are determined by CMS through rulemaking.

Historically, providers began the PI program under Stage 1 and moved consecutively through the stages. Providers met Stage 1 requirements for two to three years before they moved on to Stage 2. However, CMS eliminated this progression sequence in 2015 and instead aligns all providers to the same set of requirements for each year with options to report more advanced measures on a voluntary basis. Starting in 2019, CMS shed the "Stage"-based approach and instead establishes PI program requirements on a year-by-year basis. A brief discussion of the original three stages is provided next.

Stage 1

Stage 1 was meant to increase CEHRT adoption with a basic set of EHR functionalities. CMS revised original Stage 1 measures in 2014; thus, there were two sets of measures: the 2013 definition (original) and the 2014 definition (revised). Both definitions include objectives that measure how much data a provider collects for a patient; whether they implement a clinical decision support (CDS) intervention; perform a security risk analysis; and report public health data to a public health agency (PHA).

Table 11.4 Stage 1, Stage 2, and Modified Stage 2 Objectives[27]

Provider Type	Stage 1 2013 Definition	Stage 1 2014 Definition	Stage 2	Modified Stage 2
EH	– 12 core objectives – 5 menu from a list of 10 – 17 total	– 11 core objectives – 5 menu from a list of 10 – 16 total	– 16 core objectives – 3 menu from a list of 6 – 19 total	– 9 required objectives
EP	– 13 core objectives – 5 menu from a list of 10 – 18 total	– 13 core objectives – 5 menu from a list of 9 – 18 total	– 17 core objectives – 3 menu from a list of 6 – 20 total	– 10 required objectives

Stage 2 and Modified Stage 2

Stage 2 focuses on advanced clinical processes in three main areas: information exchange, care coordination, and patient engagement. Providers are measured on their ability to collect health information in the EHR, transmit summary of care records, report public health data to a PHA, and encourage patients to use patient portals or personal health records to view, download, or transmit their health information.

In 2015, CMS made major modifications to Stage 2 requirements to simplify program policies, reduce reporting burden, and align with Stage 3 requirements. Additionally, in November 2016 CMS eliminated certain Modified Stage 2 objectives in 2017 for Medicare EHs only, consistent with Stage 3 changes noted next.

Stage 3

Stage 3 builds upon Stage 2 and Modified Stage 2 objectives to enhance information exchange and drive data utilization to improve care delivery and outcomes. Table 11.5 presents the objectives finalized in October 2015. In November 2016, CMS eliminated certain objectives and reduced the number of required measures for Medicare EHs only. An asterisk (*) denotes eliminated objectives, and a double asterisk (**) indicates reduced measures (i.e., three of six required in CY 2017 and CY 2018).

Medicaid EPs who have remaining incentives to earn must report on Stage 3 measures starting 2019 with some adjustments to thresholds. For future years, CMS will specify the Medicare EP measures and reporting period through the annual MPFS final rule.

In contrast, Medicare EHs no longer report the original Stage 3 objectives and measures for 2019 and future years, but rather must meet updated objectives and measures based on the CMS overhaul of the PI program discussed next.

Annual Medicare EH PI Requirements (2019 Onward)

In an effort to reduce reporting burden and recast the focus of the PI program on interoperability and patient access to health information, CMS "overhauled" the Medicare EH requirements. CMS refreshed the measures and reconfigured the scoring methodology starting 2019.

Table 11.5   Stage 3 PI Objectives[27]

Stage 3 PI Objectives	Total Measures to Meet
1. Protect Patient Health Information	1
2. Electronic Prescribing	1
3. CDS*	2
4. Computerized Provider Order Entry (CPOE)*	3
5. Patient Electronic Access to Health Information	2
6. Coordination of Care Through Patient Engagement	2 of 3
7. Health Information Exchange (HIE)	2 of 3
8. Public Health and Clinical Data Registry Reporting	EPs: 2 of 5 EHs: 4** of 6

Compared to the original Stage 3 requirements, CMS reduced the total number of PI measures overall that hospitals must report. For example, they removed the requirement that measured patients' actions to view, download, or transmit their health information, but retained the measure that hospitals provide patients with access to their health information online. Table 11.6 provides the 2019 PI measures compared to the original Stage 3 requirements.

A new performance-based scoring methodology also becomes effective in 2019, instead of the previous all-or-nothing MU measure threshold requirements. As shown in Table 11.6, CMS no longer assigned a specific percentage-based threshold for each measure. Instead, hospitals earn points based on their performance across the required measures. Hospitals must report all required PI measures and additionally earn points across measures based on performance. Specifically, hospitals must meet three important measure criteria before points are scored. First, hospitals must conduct an annual security risk analysis and attest "Yes" to this measure. Second, hospitals must demonstrate that they have a numerator value of one (1) for all required measures. Third, hospitals must meet active engagement for any two out of six public health measures.

CMS establishes a different point potential for each measure. This allows Medicare EHs to focus performance on applicable measures. To satisfy 2019 PI program requirements, hospitals must earn a total of 50 or more points out of 100 to be considered a "meaningful EHR user." Another important change is the use of measure exclusions. In the past, when EHs claimed an exclusion for an applicable measure, the hospital simply skipped the measure and need not report performance. However, under the new scoring structure, when a hospital claims an exclusion, the points of the measure get shifted to other measures. For example, if an EH claims the electronic prescribing measure exclusion, the points get redistributed to both health information exchange measures, which makes each measure's point value increase to 25 total possible PI points, instead of 20. This has an important implication on a hospital's potential PI performance because they must ensure high levels of performance across fewer measures.

PI measures remain largely the same for 2020 and 2021, with only minor adjustments. CMS removed an optional measure under the electronic prescribing objective in 2020 but did not otherwise make changes to the scoring methodology or the required PI measures. Likewise, the 2021 PI measures are the same compared to the previous year, with only a small update to the name of one measure under the health information exchange objective.

For all future years of PI, CMS will specify the Medicare EH measures and reporting period requirements through the annual IPPS final rule. Thus, the measures and reporting requirements can vary from year to year, and hospitals must monitor the annual modifications to ensure compliance.

This last PI tenet requires providers to report certified electronic CQMs, which measure and track the quality of health care services in an effort to deliver high-quality care and/or meet long-term goals for quality health care (e.g., high levels of patient engagement). CMS works with organizations that endorse CQMs created by medical specialty societies and other health care industry groups. There are no performance thresholds to meet, and the CQM data must be reported exactly as generated by a provider's CEHRT. CMS establishes the number of required CQMs and the reporting period for PI each year through rulemaking.

CQM Alignment With Other CMS Programs

CQMs are included in many different CMS quality programs, not just PI. As a result, CMS has made steps to align those other reporting programs with CQM reporting requirements in PI to reduce duplicative efforts. In general, PI participants have two options to report CQM data: 1)

Table 11.6 2019 Medicare Hospital MU to PI Measure Crosswalk

Stage 3 MU Measures	MU Threshold		2019 PI Score	2019 PI Measures
Electronic Prescribing	> 25%		Up to 10 points	Electronic prescribing
			5 bonus points (optional, increases to 10 bonus points starting 2021)	Query of prescription drug monitoring program (PDMP)
			5 bonus points (optional)	Verify opioid treatment agreement (note: eliminated in 2020)
Send Summary of Care	> 10%	Meet 2 measures; attest to all	Up to 20 points	Sending health information*
Request/Accept Summary of Care	> 10%		Up to 20 points	Receiving and incorporating health information* (note: renamed to receiving and reconciling health information in 2021)
Clinical Information Reconciliation	> 50%			
Provide Patient Access	> 50%		Up to 40 points	Provide patients electronic access to their health information
Patient-Specific Education	> 10%			Removed: Patient-specific education
Immunization Registry Syndromic Surveillance Electronic Case Reporting Public Health Registry Clinical Data Registry Electronic Reportable Lab Results	Active engagement: any 3 measures		10 points Active engagement: any 2 measures	Immunization registry Syndromic surveillance Electronic case reporting Public health registry Clinical data registry Electronic reportable lab results
View, Download, or Transmit	1 patient	Meet 2 measures; attest to all	N/A	Removed: view, download, or transmit
Secure Messaging	> 5%			Removed: secure messaging
Patient-Generated Health Data	> 5%			Removed: patient generated health data

* Starting 2021, providers can report an optional bi-directional exchange measure worth 40 points, as an alternative to the two measures in the health information exchange objective *Report CQMs*

manual attestation; or 2) electronic reporting. The attestation option allows providers to meet the PI CQM reporting requirements alone, whereas the electronic option allows for the opportunity in some circumstances to receive credit for the CQM reporting component of PI as well as credit for the CQM reporting requirement for other programs, e.g., the hospital Inpatient Quality Reporting (IQR) program for EHs. CMS requires electronic CQM reporting for PI in 2018 and future years.

Reporting Periods and Attestation Deadlines

To demonstrate PI, providers must attest to the requirements previously discussed based on data from a specified timeframe and submitted by a CMS-determined deadline. The reporting period refers to the specified timeframe during each program year during which a provider must achieve the performance requirements. The attestation deadline is the last day providers can report their data to CMS or state in the submission system. The reporting period and attestation deadline vary by the provider's year of participation.

All providers in their first year of PI can choose any consecutive 90-day time frame within their program year as their reporting period. In subsequent years, providers were originally subject to a full-year reporting period. However, due to the program complexities and challenges facing providers, CMS often relaxed and reduced the reporting period requirement to less than a full year, but encouraged providers to report a full year if possible. In the years after 2011, the reporting periods varied between a full year, or program year-quarter, or continuous 90-day period. CMS determines year-specific reporting period requirements through rulemaking.

As for the attestation deadlines, from 2011 to 2014, EHs submitted attestations October 1 to November 30 for the prior FFY; and EPs January 1 to February 28 (or 29, for a leap year). For the 2015 program year and later years, EHs transitioned from an FFY basis to a CY, to align with the EP timeline. This means that the attestation window is generally January 1 to February 28 (or 29, if it is a leap year) following the PI program year. Some states have different reporting windows and associated deadlines for the Medicaid program.

PI Participation Data Trends

Since its inception in 2010 through October 2018, the PI programs have paid more than $38 billion in incentive payments to 546,644 unique providers.[28] About $22 billion are distributed to the EHs/CAHs, whereas EPs have earned more than $16 billion. Nearly 94% of the hospital incentives are allocated to EHs that participate in both the Medicare and Medicaid PI programs. In contrast, of the total incentive payments to EPs, almost $10 billion were paid through the Medicare programs, whereas $6.5 billion were paid to EPs that participate in the Medicaid program. The sequestration cut resulted in a reduction of about $121 million and $281 million from the incentive payments to EPs and EHs, respectively. Medicare incentives are no longer available and providers must continue to attest in order to avoid penalty, but there may be remaining Medicaid incentives paid to providers (based on participation timeline and eligibility) through 2021 when the Medicaid PI program sunsets.

While CMS uses providers' measure performance data in previous years to guide the modifications to measure requirements, the agency has released neither a summary nor a detailed analysis in recent years. CMS does publish general Medicare measure attestation data through the public use file (PUF) on CMS website,[26] and Medicaid attestation data is available at the state level.

Quality Payment Program

This next section describes the Quality Payment Program that subsumed legacy Medicare PI requirements. The QPP also includes several other requirements that providers must report in order to avoid financial penalties. This section includes the QPP's history, provider eligibility, the two payment tracks, and the incentive and penalty structure.

Overview

The Medicare Access and CHIP Reauthorization Act (MACRA), enacted in April 2015, established a new way to pay Medicare providers, herein referred to as eligible clinicians (ECs), who bill Medicare Part B professional services. Passed with strong bipartisan support in both the House and the Senate, this legislation repealed the outdated and flawed Sustainable Growth Rate (SGR) formula, a mechanism previously used by CMS to control growth in Medicare Part B spending on physician services. The SGR imposed a severe cut to the EC payments under the Medicare Physician Fee Schedule (MPFS). However, over the years, Congress regularly passed legislation, commonly known as a "doc fix," to temporarily avert those cuts. These "doc fixes" were unsustainable long term. As a result, MACRA, a "permanent doc fix," mandates several critical updates to Medicare Part B payments that go into effect January 1, 2019.

Specifically, MACRA creates two new payment tracks under the QPP: the Merit-based Incentive Payment System (MIPS) and Advanced Alternative Payment Model (APM) tracks. These new payment tracks incentivize the move from traditional fee-for-service payment models to value-based payment models that emphasize high quality of care and sustainable costs.

MACRA also specifies annual MPFS payment rate updates. Beginning in the second half of 2015 and through 2018, PFS payment rates updated by 0.5% annually. The 2018 Bipartisan Budget Act further reduced the 2019 update down to 0.25%. The MACRA then freezes payment rates for five years (2020–2025). Beginning in 2026, payment rates will be updated either by 0.25% annually for ECs in MIPS or by 0.75% annually for ECs in the APM track. Figure 11.1 illustrates the schedule of payment rate updates in each payment track.

Except in limited circumstances, all ECs who bill Medicare Part B professional services, regardless of their setting, are subject to the QPP – in either the MIPS or APM payment track. While the QPP policies affect Medicare Part B payments starting on January 1, 2019, CMS applies a "two-year lookback" policy to associate ECs' performance to their payment. For example, MIPS payment adjustments in the payment year 2019 are based on EC performance in the program year 2017. Thus, this is why 2017 was the first QPP participation year.

CMS anticipated that the majority of ECs will begin in the MIPS track, but the enticing financial incentives would accelerate a move into the APM track. For program year 2019, CMS estimated that approximately 165,000 to 222,000 ECs will qualify for the APM track, and nearly 800,000 ECs will participate in the MIPS track.

The APM Track

Eligibility

ECs participate in the APM track when they meet two key conditions. First, ECs must participate in an Advanced APM. CMS provides an annual list of Advanced APMs in the QPP Resource Library.[29] An Advanced APM is a payment model that:

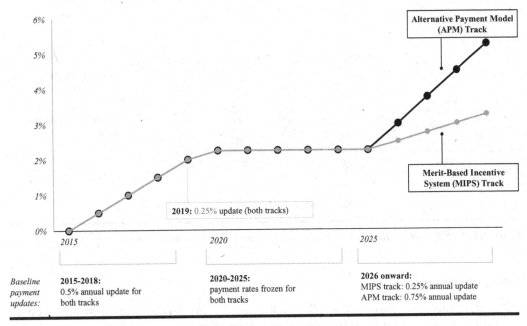

Figure 11.1   Baseline payment rate schedule under MACRA

- Incentivizes ECs to report quality measures comparable to those in MIPS;
- Requires use of CEHRT; and
- Bears more than nominal financial risk for monetary losses or be a medical home model expanded under Center for Medicare and Medicaid Innovation (CMMI) authority.

Second, Advanced APM participants must meet a volume-based requirement through either a minimum percent of payments or number of patients through the Advanced APM to be considered a Qualifying APM Participant (QP). Only after QP status is attained will that EC participate in the APM track. In the first year of the program, under the payment criterion, the QP threshold requires at least 25% of Medicare Part B payments are furnished to the attributed Medicare beneficiaries. The required threshold increases over the years, as shown in Figure 11.2.

In most cases, the QP threshold is assessed collectively across all ECs who participate in a given Advanced APM arrangement (i.e., the APM Entity). The QP threshold may also be assessed individually under some circumstances, and CMS will continue to update their policies through annual rulemaking.

If Advanced APM participants have slightly less than the required percentage of payments or number of beneficiaries, they may become "Partial QPs." For example, under the payments criteria, the Partial QP threshold requires at least 20% (but less than 25%) of Medicare Part B revenue to be furnished to attributed beneficiaries in the first year of the program.

In the first two years of the program, the APM track was reserved for Medicare Advanced APMs only. Beginning in the third program year, QP status may be earned through other types of payers with models that are considered "Other Payer Advanced APMs," in combination with volumes through Medicare Advanced APMs. This latter option is also referred to as the "All-Payer Combination Option."

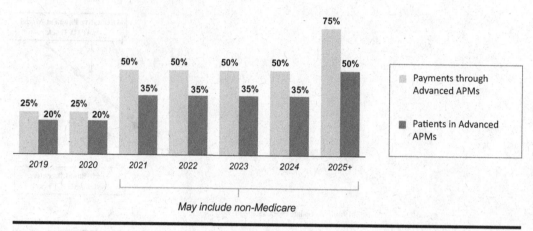

Figure 11.2 QP thresholds: percent of payments or patient counts by payment year

Financial Implications

QPs earn financial incentives in the APM track (e.g., a 5% lump-sum bonus in the first six payment years of the program from 2019 to 2024) and are exempted from MIPS reporting requirements and payment adjustments. This incentive makes participation in the APM track attractive to ECs, if they are able to meet the necessary requirements.

Incentives are paid two years after the performance year – which aligns to the MIPS payment adjustment schedule. For example, when QP status is earned in program year 2018, then across 2019, CMS calculates the APM incentive payment based on claims that year. In payment year 2020, the APM entity receives the incentive payment.

ECs who meet the "Partial QP" status do not qualify for the APM track, and thus do not earn the 5% APM payment bonus. However, they can choose to either opt into the MIPS track or do nothing. If they opt into the MIPS track, they will be subject to the reporting requirements and payment adjustments (i.e., positive, neutral, or negative) under MIPS. Partial QP ECs in many types of Advanced APMs also qualify for special scoring policies under the MIPS APM Scoring Standard, which could lead to a high MIPS final score. On the other hand, partial QP ECs who choose to opt out of MIPS need not report MIPS data, but they will neither earn incentives nor face penalties.

The MIPS Track

Eligibility

Generally, the MIPS track applies to all ECs who bill Medicare Part B professional services, regardless of setting. MIPS is the "default" payment track under the QPP, unless providers are otherwise excluded (e.g., due to qualification into the APM track).

In the first two years of the program, five types of MIPS ECs could participate: physicians, physician assistants, nurse practitioners, clinical nurse specialists, and certified registered nurse anesthetists. Beginning the third program year in 2019, CMS adds more types of ECs into the pool: physical therapists, occupational therapists, qualified speech-language pathologists, qualified audiologists, clinical psychologists, and registered dietitians or nutrition professionals. Any clinician group that includes one of these professionals may also be eligible to participate in MIPS.

CMS allows ECs to participate in MIPS as individuals, as a group (as defined by Tax Identification Number [TIN]), or both. ECs or groups that fall below the annual low-volume thresholds are ineligible to participate in MIPS for a particular program year. For example, the 2019 low-volume thresholds are:

- $90,000 or less in Medicare-covered professional services;
- 200 or fewer Medicare patients; and
- 200 or fewer Medicare-covered professional services.

The same low-volume thresholds are used to assess individual eligibility and group eligibility. There are cases in which an individual within a group is ineligible due to their own low volume. However, if the group is eligible and MIPS data is subsequently submitted for the group, the individual is opted-in to participation and subject to the adjustment the group receives.

ECs who subsequently qualify as QPs, meet Partial QP status but choose not to participate in MIPS, or are newly enrolled in Medicare are excluded from MIPS payment adjustments.

MIPS Performance Categories

The MIPS track consolidates three legacy CMS reporting programs – the Medicare EHR Incentive Program for Eligible Professionals (i.e., Meaningful Use); the Physician Value-Based Payment Modifier; and the Physician Quality Reporting System (PQRS) – into a single, pay-for-performance program. CMS has retained some components of these programs under MIPS.

The MIPS track scores MIPS ECs on four performance categories: 1) Quality; 2) Cost (formerly called Resource Use); 3) Improvement Activities (formerly called Clinical Practice Improvement Activities); and 4) Promoting Interoperability (i.e., EHR use, formerly called Advancing Care Information). MIPS data is reported to CMS annually using mechanisms of an EC or group's choice (e.g., EHR, registry, and/or claims-based reporting – depending on the type of data submitted). Generally, MIPS data are reported during the first three months of the calendar year that follows the program year. For example, program year 2019 data submission will occur for that year in the first three months of 2020. The only category that does not require data submission to CMS is the Cost category.

Quality

The requirements of the Quality category mostly align with the legacy PQRS, with annual modifications. But in contrast to PQRS, MIPS is pay-for-performance by design, whereas PQRS was a pay-for-reporting program. For most MIPS Quality data submission methods, ECs are required to report six clinical quality measures, including one outcome measure. CMS annually updates the list of available quality measures each year, and there are over 200 measures from which to choose. These measures are further segmented into various collection types and submission types (i.e., electronic CQMs, MIPS CQMs [e.g., registry-based measures], Qualified Clinical Data Registry measures, CMS Web Interface, claim-based, and Consumer Assessment of Healthcare Providers and Systems [CAHPS] survey). In addition to reporting on measures of an EC's choice, some groups may be assessed on the claims-based All-Cause Hospital Readmissions measure, if they meet the case minimum requirement.

In 2017, the Quality performance category reporting period was any continuous 90-day period. For all subsequent years, CMS has required a full calendar year reporting period for this category. Each Quality measure is assessed against peer benchmarks segmented into deciles. In general, each measure is worth up to 10 points, and the better the performance, the better the score an EC or group will earn.

Cost

Cost category performance is based on data already submitted through the Medicare administrative claims process. CMS uses claims data for the entire calendar year performance period to assess ECs' cost performance. In 2017 and 2018, CMS used two Cost measures that are based on the legacy Value Based Payment Modifier program with some modifications. The Total Per Capita Cost (TPCC) measure evaluates beneficiary costs across the entire year, and the Medicare Spending per Beneficiary (MSPB) assesses costs surrounding an inpatient admission. CMS added eight episode-based measures starting in 2019, plus another 10 episode-based measures in 2020, and may consider additional measures or other changes through future rulemaking.

In order to be scored on Cost measures, ECs must meet the required minimum number of cases. For example, the case minimum is 20 and 35 cases for TPCC and MSPB, respectively. ECs can earn up to 10 points on each Cost measure. The lower the EC's actual adjusted costs are compared to benchmarks, the more points the EC will earn. CMS establishes these benchmarks based on claims data that they receive from the current performance year.

Improvement Activities (IA)

The IA performance category measures clinical practice improvement and is a wholly new set of reporting requirements under the QPP – meaning there was no legacy program as precedent. In this category, there are over 100 activities to choose from (e.g., an EC or group can implement care coordination training and get credit toward the category).

The IA reporting period is any continuous 90-day reporting period (or as specified by the activity itself). ECs can submit IAs either manually in the QPP data submission portal or through a vendor. The available activities are not created equal because they are divided between what CMS defines as medium-weighted (10 points) or high-weighted (20 points) activities. To achieve full credit for this performance category, participants need to earn a total of 40 points through any combination of activities.

Promoting Interoperability (PI)

The requirements of the PI (formerly named Advancing Care Information) category mostly align with the legacy PI program for Medicare EPs, with annual modifications. Generally, PI requires that ECs use CEHRT to report on PI measures. ECs must select their applicable CEHRT products listed in the Certified Health IT Product List (CHPL) website to generate a specific number used during the reporting process to identify what CEHRT was in use during the reporting period. However, some providers may be eligible for an exclusion from the PI category (e.g., if they are deemed "non-patient-facing" or "hospital-based," or apply for and are granted a hardship exception).

In 2017 and 2018, ECs and groups earned points based on a mixture of a "Base Score," individual measure performance, and, if applicable, bonus points. In 2019, CMS established a new point-based scoring methodology that aligns with Medicare hospital PI requirements.

Providers must complete a Security Risk Analysis annually. Additionally, providers must report PI data for at least a continuous 90-day period on the required measures, unless exclusions apply.

Each measure has an assigned weight or maximum points that can be earned, which CMS factors against the provider's measure performance rate (i.e., numerator over denominator) to arrive at measure-specific PI points earned.

MIPS APMs

ECs who are not eligible for the APM track but participate in certain types of payment models, considered MIPS APMs, qualify for special scoring and reporting benefits. An example of a MIPS APM from the 2018 program year was Medicare Shared Savings Program Track 1.

Under the MIPS APM scoring standard, all providers in the APM Entity are assessed collectively. The APM Entity reports quality measures to CMS under the terms of the payment arrangement, and the data is used to assess the MIPS APM's Quality category performance. ECs in a MIPS APM also receive at least half credit for the IA category by CMS policy and historically have automatically received full credit so that no further reporting is required for the category. ECs in a MIPS APM are responsible for reporting PI data to CMS for the purposes of MIPS.

Starting 2021, CMS sunset the MIPS APM scoring standard that required providers to participate in MIPS through their APM Entity. Instead, providers have the option to participate as an individual, as part of a group, or through their APM Entity. At the same time, CMS established the APM Performance Pathway (APP) in 2021, which is an optional reporting framework available to MIPS APM participants. Within the APP, providers are scored on a fixed set of six measures in the quality category, and maintain the same scoring methodology for the improvement activities and promoting interoperability categories.

MIPS Performance Category Weights

MIPS performance is weighted across all four categories, which determines the relative contribution of each category toward the MIPS final score. Table 11.7 shows MIPS performance category weights under the default MIPS and the MIPS APM scoring standard, and how they change over time as established by law and through annual rulemaking.

ECs subject to the MIPS APM Scoring Standard have their MIPS performance assessed under only three performance categories: Quality, IA, and PI. Cost is not included in the MIPS APM Scoring Standard or the APP.

Table 11.7   MIPS Category Weights

MIPS Performance Category	Category Weight (%) for the Performance Year						
	MIPS						MIPS APM*
	2017	2018	2019	2020	2021	2022	N/A
Quality	60	50	45	40	40	30	50
Cost	0	10	15	20	20	30	N/A
Improvement activities	15	15	15	15	15	15	20
Promoting interoperability	25	25	25	25	25	25	30

* MIPS APM scoring standard sunset in 2021, replaced by optional APM Participation Pathway.

MIPS Scoring Methodology

MIPS participation occurs at either the individual EC or group level through the TIN, or at the APM Entity level for MIPS APM participants. CMS combines data from each performance category score to derive a MIPS final score, which ranges from 0 to 100.

This score is compared to a performance threshold (PT) set by CMS on an annual basis. For example, CMS set the PT at 3, 15, 30, 45, and 60 points for the program years 2017, 2018, 2019, 2020, and 2021 respectively. MIPS scores above the PT receive incentives (i.e., a positive payment adjustment to their future Medicare Part B professional service reimbursement rate), whereas those that fall below the PT face penalties (i.e., a negative payment adjustment). ECs with the MIPS final score equal to the PT will receive no adjustment (i.e., a neutral payment adjustment). Additionally, CMS also sets an exceptional performance threshold to reward ECs with the best MIPS final scores. Similar to PT, exceptional PT is set on an annual basis, starting at 70 in 2017 and 2018, 75 in 2019, and then further increasing to 85 in 2020 and 2021. CMS aims to increase a year-specific PT and exceptional PT over the years through future rulemaking.

Financial Implications

MIPS is a budget-neutral program, in which the penalties CMS collects from low performers and non-reporters will be paid out as incentives to high performers. An additional $500 million is also available to reward exceptional performers in the first six payment years of the program (i.e., 2019–2024). It is critical for ECs to score well under MIPS, as reimbursement will depend on their performance. The higher the score, the more incentives dollars are earned.

MACRA set maximum penalty levels under MIPS. In the 2019 payment year, the maximum penalty was a 4% reduction to reimbursements and grows to 9% in later years. Incentives paid will vary each year based on how providers perform in MIPS. Table 11.8 shows the maximum penalties and incentives (CMS estimates are published in the regulations), and the actual maximum incentive for years in which data is available.

Public Reporting of MIPS Performance

An EC's individual or group MIPS performance on each category and final score will be posted annually on the CMS Physician Compare website. The Physician Compare website was developed in 2010 by CMS to help patients make informed decisions about their health care by allowing

Table 11.8 MIPS Penalties and Incentives

Payment Year	Maximum Penalty	Actual Maximum Incentive
2019 (2017 program year)	–4%	+1.88%
2020 (2018 program year)	–5%	+1.68%
2021 (2019 program year)	–7%	+1.79%
2022 onward (2020 program year onward)	–9%	TBD

them to find and compare providers online. Public reporting may also serve as a catalyst to incentivize ECs to perform well in the MIPS program.

ECs and groups must meet a number of criteria in order to qualify for public reporting of their MIPS data. For example, they must have submitted at least one Medicare fee-for-service claim within a six-month timeframe. Towards the end of each calendar year, CMS will host a 30-day preview period for ECs to review what data will be reported on Physician Compare on the QPP website. During the preview period, ECs may also reach out to CMS in the event the preview data does not match the performance feedback report.

QPP Participation Data Trends

In the first two years, many program policies offered providers a transition period to learn about MIPS participation and avoid penalty. It was possible to avoid penalties based on a relatively low performance threshold, as previously described. CMS also implemented significant outreach efforts to bolster MIPS participation, especially among rural practices and small groups. Together, this allowed the program to achieve high levels of participation, as shown in Table 11.9 by the percentage of MIPS ECs who were at or above the PT and avoided the penalty (i.e., 95% in 2017, 98% in 2018, and nearly 100% in 2019 due to reporting flexibilities CMS established in response to the COVID-19 pandemic). However, the MIPS track will become more difficult by design, and in future years, the PT will continue to rise and result in an increase in the number of providers who are subject to penalties (along with an associated decrease in providers who earn incentives).

Meanwhile, the CMS also saw a significant surge in providers who achieved QP status to earn the APM track bonus (i.e., almost double the number from 99,076 in 2017 to 183,306 in 2018). The increase in the number of providers who qualify for QP status is expected to continue over the years, as the MIPS program becomes more challenging and additional opportunities for providers to join an Advanced APM are created.

Common PI and QPP Challenges

Some of the common challenges we have observed for providers include, but are not limited to, the following:

1. **Strategic alignment.** Successful participation in PI and/or QPP requires coordination, reliance on specific skillsets, and alignment across multiple groups within an organization. Leading organizations usually create a steering committee that incorporates multidisciplinary teams with both functional leaders and operational staff.

Table 11.9 The Number and Percentage of Providers Participating in MIPS and APM[30]

Program Year	MIPS				# QPs (APM Bonus)	# Partial QPs
	# MIPS ECs	% Above PT (Incentive)	% at PT (Neutral)	% Below PT (Penalty)		
2017	1,057,824	93.12%	2.01%	4.87%	99,076	52
2018	889,995	97.55%	0.45%	2.01%	183,306	47
2019	954,614	95.32%	4.36%	0.32%	195,564	27,995

An effective steering committee involves leaders and staff from policy and compliance, strategy, finance, quality, clinical, operations, contracting/credentialing, informatics, and information technology. This mix allows organizations to align CMS program requirements with other strategic and operational initiatives. For example, organizations that have taken on downside risk through an advanced APM can incorporate their QPP strategy as part of their overall Medicare risk strategy. That alignment may help to avoid duplicative efforts between program requirements and keep all parties in sync with evolving value-based payment policies. In an environment full of competing regulatory and value-based care priorities, it can be challenging to convene all the right parties to the table.

2. **Regulatory and legislative changes.** In addition to the annual rulemaking and occasional legislative acts that always introduce changes and modifications to CMS program policies, CMS and ONC often issue clarifications, modifications, and new policies through other sub-regulatory means, such as frequently asked questions (FAQs) or tip sheets. While the changes can be disruptive, providers must be attentive to all of them because they may impose an immediate impact on their reporting plans and/or performance. Without staff assigned and accountable to monitor for these changes, PI and/or success can be compromised.

3. **Reporting.** How and what measures providers report are also subject to annual modifications, which require providers to reassess their plan at least once a year. Reporting policies also vary within components of the same program such as the MIPS performance categories, which may make it even more difficult to keep track of what type of data needs to be submitted for which length of time. Reporting can be further complicated when data must be extracted and shared from multiple sites and EHR systems, and/or when transitioning from one EHR system to another. Additionally, providers relying on a third-party vendor to submit data on their behalf must ensure data accuracy, data completion, and submission timeliness.

4. **CEHRT implementation and upgrades.** A provider cannot demonstrate PI (either in the standalone PI program or for the MIPS PI category) without use of a CEHRT Edition required for that particular program year. For example, in 2019 a provider must use only the 2015 Edition CEHRT. This requirement can create challenges for providers who must implement an EHR system certified by ONC and subsequently upgrade their systems to meet evolving PI requirements. Providers unable to implement ONC-certified systems by defined dates could face significant financial penalties.

5. **Performance improvement and succession planning.** Providers must track performance improvement over the years. It is important to have a longitudinal improvement plan as CMS continues to raise their program requirements progressively each year. Another challenge is succession planning, when staff move on to other roles or leave the organization. Organizations need to develop a knowledge management and transition plan to minimize confusion, onboard new staff who likely face a steep learning curve, and prevent performance disruption.

6. **Audit preparation and response.** CMS and their contractors conduct data validation and audits to confirm that providers meet program requirements. CMS states that they can conduct audits at any time, and they encourage providers to keep documentation for a significant timeframe (e.g., up to ten years after MIPS data submission occurs). Providers report that audit experiences can be lengthy and labor intensive, and failure could result in hefty penalties. A systematic approach to achieve audit readiness is imperative in order to respond effectively if an audit letter is received. Organizations should establish an audit response process, conduct mock audits, and keep all necessary documentation in a centralized, accessible place.

Alignment of PI and QPP With Other Strategic Initiatives

Where there are challenges, new opportunities also exist. Seeking a sustainable solution to curtail high health care costs and improve the quality of care, the federal government and the health care industry have put emphasis on transforming payment structures, which in turn drives health systems to develop more responsive care delivery models. Embedded in health care reform is the paradigm shift from a volume-based, fee-for-service standard to a value-driven delivery environment in which providers are held accountable to their services, and patients can be selective and make an informed decision about their own health. While PI and QPP are part of the overall health care transformation, they are built on essential foundations that can be well aligned with health care organizations' strategic goals.

Leading organizations can leverage their progress in PI and the QPP to achieve success in strategic initiatives that enhance efficiency and improve outcomes. For example, health systems can focus on the new PI priorities on interoperability and patient access to health information and align them with their population health management initiative with an emphasis on care coordination across settings and patient engagement. Providers' participation in these programs fosters organizational capabilities that support and enable other goals. As providers advance through these programs, they will continue to build both human and technology assets that are necessary for health systems to thrive in the new care delivery models emerging today.

About the Authors

Anantachai (Tony) Panjamapirom, PhD, MBA, CPHIMS, is an independent consultant in healthcare management and health information technology. He was a research director with the Health Care Information Technology Advisory and Quality Reporting Roundtable research programs at the Advisory Board Company. He led strategic and best practice research, served as a subject matter expert, and provided policy analysis, strategic and operational guidance in support of hospital and health system executives. His principal areas of expertise included CMS quality reporting programs (e.g., Promoting Interoperability, Quality Payment Program, MACRA), value-based payment models, IT performance management, and IT implications in accountable care environment. He is a certified professional in Healthcare Information and Management Systems (CPHIMS).

Naomi Levinthal, MA, MS, CPHIMS, is a 15-year health information technology (IT) and medical informatics professional. Today she serves as Vice President with AVIA, the nation's leading digital transformation partner for healthcare organizations. AVIA provides unique market intelligence, proven collaborative tools across a network of 50+ leading health systems, and results-based consulting to help solve healthcare's biggest strategic challenges. At AVIA, Naomi leads AVIA's strategic partnerships business and product strategy. Previously, Naomi served as Managing Director at the Advisory Board Company for their health IT research programs serving the C-suite of hospitals and health systems and physician practices throughout the United States and overseas. Her areas of expertise are health informatics, quality reporting, digital health and innovation. Naomi received an MS from Northwestern University's Feinberg School of Medicine in Health Informatics and an MA from Loyola University Chicago, and she is a certified professional in Healthcare Information & Management Systems (CPHIMS).

Ye Hoffman, MS, CPHIMS, leads the Advisory Board's Quality Reporting Roundtable team. She provides strategic guidance to health system executives on the complex and evolving landscape of federal health IT and quality reporting requirements. Her areas of expertise include the CMS Quality Payment Program and Promoting Interoperability program, as well as the ONC health IT certification program and information blocking provision. She specializes in health informatics, quality reporting, interoperability, regulatory analysis, and IT project management. Prior to joining the Advisory Board, Ye served as IT project manager and business data analyst at the Fred Hutchinson Cancer Research Center. Ye earned a master of science from Northwestern University's Feinberg School of Medicine in health informatics and is a certified professional in Healthcare Information & Management Systems (CPHIMS).

References

1. Burns L. & V. Pauly M. Transformation of the Health Care Industry: Curb Your Enthusiasm? Transformation of the Health Care Industry, 96 *The Milbank Quarterly*. 57–109 (2018).
2. Fraser I. Ambulatory Care and Healthcare Reform, 2 *Annals Health L.* 215 (1993). Available at: http://lawecommons.luc.edu/annals/vol2/iss1/13.
3. Lave JR. The Impact of the Medicare Prospective Payment System and Recommendations for Change, 7 *Yale J. on Reg.* (1990). Available at: http://digitalcommons.law.yale.edu/yjreg/vol7/iss2/5.
4. Office of the National Coordinator for Health Information Technology. "Office-based Physician Electronic Health Record Adoption," Health IT Quick-Stat #50. https://dashboard.healthit.gov/quickstats/pages/physician-ehr-adoption-trends.php. January 2019.
5. Office of the National Coordinator for Health Information Technology. "Percent of Hospitals, By Type, that Possess Certified Health IT," Health IT Quick-Stat #52. https://dashboard.healthit.gov/quickstats/pages/certified-electronic-health-record-technology-in-hospitals.php. September 2018.
6. Medicare and Medicaid Programs; Electronic Health Record Incentive Program; 42 CFR 412, 413, 422, and 495, RIN 0938 – AP78. July 28, 2010.
7. Health Information Technology: Initial Set of Standards, Implementation Specifications, and Certification Criteria for Electronic Health Record Technology; 45 CFR 170, RIN 0991-AB58. July 28, 2010.
8. Medicare and Medicaid Programs; Electronic Health Record Incentive Program – Stage 2; 42 CFR 412, 413, and 495, RIN 0938 – AQ84. September 4, 2012.
9. Health Information Technology: Standards, Implementation Specifications, and Certification Criteria for Electronic Health Record Technology, 2014 Edition; Revisions to the Permanent Certification Program for Health Information Technology; 45 CFR 170, RIN 0991 – AB82. September 4, 2012.
10. Medicare and Medicaid Programs; Modifications to the Medicare and Medicaid Electronic Health Record (EHR) Incentive Program for 2014 and Other Changes to the EHR Incentive Program; and Health Information Technology: Revisions to the Certified EHR Technology Definition and EHR Certification Changes Related to Standards; 42 CFR 495, 45 CFR 170, RINs 0991 – AB89 and 0991 – AB97. September 4, 2014.
11. 2014 Edition Release 2 Electronic Health Record (EHR) Certification Criteria and the ONC HIT Certification Program; Regulatory Flexibilities, Improvements, and Enhanced Health Information Exchange; 45 CFR 170, RIN 0991 – AB92. September 11, 2014.
12. Medicare and Medicaid Programs; Electronic Health Record Incentive Program – Stage 3 and Modifications to Meaningful Use in 2015 Through 2017; 42 CFR 412 and 495, RINs 0938 – AS26 and 0938 – AS58. October 16, 2015.
13. 2015 Edition Health Information Technology (Health IT) Certification Criteria, 2015 Edition Base Electronic Health Record (EHR) Definition, and ONC Health IT Certification Program Modifications; 45 CFR Part 170, RIN 0991 – AB93. October 16, 2015.

14. Medicare Program; Merit-Based Incentive Payment System (MIPS) and Alternative Payment Model (APM) Incentive Under the Physician Fee Schedule, and Criteria for Physician-Focused Payment Models; 42 CFR 414 and 495, RIN 0938-AS69. November 4, 2016.

15. Medicare Access and CHIP Reauthorization Act of 2015, Pub. L. 114–10, 129 Stat. 87, 2015. Available at: https://www.congress.gov/114/plaws/publ10/PLAW-114publ10.pdf. Accessed April 18, 2015.

16. Medicare Program: Hospital Outpatient Prospective Payment and Ambulatory Surgical Center Payment Systems and Quality Reporting Programs; Organ Procurement Organization Reporting and Communication; Transplant Outcome Measures and Documentation Requirements; Electronic Health Record (EHR) Incentive Programs; Payment to Nonexcepted Off-Campus Provider-Based Department of a Hospital; Hospital Value-Based Purchasing (VBP) Program; Establishment of Payment Rates Under the Medicare Physician Fee Schedule for Nonexcepted Items and Services Furnished by an Off-Campus Provider-Based Department of a Hospital; 42 CFR 414, 416, 419, 482, 486, 488, and 495, RIN 0938-AS82. November 14, 2016.

17. Medicare Program; Hospital Inpatient Prospective Payment Systems for Acute Care Hospitals and the Long-Term Care Hospital Prospective Payment System and Policy Changes and Fiscal Year 2018 Rates; Quality Reporting Requirements for Specific Providers; Medicare and Medicaid Electronic Health Record (EHR) Incentive Program Requirements for Eligible Hospitals, Critical Access Hospitals, and Eligible Professionals; Provider-Based Status of Indian Health Service and Tribal Facilities and Organizations; Costs Reporting and Provider Requirements; Agreement Termination Notices; 42 CFR 405, 412, 413, 414, 416, 486, 488, 489, and 495, RIN 0938 – AS98. August 14, 2017.

18. Medicare Program; Hospital Inpatient Prospective Payment Systems for Acute Care Hospitals and the Long-Term Care Hospital Prospective Payment System and Policy Changes and Fiscal Year 2019 Rates; Quality Reporting Requirements for Specific Providers; Medicare and Medicaid Electronic Health Record (EHR) Incentive Programs (Promoting Interoperability Programs) Requirements for Eligible Hospitals, Critical Access Hospitals, and Eligible Professionals; Medicare Cost Reporting Requirements; and Physician Certification and Recertification of Claims; 42 CFR 412, 413, 424, 495, RIN 0938 – AT27. August 17, 2018.

19. Medicare Program; Revisions to Payment Policies Under the Physician Fee Schedule and Other Revisions to Part B for CY 2019; Medicare Shared Savings Program Requirements; Quality Payment Program; Medicaid Promoting Interoperability Program; Quality Payment Program-Extreme and Uncontrollable Circumstance Policy for the 2019 MIPS Payment Year; Provisions From the Medicare Shared Savings Program-Accountable Care Organizations-Pathways to Success; and Expanding the Use of Telehealth Services for the Treatment of Opioid Use Disorder Under the Substance Use-Disorder Prevention That Promotes Opioid Recovery and Treatment (SUPPORT) for Patients and Communities Act; 42 CFR 405, 410, 411, 414, 415, 425, and 495, RINs 0938 – AT13, 0938 – AT31, and 0938 – AT45. November 23, 2018.

20. Medicare Program: Hospital Inpatient Prospective Payment Systems for Acute Care Hospitals and the Long Term Care Hospital Prospective Payment System and Policy Changes and Fiscal Year 2020 Rates; Quality Reporting Requirements for Specific Providers; Medicare and Medicaid Promoting Interoperability Programs Requirements for Eligible Hospitals and Critical Access Hospitals; 42 CFR 412, 413, and 495, RIN 0938-AT73. August 16, 2019.

21. Medicare Program; CY 2020 Revisions to Payment Policies Under the Physician Fee Schedule and Other Changes to Part B Payment Policies; Medicare Shared Savings Program Requirements; Medicaid Promoting Interoperability Program Requirements for Eligible Professionals; Establishment of an Ambulance Data Collection System; Updates to the Quality Payment Program; Medicare Enrollment of Opioid Treatment Programs and Enhancements to Provider Enrollment Regulations Concerning Improper Prescribing and Patient Harm; and Amendments to Physician Self-Referral Law Advisory Opinion Regulations Final Rule; and Coding and Payment for Evaluation and Management, Observation and Provision of Self-Administered Esketamine Interim Final Rule; 42 CFR parts 403, 409, 410, 411, 414, 415, 416, 418, 424, 425, 489, and 498. November 15, 2019.

22. Medicare Program; Hospital Inpatient Prospective Payment Systems for Acute Care Hospitals and the Long Term Care Hospital Prospective Payment System and Final Policy Changes and Fiscal Year

2021 Rates; Quality Reporting and Medicare and Medicaid Promoting Interoperability Programs Requirements for Eligible Hospitals and Critical Access Hospitals; 42 CFR Parts 405, 412, 413, 417, 476, 480, 484, and 495. September 18, 2020.

23. Medicare Program; CY 2021 Payment Policies Under the Physician Fee Schedule and Other Changes to Part B Payment Policies; Medicare Shared Savings Program Requirements; Medicaid Promoting Interoperability Program Requirements for Eligible Professionals; Quality Payment Program; Coverage of Opioid Use Disorder Services Furnished by Opioid Treatment Programs; Medicare Enrollment of Opioid Treatment Programs; Electronic Prescribing for Controlled Substances for a Covered Part D Drug; Payment for Office/Outpatient Evaluation and Management Services; Hospital IQR Program; Establish New Code Categories; Medicare Diabetes Prevention Program (MDPP) Expanded Model Emergency Policy; Coding and Payment for Virtual Check-in Services Interim Final Rule Policy; Coding and Payment for Personal Protective Equipment (PPE) Interim Final Rule Policy; Regulatory Revisions in Response to the Public Health Emergency (PHE) for COVID-19; and Finalization of Certain Provisions from the March 31st, May 8th and September 2nd Interim Final Rules in Response to the PHE for COVID-19; 42 CFR Parts 400, 410, 414, 415, 423, 424, and 425. December 28, 2020.

24. Bipartisan Budget Act of 2018, Pub. L. 115–23, 132 STAT. 64, 2018. Available at: https://www.congress.gov/115/plaws/publ123/PLAW-115publ123.pdf. Accessed February 20, 2018.

25. Social Security Act, Payment to Hospitals for Inpatient Hospital Services. Available at: http://www.ssa.gov/OP_Home/ssact/title18/1886.htm#act-1886-d-1-b. Accessed March 12, 2011.

26. The Office of the National Coordinator for Health Information Technology. Certified Health IT Product List. Available at: https://chpl.healthit.gov/#/search. Accessed April 18, 2019.

27. Centers for Medicare and Medicaid Services. Promoting Interoperability (PI) Programs: Requirements for Previous Years. Available at: https://www.cms.gov/Regulations-and-Guidance/Legislation/EHRIncentivePrograms/RequirementsforPreviousYears.html. Accessed July 22, 2019.

28. Centers for Medicare and Medicaid Services. Promoting Interoperability (PI) Programs: Data and Program Reports. Available at: http://www.cms.gov/Regulations-and-Guidance/Legislation/EHRIncentivePrograms/DataAndReports.html. Accessed June 19, 2019.

29. Centers for Medicare and Medicaid Services. Quality Payment Programs: Resource Library. Available at: https://qpp.cms.gov/about/resource-library. Accessed June 24, 2019.

30. Centers for Medicare and Medicaid Services. Quality Payment Program (QPP) Participation in 2018: Results At-A-Glance. Available at: https://qpp-cm-prod-content.s3.amazonaws.com/uploads/586/2018%20QPP%20Participation%20Results%20Infographic.pdf. Accessed July 22, 2019.

31. Centers for Medicare and Medicaid Services. Promoting Interoperability (PI) Programs: Public Use Files. Available at: https://www.cms.gov/Regulations-and-Guidance/Legislation/EHRIncentivePrograms/PUF.html. Accessed July 28, 2019.

Chapter 12

Telebehavioral Health
Mental Health Landscape

Teresa Rufin, MPH, David Mou, and Thomas Tsang, MD, MPH

Contents

Improvements in mental healthcare continue to lag behind progress made in care for physical conditions due to barriers in accessing and affording mental health treatment. Nearly one in five adults in the United States suffers from a mental illness, yet fewer than half of those diagnosed receive treatment.[1] The Mental Health Parity Act of 2008 aimed to reduce this discrepancy by requiring health plans to provide the same level of coverage for mental health benefits as for other types of treatment, but limitations and loopholes within the legislation have allowed insurers to continue restricting their behavioral care coverage.[2]

One promising method by which healthcare organizations hope to reduce the cost burden of care for providers and patients is through the implementation of value-based payment models, which shift payments from traditional fee-for-service to prioritizing quality of care and outcomes. These alternative payment systems have gained traction among payers and providers of physical health services, but uptake has been slow in behavioral health programs.[3] Outcome measurement is particularly challenging for mental health providers due to factors such as lack of provider training and support in measuring outcomes as well as limited scientific evidence to support standardized mental health quality measures.[4]

DOI: 10.4324/9780429423109-12

Treatment accessibility in the United States is further limited by a nationwide shortage of mental health providers. Demand for mental health services has increased, but the number of practicing providers continues to shrink.[5] Nearly one in five counties in the U.S. report an unmet need for non-prescribing providers, while nearly every single county has an unmet need for psychiatrists.[5] In rural areas of the U.S., 60% of residents live in mental health professional shortage areas.[6]

Technology and Mental Health

At first glance, it would appear that the challenges facing mental health – insufficient providers, difficulty quantifying value-add, overcoming stigma – lend themselves to technological solutions. Yet, until very recently, many barriers prevented widespread adoption of technologies to enable or enhance behavioral healthcare. Tele-video technology has only recently become reliable and widespread enough for mainstream use. Mental health providers have also been reticent to embrace technology given that their training typically emphasizes the importance of in-person interactions, despite the preponderance of data suggesting non-inferiority for teletherapy and telepsychiatry.[7-8] Furthermore, health insurance companies have to establish billing procedures for technology use. Lastly, generating evidence to support the clinical and economic value of telehealth is comparatively more challenging than medical illnesses. For example, it is well known that depression screening and treatment lead to better clinical outcomes and a large reduction in total healthcare spend.[9-10] However, much of the financial benefit reaped by insurance companies and government payers occurs over the following three years. Compare this with diabetes screening, which can reduce risk of diagnosis within months, and you can appreciate why payers have historically been more reticent to commit to investments in behavioral health technologies. Despite the inertia of historical precedence, mounting evidence is suggesting that technologies in mental health are adding significant value. We will review some of the more promising ideas.

Telehealth Advantages

The use of web-based technology to deliver mental healthcare, i.e. telemental healthcare, has proliferated in recent years and shows promise in addressing current limitations facing mental healthcare cost and delivery.[7] These technologies exist in various capacities, including video-conferencing calls with providers, smartphone applications to keep patients involved and engaged in treatment, social media and digital networks to promote information transfer and communication between patients and providers, and video games providing therapeutic interventions for patients.

Studies on telemental healthcare suggest that they generate cost-savings for patients and institutions by reducing the need for in-person visits and are able to address provider shortages by delivering remote care to areas lacking in mental health providers.[7] Telehealth technologies have the capacity to facilitate more efficient data collection and dissemination, allowing for more comprehensive and accurate diagnoses and outcome measurements as well as improved communication among care providers and institutions. Many telehealth solutions are also designed to keep patients engaged with treatment outside of visits, such as through the use of smartphone apps and email or text message reminders. By creating an additional, remote point of connection between patients and their care team, these technologies enable better treatment compliance, health-promoting behaviors, and communication between patients and providers.

Research on telehealth interventions for chronic conditions have found that they yield improvements in visit attendance and medication compliance[8-10] and are associated with direct physical improvements, such as reductions in blood pressure and hemoglobin A1C among patients with hypertension and diabetes.[11-13] Among patients with behavioral health conditions, telehealth services are associated with fewer hospital admissions, suicide attempts, and symptom reduction of mental illnesses.[14-18]

The Need for Telemental Healthcare

Few events in recent history have demonstrated the necessity of telemental health services as powerfully as the ongoing COVID-19 pandemic. As regions across the United States implement increasingly stringent social isolation regulations, many healthcare providers have been forced to work remotely. Mental illness symptoms are being exacerbated by fears of disease spread, concerns about the economy and job market, stress regarding unstable financial situations, and reduced social support during isolation.[19]

The Chinese and Australian governments began providing telehealth services to address mental health needs at the start of the COVID-19 outbreak, including counseling with specialists and psychoeducation through online platforms.[19] In such times of mass panic and uncertainty, telemental health services can provide relief by connecting populations with the psychological tools needed to cope with the stress of pandemic and prolonged isolation.

Prior to the pandemic, stakeholders in healthcare had already begun to embrace telehealth as a solution to increase convenience and the reach of providers. In a way, COVID-19 served as a catalyst to further normalize the use of telehealth in general. This shift is likely to be permanent at least in part; patients who can receive care in the comfort and privacy of their own homes may prefer the new treatment modality over the in-person model.

New Methods of Delivering Care

Technology also allows for innovative approaches for care delivery. Some companies have demonstrated efficacy in providing talk therapy through asynchronous chat.[20] Therapists and patients would not meet face to face in these models, but they would chat with each other over their phones. Other companies leverage the power of peer support.[21] Some companies have connected those requesting care with 'trained listeners' who volunteer their time to help others.[22] Millions of such interactions have occurred free of charge, which serves as a sober testament to the latent demand for care and the dire inadequacy of our current mental healthcare system. Despite obvious concerns about quality, this solution appears to produce positive patient satisfaction and seems to be a net positive overall, especially if the alternative is no treatment at all.[20-21] Still other companies have supplemented human therapists with algorithms. Using artificial intelligence and machine learning, these companies have created 'chatbots' to speak with patients and triage them to the right providers.[23] For many patients, the chatbot could be sufficient by itself to deliver strategies for dealing with mild anxiety and depressive symptoms.[23-24] The user experience is still not perfect, and patients are still not accustomed to receiving care from an algorithm, but the power of this approach is that these algorithms are continually improving themselves with more practice.[24] Eventually, patients would find it difficult to differentiate between human and AI texting, though this is unlikely to take place in the short term.[24]

Such departures from orthodox treatments would be inconceivable within most healthcare organizations, but these entrepreneurial companies are intent on showing that their interventions are clinically effective, and importantly, less expensive and more easily scalable than conventional treatment. As technologies do a better job at quantifying human behaviors and linking digital interventions with positive clinical outcomes, stakeholders are beginning to listen. Increasingly, payers are paying attention to these innovative solutions, as evidenced by their heavy involvements as investors, creators, and acquirers of these companies.[25-26] Sclerotic healthcare organizations that ignore these technologies do so at their own peril; technology will inevitably become the cornerstone for mental health delivery and treatment given its convenience, low cost, and scalability.

The Advent of Digital Therapeutics

Another exciting treatment approach to mental healthcare is to rely on prescriptions, not for medications, but for smartphone apps. When a company develops a new drug, it must first show that the drug is safe in animals and humans, and then run multiple studies to demonstrate its clinical efficacy in humans. These studies are timely and expensive: taking a drug from bench to market will cost more than a billion dollars. The Food and Drug Administration oversees this process, which until very recently only included drugs and medical devices. What if you could prescribe a smartphone app instead? Given the ubiquity of smartphones, and the growing body of evidence that digital interventions are effective, the FDA is now working on creating a new framework that would allow for apps, or 'digital therapeutics,' to be approved.[27] Allowing physicians to prescribe an app would drastically improve access to digital treatments given that primary care physicians (PCPs) still serve as most Americans' gateway to care.

Companies have developed digital apps that can be prescribed for substance use disorders, insomnia, and the management of schizophrenia.[28] Importantly, many of these treatments are not stand-alone solutions and are only indicated if combined with other medications or treatment modalities. For example, for patients suffering from opioid use disorders, the therapy smartphone app can only be prescribed in conjunction with buprenorphine, an effective medication that decreases cravings.[29]

To be sure, multiple barriers remain. The logistics for onboarding technology for patients is different from filling medications at the local pharmacy. Patients without smartphones would be excluded. Insurance companies must be convinced that these apps are worth the effort to put on their formulary. Perhaps most importantly, physicians are not used to prescribing apps, and changing physician behavior has always been a trying endeavor. Yet, most of these issues have much to do with the challenge of change and habit. It may take time, but app prescriptions will likely become the norm as people become more technologically literate.

Technology Improves Care Coordination

Care coordination has always posed a great challenge for healthcare at large. A complex patient may have to coordinate care among multiple doctors and care managers. The burden often falls on patients or family members who are not adequately equipped to handle such a challenging managerial task. Some mental health technology companies have centralized care management online.[30] Care providers can share information freely within a secure communication platform.

The patient can easily access care through the smartphone or computer. All interactions are quantified, and sophisticated algorithms can determine when patients may be in need of care.[30] The goal is to make healthcare more preventative and less reactive.

Collaborative Care Case Study [MD1]

One case study published by the American Psychological Association provides first-hand evidence of how technology can promote care coordination.[31] In 2015, Montefiore Health System launched its Collaborative Care Model (CoCM), a program designed to better integrate mental healthcare with primary care. Under this model, PCPs treating patients with mental health conditions are supported by a behavioral healthcare manager and psychiatric consultant. In establishing this model, the Montefiore CoCM also piloted a smartphone application developed by Valera Health to optimize the effectiveness of the CoCM. The Valera application supported patient engagement, symptom monitoring, and timely follow-up and promoted patient self-management, allowing case managers to maintain an increased caseload. It also facilitated easier communication and collaboration among the case manager, PCP, and psychiatric consultant. Primary case sites using the application saw case managers increase their caseloads from an average of 60–70 to 90–100 patients while improving outcomes and connecting with patients in a timelier manner. Patients who used the Valera app showed higher engagement rates, follow-up rates, and satisfaction rates compared with patients not using the app.

Next Steps for Technology

After several months of lockdown, the COVID-19 pandemic shows no signs of ending soon. Countries all over the world are learning to adjust to a new reality of remote interactions and increased dependence on technology. Various factors of the pandemic have led to an explosion of demand for teletherapy services, highlighting both the promises of this industry and the barriers it faces in attaining scalability. Parity laws present a major limitation in widespread telehealth implementation.[32] While many states have expanded their statutes to require payers to cover and reimburse telehealth encounters the same as in-person visits, affordability will continue to be a deterrent for many who seek treatment.[32] Additionally, although teletherapy can ease the burden of mental health provider shortages, it will not close the workforce gap.[33] However, the challenges facing teletherapy will not inhibit its growth; rather, they will require a reckoning with how mental healthcare is viewed and prioritized.[34] It is abundantly evident that telehealth is feasible, effective, and here to stay; the question is, how quickly can healthcare systems adapt?

About the Authors

David Mou, MD, MBA, David is a psychiatrist, healthcare executive, and serial entrepreneur. He serves as the Director of MGH Psychiatry's Innovation Council. David is the Chief Medical Officer of Cerebral, one of the largest tele-health companies that has provided high quality mental healthcare to more than 300,000 patients across all 50 states. Cerebral also works with pharmaceutical companies to pioneer decentralized clinical trials, for which David serves as Principal

Investigator. Previously, David was President, Co-founder and Chief Medical Officer of Valera Health, a telehealth company that reduced unnecessary hospitalizations for patients with serious mental illness. David is on faculty at Harvard Medical School, where he has conducted research on how digital technologies can help better predict and prevent suicidal behaviors. He has been named 'Top 10 under 35 for Healthcare' by LinkedIn, as well as '40 under 40' for healthcare innovation by MedTech Boston. David graduated from Harvard College with a degree in neurobiology and earned his MD MBA from Harvard Medical School and Harvard Business School. His writings have appeared in the New England Journal of Medicine and Stat.

Thomas Tsang, MD, MPH, is the CEO and co-founder of Valera Health, a telehealth organization providing personalized team-based clinical care. His prior experiences include working as CMO of the largest FQHC network for Asian Americans, CMO at Merck's Digital Service/Solutions division, and medical director at ONC/HHS rolling out aspects of the Affordable Care Act. He was a congressional staffer on the Ways and Means Committee and helped draft legislation for the ACA and also a senior advisor to the governor of Hawaii on value-based.

Teresa Rufin, MPH, is a Program Manager at Valera Health. Prior to Valera, she worked as a behavioral health researcher at Columbia University Medical Center. She received her master's in public health in health policy at the Harvard T. H. Chan School of Public Health and holds an AB in psychology from Princeton University.

Works Cited

1. Substance Abuse and Mental Health Services Administration. 2018. Key Substance Use and Mental Health Indicators in the United States: Results from the 2017 National Survey on Drug Use and Health (HHS Publication No. SMA 18–5068, NSUDH Series H-53). Rockville, MD: Center for Behavioral Health Statistics and Quality, Substance Abuse and Mental Health Services Administration.
2. Health Affairs Policy Brief. 2014. Mental Health Parity. https://www.healthaffairs.org/do/10.1377/hpb20140403.871424/full/.
3. Center for Health Care Strategies, Inc. 2017. Moving Toward Value-Based Payment for Medicaid Behavioral Health Services. https://www.chcs.org/media/VBP-BH-Brief-061917.pdf.
4. Kilbourne, A.M., Beck, K., Spaeth-Rublee, B., et al. 2018. Measuring and Improving the Quality of Mental Health Care: A Global Perspective. *World Psychiatry: Official Journal of the World Psychiatric Association (WPA)*, 17(1): 30–38.
5. Butryn, T., Bryant, L., Marchionni, C., and F. Sholevar. 2017. The Shortage of Psychiatrists and Other Mental Health Providers: Causes, Current State, and Potential Solutions. *International Journal of Academic Medicine*, 3(1): 5–9.
6. National Institute of Mental Health. 2018. Mental Health and Rural America: Challenges and Opportunities. https://www.nimh.nih.gov/news/media/2018/mental-health-and-rural-america-challenges-and-opportunities.shtml.
7. Langarizadeh, M., Tabatabaei, M.S., Tavakol, K., Naghipour, M., Rostami, A., and F. Moghbeli. 2017. Telemental Health Care, an Effective Alternative to Conventional Mental Care: A Systematic Review. *Acta Informatica Medica: AIM Journal of the Society for Medical Informatics of Bosnia & Herzegovina: casopis Drustva za medicinsku informatiku BiH*, 25(4): 240–246.

8. Jaglal, S.B., Haroun, V.A., Salbach, N.M., Hawker, G., Voth, J., Lou, W., Kontos, P., Cameron, J.E., Cockerill, R., and T. Bereket. 2013. Increasing Access to Chronic Disease Self-Management Programs in Rural and Remote Communities Using Telehealth. *Telemedicine Journal and e-health: The Official Journal of the American Telemedicine Association*, 19(6), 467–473. https://doi.org/10.1089/tmj.2012.0197.

9. Schulze, L.N., Stentzel, U., Leipert, J., et al. 2019. Improving Medication Adherence with Telemedicine for Adults with Severe Mental Illness. *Psychiatric Services*, 70(3): 225–228. doi:10.1176/appi.ps.201800286.

10. Bingham, J.M., Black, M., Anderson, E.J., et al. 2020. Impact of Telehealth Interventions on Medication Adherence for Patients with Type 2 Diabetes, Hypertension, and/or Dyslipidemia: A Systematic Review. *The Annals of Pharmacotherapy*. 106002802095072–1060028020950726.

11. Wu, C., Wu, Z., Yang, L., Zhu, W., Zhang, M., Zhu, Q., Chen, X., and Y. Pan. 2018. Evaluation of the Clinical Outcomes of Telehealth for Managing Diabetes: A PRISMA-Compliant Meta-Analysis. *Medicine*, 97(43): e12962. https://doi.org/10.1097/MD.0000000000012962.

12. Lu, J.F., Chen, C.M., and C.Y. Hsu. 2019. Effect of Home Telehealth Care on Blood Pressure Control: A Public Healthcare Centre Model. *Journal of Telemedicine and Telecare*, 25(1): 35–45. doi:10.1177/1357633X17734258.

13. Cottrell, E., Chambers, R., and P. O'Connell. 2012. Using Simple Telehealth in Primary Care to Reduce Blood Pressure: A Service Evaluation. *BMJ Open*, 2, e001391. doi:10.1136/bmjopen-2012-001391.

14. Hilty, D.M., Ferrer, D.C., Parish, M.B., Johnston, B., Callahan, E.J., and P.M. Yellowlees. 2013. The Effectiveness of Telemental Health: A 2013 Review. *Telemedicine Journal and e-health: The Official Journal of the American Telemedicine Association*, 19(6): 444–454.

15. Kobb, R., Hoffman, N., Lodge, R., and S. Kline. 2003. Enhancing Elder Chronic Care Through Technology and Care Coordination: Report from a Pilot. *Telemedicine Journal and e-Health*: 189–195. http://doi.org/10.1089/153056203766437525.

16. Steventon, A., Bardsley, M., Billings, J., Dixon, J., Doll, H., Hirani, S., et al. 2012. Effect of Telehealth on Use of Secondary Care and Mortality: Findings from the Whole System Demonstrator Cluster Randomised Trial. *BMJ*, 344: e3874.

17. Kasckow, J., Gao, S., Hanusa, B., Rotondi, A., Chinman, M., Zickmund, S., Gurklis, J., et al. 2015. Telehealth Monitoring of Patients with Schizophrenia and Suicidal Ideation. *Suicide and Life-Threatening Behavior*, 45(5), 600–611. https://doi.org/10.1111/sltb.12154.

18. Luxton, D., O'Brien, K., Pruitt, L., Johnson, K., and G. Kramer. 2014. Suicide Risk Management During Clinical Telepractice. *International Journal of Psychiatry in Medicine*, 48: 19–31.10.2190/PM.48.1.c.

19. Pignone, M.P., Bradley, N.G., Rushton, J.L., et al. 2002. Screening for Depression in Adults: A Summary of the Evidence for the U.S. Preventive Services Task Force. *Annals of Internal Medicine*, 136(10): 765–776.

20. Valenstein, M., Sandeep, V., John, E.Z., Kathryn, B., and B. Amna. 2001. The Cost – Utility of Screening for Depression in Primary Care. *Annals of Internal Medicine*, 134(5): 345–360.

21. Zhou, X., Snoswell, C.L., Harding, L.E., et al. 2020. The Role of Telehealth in Reducing the Mental Health Burden from COVID-19. *Telemedicine and e-Health*. ahead of print. http://doi.org/10.1089/tmj.2020.0068.

22. Hull, T.D., Connolly, P., Mahan, K., and K. Yang. 2015. The Treatment Effectiveness of Asynchronous Text Therapy for Depression and Anxiety: A Longitudinal Cohort Study. https://www.talkspace.com/online-therapy/wp-content/uploads/2018/04/Talkspace-Depression_Anxiety-Large-Scale-Study.pdf.

23. Fortuna, K.L., Naslund, J.A., LaCroix, J.M., et al. 2020. Digital Peer Support Mental Health Interventions for People with a Lived Experience of a Serious Mental Illness: Systematic Review. *JMIR Mental Health*, 7(4): e16460.

24. Baumel, A., Tinkelman, A., Mathur, N., and J.M. Kane. 2018. Digital Peer-Support Platform (7Cups) as an Adjunct Treatment for Women with Postpartum Depression: Feasibility, Acceptability, and Preliminary Efficacy Study. *JMIR MHealth and UHealth*, 6(2): e38.

25. Jesus, A.D. 2019. Chatbots for Mental Health and Therapy – Comparing 5 Current Apps and Use Cases. *Emerj*. https://emerj.com/ai-application-comparisons/chatbots-mental-health-therapy-comparing-5-current-apps-use-cases/.

26. Thompson, C. 2018. May A.I. Help You? *The New York Times*. https://www.nytimes.com/interactive/2018/11/14/magazine/tech-design-ai-chatbot.html.

27. Somauroo, J. 2020. New Research Shows Global Mental Health Investment Topped $750 Million In 2019. *Forbes*. https://www.forbes.com/sites/jamessomauroo/2020/02/24/new-research-shows-global-mental-health-investing-topped-750-million-in-2019/#2396dd0f4196.

28. Hays, S. 2020. Approaching 1,000 Mental Health Startups in 2020. *What If Ventures*. https://whatif.vc/blog/approaching-1000-mental-health-startups-in 2020.

29. Food and Drug Administration. 2019. Policy for Device Software Functions and Mobile Medical Applications. *U.S. Department of Health and Human Services*. https://www.fda.gov/media/80958/download.

30. Weir, Kirsten. 2018. The Ascent of Digital Therapies. *American Psychological Association*, 49(10): 80.

31. Commissioner, Office of the U.S. Food and Drug Administration. 2018. FDA Clears Mobile Medical App to Help Those with Opioid Use Disorder Stay in Recovery Programs. https://www.fda.gov/news-events/press-announcements/fda-clears-mobile-medical-app-help-those-opioid-use-disorder-stay-recovery-programs.

32. Falconer, E., Kho, D., and J.P. Docherty. 2018. Use of Technology for Care Coordination Initiatives for Patients with Mental Health Issues: A Systematic Literature Review. *Neuropsychiatric Disease and Treatment*, 14: 2337–2349.

33. American Psychiatric Association. 2018. Leveraging Digital Technology to Improve Behavioral Health Integration with Primary Care. *Accountable Care Learning Collaborative*. https://valerahealth.com/wp-content/uploads/2018/07/Montefiore_APA_ValeraHealth_Case_Study_Website.pdf.

34. Warren, J.C., and K.B. Smalley. 2020. Using Telehealth to Meet Mental Health Needs During the COVID-19 Crisis. *The Commonwealth Fund*. https://www.commonwealthfund.org/blog/2020/using-telehealth-meet-mental-health-needs-during-covid-19-crisis.

35. Coward, K. 2020. Providers Get Creative to Address Worsening Behavioral Workforce Shortage Amid COVID-19. *Behavioral Health Business*. https://bhbusiness.com/2020/03/23/providers-get-creative-to-address-worsening-behavioral-workforce-shortage-amid-covid-19/.

36. Asar, A. 2020. Teletherapy and Digital Health Aren't Just Stopgaps – They're the Future of Mental Health Care. *Forbes Technology Council*. https://www.forbes.com/sites/forbestechcouncil/2020/07/21/teletherapy-and-digital-health-arent-just-stopgaps--theyre-the-future-of-mental-health-care/#7d3cf1f73904.

37. Hilt, R.J., Barclay, R.P., Bush, J., Stout, B., Anderson, N., and J.R. Wignall. 2015. A Statewide Child Telepsychiatry Consult System Yields Desired Health System Changes and Savings. *Telemedicine and e-Health*: 533–537.

38. Powell, A.C., Chen, M., and C. Thammachart. 2017. The Economic Benefits of Mobile Apps for Mental Health and Telepsychiatry Services When Used by Adolescents. *Child and Adolescent Psychiatric Clinics of North America, Health Information Technology for Child and Adolescent Psychiatry*, 26(1): 125–133.

[MD1]Tom

Chapter 13

Optimizing Medication Use through Health Information Technology
A Pharmacist's Perspective

Troy Trygstad, PhD, Mary Ann Kliethermes, BS, Anne L. Burns, BSPharm, RPh, Mary Roth McClurg, Pharm.D., MHS, Marie Smith, PharmD, FNAP and Jon Easter, PhD

Contents

DOI: 10.4324/9780429423109-13

KEY DEFINITIONS AND CONCEPTS:

- *Medication optimization* (MO) encompasses patient-centered activities that improve health outcomes by addressing medication appropriateness, effectiveness, safety, adherence, and access.[1]
- Historically, conveying the value of *medication optimization services* (MOS) has been challenging due to the diversity of their implementations and a lack of appreciation for the magnitude of influence that environmental factors play in determining their effectiveness.
- The Pharmacists' Patient Care Process (PPCP)[2] is a systematic approach for pharmacist provision of care, regardless of the type of service or the pharmacy practice setting. The process consists of five steps: Collect, Assess, Plan, Implement, and Follow Up: Monitor and Evaluate.
- Adoption of an *ontological approach* based on the PPCP for describing discrete MOS would serve to advance the proliferation, evaluation and overall effectiveness of these services.
- Integration and adaptation of MOS into care delivery systems through evidence-based *implementation systems* enables scalable solutions that produce consistent effectiveness outcomes.

---

[1] CMM in Primary Care Research Team. 2018. The patient care process for delivering comprehensive medication management (CMM): Optimizing medication use in patient-centered, team-based care settings. *ACCP*. https://accp.com/cmm_care_process.

[2] Joint Commission of Pharmacy Practitioners. 2014. Pharmacists' patient care process. https://jcpp.net/wp-content/uploads/2016/03/PatientCareProcess-with-supporting-organizations.pdf.

I. Introduction: Medications Are Our Principal Means of Intervention and Treatment

The use of vaccinations and medications has become and will likely continue to be the principal means of intervention and treatment used to improve the health of populations by slowing the progression of or eliminating disease. Medication-related interventions intended to improve patient outcomes encompass an innumerable set of services across the medication use spectrum. These services are provided by a wide variety of licensed and non-licensed practitioners in multiple care settings, with diverse levels of intensity and duration, often requiring differing sources of information and communication modalities to support service delivery. The potential to improve health from optimal medication use is enormous. Yet we often fail to achieve the therapeutic outcomes found in clinical trials and controlled environments owing to the additional complexities borne both by the patient and healthcare system at large when medications are deployed into real-world environments. Pharmacy informatics play an essential role in optimizing the use of vaccinations and medications to realize their value and full health producing potential.

The goals of this chapter are:

1. To provide healthcare leaders with background on the history of pharmacy practice and informatics.
2. Emphasize the need for medication optimization (MO) as a core component of quality improvement and population health management strategies.
3. Highlight emerging trends in pharmacy informatics that provide the rationale and implementation considerations for the expansion of medication optimization service lines.

II. A Short History of Pharmacy Practice and Informatics

The Profession of Pharmacy: A Product-Based Upbringing

The practice of pharmacy dates back to ancient times when the practice of "medicine" was part and parcel to the broader occupation of "healer." It wasn't until the 13th century when pharmacy and medicine were formally split into separate professions in Sicily, Italy, by Fredrick the Second by conferring certain practice responsibilities upon pharmacists. Pharmacies as places to procure medications and other household goods became prominent all over the world beginning in the 17th century, with most medicinal products compounded on site at the pharmacy. By the 20th century, modern drug development pulled the manufacturing of most prescription products from behind the pharmacy counter into manufacturing facilities.

Pharmacy Informatics: The Early Years

The simplest and most essential form of pharmacy informatics in the modern medical era has been the accurate transmission of orders from physician to pharmacy for filling and dispensing to the patient or their caregiver. Paper-based orders, written at the practice site of a physician or on site at the pharmacy and then later by other healthcare professionals, relied largely on the patient as the means of transmission for these often hard-to-interpret handwritten notes. Similarly, pharmacists inscribed handwritten instructions and labels on prescription bottles for patients to interpret. After dispensing, these quarter sheets of paper were filed in small drawers, often never

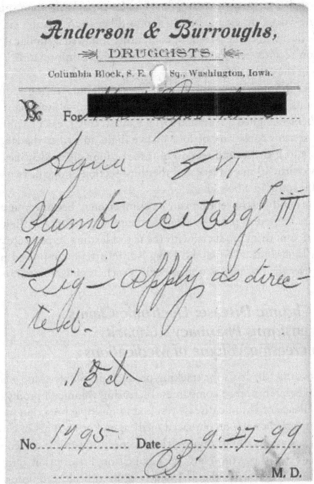

A Prescription Written and Filled at Anderson and Burroughs Pharmacy in Washington, Iowa on September 27th, 1899. Rx no. 1995.

Figure 13.1   Prescription from 1899

to be looked at again (See Figure 13.1). It wasn't until the Durham-Humphrey Amendment of 1951 to the Food, Drug, and Cosmetic Act that certain drugs required prescriptions written by authorized licensed prescribers (at the time, essentially physicians). The general lack of associated information related to diagnosis, intended effects, and continuity from one order to the next marked a general deficit in informatics for these early years.

Twentieth-Century Explosion in Medication Use Compels Digitization: Pharmacies and Payers Demand Scalable Transactions

The pharmaceutical manufacturing industry was a relatively modest industry in the earlier part of the 20th century. However, innovations in new drug discovery and approvals began to accelerate in the middle part of that century, with an average of 20 novel drug approvals per year until the early 1980s, when new drug development and approval began to steadily increase, roughly doubling in the 1990s. Meanwhile, the advent of computing followed a similar time line, and trajectory and prescription records became some of the first health information to become digitized nearly ubiquitously in the early 1990s.

As the cost of medications grew, so did the generic manufacturing industry. This resulted in many tens of thousands of different drug products becoming available in the marketplace, with each product being assigned a National Drug Code (NDC), each having ten digits in three segments. The first section consisting of four or five digits identifies the labeler (manufacturer, repackager or distributor); the second section of three or four digits identifies the drug, strength and form (e.g. atorvastatin 10 mg tablet); and the third section of one or two digits identifies the package size (e.g. 100 count in a bottle).

Importantly, this ten-digit convention can be cumbersome, because you have to account for where the sections are located to precisely identify the product. Thus, 11-digit NDCs are today's common representation of drug products, with the use of leading zeros to create unique numbering for hundreds of thousands of Food and Drug Administration approved products, both prescriptions only and over the counter, as well as devices such as glucose monitors.

From Acute to Chronic Disease: Electronic Claims Transmission Transforms Pharmacy's Capacity to Handle an Increasing Volume of Medications

In 1972 the NDC became the basis for tracking products in supply chain management and for payment to pharmacies by insurance companies. Increasing volume of product availability along with increasing prevalence of chronic disease resulted in multiple prescriptions written and filled in a given year. Pharmacy claims soon outpaced medical and other types of claims in volume.

Because pharmacies were early to digitize their records and insurance companies were keen on communicating in real time, the National Council on Prescription Drug Plans (NCPDP) put forth the TELECOM standard, the first widely utilized healthcare information technology standard in the history of healthcare administration. As the principal means by which a pharmacy communicates a prescription claim to a third-party payer, the TELECOM standard and its updates and extensions are now the basis for nearly ten billion real-time transactions per year across four billion prescription fills, drug utilization review alerts (e.g. refill too soon), prior authorization approvals and rudimentary medication management functions.

No More Scribbles: Electronic Prescribing Catalyzes the World's Largest Health Information Exchange

Though submitting claims electronically in real time became ubiquitous, handwritten prescriptions sent with the patient or printed and sent via facsimile were the norm until the SCRIPT electronic prescribing standard was created as a collaboration between NCPDP (the pharmacy plan standards entity) and Health Level 7 (HL7), the principal medical side standards entity at the turn of the century. Adoption was slow until substantial incentives were put in place, first with the Medicare Modernization Act of 2003 and then the HI-TECH portion of the Affordable Care Act. In 2018, there were approximately two billion electronic prescription transactions.[3]

---

[3] Surescripts. 2018. National progress report. https://surescripts.com/news-center/national-progress-report-2018/.

More than Dispensing: Prescription Accuracy Improves, but Suboptimal Medication Use Persists

Despite the ability to transmit prescriptions accurately from one electronic system to another with near 100% accuracy, medication errors still persist that are related to medication appropriateness, dosing effectiveness and patient safety elements in the prescribing and clinical decision-making processes. The average Medicare recipient with five or more chronic conditions will fill 51 prescriptions and have a 24% chance of experiencing at least one hospitalization during the year.[4] Medication complexity and use has grown faster than our healthcare system's ability to properly accommodate for safe and effective use. US government data indicate adverse drug events occur in two million hospital stays per year, or in 1 out of 3 patients; and in the ambulatory setting lead to over 3.5 million physician office visits, 1 million emergency department visits and 125,000 hospitalizations.[5] The cost of poorly optimized prescription medication is estimated at $528.4 billion for resulting patient morbidity and mortality.[6] Human error can lead to mis-entry or inappropriate dose, strength, form or even drug for the patients' condition(s). Patients can misinterpret instructions that are not clear or not in their native language. Multiple prescribers can contribute to polypharmacy and overuse, contraindications, drug-drug conflicts, therapeutic duplications and other errors. *None of these problems is solved by increasing the accuracy of electronic prescription transmission from prescriber to pharmacy.*

Prescription Fill History and Benefit Check: Linking Nationwide Claims Databases to Coordinate Care and Preempt Insurance Coverage Disruptions

Prescribers and other care team members are often in an information vacuum when assessing patient medication regimens for new prescriptions or for attempting to optimize existing regimens. Patient recall of medication-taking history is dependent on many factors, including cognition and health literacy, with recall of how often to take a medication or associated side effects as low as nearly 50%.[7] Additionally, the medication lists maintained in electronic medical records (EMRs) have low concordance with what has actually been filled at the pharmacy or how the patient is using actually taking the medications at home. Prior to more recent data sharing tools, a 2009 study looked at two EMRs from two large health systems and found only 65% congruence between the active medication list in their EMR and the actual prescription filling behavior in the community pharmacy.[8]

In an attempt to improve medication lists in EMRs, prescription fill history and pharmacy benefit check transactions were created and launched alongside electronic prescribing. In 2018, nearly two billion prescription fill history transactions occurred directly to EMRs and other

[4] RAND Corporation. 2017. Multiple chronic conditions in the U.S. https://www.rand.org/content/dam/rand/pubs/tools/TL200/TL221/RAND_TL221.pdf.

[5] Office of Disease Prevention and Health Promotion. 2020. *Adverse Drug Events*. US. Dept of Health and Human Services. https://health.gov/our-work/health-care-quality/adverse-drug-events.

[6] Wantanbe JH, McInnis T, Hirsh JD. 2018. Cost of prescription related morbidity and mortality. *Ann Pharmacother* 52:829–837.

[7] Backes AC, Kuo GM. 2012. The association between functional health literacy and patient-reported recall of medications at outpatient pharmacies. *Res Social Adm Pharm* 8(4):349–354.

[8] Olson MD1, Tong GL, Steiner BD, Viera AJ, Ashkin E, Newton WP. 2012. Medication documentation in a primary care network serving North Carolina Medicaid patients: Results of a cross-sectional chart review. *BMC Fam Pract* 13:83.

clinician-facing user interfaces, and more than 40 million benefits checks allow prescribers to see what medications are covered by the health plan.[9]

III. Optimizing Medication Use and the Role of Informatics

The Medication Optimization Model: Conjoint Outputs Required for Best Outcomes

The second habit in Stephen R. Covey's *Seven Habits of Highly Effective People* is "Keep the end in mind." Of all of the habits he lauded, focusing on the global objective or outcome to be produced is possibly the most difficult habit for healthcare practitioners to adopt. Care team members typically play an individual role in a complex system of care, and it is all too easy for clinicians to forget to step back from the trees and look at the forest from time to time. Perhaps this deficit stems from modern medicine's fee-for-service financing origins, which have tended to lack outcomes-based accountability and payment incentives. As a result, healthcare delivery tends to be described and defined in terms of activities rather than intended effects.

Using the outcome or the intended effect to communicate the nature of a service may be a better strategy if the objective is to provide for a more common understanding of the purpose of the service. The model illustrated below attempts to do so by separating activity from desired output. MO represents a state of ideal medication use for a given patient at a given moment in time. Medication optimization services (MOS) represent the activities or interventions deployed in order to achieve optimal medication use, which is a function of a medication regimen itself and patient use and adherence to that regimen. MOS can attempt to improve upon either or both sub-outputs of medication use.

The Need to Orchestrate Care: Increasing Therapeutic Complexity and Reliance on Patient Self-Management Cause Failure and Harm

For too long, prescribers and other health professionals have assumed that a correct diagnosis, with a well-indicated medication prescribed, filled accurately and dispensed with the correct label by the pharmacy addressed the entirety of patient need. Far too many prescribers follow clinical guidelines for prescribing and assume that so long as the right drug is prescribed, positive health outcomes will follow.

Yet the challenges associated with achieving optimal medication use are far more numerous than the rote ordering and filling of a medication. There are often many care team actors involved, including other prescribers, care managers, pharmacists, multiple pharmacies, behavioral health providers, caretakers, neighbors and friends, and of course a patient many times ill-equipped to self-manage and self-direct taking medication. Adding to the complexity of medication optimization is patient understanding of the medication label. Marginal literacy and taking greater numbers of medications leads to significant misunderstanding on appropriate medication use. A recent study found that 3 out of 4 patients filled their new prescriptions, but only 31% of new diabetes medications were filled, indicating a significant problem with adherence of medications to treat

---

[9] Surescripts 2018. National progress report. https://surescripts.com/news-center/national-progress-report-2018/.

chronic conditions.[10] In an information vacuum, the prescriber or care team member is left to make inferences about therapeutic failure or interactions with other medications that are not valid or relevant when the patient is not actually consuming the prescribed medication.

Value-Based Payments: Medicare Stars Shine a Light on Medication Non-adherence

The Medicare Modernization Act of 2003 was a seminal moment for both pharmacy informatics as well as value-based payment models and plan bonus structures. In addition to incentives for prescribers to adopt electronic prescribing, an emphasis on quality reporting and bonus programs for the newly created Part D Drug Benefit led to triple weighted Proportion of Days Covered (PDC) – often termed adherence – measures that have a disproportionate influence compared to other measures in prescription drug plan and Medicare Advantage Plan star ratings. When Medicare star ratings were implemented for the first time in 2007, awareness of both the prevalence and challenge of medication non-adherence grew from nuanced discussions among researchers to widespread recognition. The measures were a call to healthcare professionals, plans and technology providers alike to implement programs and supports for patients to achieve the 80% PDC threshold benchmark at the drug class level (e.g. oral antidiabetics) set as a label representing successful adherence by a plan member.

The PDC measurement is possible through analysis of paid prescription claims, which include the prescription fill date and the NDC (so as to know the medication dispensed but also maintain the ability to group by drug class) and the days of supply (from which the number of units per day can be determined). PDC is calculated as the number of days in a given calendar year for which the patient had possession of medication to be taken.

More than Non-adherence: Accountable Care Movement Wakes Up to the Enormity of the Challenge

With Part D also came formal medication therapy management (MTM) programs to be administered by Part D plans via comprehensive medication reviews (which are single weighted) and gap in care closures such as statin use with diabetes. The gap in care measures are typically prescription claims based and do not consider medical claims, humanistic or clinical outcomes, despite medications being the primary means by which we achieve these healthcare goals.

Without Part D plan access to medical claims and without incentives to improve clinical measures such as blood pressure and glycated hemoglobin, pharmacy quality measurement has been somewhat limited to a narrow set of measures related to ensuring prescriptions are filled regularly. Yet, Medicare Advantage, Health Effectiveness Data Information Set (HEDIS) and other medical side quality and value-based purchasing measures are heavily influenced by optimizing medication use. In fact, 29 of the 44 HEDIS measures in 2020 are directly or indirectly influenced by medication use.[11] Ironically, the healthcare professionals and settings of care that most influence actual patient use of medications and attainment of clinical goals are the pharmacist and the

---

[10] Fischer MA, Stedman MR, Lii J, et al. 2010. Primary medication non-adherence: Analysis of 195,930 electronic prescriptions. *J Gen Intern Med* 25(4):284–290.

[11] NCAQ. 2020. HEDIS measures and technical resources. www.ncqa.org/hedis/measures/.

pharmacy, yet both are either implicitly or explicitly excluded from direct measurement of outcomes emanating from pharmacotherapies.

Accountable care organizations (ACOs) and other manifestations of clinical integration and provider-led quality organizations have invested greatly in population management resources both technical with EMR installations and care management systems as well as the human resources to accompany them. At-risk contracting and bonus or penalty programs, such as 30-day readmission penalties and bundled payment for joint replacements, require patient check-ins and supports outside the traditional encounter or surgery. Medication adherence and associated regimen optimization and consumption are manifest during periods of time between encounters with physicians and other healthcare providers. Thus patients, especially complex patients with multiple co-morbidities and medications, who influence disproportionately clinical and global measures such as hospitalizations and total cost of care in shared savings arrangements, greatly influence these payment models.

Medication Optimization: A Holistic Approach to Getting the Most from Our Medications

Medication optimization (MO) encompasses patient-centered activities that improve health outcomes by addressing medication appropriateness, effectiveness, safety, adherence and access. The appropriate, safe, and cost-effective use of medications is fundamental to achieve the triple aim: better patient care, healthier populations and smarter healthcare spending. Medication optimization services (MOS) can be thought of as a broad and diverse set of services provided by care team members to achieve MO and supported by technology and informatics to address patient-specific medication use needs. MOS can be provided by multiple disciplines of licensed and non-licensed professionals as well as by consumers through self-care efforts. Although the pharmacists often have primary responsibility for optimizing medications given their pharmacotherapy expertise, some MOS may also be addressed by other licensed providers. Examples of MOS where others participate in the process may include medication reconciliation activities by medical assistants or discharge planners, drug pours and related drug administration supports by home health aides, parts of MTM services or chronic care management services by pharmacy technicians or medical assistants by phone. MOS may also occur in any healthcare setting, such as drug regimen reviews by pharmacists in long-term care or diabetes self-management coaching by an educator or pharmacotherapy services staffed by a co-located pharmacist in an outpatient clinic. The spectrum of MOS has expanded over the past decade in both volume and variety in response to increasing complexity of medication regimens. An emphasis on MO encompasses patient-centered activities that improve health outcomes by addressing medication appropriateness, effectiveness, safety, adherence and access on value-driven processes and payment, and the reliance on optimal medication use to improve patient health outcomes and overall population health metrics. Modern pharmacy informatics systems must account for the plethora of product, service and biomarker data flows that emanate from these multiple therapies, interventionists, support staff, laboratory tests and devices meant to support optimal medication use.

The Medication Optimization Model: Conjoint Inputs Required for Effective Intervention and Care Delivery

Achieving optimal increases in health outputs from medications requires the conjoint inputs of an optimal medication regimen that addresses all of the conditions being treated as well as optimal consumption by the patient, through either self-administration or administration by care team

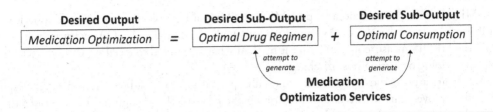

Figure 13.2   Medication Optimization Model

members, caretakers or even machines. Both optimal regimen and optimal consumption often require patient-specific considerations owing to personal and environmental factors (See Figure 13.2).

Successful MOS requires information technology systems that can account for efforts to optimize a patient-specific drug regimen alongside efforts to optimize medication-prescribing and patient adherence. A multitude of considerations are needed to optimize medications, from genetics that may affect metabolism to lack of transportation to pick up medications regularly. The informatics sequence of making the diagnosis to prescribing to prescription filling/re-filling to patient adherence in a chronic disease model to inform new prescribing and new filling is critical to getting the most health return out of our medication armament and MOS efforts.

Medication misadventures are common and often result in polypharmacy and the need to de-prescribe.[12] The origins of these misadventures can often be traced back to lack of information about other prescribing, side effects and adverse drug events not reported, non-adherence, improper or ineffective administration or consumption, or other patient-specific circumstances.

Beta-Blocker Use After Myocardial Infarction Highlights the Need for Dual Focus on Optimal Drug Regimen and Consumption

The first beta-blocker (propranolol) was discovered in 1964 by Sir James Black[13] and offered great promise for the treatment and prevention of heart diseases. Over the course of the ensuing decades, a number of beta-blockers were discovered that came to market, and they found their way into clinical pathways soon thereafter for the treatment of high blood pressure and even headaches for a period of time. By the 1980s, it became clear that beta-blockers were the clear choice for prevention of complications and future events following a prior myocardial infarction (MI). But it was not until the 1990s that beta-blockers became a staple of post-MI quality of care measurement, when HEDIS published its set of quality measures for health plans in 1997.[14] Prescribing a beta-blocker post-MI was abysmally low at the time (62%) for managed plans and an even worse 25% for Medicare fee for service, despite being widely acknowledged as best practice to prescribe

[12] Page AT, Clifford RM, Potter K, Schwartz D, Etherton-Beer CD. 2016. The feasibility and effect of deprescribing in older adults on mortality and health: a systematic review and meta-analysis. *Br J Clin Pharmacol* 82(3):583–623.

[13] Stapleton MP1. Sir James Black and propranolol. 1997. The role of the basic sciences in the history of cardiovascular pharmacology. *Tex Heart Inst J* 24(4):336–342.

[14] National Committee for Quality Assurance. 2006. *The State of Health Care Quality*. Washington, DC: National Committee for Quality Assurance.

post-MI.[15] [16] Over the next decade, post-MI prescribing of beta-blockers improved dramatically, until the point that the National Committee for Quality Assurance (NCQA) essentially "graduated" the HEDIS measure in 2007 after it reached what amounted to a ceiling with greater than 95% prescribing occurring post-discharge.[17]

Yet, heart attacks did not go away, and sub-optimal use of beta-blockers continues despite marked improvements in the rate of prescribing them post-MI. For optimal use, consideration of the beta-blocker's role alongside other medications in a patient's regimen, its dose, potential duplications and interactions, and needed adjustments from side effects are necessary to optimize a given patient's drug regimen. Additionally, consideration of patient-specific and often idiosyncratic drug-taking behavior and patient belief systems require adherence coaching, co-payment assistance, disease-state education and other MOS to optimize consumption of beta-blockers. Prescribers became aware during the advent of accountable care efforts that prescribing or ordering a beta-blocker post-MI is only one small (and relatively easy) activity that requires concomitant MOS to maximally effectuate the drug's potential.

Subsequent to emerging evidence of high levels of prescribing beta-blockers alongside low rates of prescription filling by the patient in the 2000s, HEDIS revised the prior measure to include both components of the MOM model: optimal regimen and optimal consumption. As of 2019, the HEDIS measure for beta-blockers post-MI is "Persistence of Beta-Blocker Treatment after a Heart Attack," and is measured by

> [the] percentage of members 18 years of age and older during the measurement year who were hospitalized and discharged from July 1 of the year prior to the measurement year to June 30 of the measurement year with a diagnosis of AMI and who received persistent beta-blocker treatment for six months after discharge.

This acknowledgement of a need for a dual focus toward prescribing the right medications and having those medications optimally consumed is becoming more and more commonplace. And though it seems simple to achieve on its face, MO is stubbornly difficult to achieve, especially in the 35% of Americans with multiple chronic diseases who are responsible for 70% of our healthcare system's cost.[18] Fully 80% of patients with heart attacks have co-morbidities, such as diabetes and chronic obstructive pulmonary disease,[19] complicating the seemingly easy task of optimizing the patient's full complement of medications, including over the counter, herbals, and supplements.

Unfortunately, only the beginnings of integrated data systems exist between prescribers and their EMRs and ordering systems, pharmacies and their dispensing and filling systems, and MOS providers and their various information technology systems. Active medication lists in clinical

---

[15] Dalzell MD. 1997. NCQA's quality compass points to plan differences. *Managed Care* 52A, 52G, 52H. www.managedcaremag.com/archives/9711/9711.compass.shtml.

[16] Howard PA, Ellerbeck EF. 2000. Optimizing beta-blocker use after myocardial infarction. *Am Fam Physician* 15;62(8):1853–1860, 1865–1866.

[17] Curtiss FR. 2008. HEDIS, beta-blockers, and what more can be done to improve secondary prevention in ACS. *J Manag Care Pharm* 14(3):316–317.

[18] Agency for Healthcare Research and Quality. 2010. Multiple chronic conditions chartbook. Medical Expenditure Panel Survey Data. https://www.ahrq.gov/sites/default/files/wysiwyg/professionals/prevention-chronic-care/decision/mcc/mccchartbook.pdf.

[19] Ellerbeck EF, Jencks SF, Radford MJ, Kresowik TF, Craig AS, Gold JA, et al. 1995. Quality of care for Medicare patients with acute myocardial infarction: A four-state pilot of the cooperative cardiovascular project. *JAMA* 273:1509–1514.

documentation systems are incongruent with pharmacy dispensing data, which is entirely removed from care management systems' coaching and medication plan of care reinforcement efforts.

A Team Sport: Medication Optimization Requires Coordination across Settings and Disciplines

Achieving optimal medication use for a given patient is challenging for both patients and the care team members charged with guiding their therapies. Medicare beneficiaries with multiple chronic illnesses see an average of 13 different physicians, have 50 different prescriptions filled per year, account for 76% of all hospital admissions and are 100 times more likely to have a preventable hospitalization than those with no chronic conditions.[20] Yet even patients having single-medication regimens that treat a single condition may fail to reach a therapeutic objective even when the medication is known to be highly efficacious owing to deficiencies in regimen (e.g. sub-optimal dosing) or deficiencies in sub-optimal consumption (e.g. failure to administer the drug on an empty stomach).

MOSs are too essential and too intertwined with the entire system of care to exclude any one care team member or discipline. Further, no single discipline in any single setting of care is likely to be able to effectuate continuously optimized medication use for the majority of patients. At any given moment in a panel of patients, a large subset will maintain an ever-changing need for regimen evaluation and adjustment, adherence coaching, education on administration, procurement assistance or other MOS that would be pragmatically impossible for any given physician, pharmacist, nurse or other care team member to tackle alone. The nearly impossible challenge of a single type of practitioner or allied healthcare provider achieving optimal medication use across an entire patient population is arguably the single most apt example of the need for healthcare delivery to be a team sport, inclusive of both professional and non-professional team members.

The Pharmacy Home Project: Highlighting the Need to Get on the Same Page

In an effort to achieve a model of team-based MO, Community Care of North Carolina, a primary care network of more than 2,000 practices, implemented the Pharmacy Home Project in 2007 on the theory of shared care team informatics and shared care team responsibilities. The more than 4,500 users of all types of skill sets and practice locations using an internally modified care management system had access to multiple medication lists across multiple settings of care, and detailed tasking and MOS intervention histories for multiple types of licensed and credentialed users. Different list contexts were created for each MOS provider type and setting of care. Examples included care manager at discharge, pharmacist in the pharmacy, care manager at home and physician in the clinic. More than 50 different provider and setting combinations of medication list sources and contexts were modeled in the database. Each time a user modified the unified pharmacy informatics profile of a patient, a matrix was created (See Figure 13.3).

This was possible through the deployment of widely utilized pharmacy reference databases. Available for many decades, commercial entities created listings of medications and various levels of aggregation and naming conventions. With NDC, the most granular means of identification, logical groupings of higher orders can aid in both pharmacy administration and claims

---

[20] Anderson GF. 2007. Testimony before the senate special committee on aging. The future of Medicare: Recognizing the need for chronic care coordination. Serial No. 110–7, pp 19–20.

Access II Care of Western North Carolina
Medication Reconciliation
Dana Kinney, PharmD

Date: 4/9/2008
Patient Name: _____
PCP: _____

Referral Source: Bethany Brown, Chronic Care Case Manager
DOB: _____   MCD# _____
Practice: Community Family Practice   Primary CM: Greg McCoy

Past Medical History: Type 1 DM, h/o DKA, HTN, Renal Disease, Retinopathy, Migraines, Glaucoma, GERD, Hyperlipidemia

Med Reconciliation:

Rx Claim History 5/07-2/08 from Medicaid Rx Claims Data	PCP Med List from OV 2/22/08	Admin Med List from Mission 3/1/2008 (per pt)	Discharge Med List from Mission 3/7/2008	PCP Med List from most recent OV 3/26/08	Med Review with Pt's Mother 4/10/08
Alphagan P 0.15% 11/27/07, 15 mL		Alphagan	Alphagan 1gtt os BID		
Amlodipine 10mg QD 1/22/08 #30, adherent	Amlodipine 10mg QD	Amlodipine 10mg QD	Amlodipine 10mg QD	Amlodipine 10mg QD	Amlodipine 10mg QD
OTC	Aspirin 81mg QD	Aspirin 81mg QD	Aspirin 81mg QD	Aspirin 81mg QD	Aspirin 81mg QD
	Atropine 1% QD			Atropine 1% ou BID	Atropine 1 gtt ou QD
	Azopt QD			Azopt ou BID	Azopt 1 gtt ou BID
Benicar HCT 20/12.5mg BID 3/5/08 #62	Benicar HCT 20/12.5mg QD	Benicar HCT 20/12.5mg QD	Benicar 20mg BID	Benicar HCT 20/12.5mg QD	Benicar HCT 20/12.5mg QD
Clonidine 0.1mg BID 1/22/08 #60	Clonidine 0.1mg QD	Clonidine 0.1mg BID	Clonidine 0.1mg BID	Clonidine 0.1mg BID	Clonidine 0.1mg BID
Combigan QD	Combigan QD	Combigan BID		Combigan BID	Combigan 1 gtt OU BID
Diamox 500mg 1/5/08 #20, only fill					
Cosopt 1/11/08, 10 mL			Cosopt 1gtt os BID		
OTC	Docusate 100mg BID	Docusate 100mg BID	Docusate 100mg BID	Docusate 100mg BID	
OTC	Ferrous Sulfate 325mg BID	Ferrous Sulfate 325mg BID	Ferrous Sulfate 325mg BID	Ferrous Sulfate 325mg BID	Poly-Iron 150mg BID
Furosemide 20mg QD 11/5/07 #31, only fill		Furosemide 40mg QD	Furosemide 40mg QAM	Furosemide 40mg QD	Furosemide 40mg QD
			Gabapentin 900mg QHSx3nights	Gabapentin 900mg QHS	
Humalog: 2 vials approx. every 2 months	Insulin Pump	Insulin Pump, no recent changes	Humalog: Insulin Pump at levels ud Dr. Speed	Insulin Pump	Humalog 1 unit/15 carbs
Lexapro 20mg QD 1/22/08 #31	Lexapro 20mg QD	Lexapro 20mg QD	Lexapro 20mg QD	Lexapro 20mg QD	Lexapro 20mg QD
			Lipitor 10mg QD	Lipitor 20mg QHS	Lipitor 20mg QD
Lisinopril 5mg 9/22/07 #30, nonadherent		Lisinopril 20mg QD (per pt)		Lisinopril 5mg QD	Lisinopril 25mg QAM and 5mg QHS

Dana Kinney, Clinical Pharmacist
dkinney@accessiicare-wnc.org

Access II Care of Western North Carolina
Phone: (828) 259-3879
Fax: (828) 259-3875

Bethany Brown, Nurse Case Manager
bbrown@accessiicare-wnc.org

Figure 13.3   Pharmacy Home Project Medication Matrix

adjudication (using the TELECOM transaction from NCPDP) as well as medication reconciliation efforts. While an NDC may identify a medication product like "atorvastatin 10 mg tablet in a 1000 count bottle from manufacturer A," a drug strength and form identifier such as "atorvastatin 10 mg tablet" might account for the many hundreds or even thousands of available supplied products containing that drug, strength and form, whereas a drug class identifier may aggregate this record as an "HMG CoA reductase inhibitor" or "statin." Pharmacy reference databases are essential for the successful translating, grouping and transacting of data for functions such as electronic prescribing, medication reconciliation, decision support, and quality and performance analytics.

Bringing together multiple list contexts, and with over a half a million matrices created for patients receiving care management and targeted primary care support services, not a single patient had complete congruence across lists in over a decade of MOS services. Among patients receiving matrix reviews by a pharmacist, more than five drug therapy problems per review were discovered, and the more medication lists that were available for the care team member, the more meaningful opportunities to optimize medication use discovered.

Medication Use Follows the Patient through Many Settings of Care

Unlike most healthcare service procedures and interventions, medication use follows the patient wherever they go. Medication regimens and the consumption of those regimens are ever changing and often never-ending. For complex patients, it would not be uncommon to experience multiple hospitalizations and visits to skilled nursing facilities, with multiple home health and care management interventions and touch points both at home and in the community, and with multiple visits to the pharmacy to fill medications from multiple primary care and specialty care prescribers. All of those touch points require some level of MOS in order to optimize medication use. Pharmacy informatics vendors need to account for this dynamicity, and users of these systems must resist the idea that any medication list should be considered a reference list or gold standard reconciled list. Rather, through the multiple streams of context and the patient's journey throughout the system and their personal interactions with medications, a drug use narrative should form that helps the care team member achieve both optimal regimen and optimal consumption.

Patients Are Consumers with Varying Wants, Needs, Desires and Self-Care Capabilities

To further complicate matters, patients respond to different modalities and means of MOS implementation. They also have diverse needs ranging from lack of transportation, to forgetfulness, to lack of understanding and cultural aversions to medical interventions. Some patients seek convenience, whereas others seek reassuring conversation with a trusted clinician. Patients also have varying levels of self-care capability, sometimes matching well with their medication regimen and sometimes not. Use of motivational interviewing or the addition of technology may be needed to effectively deploy MOS services depending on the unique patient circumstance and represent a distinct and important subset of MOS that are quite agnostic to practitioner and can even be deployed without human participation.

"The care team member that relies on medication history taking as a simple medication list based on patient recall or EMR entry alone, without associated semantic contexts of who ordered, where they procured the medication, why they received it, the patient's response to those therapies to date and how their medications relate to their health concerns and health goals, is likely to provide a superficial reflection of medication use that leads to failure of therapeutic objectives, or worse - harm."

IV. Pharmacists as Providers of Healthcare Services

If the Shoe Fits: Pharmacist Education and the Pharmacist Care Process

MOS that attempt to improve upon an existing patient medication regimen may address suboptimal circumstances such as untreated or undertreated conditions, non-adherence to best evidence, problematic combinations of medications, difficult to follow dosing schedules or even affordability. Services that attempt to improve consumption may involve patient education on proper medication storage and administration or even coaching on the importance of regimen adherence, providing reminder utilities, home delivery or even copayment assistance. The MOS umbrella (See Figure 13.4) covers an array of services that combine ideal regimen and ideal consumption that lead to ideal medication use and subsequently better patient outcomes. Both components of optimal medication use are patient specific and dynamic, particularly for patients with multiple chronic conditions, unstable conditions, complex medication regimens from multiple prescribers, and those who use multiple pharmacies and have care team members in different health systems or networks.

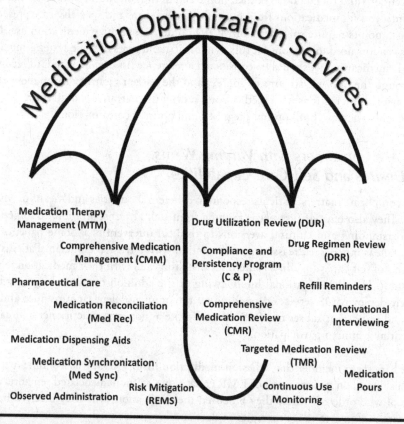

Figure 13.4   Medication Optimization Services Umbrella

Pharmacists are well trained to address both suboptimal regimens and needed adjustments as well as the investigation and resolution of suboptimal consumption (whether through caretaker administration or poor patient self-administration). Since 2002, all pharmacists graduate with a doctor of pharmacy (PharmD) that consists of a minimum of six years of training. The rigorous science and clinically based curriculum includes hours of advanced therapeutics and patient behavior with an emphasis on optimizing drug use in both acute and multiple chronic condition circumstances. PharmD training includes a year's worth of experiential rotations in multiple settings of care with an emphasis on interprofessional care, and oftentimes pharmacy graduates go on to complete one or two years of residency akin to physician residency training.

Accessible and Goal Oriented: A Pharmacist's Approach to Population Health

As the American Pharmacists Association puts it, "the equivalent of the entire population of the United States visits a pharmacy every week." Pharmacists are not only accessible providers in pharmacies, but they also practice in almost every healthcare setting, including hospitals, clinics, physician office practices, long-term care and managed care. Throughout pharmacist training, patient cases and therapeutics classes emphasize assessing the patient's medications, choosing the optimal regimens in setting goals of therapy and the use of markers to determine if therapeutic endpoints are being achieved. Comprehensive history taking and a patient-centered care plan for each medication specific to each patient are core components of pharmacists' patient care.

Patients are especially vulnerable during care transitions, often experiencing medication errors. Recent innovations have shown that the "pharm-to-pharm" model is particularly effective, especially for patients with multiple chronic conditions, multiple prescribers, multiple care team members and serious acute events. Having a pharmacist in a hospital communicate a medication list and plan of care to a pharmacist within the community resulted in a 36.5% drop in medication-related readmissions.[21] Pharmacists providing MOS who have similar training, educational and experiential backgrounds can work very effectively and efficiently across settings of care and special needs populations that drive most of the performance metrics in accountable care and value-based purchasing contracts.

The Pharmacist Care Process: Universal in Approach, with Emphasis on Optimizing Medication Use

The Pharmacist Care Process (Figure 13.5) was developed by the Joint Commission of Pharmacy Practitioners (JCPP) and released after being adopted by the group in May 2014. The goal of the JCPP was to apply a common care process executable across the spectrum of pharmacist-provided patient care services, including MOS. Regardless of the type of MOS provided or the patient need, the steps remain the same: (1) collecting the required data necessary to perform the service; (2) assessing for sub-optimal regimen (each medication is assessed for appropriateness, effectiveness, safety and adherence) and sub-optimal consumption; (3) taking the findings from the assessment and creating a new medication-related care plan (or altering an existing medication-related plan); (4) implementing that plan; and (5) focusing on follow-up to monitor and evaluate the medication regimen and overall health outcomes.

---

[21] Pellegrin KL, Krenk L, Oakes SJ, et al. 2017. Reductions in medication-related hospitalizations in older adults with medication management by hospital and community pharmacists: A quasi-experimental study. *J Am Geriatr Soc* 65(1):212–219.

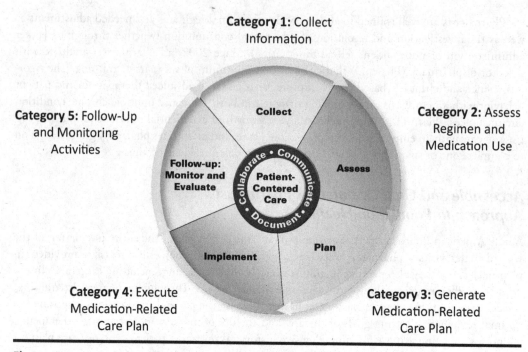

Figure 13.5   An overlay of ontological categories on the Pharmacist Care Process

Product-Based Upbringing and Service Line Provisions Absent Payment Have Stunted Pharmacy Practice Evolution and Pharmacy Informatics

As early as the 1970s, the need for pharmacist-provided MOS was evident in select pharmacy circles. The following excerpt from Millis's report[22] on the role of pharmacists in the optimal use of medications provides a rather matter-of-fact view about the distinction between the capabilities of a given medication and the reality that challenges it to be optimally used:

> Pharmacy is a knowledge system in which chemical substances and people called patients interact.

Chemicals may be well understood, and their properties remain the same over time, but patients and disease states are far more complex and require continuing attention. In 1990, Hepler and Strand gave appreciation to this phenomenon and coined (yet another) term: pharmaceutical care:[23]

> Pharmaceutical care is the direct, responsible provision of medication-related care for the purpose of achieving definite outcomes that improve a patient's quality of life.

---

[22] Millis JS. 1976. Looking ahead–the report of the study commission on pharmacy. *Am J Hosp Pharm* 33(2):134–138.
[23] Hepler CD, Strand LM. 1990. Opportunities and responsibilities in pharmaceutical care. *Am J Hosp Pharm* 47(3):533–543.

Unfortunately, as pockets of advanced pharmacy practice evolved over the ensuing decades, no explicit ubiquitous payment mechanism or fee schedule emerged for pharmacists or any other healthcare professional wishing to provide robust MOS. Had one emerged, it is likely that payers would have required more granularity of billing description and subsequent documentation, thereby aiding the evolution of service definitions and the ability to discriminate between various and sometimes nuanced MOS. The slow evolution of payment for pharmacist-provided MOS, in combination with much needed multi-professional participation in MOS, has stunted the proper evolution of MOS definition and subsequent coding ontologies that have become common in medicine, physical therapy, occupational therapy, home health, and other professional and paraprofessional lines of service. The result has been an amalgamation of informal, often undocumented, rarely translatable, side-car-to-billable-time efforts to optimize medication use developed through use cases and circumstantial need often created by principled clinicians who have frequently elected to provide MOS without requirement or remuneration. And without remuneration and payment comes lack of standardization and consistency of MOS delivery along with a lack of interoperable pharmacy informatics related to care delivery and service provisions.

V. Moving toward a Common Language: Developing Cross-Cutting Informatics to Support the "Team"

Medication Optimization Requires That Everyone Know the Play Call and Their Role in the Play

Members of a high-performing team have a precise understanding of each other's training, capabilities, roles and tasks.

Medication handoffs (or lack thereof) are extremely common in our modern healthcare system and require a high level of operational coordination, yet we lack a common lexicon that is universally accepted or understood when engaging in team-based, multi-setting, multi-modality MOS. Conventional use of the term "medication reconciliation" is an unfortunate but salient example of a set of MOS that have generally failed to live up to their potential to prevent harm and produce better patient outcomes owing to a lack of clarity about the intended activities and environmental factors required for successful execution. Current deployments of medication reconciliation range from the application of a software-based algorithm implementing cursory review of a single medication list in a computerized prescription order entry system, to comparing and evaluating an admitted patient's self-proclaimed list of medications, to the discharge list of medications to the home health's report of medication use, to the active medication list in the ambulatory clinic's electronic medical record. Both are broadly considered medication reconciliation and are valuable in their own right when called for, but they vary dramatically in their intensity, depth and appropriateness for a given patient circumstance or situation.

More recently, another MOS, comprehensive medication management (CMM), was the focus of research that sought to explicitly define the MOS so that a common lexicon could be created to enhance understanding of the activities that define the CMM service. Building off of the JCPP PPCP, a common language was developed for the delivery of CMM that provides granularity around all steps of the CMM patient care process.[24]

---

[24] CMM in Primary Care Research Team. 2018. The patient care process for delivering comprehensive medication management (CMM): Optimizing medication use in patient-centered, team-based care settings. https://accp.com/cmm_care_process.

As with the Pharmacy Home Project goals, regardless of which type of practitioner, non-practitioner or technological aide conducts the MOS, each person (or aide) involved in that patient-consumer's care needs a clear understanding of the activities, intentions and findings of the patient's prior MOS, as well as a high level of confidence that the activities, intentions and findings of the MOS they are providing are well understood by the person or utility providing ensuing MOS. Technology solution providers must not only bring together data relevant to MO but also the self-directed tasks and tasking others with descriptions of care team activities. Yet, without cross-cutting clear and unambiguous terminology, care team members cannot efficiently or effectively work together toward a common MO goal. Medication reconciliation must mean the same thing to everyone involved.

Terms of Art Lead to Ambiguity and Inconsistency of Medication Optimization Service Line Delivery

Terms of art are words or phrases that have ubiquitous understanding within a field of work or in a small community of collaborators, working groups or institutions. An example term of art in the legal field is "specific performance," which for most anyone outside of the legal field may have a different meaning (or no meaning at all), but in a legal context means an order of the court (typically in the performance of a real estate contract). Terms of art typically arise out of a need to speak to a particular audience with technical meaning that requires very specific interpretation. Unless they are able to achieve ubiquitous and specific interpretation from the intended audience or group, terms of art are susceptible to frequent misinterpretation rather than bring clarity of interpretation. Terms of art such as "medication reconciliation" or "medication management," which have different meanings for different audiences, are the most problematic.

Pharmacy is riddled with terms of art and shorthand descriptors as well as symbology. Instead of saying "right ear," "left ear" or "both ears," we have a tradition of "a.d.," "a.s." (or "a.l.") and "a.u." "MTM" and "med rec" are exemplars of shorthand terms of art that are simply high-level labels. They possess little meaning or reference to more granular descriptors and thus result in confusion and misinterpretation to those outside of healthcare, and multiple meanings across fields of study and within healthcare professions. For MOS services to thrive and for MO to be achieved, a clear and consistent understanding of the persons and/or utilities involved and environmental factors, such as setting and data use, as well as ubiquitous explanations of findings and intentions must be communicated with granularity; otherwise, ambiguity ensues across collaborators.

The natural by-product of ambiguity is inconsistency both in the delivery of MOS and the interpretation of MOS findings by other care team members. Ambiguity and inconsistency then become anathema to health services researchers trying to understand the nature of the service and its clinical and economic effects, as well as policy makers that may depend on valid and reliable findings to provide support and funding for MOS.

In computer programming, a "label" (a term of art itself) is used to represent a specific part of the code that has particular function with a particular intention when executed. If a label were executed in a computer program that referred to overlapping code, the program would break. Computer programming labels are not interchangeable.

Similarly, if MTM, comprehensive medication review, medication synchronization and the like have overlapping elements such as "review for therapeutic discrepancies," with overlapping interventionists and overlapping outputs, then the use of those terms of art as labels will have little meaning and only serve to frustrate the MOS activity and promotion efforts of care team members, patients, researchers and policy makers alike. Until recently, few efforts have been made to more granularly define and describe all of the services under the MOS umbrella.

Granularity Matters: Ontological Frameworks Bring Order and Clarity of Interpretation across Many Participants and Stakeholders in a Domain

Ontologies are the discrete and explicit specifications of a representational vocabulary for a shared domain of discourse that includes definitions of classes, relations, functions and other objects.[25] In other words, they categorize terms unambiguously and provide an understanding of the relationships between those terms. Ontologies also enable the aggregation of granular components from different branches within the ontology to provide a composite view of those elements. Ontologies are becoming widely adopted in many industries and research communities, as they bring efficiencies to cross-entity collaboration and domain development because they act to reduce the time and energy required to translate findings and activities from one project, activity or entity to the next.

Ontological Use in Current Medical Practice and Payment

Classification systems and ontologies are not foreign to the healthcare domain. They have evolved in healthcare alongside our ever-increasing ability to discover and distinguish disease and pathology as well as the ever-increasing number of procedures and services that may be deployed to address those diseases. Examples of widely recognized classification systems include the International Classification of Diseases (ICD), currently in its 10th edition, for terming and classifying diseases, with its sister ICD-PCS for procedure coding maintained by the World Health Organization.[26] In the United States, Current Procedural Terminology (CPT) code sets maintained by the American Medical Association are principally used to report medical, surgical and diagnostic procedures using a coding classification system.

The Unified Medical Language System (UMLS) is sponsored by the National Library of Medicine (NLM) and has focused its efforts of late on enabling interoperability between often disparate proprietary and non-proprietary classification systems embedded within electronic medical and other health records systems. In addition to classifying diseases and procedures, relationships are defined between terms to create ontological structures. The Systematized Nomenclature of Medicine-Clinical Terms (SNOMED-CT), maintained by the International Health Terminology Standards Development Organization (IHTSDO), and RxNorm, produced by the (NLM) itself, are probably the most well-known and widely used ontologies in the US healthcare system, with the latter being used to classify pharmaceuticals to aid interoperable functions such as electronic prescribing and computerized physician order entry systems.

Ontological Use in Current and Future MOS and Payment

Historically, the creation and widespread adoption of an ontology such as SNOMED-CT for describing MOS has been met with a lack of enthusiasm owing to its perceived limited value

---

[25] Gruber TR. 1993. A translation approach to portable ontology specification. *Knowledge Acquisition* 5:199–220.

[26] World Health Organization. 2014. International statistical classification of diseases and related health problems, 10th revision (ICD-10)-2014-WHO version. https://icd.who.int/browse10/2014/en#!/XIV.

proposition for pharmacy management system vendors, pharmacist practitioners and payers alike because MOS have been largely voluntary and perfunctory regulator-mandated services, often without explicit payment.

Yet lack of adoption of ontological frameworks for MOS may be the very reason widespread acknowledgment of the need and value of MOS has struggled for these many decades. Because there has not been a long history of payment for MOS, regulators have often had the privilege (or burden) of coming up with terms, such as drug utilization review, drug regimen review and MTM, that act as labels for a set of activities that met the specific needs of the proposed regulation. Because SNOMED-CT or other classification systems for MOS either did not exist or were not acknowledged in policy formation and rulemaking, regulatory-based definitions and terms (labels) evolved in their own silos with their own purposes, without a unifying ontology. Unfortunately, when considering the diversity of health professional competencies, settings, information sources, levels of intensity and duration, and modalities that can (and should) be used to optimize the use of medications for a given patient or system of care, no small number of labels can adequately describe the various combinations of those service components.

Adoption of a widely accepted and universally applicable MOS ontology that is integrated across professions, payers, information technology systems and researchers alike would bring the necessary systemization features required for mechanically efficient implementation as well as socialization and acceptance of MOS as part of a core set of healthcare services and utilities upon which we rely to produce better health.

Bringing It All Together: The Emergence of Broadly Accepted MOS Ontological Frameworks

The JCCP PPCP is widely applicable to MOS and durable across many care team members and settings of care. The distinguishing characteristic of the PPCP is that it subdivides activities into the five aforementioned categories of activities based on sequential requirement and function. Because ontologies are classification systems that include functions and relationships between those functions, the PPCP provides and elegant framework for MOS ontologies.

Applying an Ontological Framework to Medication Optimization Service Lines across Roles, Settings, and Skill Sets

For an MOS ontological framework to be useful and enduring, it requires order and logic that enable straightforward, consistent and widely understood execution of MOS service lines. The fundamentally important result of adopting an MOS ontological framework is consistency in the process and delivery of MOS. When another provider delegates or refers for MOS (e.g. CMM), or a patient participates and receives MOS, or the payer reimburses for a specific MOS, the MOS delivered by the responsible healthcare provider needs to be known, familiar and expected. The MOS service line should not deviate from its explicitly characterized combination of descriptors or elements, and when broadly consistent throughout the entire healthcare system, inclusive of providers, payers and patients. Figure 13.6 provides an example of a high-level ontological framework of MOS activities (e.g. comprehensive medication management) overlaid on the PPCP.

Activities performed within each of the five steps can be further described in more granular terms and in hierarchical fashion using the PPCP framework. For example, in category one, the collection of information necessary to perform an assessment for a particular MOS implementation may or may not involve collecting one or more medication lists or laboratory results, social history, conditions or other class of information relevant to the service. Some medication

Activity
Category 1: Collect Information
      1.1 Collect Medication Lists
           1.1.1 Collect Patient Report of Medication List
           1.1.2 Collect Prescription Fill History Medication List
           1.1.3 Collect Hospital Discharge Medication List
           1.1.4 Collect Active Medication List from Primary Care
           1.1.n. . .
      1.2 Collect Vitals
      1.3 Collect Laboratory Results
      1.4 Collect Conditions
      1.n. . .
Category 2: Assess Regimen and Medication Use
      2.1 Assess Adherence to Medications
      2.2 Assess for Contraindications
      2.3 Assess for Therapeutic Duplications
      2.4 Assess for Untreated Conditions
      2.n. . .
Category 3: Generate Medication-Related Care Plan
      3.1 Plan for Timing of Medication Administration(s)
      3.2 Plan for Responding to Adverse Events
      3.3 Plan for Laboratory Monitoring
      3.4 Plan for Coaching and Motivating Medication Taking
      3.5 Plan for Procuring Medications
      3.n. . .
Category 4: Execute Medication-Related Care Plan
      4.1 Communicate Care Plan to Patient
      4.2 Communicate Care Plan to Care Team Member(s)
      4.3 Communicate Care Plan to Caretaker(s)
      4.4 Administer Medications to Patient
      4.n. . .
Category 5: Follow-Up and Monitoring Activities
      5.1 Monitor for Medication Regimen Changes
      5.2 Monitor for Disease Progression and Resolution
      5.3 Monitor for Adherence to Medication-Related Care Plan
      5.n. . .

Figure 13.6 Example of a high-level ontology of medication optimization activities overlaid on the Pharmacist Care Process

reconciliation MO services may only require collecting medication lists to implement the MOS, whereas other MO service lines such as comprehensive medication management may require collecting laboratory results, social history and conditions. It is helpful to all stakeholders to know what categories of information are gathered when referring, reporting or communicating the MOS taking place and its findings.

Pharmacy Organizations Begin to Develop Ontologies for Medication Optimization Services that Cross Care Team Member Boundaries

Within the last few years, professional pharmacy associations, technology solution providers and efforts emanating from the Centers for Medicare and Medicaid Innovation (CMMI), supported by the Office of the National Coordinator (ONC) have attempted to create opportunities for pharmacists to participate in value-based purchasing and accountable care efforts alongside the harmonization of pharmacy informatics with medical informatics and related systems. The Pharmacy Health Information Technology Collaborative (PHIT Collaborative) maintains stakeholders from most of pharmacies' professional associations as well as technology solution providers. Their focus is bridging the gap between pharmacy information technology (IT) systems and medical and care team IT systems. Additionally, NCPDP's efforts around prescription-filling standards has also evolved to interoperable transactions between EMR, pharmacy and insurer as well as the adoption of care planning standards as they relate to MOS.

VI. Pharmacy Informatics in 2020 and Beyond

Ongoing Efforts to Improve Pharmacy Informatics and Medication Optimization Dependent on Payer and Regular Influence and Support

Today, a number of efforts are ongoing to improve the sharing of information related to medication prescribing, coverage, use and ultimately the consumption of medications. Payer support is critical to sustainable innovation and adoption of more advanced pharmacy informatics. The Centers for Medicare and Medicaid (CMS) continues to promote and reward interoperability through efforts like Meaningful Use, Blue Button, and a large emphasis on medication-related, value-based purchasing programs. The CMMI Enhanced Medication Therapy Management (EMTM) program requires the use of SNOMED-CT concepts to be incorporated into program administration and encourages interaction with community-level EMTM providers. In states like Washington and California, legislation creating provider recognition and payment for pharmacists' services has stimulated pharmacists to adopt IT systems that are able to bill CPT codes and X12 transactions in the same payer systems using the same credentialing and claims administration as those of other care team members. These governmental efforts, in combination with efforts in the private insurance space to better allocate clinician and support resources, have also created a robust and growing technology solution provider vendor community of pharmacy analytics, decision support tools and user interfaces that help care team members sort through the now copious number of records and data elements available at the point of care.

A Place to Call Home: An Effort to Enable Pharmacist EMR Capabilities

Pharmacists and pharmacy technicians have rarely had an electronic documentation system for MO service lines. In the community pharmacy, IT systems have been historically designed for product inventory management, prescription filling and billing, not clinical or MOS activities, oftentimes not having a place to even record an mm Hg or A1c reading. For pharmacists providing patient care on the floors at the hospital or in an ambulatory care environment within an outpatient clinic, the traditional EMR is the principal means of documentation. However, EMRs have also historically never had MOS modules or histories or encounter documentation for pharmacist-provided services, and thus pharmacists adapt their documentation to other care team members' templates. In long-term care pharmacy, some clinical documentation systems have emerged owing to the regulatory requirement for drug regimen reviews at specified intervals in facilities. However, those systems are almost never integrated with other care team members such as the medical director's or the nursing facilities' system of record. In the MTM industry, software has been developed to meet a particular MOS, such as Medicare Part D MTM, but it is not broadly applicable and is designed more for call centers not heavily staffed by pharmacists.

However, within the past few years, much progress has been made towards giving pharmacists and those providing MOS services clinical documentation and MO-related care coordination their own user interfaces, database structures and standardized system-to-system transactions. In 2020, EMRs released MOS templates and pharmacist spaces for clinical documentation. Community pharmacy management systems are adopting care planning user interfaces and entry capabilities for clinical data. Long-term care environments are newly subject to interoperability requirements that include medication-related information. The year 2022 may end up becoming the turning point towards more advanced and sharable pharmacy informatics for practitioners and their extended care teams after a three-decade dominance of pharmacy informatics advancement in medication product distribution only.

The Missing Link(s): Bridging the Medical and Pharmacy Informatics Divide Using Interoperable Standards and Registries

A number of seminal advances have occurred in recent years to bridge pharmacy informatics with medical and other care team informatics, such as care management systems. These capabilities are critical for achievement of MO given the multiple settings and skill sets omnipresent with patient need. Among them are the updated capabilities NCPDP SCRIPT version 2017071 standard for electronic prescribing, which includes laboratory values and notifications for canceling or discontinuing prescriptions. Prescription drug monitoring programs, which are accessed by pharmacists and prescribers for controlled substance filling and monitoring that includes cash prescription fills, previously were challenged to capture for prescription fill history solutions where there was no claim to reference. New in-home dispensing devices provide data streams for continuous monitoring of medication taking, consumption and administration for prescribers, pharmacists and care management teams alike. For pharmacists and pharmacies who wish to engage in MOS activities and share their findings and activities with payers and care team members, the HL7 Pharmacist Electronic Care Plan (PeCP) standard has been adopted by more than a dozen pharmacy management and care management system vendors and clinically integrated networks of community pharmacies.

Increasing the Breadth of the Data Payload: Electronic Prescribing and the Pharmacist Electronic Care Plan Evolve to Serve Team-Based Care

The PeCP was created under a collaboration between the US pharmacy standards bearer of NCPDP and the international medical standards bearer HL7. It was tested under a CMMI and

ONC joint experiment with Collaborative Care of North Carolina (CCNC) following the successful decade-long implementation of their Pharmacy Home Project. The PeCP contains many different elements, much like its sister transaction the HL7 Care Plan Standard, but it has been modified to build up many of the elements needed to implement MOS. Key elements that are meant to be included in all care plans transacted include health concerns, patient goals, drug therapy problems, active medication list, plan of care, intervention through SNOMED coding, vitals and laboratory findings. This is the type of transaction information payload that has never been collected by or utilized by pharmacists or pharmacies specific to their MOS activities. Other, non-pharmacist workforces such as care managers and pharmacy technicians have started to adopt and utilize the PeCP transaction. As the PeCP gains adoption, so too are the user interfaces and underlying databases for technology solution partners beginning to evolve based on the standard for the free flow of that valuable information payload.

Conveying the Value of MOS through Reliable, Granular, and Testable Descriptor Sets that Include Environmental Considerations

The value of a service is equal to its benefit in relation to its cost. Increasingly, a focus on delivering value in healthcare manifested through measurement and payment is being held up as the means by which the healthcare system achieves sustainability. Optimizations of products and services are attempts to increase the value of those products and services through activities that maximize their intended effects or benefits. For medications, our system of care has failed to realize the full benefit of life-saving, life-extending and life-enhancing medications for lack of supporting MOS that are essential to achieve optimal use.

Current use of labels that inadequately describe MOS most often lead to unreliable, inadequate or cost-ineffective implementations that do not meet the needs of the value purchaser. Without granular descriptors of the MOS that include environmental considerations, such as setting of care, access to information, proximity of care delivery and maturity of relationship with other care team members, it becomes a daunting task to determine value in such a manner that is testable and repeatable. With an established MOS ontology, a rubric of program elements and practice environment can be created to aid in comparing and contrasting MOS services. Reliable, granular and testable descriptor sets that include environmental considerations give rise to program evaluation and comparative research that serves to both elucidate best practices and high-value streams as well as to provide higher face-value representations of the effectiveness of the evaluated MOS.

VII. Ensuring Provider Adoption and MOS Evidence Generation

Workflow-Enabled Capabilities Are Essential to Adoption

The healthcare delivery system is an incredibly complex, diverse and oftentimes fragmented environment. It is not surprising, then, how often we hear that technology or software systems are challenging to implement. Common feedback from clinicians is that most solutions do not "fit within our workflow" or "our system does not talk to other systems." Challenging implementations are also true for MOS interventions, where the conclusion from a landmark meta-analysis showed insufficient evidence because of inconsistency and imprecision in part from heterogeneity in populations and interventions.[27] Yet the effects of interventions themselves may not have been reflected in the data as authors could not assess whether the intervention itself did not work or whether the interventions were not properly implemented.[28] In other words, inconsistent uptake of an intervention or technology or the lack of fidelity to that intervention often contributes to lower effectiveness, which then falls short of the desired outcome.

As discussed throughout the chapter, MOS are far-ranging technology solutions that seek to address everything from identifying ideal regimens to working with patients on ideal medication consumption. As a result, healthcare leaders should ask three critical questions as they work with vendors, pharmacists and clinicians to implement MOS technology solutions. First, are the proposed service lines and interventions patient centered? Engaging the patient through enhanced communication, education and coordination with a goal of eliminating medication therapy problems should be the initial requirement. Second, is there any evidence to suggest that the proposed MOS interventions are effective at improving the desired outcomes? Third, what is the implementation plan for the MOS intervention to ensure a reasonable pathway to scalability within their environment? MOS providers need to provide this evidence to the purchaser, just as the interventions need to be built with standardized ontologies that clearly define the intervention and clinician activities.

A Model for Evaluating Technology Solutions and Cultivating Sequent User Adoption

To answer the scalability question, healthcare providers and leaders should vet the vendor implementation process through the lens of a synergistic technology testing process.[29] The goal of the process is to ensure the technology solution has gone through a traditional testing process like functional validation and usability testing, but also that it has undergone implementation and scalability testing. To fully vet a MOS technology solution, the purchaser should gauge the commercial readiness of the product against four key tenets that will enable healthcare leaders to establish the likelihood of success for the solution in their environment.

Core tenet 1: Is the MOS technology solution a usable innovation? Has it been designed to be easy to use with simple design features, including necessary ontologies and user rubrics to document activities and define user roles? Vendors should be able to produce data on related usability testing.

Core tenet 2: Does the MOS technology attend to contextual influences? As discussed earlier in the chapter, understanding the environment in which the MOS intervention will be implemented is critically important. This might be in a primary care clinic, a community pharmacy or the patient's home. Vendors should have data here on feasibility testing and perhaps have performed contextual assessments, which all roll up into an implementation roadmap or holistic plan.

[27] Viswanathan M, Kahwati LC, Golin CE, et al. 2015. Medication therapy management interventions in outpatient settings a systematic review and meta-analysis. *JAMA Intern Med* 175(1):76–87.

[28] Agency for Healthcare Research and Quality. 2010. Multiple chronic conditions chartbook. Medical Expenditure Panel Survey Data. https://www.ahrq.gov/sites/default/files/wysiwyg/professionals/prevention-chronic-care/decision/mcc/mccchartbook.pdf.

[29] Livet, M, Easter J. 2019. Optimizing medication use through synergistic technology testing process. *JAPhA* 59:S71–S77.

Core tenet 3: Studying the implementation process. Is thorough coaching and training with iterative course corrections provided? This allows the organization to learn and adapt to different environments. It is critical for vendors to partner with healthcare organizations around training to ensure you can monitor the fidelity of the services and interventions.

Core tenet 4: Assessing scalability of the MOS technology. The first three tenets are the building blocks to scaling a MOS technology. However, the organization needs to think through various components of scale as to whether they should "scale up" the solution in similar settings or "scale out" the solution in different settings of care or environments. If you are scaling out, adaptations must be considered for these new environments. Vendors should be able to assist with scalability assessments.

For healthcare leaders, a key pathway to success with MOS-centric informatics solutions and the interventions they support means holding developers and vendors accountable to produce defined MOS interventions along with an ontological framework for reimbursement and evaluation purposes. Vendors should also partner with healthcare organizations to produce implementation and scalability data, and then reinforce with a solid training and coaching implementation roadmap that ensure success with an organization's ultimate goals of enhanced outcomes and patient-centered care through the optimization of medications.

Splitting Preferred over Lumping for Clarity of Intervention

As more scrutiny is given to fee-for-service payment methodologies and CMS continues to forge a pathway for value-driven models of service remuneration, it will become increasingly important to be able to distinguish high-value versus low-value services. It will also become important for providers and MOS to be able to very specifically describe the MOS service offering (i.e. usable innovation) and environmental conditions (i.e. context) within which it is being offered and be able to trust that the MOS offering is consistently and reliably delivered (i.e. fidelity) across the provider and vendor community. A healthcare service line is only as appealing to providers and value purchasers as the sum of its value across different vendors and providers within their orbit. In some cases, the more intensive, more comprehensive MOS with close proximity to patients and other care team members with frequent follow-up are valued and valuable (cost-effective) at producing the outcome(s) of interest to the provider and value purchaser. In other instances, the low-intensity focused effort by telephonic outreach (or perhaps even the use of a technology such as an adherence aide) will suffice to produce the outcome of interest at lower cost.

Evidence Generation

As pharmacy informatics evolves both in its ability to granularly describe MOS lines and in its ability to communicate critical data elements across multiple settings of care and care team members, health services researchers gain access to critical data elements and interactions not previously available for their analyses. While research related to MO has generally resulted in positive findings, it has been subject to scrutiny related to the lack of ability to parse structured data about MOS interventions that better describe the environment, activities and clinical findings. New transactions and health information exchange capabilities and integrations of pharmacy informatics with non-pharmacy informatics are likely to bring about a rich and more instructive body of literature relating to MO and MOS.

About the Authors

Troy Trygstad, PharmD, MBA, PhD, is the Executive Director of CPESN USA, a clinically integrated network of community-based pharmacy networks that endeavors to improve the quality and effectiveness of enhanced services provided by participating pharmacies and align them with the workflows and payment reform incentives of physicians, their support staff, and other healthcare providers. He also serves as the Vice President of Pharmacy Provider Partnerships for Community Care of North Carolina, an organization providing wrap-around population health management supports for nearly 2,000 primary care practices.

Troy possesses over 20 years of experience with multidisciplinary care teams and intervention development under alternative payment and support models. He was the project director for a Center for multi-year Medicare and Medicaid Innovation Award that tested new models of payment and pharmacy connectivity to primary care providers. Troy co-founded the Pharmacy Home Project in 2007 and a web application to accompany that combined more than 50 different medical list contexts into a single portal utilized by multiple care team members and care managers, including pharmacists in multiple settings of care.

Troy proudly practices in a community pharmacy setting on nights and weekends and served recently as a board member for the American Pharmacists Association Foundation and the Pharmacy Quality Alliance, as well as editor in chief of *Pharmacy Times*. Troy received doctor of pharmacy and master's in business administration degrees from Drake University and a PhD in pharmaceutical outcomes and policy from the University of North Carolina at Chapel Hill.

John Easter BS Pharm, RPh, PhD, joined the UNC Eshelman School of Pharmacy in January 2016 as a Professor of the Practice and Director, Center for Medication Optimization (CMO). CMO conducts applied research that implements and evaluates medication optimization interventions to inform value-based payment models. Jon also directs the US healthcare course and leads the pharmacy practice domain within the global PharmAlliance collaboration. Jon previously spent 19 years at GlaxoSmithKline (GSK), where he led a health policy team focused on quality measurement and medication management policy development. Jon has a BS in pharmacy from the University of Georgia and is a registered pharmacist.

Anne L. Burns, BSPharm, RPh, is Vice President, Professional Affairs, at the American Pharmacists Association (APhA). She is responsible for the association's strategic initiatives focused on advancing pharmacists' patient care services in team-based care delivery models, as well as payment for pharmacists' services, collaboration with other healthcare practitioners, and healthcare quality. She leads the association's practice initiatives on pain management and the opioid crisis, and also works on AphA's medication management, health IT, medication safety, and credentialing and privileging programs. She has served on many medication management, quality, and prescription drug misuse and abuse advisory councils. She currently serves on the board of directors for the Pharmacy Quality Alliance and the Council for Credentialing in Pharmacy, the national advisory board for the National Rx Drug Abuse and Heroin Summit, and is Chair of the Pharmacy HIT Collaborative Workgroup on Professional Service Claims and Codes. Ms. Burns joined AphA in 1997. Prior to AphA, she served on the faculty at The Ohio State University (OSU) College of Pharmacy. She received her BS in pharmacy from OSU and completed the Wharton Executive Management Program for Pharmacy Leaders.

Mary Ann Kliethermes, BS Pharm, Pharm. D., FAPhA, FCIOM, received a BS in pharmacy from the University of Michigan in 1977 and her doctor of pharmacy from the Philadelphia College of Pharmacy and Science in 1981. Her career includes clinical practice and management in hospital, home infusion, ambulatory practice, and academia. Her current position is Director of Medication Safety and Quality at the American Society of Health-System Pharmacists. Her expertise is in pharmacist reimbursement, medication optimization, safety, and quality attainment associated pharmacist services, particularly in new healthcare models and value-based payment systems.

She has served as chair of the Section of Ambulatory Care for ASHP, represented ASHP at the Joint Commission Ambulatory Professional and Technical Advisory Group, the Care Transitions Work Group of the PCPI, and the Ambulatory Patient Safety Technical Advisory Panel for ASPE/ HHS. She has served as chair of the executive committee and board member, and on numerous committees for the Pharmacy Quality Alliance (PQA). She is past chair for the AphA PCMH/ ACO SIG. Mary Ann has been awarded Pharmacist of the Year, Shining Star Award, and the Amy Lodolce Mentorship Award from ICHP, the Distinguished Service Award and Distinguished Leadership in Health-System Pharmacy Practice from ASHP, CCP Outstanding Faculty Award, and the Daniel B. Smith Practice Excellence Award from AphA.

Marie Smith, PharmD, FNAP, is the Henry A. Palmer Endowed Professorship of Community Pharmacy Practice and, Assistant Dean for Practice and Public Policy Partnerships at the University of Connecticut School of Pharmacy. In 2013, she served as senior adviser to the CMS Innovation Center (CMMI) in Baltimore, MD, to develop a national strategy and implementation plan to integrate pharmacist-provided medication management services in the Comprehensive Primary Care Initiative. Dr. Smith has worked with multiple state-level and national healthcare reform policymakers and stakeholders to address healthcare delivery issues that involve medication management programs, patient safety, performance measures, health information technology, and integration of clinical pharmacists in advanced primary care practices (workforce development).

Prior to joining the Uconn School of Pharmacy faculty, Dr. Smith was vice president, e-strategy and integration, at Aventis Pharmaceuticals, and was on the senior management staff at the American Society of Heath-System Pharmacists, where she led business development, publishing and software development teams. Dr. Smith is a graduate of the University of Connecticut and Medical College of Virginia Schools of Pharmacy, and completed a hospital pharmacy residency at Thomas Jefferson University Hospital in Philadelphia. In addition, she completed a Fellowship in Change Management at Johns Hopkins University and post-graduate work in global leadership executive education at the Wharton School (University of Pennsylvania) and INSEAD (France).

Mary Roth McClurg, Pharm.D., MHS, is Professor and Executive Vice Dean-Chief Academic Officer at the UNC Eshelman School of Pharmacy. Roth McClurg practiced for 12 years as a clinical pharmacist in primary care practice within the VA Health System and in the interdisciplinary geriatric clinic within the Department of Geriatrics at UNC Healthcare, providing direct patient care as part of an interprofessional care team. Roth McClurg has focused her research efforts on advancing comprehensive medication management and the role of the clinical pharmacist as an integral member of the primary care team, with the goal of optimizing medication use and improving care in patients with multiple chronic diseases. Roth McClurg is a fellow of the American College of Clinical Pharmacy.

References

Agency for Healthcare Research and Quality. 2010. Multiple chronic conditions chartbook. Medical expenditure panel survey data. https://www.ahrq.gov/sites/default/files/wysiwyg/professionals/prevention-chronic-care/decision/mcc/mcccchartbook.pdf.

Anderson GF. 2007. Testimony before the senate special committee on aging. The future of Medicare: Recognizing the need for chronic care coordination. Serial No. 110–7, pp. 19–20.

Backes AC, Kuo GM. 2012. The association between functional health literacy and patient-reported recall of medications at outpatient pharmacies. *Res Social Adm Pharm* 8(4):349–354.

CMM in Primary Care Research Team. 2018. The patient care process for delivering comprehensive medication management (CMM): Optimizing medication use in patient-centered, team-based care settings. *ACCP*. https://accp.com/cmm_care_process.

Curtiss FR. 2008. HEDIS, beta-blockers, and what more can be done to improve secondary prevention in ACS. *J Manag Care Pharm* 14(3):316–317.

Dalzell MD. 1997. NCQA's Quality Compass points to plan differences. *Managed Care* 52A, 52G, 52H. www.managedcaremag.com/archives/9711/9711.compass.shtml.

Ellerbeck EF, Jencks SF, Radford MJ, Kresowik TF, Craig AS, Gold JA, et al. 1995. Quality of care for Medicare patients with acute myocardial infarction: a four-state pilot of the cooperative cardiovascular project. *JAMA* 273:1509–1514.

Fischer MA, Stedman MR, Lii J, et al. 2010. Primary medication non-adherence: Analysis of 195,930 electronic prescriptions. *J Gen Intern Med* 25(4):284–290.

Gruber, TR. 1993. A translation approach to portable ontology specification. *Knowledge Acquisition* 5:199–220.

Hepler CD1, Strand LM. 1990. Opportunities and responsibilities in pharmaceutical care. *Am J Hosp Pharm* 47(3):533–543. Opportunities and responsibilities in pharmaceutical care.

Howard PA, Ellerbeck EF. 2000. Optimizing beta-blocker use after myocardial infarction. *Am Fam Physician* 15;62(8):1853–1860, 1865–1866.

Joint Commission of Pharmacy Practitioners. 2014. Pharmacists' patient care process. https://jcpp.net/wp-content/uploads/2016/03/PatientCareProcess-with-supporting-organizations.pdf.

Livet, M, Easter J. 2019. Optimizing medication use through synergistic technology testing process. *JAPhA* 59:S71 S77.

Millis JS. 1976. Looking ahead – the report of the study commission on pharmacy. *Am J Hosp Pharm* 33(2):134–138.

National Committee for Quality Assurance. 2006. *The State of Health Care Quality*. Washington DC: National Committee for Quality Assurance.

NCAQ. 2020. HEDIS measures and technical resources. www.ncqa.org/hedis/measures/.

Office of Disease Prevention and Health Promotion. 2020. *Adverse Drug Events*. US. Dept of Health and Human Services. https://health.gov/our-work/health-care-quality/adverse-drug-events.

Olson MD1, Tong GL, Steiner BD, Viera AJ, Ashkin E, Newton WP. 2012. Medication documentation in a primary care network serving North Carolina Medicaid patients: results of a cross-sectional chart review. *BMC Fam Pract* 13:83.

Page AT, Clifford RM, Potter K, Schwartz D, Etherton-Beer CD. 2016. The feasibility and effect of deprescribing in older adults on mortality and health: A systematic review and meta-analysis. *Br J Clin Pharmacol* 82(3):583–623.

Pellegrin KL, Krenk L, Oakes SJ, et al. 2017. Reductions in medication-related hospitalizations in older adults with medication management by hospital and community pharmacists: A quasi-experimental study. *J Am Geriatr Soc* 65(1):212–219.

RAND Corporation. 2017. Multiple chronic conditions in the U.S. https://www.rand.org/content/dam/rand/pubs/tools/TL200/TL221/RAND_TL221.pdf.

Stapleton MP1. Sir James Black and propranolol. 1997. The role of the basic sciences in the history of cardiovascular pharmacology. *Tex Heart Inst J* 24(4):336–342.

Surescripts. 2018. National progress report. https://surescripts.com/news-center/national-progress-report-2018/.

Viswanathan M, Kahwati LC, Golin CE, et al. 2015. Medication therapy management interventions in outpatient settings a systematic review and meta-analysis. *JAMA Intern Med* 175(1):76–87.

Wantanbe JH, McInnis T; Hirsh JD. 2018. Cost of prescription related morbidity and mortality. *Ann Pharmacother* 52:829–837.

World Health Organization. 2014. International statistical classification of diseases and related health problems 10th revision (ICD-10)-2014-WHO version. https://icd.who.int/browse10/2014/en#!/XIV

Chapter 14

Nursing Informatics Today and Future Perspectives for Healthcare

Victoria L. Tiase, PhD, RN-BC, FAMIA, FAAN and
Whende M. Carroll, MSN, RN-BC, FHIMSS

Contents

DOI: 10.4324/9780429423109-14

Introduction

Since the passage of American Recovery and Reinvestment Act of 2009 (ARRA) and Health Information Technology for Economic and Clinical Health (HITECH), the use of technology in healthcare in the last decade has consistently advanced across all care settings to include patient and consumer engagement. Healthcare payment reform and new care delivery models have created increasing demands for information and access to information. Amid COVID-19, telehealth and remote patient monitoring have become critical tools to increase the access of care to individuals from the safety of their homes.[1] Providing data and information to healthcare providers and patients is needed now more than ever. This rapid transformation of healthcare delivery is creating new demands for both the types of technology and the way technology is used as well as emerging roles to support the changing environment. The need to bridge between clinical workflow and care settings with technology continues to create opportunities for clinical informatics and, specifically, nursing informatics. Nurse informaticists are necessary to facilitate information processes that support healthier individuals, communities, and population health, including connections with patients and families. This chapter outlines the state of the profession, influencing trends, and opportunities for future growth.

Nursing Informatics Defined

Nursing informatics (NI) is defined by the American Nurses Association[2] as an applied science that:

> integrates nursing science, computer science, and information science to manage and communicate data, information, and knowledge in nursing practice. Nursing informatics facilitates the integration of data, information, knowledge, and wisdom to support patients, nurses, and other providers in their decision making in all roles and settings. This support is accomplished using information structures, information processes, and information technology.

The foundational concepts of NI are derived from the data, information, knowledge, and wisdom framework by Nelson (Figure 14.1).[3] In this conceptual model, data are processed to produce information. In turn, data and information are used to generate knowledge. In clinical practice, nurses demonstrate wisdom by applying data, information, and knowledge to care decisions to meet the needs of patients and families.

By utilizing the DIKW model, NI closes the gap between information technology and clinical practice. The consistent growth of NI can be attributed to the applied skills and expertise that NI brings to technology, as well as data initiatives that are so vital to healthcare transformation.

The Current State of NI

NI Roles and Structures

Many healthcare organizations are in the process of implementing and optimizing electronic health records (EHRs) and other informatics innovations as a core strategy to advance healthcare delivery. In many organizations, nurses perform much of the her system configuration work, such as workflow analyses and content design, which require clinical knowledge and expertise. NI

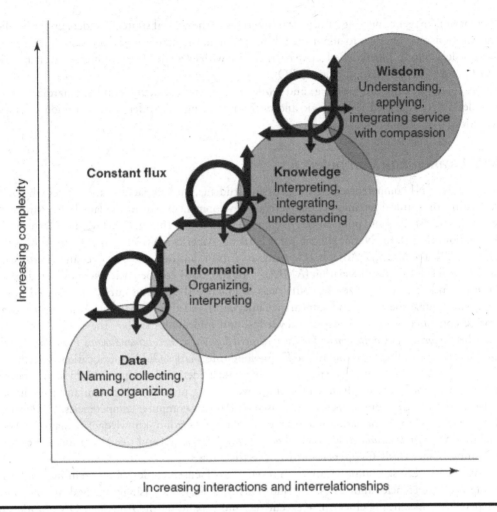

Figure 14.1   Revised data information knowledge wisdom model – 2013 version

Source: Figure reprinted with permission from Ramona Nelson. Copyright © 2013, Ramona Nelson Consulting at ramonanelson@verizon.net. All rights reserved.

competencies are a critical component of successful interprofessional clinical informatics practice within healthcare delivery organizations. Established leadership roles include chief nursing officer (CNO), chief nursing information officer (CNIO), director of nursing informatics, and nurse informaticist. Although nurses enter the NI specialty from a variety of educational backgrounds, expectations for these roles include advanced education at the master's or doctorate level. Collins et al. defined the CNO's clinical informatics role as an executive strategic leader who values, invests in, and supports interprofessional informatics practice approached from the perspective of nursing strategy and nursing practice needs.[4] The CNIO functions as a centralized and strategic leader with decision making authority and operational oversight.[4] The CNIO and chief medical information officer (CMIO) are independent yet collaborative and partnered roles with established practice in organizations that have served as pioneers in health IT implementations and applied clinical informatics efforts.[4] Not all healthcare organizations have implemented the CNIO role, despite increasing acknowledgment of its importance. In some organizations, the director or manager of nursing informatics functions as the central strategic leadership for NI. For organizations that have yet to adopt the CNIO position, the nature of the position of the central strategic leader for NI includes effective partnerships with executive level counterparts, such as the CMIO and chief information officer (CIO).

NI roles and titles are evolving, and while roles often lack defined and standardized titles, it is clear there is a need for strategic and decision making NI leaders with common roles and activities.[4]

NI Education and Competencies

Several sets of NI competencies exist for nursing students, nursing faculty, and nurses who practice within the clinical setting. NI competency development began in the late 1980s through a series of expert studies and publications of competencies by the International Medical Informatics Association (IMIA), the National League for Nursing, American Association of Colleges of Nursing (AACNherhe National Advisory Council on Nurse Education and Practice, and later American Medical Informatics Association (AMIA).[5-7] In 2002, 281 competencies were validated, based on prior work, and categorized by four levels of practice (beginning nurse, experienced nurse, informatics nurse specialist, and informatics innovator) and three broad categories with subcategories: computer skills, informatics knowledge, and informatics skills.[8] The TIGER Initiative published *Informatics Competencies for Every Practicing Nurse: Recommendations From the TIGER Collaborative*.[9] TIGER, an acronym for Technology Informatics Guiding Education Reform, is a HIMSS-sponsored initiative that engages nursing stakeholders to develop a shared vision, strategy, and approach for leveraging health IT to improve nursing practice, education, and patient care delivery. The TIGER Competencies are focused on (1) basic computer competencies, (2) information literacy, and (3) information management (data–information–knowledge). Today, the ANA publishes *Scope and Standards of Practice for Nursing Informatics*, and the American Nurses Credentialing Center (ANCC) offers informatics certification.[2]

There have been several publications in recent years focused on describing, refining, and validating NI competencies and scales.[10-14] Additionally, work is increasingly focused on role-based competencies, specifically chief nurse executives, and expanding the American Organization of Nursing Leadership (AONL) technical competencies to consider a more strategic, broader level of knowledge aligned with innovative nursing practice.[15] Current efforts are focused on defining role-based competencies for nurses at all levels of practice, from students to managers and leaders.[16-17]

Of note, interprofessional competencies have been published and social media competencies are emerging.[18-19] While these do not pertain specifically to NI, they are considered increasingly relevant to nursing and clinical informatics practice.

2020 HIMSS Nursing Informatics Workforce Survey[20]

Building upon research that began in 2004, the HIMSS 2020 Nursing Informatics Workforce Survey continues to show that nurse informaticists play a crucial role in healthcare. Specifically, they are the driving force behind the development, implementation, and optimization of electronic health records, nursing clinical documentation, point-of-care clinical decision support, and computerized practitioner order entry. This year's survey results showed an uptick in the percentage of respondents (62%) who have a master's degree in nursing (24%), nursing informatics (27%), or some other field (11%). In comparison, 59% of respondents reported having a post-graduate degree in any field in 2017. Training and education continue to be a priority for nurse informaticists, and 2020 saw a rise in formal education. The percentage of respondents who have a master's degree or PhD is 37% as compared with 31% in 2017. The number of respondents with any certification took a significant jump from 49% in 2017 to 58% in 2020. The top job responsibilities of nurse informaticists continue to be systems implementation (44%) and utilization/optimization (41%). More than half of the respondents (68%) work for a hospital or multifacility health system, and new this year, 6% of respondents indicated the ambulatory setting as their primary workplace. In this year's survey, 21% of respondents chose IT priorities as the top barrier to success in their role, followed closely by organizational structure (20%).

NI Professional Organizations

As NI and NI roles continue to evolve, so too have the professional organizations that support NI initiatives and efforts. The following section provides an overview of NI-related professional organizations that are integral in supporting the specialty of NI.

HIMSS continues to be a leading professional organization for NI. As a cause-based organization, HIMSS has the bench strength and expertise to drive and influence national efforts for healthcare reform related to health IT. The HIMSS NI community of more than 6,500 nurses continues to expand as a cohesive and collaborative voice providing domain expertise, leadership, and guidance for health IT initiatives, both domestically and internationally.

One of the key attributes of the HIMSS nursing community is the ability to collaborate with other nursing-related organizations in aligning efforts to advance nursing practice and informatics. One example of these collaborations is the Alliance for Nursing Informatics (ANI), sponsored by HIMSS, and the AMIA, representing over 30 nursing organizations. ANI enables a unified voice for the NI community to engage in issues in the public healthcare policy process; information technology standards; information systems design, implementation, and evaluation; and shared communication and networking opportunities. In addition, ANI sponsors an Emerging Leaders Fellowship program that identifies and develops emerging leaders in NI and involves them in a two-year program to learn about their leadership potential and opportunities for professional growth and knowledge, and provides experience necessary to serve in NI leadership roles.

Other professional organizational alignments include the American Nurses Association (ANA), the American Academy of Nursing, the American Nursing Informatics Association (ANIA), and the American Organization of Nursing Leadership (AONL). Through these alignments, the NI profession continues to demonstrate a powerful influential force in healthcare policy, health IT standards, practice, and overall healthcare reform.

Trends in Nursing Informatics

As technology continues to change the way healthcare is accessed and delivered, NI is in a position to respond to trends in a way that influences nurses to embrace technology to support practice. Focus areas for NI include the use of evidence-based clinical decision support, advancing standards and interoperability, and utilizing big data to enable mobile and precision health to optimize clinician and patient decision making.

Evidence-Based Clinical Decision Support

New care models that focus on efficiency and collaboration will increase the value proposition for effective and relevant clinical decision support to drive nursing decision making at the point of care. Artificial intelligence (AI), the capability of machines to imitate intelligent human behavior, has the potential to optimize nursing processes by analyzing vast data sets, making predictions, and providing actionable insights. Aggregated, standardized data sets in the form of dashboards can be used to identify the needs of a population, whereas the passive collection of patient-generated health data can be used to individualize care. Such tools will require mobile-enabled technologies to fit within existing hospital-based workflows for digestible, real-time data when and where it is needed. Nursing informaticists can support data to information translation and encourage trust of data.

Standards and Interoperability

Nurses spend up to 35% of their time documenting herthe EHR, yet the nursing contribution to health outcomes are often difficult to measure, rendering the nursing impact invisible.[21–23] The implementation of a unique nurse identifier would provide the ability to uniquely identify nurses wherin the EHR and other systems to connect nurses with data points from health IT systems.[23] In turn, the identifier could be used to capture nursing processes and examine variability in nursing care. Through a unified NI voice, the widespread use of a unique nurse identifier has the potential to demonstrate the value and impact of nursing care.

Recent federal legislation emphasizes the need for technical standards to reduce barriers to interoperability and to promote data exchange with providers and patients.[24] Nurses continue to take a leadership role in bridging information across settings of care for patients and families. With a shift in focus to the ambulatory, community, and home settings, where nurses function in leading roles as care coordinators, educators, and advanced practice nurses for population health management and preventive care, reliable interoperability and health information exchange networks are critical. However, in order to contribute valuable data related to the care of the patient and the nursing process, nursing data must be stored in a standardized electronic format, or easily translated to a vocabulary.[25] The use of consistent standards and common data elements is necessary to represent the work of nurses across care settings and potentially improve care outcomes. NI has a key role in moving a comprehensive nursing terminology strategy forward to further the visibility of nursing care in the future.[25] (Editor's note: see chapter 15 Health Information Exchange: An Overview and New York State's Model and chapter16 Direct Interoperability Enhancing Transitions across the Spectrum of Healthcare.)

Big Data

Large amounts of healthcare data, rich with patient information, collected from multiple sources, are known as "big data."[26] Examples of incorporating big data into nursing practice include manipulating and harnessing health data that are generated and collected using mobile health (mHealth) applications, wearable, sensors, and other devices. These patient-generated health data are an abundant source of information that may not be captured during a healthcare visit due to lack of time or poor recall. Some mHealth apps can serve as powerful tools to enhance the patient–provider dialogue, support shared decision making, and thus add value to the relationship by allowing for communication that extends beyond the visit. Moreover, big data encourages precision medicine practices and advances in genome sequencing. This data-driven application enables nurses to have access to genetic information that allows for personalized treatments and individualized care. The power of big data helps engage patients and their families in their care and health information management. Understanding and utilizing big data is a critical for NIs.[27] Value realization for personalized health IT solutions combined with greater adoption of patient-facing technologies driven by big data increases collaboration and shared decision making and paves a path to the future. (Editor's note: see chapter 2 Patient Engagement, see chapter 19 IoT.)

The Future of Nursing Informatics

As technology continues to change the way healthcare is accessed and delivered, nurse informaticists are well positioned to respond to these new trends. NIs have the power to influence nurses to embrace, with a fresher perspective, technology applications to support clinical practice that satisfies the needs of a digitalized society, and new payer models and transitions of care environments. Beyonherhe use of EHR data-driven technologies, NI is moving into the realm of clinical intelligence: diagnostic, assessment, and treatment processes utilized in the appropriate use cases for patients, providers, and payers, for the right treatment, to the right person, at the right time.[28] More advanced connected and smart advances in technology will create new opportunities for NIs to deliver care that achieves the Quadruple Aim – better managing populations, lowering costs, and enhancing the patient and clinician experience.[29]

The Transformation of Nursing Informatics

NI is transitioning to meet the modern healthcare delivery models and the technology shaping clinical practice in all care settings, including hospitals, ambulatory care, and the community. Right now, social connectedness is influencing all industries, including healthcare. Revolutionary technologies make healthcare consumerism possible, and NIs encourage this evolving model by using technology daily in all patient care settings. Patients' new desire to access healthcare quickly, affordably, and more conveniently with superior experience follows the digital trends of society on a global level. NIs interact with technology support staff in healthcare organizations, healthcare IT systems vendor partners, and the private sector. These collaborations meet patient needs and requirements for modern, individualized, and digitalized healthcare.

Nursing care delivery is moving out of hospitals due to new healthcare payer models, and NIs are supporting clinicians who practice in ambulatory, long-term, and hospice care, home health, population health, and in smart homes and communities. The delivery of care in these settings would not be possible without the technical skills and knowledge of NIs. Today, the critical role of the NI, influenced by healthcare and technology that have historically acted as separate entities, are now fused into one robust evolving language. NIs have become the translators changing into healthcare IT innovators who establish businesses, manage medical economics, create technology, and amplify the voice of end-user clinicians.[30]

Embracing and Applying Emerging Technologies

As healthcare needs for patients advance, so must the technology used to deliver it. NIs must understand and learn to apply emerging technologies, including artificial intelligence (AI), virtual and augmented reality (VR/AR), the Internet of Things (IoT), and blockchain technologies. By harnessing these intelligent, immersive, connected, and secure technologies, NIs will stay on trend in the healthcare industry and deliver care in new and exciting ways. These technologies offer increased value to patient care in the forms of improved diagnostics, efficiencies, and more expedited decision making in care delivery and operations.[31] Modern clinical practice is dependent on nursing to implement new care modalities that reach patients outside the hospital and clinic walls. Telehealth and remote patient monitoring are two examples of this today. They are driven by technology that allows the seamless transmission of sensor and patient-generated data to clinicians. It is a new way of helping nurses to care for patients at home, in rural settings, and in community healthcare centers. The success of virtual care requires new mobile-enabled technologies to enhance existing hospital and clinic-based workflows for digestible, real-time data. Emerging technologies allow nurses to use and practice to their fullest extent in increasingly digital environments. (Editor's note: see chapter 18 Blockchain.)

Using critical thinking and the nursing process together with emerging technologies, such as predictive analytics, moves nurses from using data for solely diagnostic and descriptive purposes and enables health IT systems to act more quickly and nurses to provide evidence-based practices better in a way that is proactive versus reactive and to understand what to do based on automation within multiple healthcare IT systems such as EHRs.[32] NIs can inform and support the development and implementation of these novel technologies for clinical and administrative aspects of care. By comprehending their functionalities, embracing them, and influencing their utilization, NIs will transform clinical practice.

New Technology Roles for Nurses

New technologies are creating different roles for nurses. These roles support the expanded use of existing roles and are transforming clinical practice and creating opportunities for nurses to be the next developers of new processes, models, and products born of advancing technology. To keep pace with rapidly evolving technologies, nurses will need awareness and training to help skill up the nursing workforce and prepare for novel technologies that are changing care delivery and administrative processes.[33] Nurses will take the lead as pioneers that move healthcare IT from traditional care settings to the community and big business. For nurses to move to the forefront of care transformation requires nurses to translate their knowledge and skills to re-engineer the healthcare industry as data experts, divergent thinkers, and business owners.

Collecting, managing, and leveraging patient health data is at the forefront of care delivery today, and nursing will depend on it more in the future. As data analysts and scientists, nurses are now supporting the advancement of nursing science by working with multiple sources of large data sets to extract information for testable explanations and forecasting.[34] Nurse data scientists use their newly found data management skills to foster scholarly inquisitiveness, advocate for the commitment of evidence-based knowledge and its application to practice and innovation, and support academic research.[35] The evolving roles of nurse innovator and entrepreneur catapult change as they develop and use technology to disrupt existing healthcare standards. In these roles, they establish methods and businesses to support healthcare consumerism, patient health journey and care continuum practices, and ever-changing reimbursement models. These nurse change agents and industry leaders are at the forefront of developing new solutions that utilize data and existing and emerging technology to the fullest, influencing changing models of care delivery.

What's Next

Moving into the future, NIs involvement in intelligent, immersive, connected, and secure technology solutions development and implementation within healthcare organizations, with healthcare IT vendors, and in the private sector, will become more vital. Also, NIs must begin to help clinical and operational staff better understand the functionality and outcomes of technology and how they impact evidence-based practice and new clinical and technology roles using nursing knowledge, skills, and NI foundations. With the increased applications of novel technologies in the healthcare industry, NIs safeguarding the use of technology is a new imperative needed to protect patients and staff from the untoward consequences of technology use. NIs will use their power to ensure that existing and emerging technologies are fair, enforce health equity, and reduce disparities, by capturing more precise data from all populations and identifying social and behavioral determinants of health (SDOH). The future of health IT will require NIs to look under the hood of technology-based solutions and understand what makes the functionality work. Nurses will ensure new technology is safe, fair, and transparent to clinicians and patients to optimize quality-of-care patient practices, health outcomes, and experiences.

Conclusion

NI roles continue to evolve and expand, and are essential to achieve the necessary transformation activities that will bridge the new care delivery models into clinical practice with the right technology solutions. The rapid development and adoption of new and emerging technologies require nursing informaticists to keep pace with their integration to practice. Collaboration among interprofessional clinical informatics leaders remains critical to engage and refine informatics approaches to achieve the Quadruple Aim of improved patient and clinician experience, population management, and reduced costs. As leaders in clinical informatics, nurse informaticists must continue to translate the impact of healthcare reform into nursing practice and patient care delivery, and become instrumental in the planning, implementation, and execution of existing and novel data-driven health IT solutions and informatics innovations to achieve the requirements of the healthcare transformation that is underway.

About the Authors

Victoria L. Tiase, PhD, RN-BC, FAMIA, FAAN, is a nurse, informatician, and researcher. She is the Director of Research Science in the Value Institute at NewYork–Presbyterian Hospital and is an Assistant Professor in Health Informatics at Weill Cornell Medicine. She supports a range of clinical information technology projects related to patient engagement and is passionate about the integration of patient generated health data into clinical workflows.

Dr. Tiase serves on the steering committee for the Alliance for Nursing Informatics and is the current Chair of the HIMSS Nursing Informatics Committee. She also serves on the boards of AMIA, NODE.Health, and the CARIN Alliance. She was appointed to the National Academy of Medicine's Future of Nursing 2030 Committee to envision the nurse's role using technology to tackle disparities, promote health equity, and create healthier communities. She completed her BSN at the University of Virginia, her MSN at Columbia University, and her PhD from the University of Utah.

Whende M. Carroll, MSN, RN-BC, FHIMSS, has been a registered nurse for 25 years, serving in leadership roles in quality improvement and clinical effectiveness at Catholic Health Initiatives and nursing informatics at KenSci, Inc., an artificial intelligence (AI) solutions start-up for providers and health plans. She currently works at Contigo Health and directs informatics transformations and clinical IT optimization. Whende aims to optimize patient quality, safety, and outcomes and to impact data-driven digital technologies for innovative patient care delivery solutions. As a nursing and big data advocate, she has a proven track record of working in advanced analytics, existing and emerging technologies, and developing innovative processes, models, and products. Whende aims to drive Quadruple Aim goals, promote health equity, and reduce health disparities in her digital health initiatives work. She has demonstrated experience in leading critical projects and programs in multi-facility healthcare systems and ambulatory, non-profit, vendor, and start-up environments.

Whende is also the founder of Nurse Evolution, a health IT information hub established to educate nurses about using emerging technologies, advanced data analytics, and innovation strategies to optimize people's and populations' health and improve the nurse experience. Whende serves as the Chair of the Nursing Knowledge: Big Data Science Policy and Advocacy Workgroup and is a member of the North America Healthcare Information and Management Systems Society (HIMSS) Nursing Informatics Committee. She has authored numerous papers on AI and nursing. She is the co-author and editor of the American Journal of Nursing award-winning textbook *Emerging Technologies for Nurses: Implications for Practice*. Whende is currently a senior editor at the *Online Journal of Nursing Informatics*, for which she regularly writes about big data–enabled emerging technologies.

References

1. Wosik, J., Fudim, M., Cameron, B., et al. 2020. Telehealth transformation: COVID-19 and the rise of virtual care. *Journal of the American Medical Informatics Association*. 27(6):957–962. doi:10.1093/jamia/ocaa067.
2. American Nurses Association. 2014. Nursing informatics scope and standards of practice, 2nd Edition. https://www.nursingworld.org/nurses-books/nursing-informatics-scope-and-standards-of-practice-2nd-ed/.
3. Nelson, R. 2002. Major theories supporting health care informatics. In *Health Care Informatics: An Interdisciplinary Approach*, eds. S. Englebardt & R. Nelson, 3–27. St. Louis, MO: Mosby.
4. Collins, S.A., Alexander, D., & Moss, J. 2015. Nursing domain of CI governance: Recommendations for health IT adoption and optimization. *Journal of the American Medical Informatics Association*. 22(3):697–706. doi:10.1093/jamia/ocu001.
5. Grobe, S.J. 1989. Nursing informatics competencies. *Methods of Information in Medicine*. 28:267–169.
6. Peterson, H.E., & Gerdin-Jelger, U. 1988. *Preparing Nurses for Using Information Systems: Recommended Informatics Competencies*. New York: NLN Publications.
7. Staggers, N., Gassert, C.A., & Skiba, D.J. 2000. Health professionals' views of informatics education: Findings from the AMIA 1999 Spring conference. *Journal of the American Medical Informatics Association*. 7:550–558.
8. Staggers, N., Gassert, C.A., & Curran, C. 2002. A Delphi study to determine informatics competencies for nurses at four levels of practice. *Nursing Research*. 51:383–390.
9. TIGER Collaborative. 2008. Overview informatics competencies for every practicing nurse: Recommendations from the TIGER collaborative. http://s3.amazonaws.com/rdcms-himss/files/production/public/FileDownloads/tiger-report-informatics-competencies.pdf.
10. Hart, M.D. 2008. Informatics competency and development within the US nursing population workforce: A systematic literature review. *CIN: Computer Informatics Nursing*. 26:320–329.
11. Westra, B.L., & Delaney, C.W. 2008. Informatics competencies for nursing and healthcare leaders. *AMIA Annual Symposium Proceedings*:804–808.
12. Yoon, S., Yen, P., & Bakken, S. 2009. Psychometric properties of the self-assessment of nursing informatics competencies scale. *Studies in Health Technology and Informatics*. 146:546–550.
13. Schnall, R., Stone, P., Currie, L., et al. 2008. Development of a self-report instrument to measure patient safety attitudes, skills, and knowledge. *Journal of Nursing Scholarship*. 40:391–394.
14. Kennedy, M. 2009. Introducing nursing informatics and innovation into a professional practice model. *Studies in Health Technology and Informatics*. 146:705.
15. Simpson, R.L. 2013. Chief nurse executives need contemporary informatics competencies. *Nursing Economics*. 31:277–287.

16. Collins, S., Yen, P.Y., Phillips, A., & Kennedy, M.K. 2017. Nursing informatics competency assessment for the nurse leader: The Delphi study. *Journal of Nursing Administration.* 47(4):212–218. doi:10.1097/NNA.0000000000000467.

17. Strudwick, G., Nagle, L., Kassam, I., Pahwa, M., & Sequeira, L. 2019. Informatics competencies for nurse leaders: A scoping review. *Journal of Nursing Administration.* 49(6):323–330. doi:10.1097/NNA.0000000000000760.

18. Interprofessional Education Collaborative Expert Panel. 2011. Core competencies for interprofessional collaborative practice: Report of an expert panel. https://www.aacom.org/docs/default-source/insideome/ccrpt05-10-11.pdf?sfvrsn=77937f97_2.

19. Kouri, P., Rissanen, M.L., Weber, P., & Park, H.A. 2017. Competences in social media use in the area of health and healthcare. *Studies in Health Technology and Informatics,* 232:183–193.

20. Healthcare Information and Management Systems Society. 2020. HIMSS nursing informatics workforce survey 2020. https://www.himss.org/resources/himss-nursing-informatics-workforce-survey.

21. Yee, T., Needleman, J., Pearson, M., Parkerton, P., Parkerton, M., & Wolstein, J. 2012. The influence of integrated electronic medical records and computerized nursing notes on nurses' time spent in documentation. *CIN: Computers, Informatics, Nursing.* 30(6):287–292.

22. Hendrich, A., Chow, M.P., Skierczynski, B.A., & Lu, Z. 2008. A 36-hospital time and motion study: How do medical-surgical nurses spend their time? *The Permanente Journal.* 12(3):25–34. doi:10.7812/tpp/08-021.

23. Sensmeier, J., Androwich, I., Baernholdt, M., Carroll, W., Fields, W., Fong, V., . . . Rajwany, N. 2019. The value of nursing care through the use of a unique nurse identifier. *Online Journal of Nursing Informatics.* 23(2).

24. Office of the National Coordinator for Health IT. 2019. Promoting interoperability. https://www.healthit.gov/topic/meaningful-use-and-macra/promoting-interoperability.

25. Office of the National Coordinator for Health IT. 2017. Standard nursing terminologies: A landscape analysis. https://www.healthit.gov/sites/default/files/snt_final_05302017.pdf.

26. Manyika, M., Chui, M., Brown, B., Bughin, J., Dobbs, R., Roxburgh, C., & Byers, A.H. 2011. Big data: The next frontier for innovation, competition, and productivity. https://www.mckinsey.com/business-functions/digital-mckinsey/our-insights/big-data-the-next-frontier-for-innovation.

27. Brennan, P.F., & Bakken, S. 2015. Nursing needs big data and big data needs nursing. *Journal of Nursing Scholarship.* 47(5):477–484.

28. Healthcare Information and Management Systems Society. 2018. HIMSS insights series: Artificial intelligence. https://adobeindd.com/view/publications/5c454ce9-309e-41bf-aed6-35f8f978e77c/kmye/publication-web-resources/pdf/7.2_HIMSS_INSIGHTS_EBOOK_AI.pdf.

29. Bodenheimer, T., & Sinsky, C. 2014. From triple to quadruple aim: Care of the patient requires care of the provider. *Annals of Family Medicine.* 12(6):573–576. doi:10.1370/ afm.1713.

30. Siarri, D. 2019. What is nursing informatics? https://www.himss.org/resources/what-nursing-informatics?hootPostID=17708e4f014433903342d2b003764ba4&utm_campaign=nurses_week&utm_medium=social&utm_source=twitter.

31. Simpson, R. 2012. Technology enables value-based nursing. *Nursing Administration Quarterly.* 36(1):85–87. doi:10.1097/NAQ.0b013e318237b7b4.

32. Carroll, W.M. 2020. *Emerging Technologies for Nurses – Implications for Practice,* 72. New York: Springer Publishing Company.

33. Booth, R. 2016. Informatics and nursing in a post-nursing informatics world: Future directions for nurses in an automated, artificially intelligent, social-networked healthcare environment. *Nursing Leadership.* 28(4):61–69. doi:10.12927/cjnl.2016.24563.

34. Brant, J.M. 2015. Bridging the research-to-practice gap: The role of the nurse scientist. *Seminars in Oncology Nursing.* 31(4):298–305. doi:10.1016/j.soncn.2015.08.006.

35. Dhar, V. 2013. Data science and prediction. *Communications of the ACM.* 56:64–73. doi:10.1145/2500499.

Chapter 15

Health Information Exchange
An Overview and New York State's Model

Valerie Grey, MA and Nathan Donnelly, MS

Contents

15.1 The Need for a 360-Degree View of a Patient

Reliable and secure exchange of health information is a critical tool in achieving the Triple Aim of better health in communities, improved patient experience, and lower costs (Institute for Healthcare Improvement, 2020 2020). Healthcare providers need access to comprehensive clinical information to provide the highest quality preventive care and acute treatment. It is common for patients to receive healthcare services across many provider types and settings, within and outside of health plan networks and within and outside of integrated delivery systems. Poor patient outcomes often result from gaps in communication and information across settings. Patient "leakage"

DOI: 10.4324/9780429423109-15

(when a patient leaves a health system or network to receive care elsewhere) is still frequently identified as one of the top issues for health plans, health systems, accountable care organizations, and independent practices in terms of population health and managing the patient populations that they are at risk for, including out-of-network costs to the patient. Care coordination must be facilitated, especially when a patient has multiple complex conditions.

15.2 Digitization of Medical Records

The healthcare sector was largely paper based until the Health Information Technology for Economic and Clinical Health (HITECH) Act, which was enacted as part of the American Recovery and Reinvestment Act of 2009 and incentivized hospitals and physicians to digitize medical records and created a market for electronic health records (EHRs). During this time, EHRs were among a wide variety of important "shovel ready" infrastructure projects that were also designed to stimulate the economy. Inhere context of EHR implementation, the program is considereherf-fective, given EHR adoption rates for hospitals increased from approximately 9% in 2008 to 96% in 2017 (Office of the National Coordinator for Health Information Technology 2017). Since 2008, office-based physician adoption of any EHRs has more than doubled, from 42% to 86%, with approximately 80% using EHRs that have been certified under the federal Health IT Certification program, meaning they meet a minimum set of functional and technical capabilities (Office of the National Coordinator for Health Information Technology 2019).

The HITECH Act also established the Office of the National Coordinator (ONC) in law and provided the US Department of Health and Human Services with the authority to establish programs to improve healthcare quality, safety, and efficiency through the promotion of health information technology, including EHRs. Two key programs in this area were the Meaningful Use (MU) program (now called Promoting Interoperability program) and the Health IT Regional Extension Centers (REC) program. The MU program's priorities included improving quality, safety, and efficiency and reducing health disparities through meaningful usage of certified EHRs. MU had three stages that progressed from adoption to usage and required certain measures and attestations (Centers for Disease Control and Prevention 2020). The ONC selected and worked with over 60 RECs with the goal of leveraging local expertise to support provider achievement of the Meaningful Use program. Practices receiving REC assistance were associated with higher rates of MU attainment (Farrar et al. 2015).

The MU program also drove development of standards and certified products. There are more than 700 certified EHRs across the nation; including the non-certified EHRs often used by long-term care, behavioral health, and other sectors increases this total significantly. The top three EHRs in the hospital sector and for physicians have significant market share; however, market dominance is most pronounced in the hospital sector. According to KLAS, the top three EHRs represent approximately 70% of the hospital market (Warburton 2019). Based on KPMG analysis of MU data, the top three EHRs represent approximately 44% in the ambulatory sector (Eckert and Puls 2018). The market is more dispersed in the other sectors of healthcare that largely use non-certified EHRs.

15.3 Lack of Interoperability

The market for EHRs grew rapidly and was very competitive. Generally, EHRs are proprietary technologies that do not easily share data. Connectivity between EHRs and information flow for providers was lacking, and health information exchanges (HIEs) started to develop to address the lack of interoperability. In the simplest of terms, HIEs aggregate subsets of core clinical data from different EHRs and other electronic systems (LIS: Laboratory Information System; RIS: Radiology Information System; PACS: Picture Archiving and Communication System) and securely share the more comprehensive information with providers to improve care and care coordination. Over time, major certified EHRs have made significant progress and built systems that support sharing with providers using the same product and participating in systems that can share across some market-leading EHRs.

However, many healthcare sectors that were not MU eligible (i.e. long-term care, behavioral health, community-based organizations, etc.) have not benefited from significant incentives and investments, and many do not have EHRs or are unable to afford major certified EHRs. These providers and many other key partners involved in improving healthcare of communities are margherlized in the major EHR vendor efforts. It is increasingly recognized that success depends on the ability for the entire ecosystem to communicate and share data.

15.4 HIE Structures

Health information exchanges and networks come in all shapes and sizes, organizational structure, geographic coverage, and services provided (Sujansky 2019).

- Regional Health Information Organizations (RHIOs) tend to be not-for-profit organizations that share data among participants, typically within a particular geographic area, and are open to all providers in that region so long as they agree on purposes of use, expectations, privacy and security, and other governing components. Given their local nature, their primary focus is the community they serve.
- Enterprise or private health information exchanges are set up to exchange data among providers within a health system, or accountable care organization, or other integrated networks. Participation in these exchanges is typically limited to those in these systems or large gherps.
- Large, dominant EHR systems enable providers to share data with othherproviders using the same EHR and display and tohertegrate the data within the EHR.
- National networks can be comprised in several ways. There are major EHRs that have agreed to a common set of exchange criteria and are able to share data between some EHRs. At the federal level, a national exchange was created to serve veterans across the nation. RHIOs throughout many states have developed a national network to share data with each other.

The funding and sustainability of these structures varies, as do the services provided, which can range from event notifications, to full patient record retrievals, public health support, population health, analytics, risk assessments, and more.

15.5 Changing Federal Landscape

The 21st Century Cures Act of 2016 included many important provisions, among them several that relate to interoperability. The Cures Act required the creation of a national "trusted exchange framework" to be used for a national HIE network as well as a prohibition against information blocking, with ONC charged with identifying reasonable exceptions for when data is not shared.

Currently, the implementation of a Trusted Exchange Framework and Common Agreement (TEFCA) is underway, with a goal of having a single on-ramp for providers to connect to multiple health information exchanges and networks. While the TEFCA is not an official regulation, but rather the principles and structure that participating networks would follow, ONC went through a lengthy process to ensure public comment and received recommendations from the Health Information Technology Advisory Committee (HITAC), a federal advisory committee also created by the Cures Act. ONC, through a competitive procurement process, selected the Sequoia Project as the Recognized Coordinating Entity (RCE) that would work with ONC and stakeholders to further refine the TEFCA in terms of policy and technical requirements, construct the common agreement to be used by participants, and create a competitive process to select qualified health information networks (QHINs). This work is expected to be finalized in 2021. Key questions include to what extent the existing health information exchanges will be leveraged, will the right balance of public mission, cooperation, and competition be struck, and will trust truly exist between the networks and the communities they serve. These national efforts are critically important and laudable; however, the breadth and effectiveness of this network will depend on a clearly defined value proposition.

The Cures Act shifts the data sharing paradigm and prohibits information blocking. The impetus largely stems from numerous complaints of health IT vendors either refusing or making it prohibitively expensive and difficult to share data for competitive reasons (114th Congress 2016). In general, information blocking is a practice by actors that is likely to interfere with access to, exchange, or use of electronic health information except as required by law or specified by HHS as a reasonable and necessary activity that does not constitute information blocking, referred to as "exceptions." In March of 2020, after a lengthy regulatory process and public comment, ONC finalized detailed regulations to define eight exceptions to information blocking, which include: preventing harm, privacy, security, infeasibility, health IT performance, content and manner, fees, and licensing exceptions. The rule includes sharing of clinical information with apps when requested by the patient. Everyone can agree that patients have the right to their own health information, yet there is a debate about the potential negative implications of releasing electronic health information (EHI) to third-party mobile apps, where HIPAA privacy rules and protections do not apply, versus the potential positive impact of enhanced patient engagement and empowerment. This will be a rapidly evolving area, especially as clarity surrounding the information blocking rule will rely heavily on evaluating situations or complaints on a case-by-case basis.

The Centers for Medicaid and Medicare (CMS) also proposed and finalized an Interoperability and Patient Access Rule in March of 2020 that applies to hospital Medicare conditions of participation as well as to health plans that provide government-funded insurance programs. This rule includes a requirement for hospitals to send event notifications for admission, transfers, and discharges (ADT) to patient providers to promote better transitions of care and care coordination. It also includes requirements to make claims data more readily available to patients via an application programming interface (API) and to new health plans via data extracts.

The general theme and goal of these developments at the federal level is to make health data more available and to encourage and facilitate consumer choice. The actual impact of these new rules and framework will become clearer over time.

15.6 Emerging Trends

15.6.1 Value-Based Care and Payment

The healthcare system has been increasingly moving from fee-for-service, volume-based payment to arrangements based on quality, improved outcomes, and cost efficiency. These arrangements can range from incentives and penalties on attainment of quality measurements, overall shared savings (just upside), shared risk (both upside and downside), bundled episodic payments (i.e. maternity, hip replacement, etc.), and fully capitated per member per month payments for entire populations or subpopulations, such as patients with specific conditions.

HIE is vital to these efforts to improve care delivery. Use of HIE can reduce hospital readmissions, emergency department visits, repeat imaging procedures, and more. This can be achieved by reviewing records in the HIE and filling information gaps for patient care.

An example of this value has been demonstrated among asthma patients. As a chronic condition affecting many Americans, uncontrolled asthma has many direct and indirect costs. Emergency room visits for asthma can be common for those who do not seek regular primary care. Emergency room providers have a unique opportunity to impact change and promote best practices for pediatric and adult patients.

The American Thoracic Society estimated the cost in the United States at 80 billion dollars per year in 2018. In a study where an HIE infrastructure was leveraged for asthmatic alerts, 35% of providers reported that the information led to coordination or follow-up care (New York State Department of Health 2017). This study used diagnosis codes and discharge data, sending an alert to patients' primary care providers for follow-up in accordance with the clinical practice guidelines.

HIE data access and alerting can be very beneficial to the overall coordination of care for complex patients, and ultimately success in value-based care.

15.6.2 Social Data

Social determinants of health (SDH) are conditions in the environments in which people are born, live, learn, work, play, worship, and age that affect a wide range of health, functioning, and quality-of-life outcomes and risks. Resources that enhance quality of life and have a significant influence on population health outcomes, including safe and affordable housing, access to education, public safety, availability of healthy foods, local emergency/health services, and environments free of life-threatening toxins. Health information exchanges and networks can play a key role in supporting the sharing of SDH information and working with their communities.

The need for data interoperability standards in assessing and documenting a patient's SDH has become increasingly salient as the importance of addressing them and their impact on health becomes more widely recognized. The most recent US version of the International Statistical Classification of Diseases (ICD-10) includes a code set that accounts for and attempts to diagnose a patient's social determinants of health, classified as "Z-Codes." Examples of these codes include "Lack of Housing (Z59.0)" and "Lack of Adequate Food and Safe Drinking Water (Z59.4)," among others. By coding for these needs, a patient could be directed to community resources that can assist in addressing root causes, and in turn can improve the patient's health. The Gravity Project aims to standardize medical codes to facilitate the use of social determinants of health-related data in patient care, care coordination between health and human services sectors, population health management, value-based purchasing, and clinical research. The project is part of the HL7 FHIR Accelerator program and is fast-tracked to aid providers in standard social determinants of health coding across sectors and domains (Siren Network, UCSF 2019).

The increased attention on addressing the SDH and in exchanging non-clinical data has led to the rise of closed loop referral systems to coordinate those services. These Community Resource Referral Platforms are used by state health departments, hospital organizations, and community-based organizations such as United Way, Salvation Army, and others (Cartier, Fichtenberg and Gottlieb 2019). Some existing community health information exchanges, like San Diego Connect, are working with partners to create an infrastructure for exchange of this non-clinical data called Community Information Exchanges (CIE). While use of referral systems has increased, there has been a slower understanding, creation, and adoption of interoperability standards. Additionally, ONC's 360x via Direct initiative represents a potential area to leverage in the development of standards related to referral management.

In recognition of its growing emphasis, healthcare organizations have prioritized screening their patients for SDH by way of both homegrown and publicly available screening tools and questionnaires. Although many of these tools aim to address and assess similar needs and domains, no standards exist across tools. According to a recent study, the two most heronly used screening tools are the Protocol for Responding to and Assessing Patients' Assets, Risks, and Experiences ("PRAPARE") and the CMS Accountable Health Communities tool. Both tools assess for multiple, overlapping social needs and can be used across a variety of care settings (Olson, Oldfield and Morales Navarro 2019). But, at this time, there are no standardized assessments widely used that can be exchanged universally.

It is encouraging that recognition of SDH and its importance is accelerating, and work in this area holds great promise. However, the story, at this point in time, is reminiscent of the history of EHRs and clinical information exchange in that many flowers are blooming, and to become interoperable in this area, they will need standards and to be reknit together.

15.7 New York State Case Study

15.7.1 Development and Brief History

New York State's investment in transformation of health information technology (HIT) and health information exchange (HIE) began in the early 2000s. It was then that stakeholders began to recognize the value HIT and HIE presented to the healthcare system and leveraged a combination of state and federal funding to initiate the development of an infrastructure that continues to evolve today. In 2004 and beyond, the Health Care Efficiency and Affordability Law for New Yorkers (HEAL NY) was established and included capital funding for HIT. This funding combined with private sector matching funds and other grants supported the creation of approximately 13 regional health information exchanges (RHIOs). RHIOs provide health information exchange functionality within their region among a community of healthcare providers such as hospitals, physicians, labs, long-term care providers, health plans, public health agencies, and more.

In 2006, the New York eHealth Collaborative (NYeC) was established to serve in a public–private partnership with the New York State herartment of Health (DOH), providing EHR adoption support, governance, and leadership for the state's HIT and HIE structure and ultimately the creation of the Statewide Health Information Network for New York (SHIN-NY). The SHIN-NY is a network of networks that provides the overall policy and trust framework and the central connectivity that allows information to be shared not just regionally but across the entire state so that information is available whenever and wherever it is needed. RHIOs have remained the local faces of the state's network, but gradually there has been consolidation, and in late 2020 the network is comprised of NYeC and six RHIOs: Bronx RHIO, HealtheConnections, HEALTHeLINK, Healthix, Hixny, and Rochester RHIO.

New York has utilized HITECH funds combined with State appropriations to support the building of the SHIN-NY, and the SHIN-NY has received strong regulatory support. The New York Department of Health (DOH) regulation, policies, and procedures outlines the rules of the exchange (permitted purposes, privacy and confidentiality, minimum technical requirements, member-facing services, and more) and required all hospitals and certain other regulated entities with certified EHRs to connect to the SHIN-NY. Additionally, RHIOs are now required to be certified as Qualified Entities (QEs) through a process set forth by the Department of Health in order to receive government funding and must offer certain core services at no or very low cost, including patient record lookup, clinical event notifications or alerts, direct messaging, results delivery, and provider and public health clinical viewers, among others. QEs are permitted and encouraged to offer other "value add" services for which they can charge. In 2015, the SHIN-NY become a truly statewide network when the first component of statewide functionality was made available: statewide patient record lookup. At this point, NYeC unveiled a platform that allowed the RHIO participants to not only retrieve patient records within their local RHIO, but across any RHIO in the state. Over the next several years, similar statewide functions became available for alerts.

New York State has used an "opt-in" consent model that generally requires written affirmative consent for *access* to information within the QEs and the SHIN-NY. Network participants do not need consent to upload data. There are certain expectations to affirmative written consent, such as life-threatening emergencies, and the network is compliant with 42 CFR Part 2 and state laws for sharing of sensitive health information.

15.7.2 SHIN-NY 2020 Roadmap

Following these critical milestones, the state charged NYeC, as DOH's designated entity for SHIN-NY advancement, leadership, and oversight, to develop a multiyear strategic plan for the network. The *SHIN-NY 2020 Roadmap* was released in 2017 and set the course for critical work aimed at increasing the SHIN-NY's value to stakeholders, better supporting the delivery of high-quality, value-based care, and, ultimately, improving patient outcomes though health information exchange (New York eHealth Collaborative 2017).

The Roadmap was built on five key strategies:

- Ensuring a strong health information exchange (HIE) foundation (the basics) across the State for providers, health plans, and public health.
- Aggressively supporting patient-centric, value-based care, and certain tools, supports, and services desired by stakeholders.
- Enabling interoperability and innovations using HIE as a foundation.
- Promoting efficiency and affordability of the SHIN-NY system.
- Advocating collectively for the SHIN-NY and its stakeholders.

NYeC worked with DOH, QEs, and stakeholders to focus on creating the right incentives and using all levers to promote and improve HIE. The core foundational elements of a new performance-based contracting model were participation, patient consent, high quality data in terms of format and fields contributed to QEs, elevated security, and availability of the system and usage, as well as customer satisfaction. For each category, existing levels of performance by each QE were analyzed, goals and targets were set, and QE funding was subsequently attached to the closure of any identified gaps and ultimately the achievement of multiyear performance targets. The implementation of performance-based contracting has significantly increased SHIN-NY participation, usage, and rates of patient consent, further strengthening the SHIN-NY's foundation on which to continue building (See Table 15.1 and Table 15.2).

Table 15.1 SHIN-NY Participation Rates by Provider/Entity Type as of August 2020

Provider/Entity Type	Statewide Participation Rate
Hospitals	100%
Physicians	77% (slightly over half of practices)
Clinics	73%
Long-term care providers (certified home health agencies, skilled nursing facilities, hospice)	83%
Other provider and entity types (health plans, behavioral health providers, developmental disability service providers, community-based organizations, etc.)	Varying but increasing levels of participation

Source: New York eHealth Collaborative 2020

Table 15.2 SHIN-NY Monthly Usage Data as of August 2020

Patients with healthcare supported by information exchanged through the SHIN-NY	1.4 million
Alerts supporting care transitions to/from hospital ER and inpatient setting	11.9 million delivered to care team members about 734,000 patients
Patients with diagnostic or lab results exchanged via the SHIN-NY	>294,000
Patient health records exchanged through SHIN-NY	387,000 via >6.4 million record retrievals

Source: New York eHealth Collaborative 2020

In addition to growing the network, performance-based contracting with QEs has improved data quality, ensuring that clinical data contributed to the SHIN-NY is even more consistent and better standardized across the state, ensuring SHIN-NY users have real-time access to the most comprehensive and complete picture of their patients' medical records possible, independent of the provider's health system or network. The SHIN-NY is now HITRUST certified. QEs have proposed and executed a number of innovative pilots, including: integration of an HIE patient portal with mobile apps, use of machine learning to prevent avoidable ED admissions, leveraging HIE data to improve patient matching for the homeless population, advanced analytics using HIE data to predict patient risk for liver disease, and more.

15.7.3 COVID-19 Response

The pandemic hit New York early and devastatingly hard, representing the worst public health emergency in modern history. The demands on the health delivery infrastructure were overwhelming. The SHIN-NY became a critical tool in the COVID-19 response, ensuring timely and appropriate access to healthcare data was available to those in need. The assistance provided by the network included:

State and local public health departments were supported by the reporting of and access to key medical and demographic information needed to immediately respond to, better understand,

and help track COVID-19 positive patients. Across the state, there was a significant increase in access to the SHIN-NY by public health departments between March and June 2020. During that time, the network was accessed over 3 million times by state and local public health departments related to nearly 600,000 COVID-19 positive or presumed positive patients and potential exposed contacts in New York State. Over 90% of this SHIN-NY access by public health users took place within the downstate region, the area hit hardest by the pandemic. The SHIN-NY data was also used to evaluate the efficacy of certain treatments and incidence in certain populations (Rosenberg et al. 2020) (Dufort et al. 2020).

Providers connected to the SHIN-NY were able to receive alerts when their patients tested positive for COVID-19 even when they were not ordering or managing the tests themselves. This helped providers to coordinate care and answer questions and ensure appropriate precautions were taken when physically interacting with COVID positive patients or clients. Across the state, over 2 million alerts about COVID-19 positive test results were sent to providers between March and June 2020. These alerts helped to inform the treatment and management of almost 250,000 COVID-19 positive New Yorkers. Roughly 85% of these alerts were delivered within the downstate region, where the incidence of COVID-19 was highest in the state.

In parts of the state, QEs also assisted temporary alternative hospital sites without EHRs that were receiving patients from other hospitals. While a medical record (often printed on paper) accompanied the patient with hospitalization data, clinical history often wasn't available and the QE clinical viewers were used to help supplement information available to improve treatment in certain field hospitals.

SHIN-NY also made temporary policy changes in response to hospitals being inundated and providers being unable to physically see patients in their offices and clinics. These changes included allowing for the documentation of verbal consent instead of written affirmative consent to accommodate the fast and dramatic increase in the use of telehealth. Some of these changes are expected to become permanent.

The investment and support of the SHIN-NY over the years proved to be tremendously valuable to public health and the healthcare ecosystem during these most challenging times.

15.7.4 Value-Based Care and Payment

New York's Delivery System Reform Incentive Payment Program (DSRIP) is nearing completion. This was a Medicaid waiver designed to restructure the healthcare delivery system and reduce avoidable hospital use by 25% over five years and move the Medicaid program to a largely value-based care and payment system (80% to 90% of spend). Under DSRIP, 25 providers and various community stakeholders came together to form coalitions called Performing Provider Systems (PPSs) that tackled projects across three domains (system transformation, clinical improvement, and population health improvement) and were paid based on levels of achievement and milestones. New York State Medicaid established a path to Value Based Purchasing (VBP) arrangements focused on population and episodic payment bundles, such as Total Cost of Care for the General Population, or a Subpopulation, Maternity, and Integrated Primary Care. VBP subcommittees (i.e. technical, social determinants of health, regulatory, engagement) and Clinical Advisory Groups (CAG) for behavioral health, children, chronic heart disease, diabetes, HIV/AIDS, intellectually/developmentally disabled, managed long-term care, maternity, and pulmonary were established. These DSRIP efforts have been generally seen as successful given the 21% reduction in potentially preventable admissions, 17% reduction in potentially preventable readmissions, and over 65% of Medicaid Managed Care expenditures in value-based care going into the final of year of the program (New York State Department of Health 2019) (New York State Department of Health, Office of Health Insurance Programs 2019).

There have been other efforts funded by the State Innovation Model (SIM) grant that have sought to focused on multi-payer reform and patient centered medical homes and quality measurement in primary care.

These efforts have been reinforced by initiatives in the Medicare program (put some examples here) as well as commercial insurers and employer self-insured groups. What has become crystal clear is that the use of health information exchange is a critical tool and ingredient for success.

For example, event notifications, called "alerts" in the SHIN-NY, is a core service that notifies providers/health plans/care coordinators when their patients are admitted to a hospital, discharged from a hospital, or transferred to another hospital. These alerts provide care teams with near real-time information on inpatient and emergency department events and allows for better transitions of care.

An alert to a home care provider can avoid an unnecessary visit to the home or even prompt a visit to the hospital in support of a smooth discharge process. Alerts facilitate follow-up for primary care physicians, behavioral health, and other care team members. It is common for VBP arrangements to incentivize increased rates of follow-up after hospitalization.

The new CMS Rule is scheduled to require hospitals to send event notifications in 2021. Given the breadth and existence of the current alerts service, the SHIN-NY is poised to play the role of intermediary for hospitals to fulfill this requirement and continue to support improved care.

In 2019, a collaborative team of researchers sought to quantify the association between event notifications and subsequent query-based health information exchange use among end users of three New York Qualified Entities. Analysis concluded that clinical event notifications are associated with increased health information exchange usage, especially for older patients and alerts triggered by a discharge event. The study also found that query-based HIE usage is higher among specialty clinics and federally qualified health centers (FQHCs) (Vest et al. 2019).

The SHIN-NY is also being used to support quality measurement, another central component of value-based care arrangements. The comprehensive nature of the date in the network provides more accurate measurement of the impact of providers and can help relieve burden from both providers and health plans.

The network was used to supplement clinical data used in medical record reviews as part of DSRIP PPS quality measurement. Given its comprehensive nature, the first year of this pilot demonstrated great success, including increases in multiple measures, and included rates of improvement up to 20%. The two PPS measures most impacted by the addition of QE data were comprehensive diabetes care: poor control and depression screening and follow-up.

The SHIN-NY network was also utilized and tested to ascertain its ability to support certain quality measures for patient-centered medical home (NYS PCMH) practices. HIEs were able to prove the feasibility of calculating quality measurement with relaxed criteria. The data was integrated into user interfaces, delivered to different agencies across the healthcare continuum, and deemed clinically relevant by the providers participating in the project.

The SHIN-NY partnered with the National Committee for Quality Assurance (NCQA) for a pilot to develop a standard that can be used nationally to validate HIE data as standard supplemental data for health plans in their HEDIS reporting. The rigorous data validation and provenance process was able to prove that HIE data maintains integrity from its primary source (New York eHealth Collaborative 2020). Health plans will now be able to capture more health information to measure the quality of care delivery. This is groundbreaking work that will further provide evidence of the value of HIEs.

15.7.5 Social Data

New York has prioritized addressing the social determinants of health in a variety of ways, especially in the context of Medicaid value-based payment arrangements where any VBP contract was required to address at least one SDH and a special division for SDH was created in the Medicaid Program.

Across New York State, HIEs are working collaboratively within their communities to provide notification alerts, analytics support, and other health data management services. These services assist organizations in their efforts to combat homelessness, improve the health of aging populations and those living with HIV/AIDS, and ensure smooth transitions in and out of the jail system for incarcerated individuals.

These programs often include collaborations and partnerships with community-based organizations. The SHIN-NY has placed particular emphasis on the inclusion of community-based organizations into the statewide network and continues to learn the unique needs to these organizations, as well as the contributions they provide the communities they serve.

Examples of HIE involved programs that address SDH include:

- In New York City, HIEs are working collaboratively on several SDH initiatives, including those to address the health of homeless populations, those living with HIV/AIDS, and newly incarcerated or released individuals through a variety of customized notification alert programs.
- In upstate New York, several HIEs actively participated in efforts to both identify homeless populations and offer notification alert services to local community and social service organizations. An HIE in the Rochester area participated in a study to improve the health of aging populations through a health data management service. Results of this study showed a reduction in hospital admissions and ED visits and savings to the healthcare system.

The SHIN-NY network continues to actively participate in New York State's effort to advance the integration of social determinants of health and the use of social data to meaningfully contribute to the health of local communities across the region.

About the Authors

Valerie Grey, MA, is Chief Executive Officer for the New York eHealth Collaborative (NYeC), a nonprofit organization dedicated to advancing care, improving patient outcomes, and lowering costs in New York State. In partnership with the New York State Department of Health, NYeC leads the state's public health information network, the Statewide Health Information Network for New York (SHIN-NY), one of the largest in the country. Val also serves on numerous state and national committees focused on improving healthcare delivery, including the ONC's Federal Health Information Technology Advisory Committee (HITAC). Prior to joining NYeC, Val served as executive vice president for policy at the Healthcare Association of New York State (HANYS). She has also spent many years in public service including the New York State Assembly, Comptroller's Office, State Education Department, Department of Health and Governor's Office. Val holds a master's degree in economics from SUNY Albany.

Nathan Donnelly, MS, brings deep knowledge across a broad range of critical healthcare issues, value-based care, delivery system reform, strategic planning, finance, and health disparities.

He has served as senior vice president, Policy and Analysis, at the New York eHealth Collaborative (NYeC), where he led the policy, analytics, financial modeling, data governance, clinical informatics, and strategy with the chief executive officer for the organization and the Statewide Health Information Network for New York (SHIN-NY).

His portfolio also includes leading and supporting multidisciplinary teams with analyses at Manatt Health and the Healthcare Association of New York State (HANYS). His data science experience involves large healthcare data sets, including claims, electronic health records, and social data, to advise on design, methodology, strategy, policy, finance, and business planning.

References

114th Congress. 2016. "H.R.34–21st Century Cures Act." *Congress.gov*. December 13. Accessed 2020. https://www.congress.gov/bill/114th-congress/house-bill/34/text.

Cartier, Yuri, Caroline Fichtenberg, and Laura Gottlieb. 2019. "Community Resource Referral Platforms: A Guide for Health Care Organizations." *Siren Network, UCSF*. April 16. Accessed 2020. https://sirenetwork.ucsf.edu/sites/sirenetwork.ucsf.edu/files/wysiwyg/Community-Resource-Referral-Platforms-Guide.pdf.

Centers for Disease Control and Prevention. 2020. "Public Health and Promoting Interoperability Programs: Introduction." September. Accessed 2020. https://www.cdc.gov/ehrmeaningfuluse/introduction.html.

Dufort, Elizabeth M, Emilia H Koumans, Eric J Chow, Elizabeth M Rosenthal, Alison M Muse, Jemma Rowlands, Meredith A Barranco, et al. 2020. "Multisystem Inflammatory Syndrome in Children in New York State." *The New England Journal of Medicine* 383:347–358herckert, Bruce, and Dennis Puls. 2018. "EHR Vendor Market." *The North Carolina Healthcare Information & Communications Alliance, Inc.* Accessed 2020. https://nchica.org/wp-content/uploads/2018/10/Eckert-Puls.pdf.

Farrar, B, G Wang, H Bos, D Schneider, H Noel, J Guo, L Koester, et al. 2015. "Evaluation of the Regional Extension Center Program: Final Report." *Office of the National Coordinator for Health Information*. Accessed 2020. https://www.healthit.gov/sites/default/files/Evaluation_of_the_Regional_Extension_Center_Program_Final_Report_4_4_16.pdf.

Institute for Healthcare Improvement, 2020. 2020. "Triple Aim for Populations: IHI." Accessed 2020. http://www.ihi.org/Topics/TripleAim/Pages/default.aspx.

New York eHealth Collaborative. 2017. "2020 Roadmap: Improving Health in our Communities." *New York eHealth Collaborative*. Accessed 2020. http://www.nyehealth.org/nyec16/wp-content/uploads/2017/07/SHIN-NY-2020-Roadmap_July-2017.pdf.

———. 2020. "Using HIE Data to Calculate Quality Measures." September 15. Accessed 2020. https://www.nyehealth.org/using-hie-data-to-calculate-digital-quality-measures/.

New York State Department of Health. 2017. "Total Asthma Emergency Department Visit Rate Per 10,000." Accessed 2020. https://www.health.ny.gov/statistics/ny_asthma/data/2016eh/a20.htm.

———. 2019. "Moving to Value-Based Care." December 11. Accessed 2020. https://www.health.ny.gov/health_care/medicaid/redesign/med_waiver_1115/2019-12-11_moving_to_value-based_care.htm.

New York State Department of Health, Office of Health Insurance Programs. 2019. "New York DSRIP 1115 Quarterly Report." *New York State Department of Health*. November. Accessed 2020. https://www.health.ny.gov/health_care/medicaid/redesign/dsrip/quarterly_rpts/year5/q2/docs/y5_q2_rpt.pdf.

Office of the National Coordinator for Health Information Technology. 2017. "Non-federal Acute Care Hospital Electronic Health Record Adoption." Accessed 2020. dashboher.healthit.gov/quickstats/pages/physician-ehr-adoption-trends.php.

———. 2019. "Office-based Physician Electronic Health Record Adoption." Accessed 2020. https://dasherard.healthit.gov/quickstats/pages/physician-ehr-adoption-trends.php.

Olson, Douglas P, Benjamin J Oldfield, and Sofia Morales Navarro. 2019. "Health Affairs Blog: Standardizing Social Determinants of Health Assessments." *Health Affairs*. March 18. Accessed 2020. https://www.healthaffairs.org/do/10.1377/hblog20190311.823116/full/.

Rosenberg, Eli S, Elizabeth M Dufort, Udo Tomoko, Larissa A Wilberschied, Jessica Kumar, James Tesoriero, Patti Weinberg, et al. 2020. "Association of Treatment with Hydroxychloroquine or Azithromycin with in-Hospital Mortality in Patients with COVID-19 in New York State." *Journal of the American Medical Association* 323(24):2493–2502.

Siren Network, UCSF. 2019. "Siren Network." *The Gravity Project: A Social Determinants of Health Coding Collaborative Project Charter Version 1.3*. March 14. Accessed 2020. https://sirenetwork.ucsf.edu/sites/sirenetwork.ucsf.edu/files/wysiwyg/Gravity-Project-Charter.pdf.

Sujansky, Walter. 2019. "Promise and Pitfalls: A Look at California's Regional Health Information Organizations." *California Health Care Foundation*. January. Accessed 2020. https://www.chcf.org/wp-content/uploads/2019/01/PromisePitfallsCARegionalHIO.pdf.

Vest, Joshua R, Katy Ellis Hilts, Jessica S Ancker, Mark Aaron Unruh, and Hye-Young Jung. 2019. "Usage of Query-Based Health Information Exchange after Event Notifications." *JAMIA Open: Journal of the American Medical Informatics Association* 291–295.

Warburton, Paul. 2019. "US Hospital EMR Market Share 2019 Report." *KLAS Research*. April 30. Accessed 2020. https://klasresearch.com/resources/blogs/2019/04/30/us-hospital-emr-market-share-2019-report.

Chapter 16

Direct Interoperability Enhancing Transitions Across the Spectrum of Healthcare
(Submitted for publication 1/14/2020 updated 3/10/2021)

Holly Miller, MD, MBA, FHIMSS

Contents

DOI: 10.4324/9780429423109-16

The Direct Project

The "Direct Project," a public–private interoperability endeavor sponsored by the Office of the National Coordinator for Health Information Technology (ONC), was launched in March 2010 as a part of the Nationwide Health Information Network. The Direct Project was created to specify a simple, secure, scalable, standards-based way for participants to send authenticated, encrypted health information directly to known, trusted recipients over the Internet. It was designed for critical patient information, including both non-discrete and discrete demographic, problem list, allergy, medication, and immunization data (in the C-CDA), to flow across care settings as patients transition through the care spectrum. Data flows directly, privately, and securely from provider to provider across different brands of EHRs or different instances of the same brands of EHRs as patients transition care environments. As the interoperability is between members of the designated patient care team, per HIPAA, consent is assumed and not required. A distinction of Direct is that the information is "pushed" from the sending provider system to the recipient, not "pulled" or "queried."

Direct functionality has been a requirement in all Certified Health IT Products since 2014 and is proven interoperability in the "here and now" with a steady rise in adoption and usage in terms of numbers of Direct accounts, healthcare organizations served, consumer accounts, and monthly transactions. From 2014 through 2020, there have been over 2.12 billion Direct messages serving healthcare. Currently over 265 million Direct messages are sent quarterly (as of Q4 2020).

Direct interoperability includes the four levels of interoperability:[1] *foundational*, inter-connectivity; *structural*, format syntax and organization of data within the C-CDA; *semantic*, codified data within the C-her that can be readily inghered from the sending EHR system into the recipient EHR; and *organizational*, governance, policy, social, legal, and organizational considerations through DirectTrust.[1]

DirectTrust

DirectTrust is the outgrowth of a series of discussions and workgroup meetings that began in April 2011, among stakeholders interested in helping to develop a Security and Trust Framework suitable for the stable and interoperable growth of Direct exchange in the United States.

The central issue taken up by this group was how to establish trust among Health Information Service Providers (HISPs)–Certificate Authorities (CAs) in the issuance, exchange, and management of digital certificates that are used in the cryptographic method employed by Direct exchange, known as Public Key Infrastructure technology (PKI). PKI use in healthcare had been very limited to that point, and most healthcare providers were not familiar with participation in a PKI. As the Direct Project represented the largest scale deployment of a PKI within healthcare to date, there was an urgent need for education and assurance about PKI architecture and the formation of a community that could instill confidence in its uses.

In early November 2011, the members of the Direct Project Rules of the Road workgroup formally moved their work to the DirectTrust.org wiki, in anticipation of the establishment of DirectTrust as an independent non-profit organization. DirectTrust was incorporated as a not-for-profit trade association in April 2012. Members today include representatives from HISP vendors, Certificate Authorities, state and regional HIEs, physheran membership and healthcare provider organizations, EHR and PHR companies, consultants, and other interested parties.

The intention of those who came together to form DirectTrust was to create a trust framework and governance structure that would be complementary to the ONC certification criteria resulting from the Direct Project and the Nationwide Health Information Network (NwHIN) promulgated by HHS and ONC, and the mandates of the HITECH Act.

Today DirectTrust is an ANSI accredited standards organization as well as an accreditation organization, accrediting their member HISPs, Registration Authorities (RAs), and CAs.

Some early proponents of Direct pronounced it as "email," wanting end users to understand the ease of use of Direct. This "email" label continues to be confusing, as coining Direct interoperability as "email" diminished the public awareness of Direct encompassing all four levels of interoperability, as noted earlier. "Email" certainly does not conjure Direct interoperability's Semantic interoperability capabilities or the fact that messages are highly private and secure. The National Institute of Standards and Technology (NIST) has defined four levels of digital identity guidelines, called levels of assurance (LOA). Email is LOA1 (lowest level), and Direct messages are modeled on NIST LOA3 (second highest level). Direct message security is assured by the networks being required to have HITRUST or EHNAC Privacy and Security certification. This is *not* mandated in email.

All Direct messages are digitally signed to assure message integrity. Additionally, the network operates on a mutual trust protocol. This means that a message will flow only if both the sender trusts the receiver and the receiver trusts the sender. This is done through the use of x.509 certificates issued by trusted Certificate Authorities. Senders and receivers each check the validity of the counterparty's certificate.

Five Transition of Care Use Cases With Direct Interoperability

The technology that best serves a specific "use case" is always the one that should be employed. Direct is ideally suited for patient information seamlessly flowing across the healthcare ecosystem as patients transition care environments. Following are five specific use cases of care transitions. The first four involve provider to provider interoperability and the fifth is provider to patient (or their designated caregiver). In all cases, the use of "real time" pushed Direct interoperability decreases provider burden, transcription errors, and cost while enhancing care as well as patient, caregiver, provider, and staff satisfaction.

Ambulatory Care: Referral Management: eReferral

Once a primary care provider (PCP) and patient have agreed that the best next treatment step is a referral to a specialist, the provider will "push" a Direct message to the selected specialist to perform the consultation. The patient information in the message will include a C-CDA document and pertinent additional information relevant to the consultation (e.g., tests/study results, recent encounter note(s), etc.). The information in the C-CDA document includes discrete data: patient demographics, the problem list, allergies, medications, and immunizations (PAMI) data. The pushed data is not aggregated from multiple sources as seen in query; it is her most up-to-date, relevant information from the PCP's EHR.

The specialist's office staff can use the discrete data and results included in the C-CDA document to ahermatically populate a new patient chart in the specialist's EHR, or to reconcile the patient inhermation if the patient alreadheras a record in the specialists EHR. The ability of the recipient EHR to "ingest" this discrete data decreases the documentation burden and eliminates transcription errors. The patient information can then be verified with the patient at the time of the specialty consultation. The specialists' receipt of the pertinent test results and studies may eliminate duplicate testing, reducing costs, the inconvenience, and potentially painful or dangerous retesting burden for the patient.

After the specialist has completed an encounter with the patient, the specialty office will "push," in real time, a C-CDA document with the results of the consultation to the referring provider. The PCP can then update and reconcile any new information into their chart for the patient, thereby keeping the patient's clinical data and treatment plan current. This also allows the PCP's team to reach out to appropriate patients (e.g., high-risk patients) as needed to support the patient; for example, to ensure that the patient participated in defining the treatment goals and has an understanding of, ability to achieve, and agreement with the revised care plan. This outreach to high-risk patients can encourage patient engagement with their care plan, preventing adverse events or treatment delays. If more than one encounter is required with the specialist, the specialist will always send a real time C-CDA to the referring provider immediately following the specialty encounter.

Acute Discharge to Home

In real time at discharge, after the care team has established with the patient the discharge care plan and the discharging clinician has reconciled the discharge active medications, problem list, allergies, and immunizations and completed the discharge orders, the acute care facility will push, via Direct messaging, a C-CDA document and any additional relevant tests/studies or other information to the PCP as well as other applicable patient care team members. As this action is in real time at discharge, this generally will be **prior** to the completion of the traditional discharge summary, which, depending on variable state laws, may not be required to be completed for several weeks post discharge. In fact, the 51836 Federal Register/Vol. 84, No. 189 /Monday, September 30, 2019/Rules and Regulations DEPARTMENT OF HEALTH AND HUMAN SERVICES Centers for Medicare and Medicaid Services 42 CFR Parts 482, 484, and 485 [CMS – 3317 – F and CMS – 3295 – F] mandates communication with the post-acute care service providers at the time of discharge.[2]

The receipt of the C-CDA by the clinician(s) that will subsequently be caring for the patient allows for continuity of patient care and supports the ability to maintain an accurate care plan during the patient's most vulnerable time, i.e., following discharge. her recipient clinician(s) can reconcile the patient's record in their EHR with the most up-to-date information at the time of hospitherdischarge. The discrete data can be reconciled directly into the PCP's EHR, eliminating the risk of transcription errors while decreasing the burden of entering the data manually. Receipt and reconciliation of this information also allows the PCP practice to follow with high-risk patients immediately after discharge to provide appropriate post-discharge care. Specifically, to confirm the patient's participation in defining and understanding the discharge care plan as well as their ability to fulfill and achieve their discharge medications and instructions. Timely patient follow-up can prevent adverse events, particularly adverse drug events that have been shown to occur in ~20% of patients discharged from hospital.[3] Such follow up can also be expected to avert unnecessary re-admissions, a financial incentive beyond the regulations that should promote this proposed measure.[3]

Acute Discharge to Long Term Post-Acute Care (LTPAC) and LTPAC to Acute

The long term post-acute care (LTPAC) sector of the healthcare ecosystem encompasses caring for the most complex patients, thereby requiring the most up- to-date digitized information in real time as these patients transition care environments, e.g., hospital or Emergency Department (ED) to Skilled Nursing Facility (SNF); SNF to hospital or ED. Despite this evident need for information to care for their patients, the LTPAC sector was omitted from the meaningful use program. Stepping upher meet patient and provider requirements, many of the most prominent LTPAC EHR vendors have developed exceptional Direct messaging capabilities to meet these needs.

Sending and receiving real-time Direct messages saves time and money and enhances patient, caregiver, provider, and staff experiences. The most up-to-date discrete data pushed in real time in a C-CDA can be used to create a new patient chart or reconcile the information in an existing patient chart, avoiding transcription burden while preventing errors. The ability to include additional attached test and study herults avoids the expense of duplicate testing. Several of the prominent LTPAC EHR vendors now encomhers these capabilities with user-friendly interfaces. Please see the Leading Age EHR Selection Matrix.[4]

Despite these huge advancements in LTPAC EHR software capabilities, the acute facilities that have these capabilities (required for their certification) have not stepped up to ensure that these messages are regularly sent in "real time" at the time the patient is transferred, leaving the recipients scrambling with sending and receiving faxes and performing manual data entry, rather than devoting time to patient care. Dr. Terry O'Malley, a LTPAC subject matter expert, points out,

> We have this life saving, error preventing capability to care for patients **today**, there is no excuse for acuherand LTPAC facilities to not send real time Direct transition of care messages, or for EHR vendors not to optimize their Direct interoperability capabilities or help their clients with this deployment.

The September 2019 CMS Regulations should strongly encourage acute to LTPAC and ambulatory interoperable communication. Ideally, LTPAC to acute and ambulatory will also become the best practice standard.

Ambulatory to Hospital or ED Admission

When a patient is admitted to an acute facility, in order for the patient to receive the best possible care and to prevent medical errors and adverse events, the treating clinicians must have the most up-to-date clinical information about the patient. Imagine the potential for harming a patient with no information about their health conditions, medications, or allergies. When a patient has a planned admission to an acute facility, prior to the admission, the patient's ambulatory treating clinician can push an up-to-date C-CDA as well as other pertinent information to the acute facility. Under HIPAA law, this "pushed" information does not require additional consent as it is being passed to the patient's next treating clinician. If the patient is new to the hospital, the discrete data from the C-CDA can be used to create a new patient chart. If the patient has had prior admissions, the pushed information can be used to update and reconcile the existing patient chart. In all cases, this prevents errors and decreases provider and staff burden. At least one healthcare aherlatory group has configherd an automated Direct "push" of patient information from their EHR to the acute environment EHR once they receive an Admission/Discharge/Transfer (ADT) notification that their patient has been admitted to a hospital or ED.

For unplanned acute admissions to a hospital or emergency department, in some cases, patient summary information can be provided by querying health information exchanges (HIEs) or networks such as CommonWell or Carequality. For this information to be available for query, the patient must have either consented by "opting in" or not "opting out" to having their information available. HIEs even offer summary information that has undergone automated de-duplication, eliminating the duplication of information within the problem or medication lists, for example.

Table 16.1 Comparison of Interoperability Networks

Network	Push/Pull	Consent	Trust Framework	Record Locator Service	Documents	Use Case
Carequality	Query-based pull	Yes	Carequality Trust Principles Agreement and Carequality Connected Agreement	Yes	Aggregated Record	Finding available patient data
CommonWell™	Query-based pull	Yes	Data Privacy and Security Policy and CommonWell Member Services Agreement	Yes	Aggregated Record	Finding available patient data
Direct	Push	No	Registration Authority, Certificate Authority, HISP Trust Framework, Federated Services Agreement	No, not required as point to point push	Curated from sender to receiver	Transition of care
Regional/State HIE	Pull	Yes	Via Participation Agreement (business associates of their covered entities) HIE can produce an audit log	No, MPI and data clean-up algorithms	Aggregated Record for specified region	Finding available patient data
SHIEC	Pull	Yes	Patient-Centered Data Home Model (PCDH) Trust Framework	No, each HIE's MPI identifies patient PCDH routing of ADT alerts are based on patient's home address(es)	Aggregated Record across regional and state HIEs	Finding available patient data

Comparison of Interoperability Networks

Table 16.1 demonstrates some of the similarities and differences of the existing interoperability networks. This is a very basic description. Some HIEs have their own HISPs and are able to "push" Direct messages beyond their query capabilities.

Patients

The federal regulations cited earlier now mandate the patient's right to access their medical records in the form and format requested by the individual. For patients (or their designated caregivers) that have Direct accounts, C-CDA documents pushed in real time via Direct interoperability following any encounter would meet this requirement and greatly enhance patient satisfaction and ability to follow their care plan.

In all cases, the patient, or their designated caregiver, must be included in defining the goals and activities of the plan of care, and the transitioninherrovider must ensure that the patient information has been updated and reconciled in her or his EHR prior to sending the Direct message. The PCP following an encounter, the consulting specialist, and the discharging physician from the acute or LTPAC facility will reconcile the patient's problem list, allergies, and active medications and immunizations and include all pertinent information, such as their agreed-upon, updated care plan and instructions, relevant final or pending results, etc., prior to sending the patient/caregiver the C-CDA via Direct interoperability.

This provides patients with electronic access to their data, if so desired, following care transitions, the time when they are most vulnerable to miscommunication and resultant adverse events. This sharing of data will facilitate enhanced patient/provider communication and patient engagement in their care.

These use cases promote interoperability, health information exchange, and continuity of care while decreasing the costs of provider/staff documentation burden, eliminating transcription errors and faxing, and decreasing duplicate testing.here ability to incoherrate the latest accurate discrete data received in real time from the sending EHR into the recipient EHR for reconciliation, or to create a new patient chart, decreases clinician documentation burden and eliminates transcription errors.

Timely pushed information enables caregivers to best prepare and manage patient care and to reach out to their highest risk patients to identify and eliminate barriers to care. Pushed information eliminates therstaff burden of manually searching and "pulling" their patient information from outside resources.

Many EHR vendors have enhanced their Direct capabilities, configurability, functionality,herd user interfaces. As Direct message adoption and usage continues to increase, it is hoped that all of the EHR vendors will step up and continue to enhance their products.

Future

360X via Direct

Background

All five clinical use cases discussed previously involve current Direct interoperability technology that is readily available in all 2015 Certified Health IT Products. Future enhancements to patient transition of care workflows are offered through the 360X project. In 2012, 360X launched as an initiative of ONC's State Health Information Exchange Cooperative Agreement Program, a component of the Health Information Technology for Economic and Clinical Health (HITECH) Act, enacted as part of the American Recovery and Reinvestment Act of 2009 with a goal of supporting states' efforts to rapidly build capacity for exchanging health information within and across state lines. Specifically, the mission of 360X using Direct and other proposed Meaningful Use Stage 2 standards (now the Promoherg Interoperability program) was to enable providers to exchange patient information for referrals from their EHR workflow, regardless of the EHR systems and/or HISP services used (i.e., allowing information to move point to point between unaffiliated organizations, differing EHRs, and differing HISPs) and with herleast the same quality of workflow integration providers currently experience when referring between homogeneous EHR systems.

While the State HIE Program has ended, and Meaningful Use Stage 2 requirements have been eclipsed by newer iterations of CMS incentive programs (Promoting Interoperability), the work of the 360X community continues toward meeting the mission established in 2012.

Since its inception, the 360X project has had input from a broad representation of stakeholders throughout the public and prherte sectors. This dedicated group has included clinicians and technical experts, including representation from many EHR, HIT, and HISP vendors and ONC representatives among its members.

The project has focused on using existing proven industry standards only, including: C-CDA for clinical content, Direct protocols for transport, XD for establishing context (metadata), and HL7 V2 messages for referral/transfer status messages across care environments. The use cases to date have focused on "closed loop referrals" and "transfer from acute to skilled nursing facility (SNF)," both of which have been balloted and approved as IHE Patient Care Coordination domain profiles.

Clinical Overview

The initial focus of 360X was the creation of technical specifications and protocols to address the specific clinical use case of referral management via Direct exchange. The initial goals were to:

- standardize the type of data exchanged (C-CDA and other pertinent study and test result documents) and method of transport (Direct exchange)
- have transparency between the PCP and specialty offices regarding the progress of the consultation and gaps in care (HL7 V2 messages, such as "accept," "decline," "no show," "cancel,"herc.)
- create a process with a low technical bar for entry and for implementation to create broad rapid adoption across EHR vendors and clinical practices
- add value to patients, clinicians, office staff, and overall clinical workflows

360X via Direct builds on the ability of certified health IT systems to exchange C-CDA documents containing discrete data using standardized vocabularies as required previously by Meaningful Use and now by the Promoting Interoperability program as well as other CMS incentive programs. This enables the receiving system/end user to pull the discrete data into the chart, reducing clinician transcription burden and eliminating transcription errors.

hersed Loop Referral Use Case

The 360X closed loop referral process begins with the clinician ordering a referral from their EHR and the stafheranaging the referral per office protocol, which includes sending a "referral request" via Direct message to the specialist's EHR along with the C-CDA and any patient information deemed pertinent to the referral request. The recipient office staff can either "accept" or "decline" the request. Along with an accepted request, the recipient office can return the patient's scheduled appointment. A declined request will result in all the patient information being purged by the recipient's system, and the requesting office will continue sending requests to other specialists until the request is accepted and an appointment is scheduled. This process can occur while the patient is still in their PCP's office at the time of check out. Patients no longer leave the office with a "do it yourself" process to tackle; through 360X, they can leave with a specialty appointment in hand. Until the final visit, which closes the referral loop, standardized status messages and key clinical information can be exchanged between the two offices. Examples of status and clinical messages include "no show," "canceled," "appointment rescheduled," and other interim consultation notes.

A key feature of 360X via Direct is that once the initial order is entered and the process is started, the order is assigned a specific globally unique referral ID number, which persists achers all transactions until the referral loop is completed and the referral order closed. This specific referral number allows the EHR systems to readily identify and associate the communication across systems with the relevant patient.

Acute to Skilled Nursing Facility (SNF) Transfer Use Case

The 360X acute to SNF (or SNF to acute) transfer use case begins as the patient and the discharging team are determining the best next steps for the patient's ongoing care as part of the discharge planning process. If it is determined that the patient requires transfer to a SNF, the acute facility can send several SNFs transfer of care requests along with the patient's most up-to-date information in a C-CDA as well as other relevant care, test, or study documents to the multiple SNFs selected. The SNFs can then review the documents received, allowing the SNFs to determine if they have the capability to properly care for the patient. Depending on this assessment on the part of the SNFs that have received the request, the SNF organizations can respond to the acute facility with "accept" or "decline" messages. Once the acute facility receives these messages, they can review the organizations that have "accepted" with the patient and their caregivers. The acute facility will provide the patient with information about the SNFs that have accepted (per the federal regulations cited earlier), and the patient can select the SNF from these. Once the patient has selected the SNF, the acute facility will send the selected facility a "confirm accept patient transfer" notification and to all non-selected SNFs that sent "accept patient" notifications, the acute facility will return "discontinue request patient transfer" notifications. The final step at the time of transfer will be the acute facility sending a C-CDA and additional relevant documents to both the SNF and to the patient's PCP at the time of discharge from the acute facility and transfer to the SNF. This closes the transfer loop. Once the SNF has admitted the patient, the SNF will send a C-CDA to the patient's PCP.

Again, once the initial transfer request is sent to the SNFs and the patient transfer process is started, the transfer request is assigned a specific globally unique ID number that persists across all transactions (acute facility and all involved SNFs) until non-selected SNFs receive a "discontinue transfer request" and the selected SNF receives a "confirm accept patient transfer" and the C-CDA aherhe time of discharge, and the patient transfer is completed closing the transfer loop. This specific ID number facilitates all the EHR systems involved in the process to readily identify and associate the communication across systems pertaining to the relevant patient.

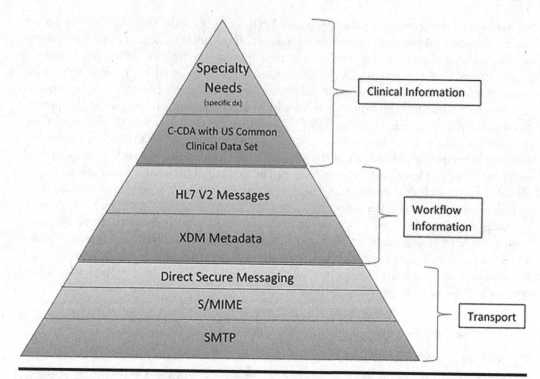

Figure 16.1   360X layers of interoperability

Technical Overview

The 360X implementationheride is built on several layers of interoperability standards and specifications, most of which are already in established use by many EHR and other health IT systems. This is illustrated in Figure 16.1.

In the process of developing the specification, the 360X via Direct project focused on the workflow information components in order to provide a base set of capabilities for the referral initiator/acute transfer initiator and the referral recipient systems/SNF recipient. These base capabilities are listed in Figure 16.2.

Indeed, the 360X community has also completed the work on the LTPAC use case of acute to SNF transfer, with many members of the LTPAC community joining the 360X project and contributing to the community's knowledge in this area.

Currently, the 360X workgroup is focused on the pandemic relevant use cases of SNF to ED transfer and social determinants of health (SDOH) needs based referrals to community-based organizations (CBOs).

Direct Paired With Additional Technologies to Best Fit Each Use Case

Current 360X work has also contemplated pairing additional technologies with 360X at the appropriate points in the clinical workflow, as philosophically the group firmly believes that the use case should diherte the best fit technology. For example, using Direct messaging for the pushed transition of care information and FHIR scheduling across EHR systems triggered with a

Referral Management	
Referral Initiator	**Referral Recipient**
■ Ability to send referral information in addition to the C-CDA clinical summary, including patient and referral identifiers	■ Ability to receive a referral request
■ Ability to process a decline of a referral	■ Ability to properly manage the patient identifier and referral identifier as sent by the initiator
■ Ability to process an accept of the referral	■ Ability to create and send accept or decline for a referral request
■ Ability to detect that a response to the request has not been received in a timely manner	■ Ability to process a referral cancel request
■ Ability to request a cancel for an existing referral	■ Ability to send a referral outcome, including the referral information such as the proper patient and referral identifiers
■ Ability to process the referral outcome (link C-CDA to the correct referral and patient)	
■ Ability to detect that a referral outcome has not been received in a timely manner	
Acute to SNF Transfer	
Acute Transfer Initiator	**SNF Transfer Request Recipient**
■ Ability to send transfer information in addition to the C-CDA clinical summary, including patient and transfer identifiers	■ Ability to receive a transfer request
■ Ability to process a decline of a transfer	■ Ability to properly manage the patient identifier and transfer identifier as sent by the initiator
■ Ability to process an accept of the transfer	■ Ability to create and send accept or decline for a transfer request, including the transfer information such as the proper patient and referral identifiers
■ Ability to send a "confirm accept patient transfer" or a "discontinue request patient transfer" with information in addition to the C-CDA clinical summary, including patient and transfer identifiers	■ Ability to process a "confirm accept patient transfer" or a "discontinue request patient transfer"

Figure 16.2 360X workflow components and capabilities

specialist referral acceptance or using FHIR pre-authorization between the provider and the payer as required in the process of care. The group anticipates always using the best technology available to fit the use case.

This chapter was written well over 2 years prior to publication of this book. Over the last two years there have been huge advances and innovations in health information technology (HIT).

Among them is progress made by the Trusted Exchange Framework and Common Agreement (TEFCA) that may lead to a national interoperability superhighway with Quality Health Information Networks (QHINs) being the on-ramps. Direct Secure Messaging (DSM), however, continues to be a primary tool in the HIT armamentarium particularly for clinical care transitions with continued growth each quarter. In the fourth quarter of 2021, there were well over 250 million DSM transactions between trusted endpoints.

About the Author

Holly Miller, MD, MBA, FHIMSS. For over 10 years, Dr. Miller has been the Chief Medical Officer of MedAllies, a company that leverages HIT and clinical practice transformation to improve healthcare value. MedAllies operates one of the leading Health Information Service Provider (HISP) networks in support of interoperability. At MedAllies, Dr. Miller provides operational, tactical, and strategic collaborative leadership.

Dr. Miller is currently a co-chair or member of many Health Information Technology (HIT) interoperability–related committees and workgroups engaged in enhancing healthcare value. These include committees within the following organizations: Carequality; DaVinci; HL7; CMS: PACIO; ONC and Integrating the Healthcare Enterprise (IHE): 360X; DirectTrust; NCQA; HIMSS; and KLAS. She continues to be a frequent speaker at national conferences.

Dr. Miller was formerly a vice president and the CMIO of University Hospitals and Health Systems (UH), a community-based system with more than 150 locations, seven wholly-owned and four affiliated hospitals throughout Northern Ohio. Prior to joining UH, she worked as an HIT Managing Director for the Cleveland Clinic, where she also maintained a clinical practice in general internal medicine. She has been active in healthcare informatics research and has been a co-investigator on multiple grants.

As a member of HIMSS since 1999, Dr. Miller is a past vice chair of the HIMSS Board and a past inaugural member of the HIMSS World Wide Board. Her past roles within HIMSS also included being a physician leader of the HIMSS/AMDIS Physician Community and serving as the board liaison to HIMSS Europe for four years. She was also active in a variety of previous S&I ONC committees and other state and government HIT committees.

References

1. HIMSS. 2021. Interoperability in Healthcare. What is Interoperability? Four Levels of Interoperability. https://www.himss.org/resources/interoperability-healthcare#Part1.
2. Centers for Medicare & Medicaid Services (CMS), HHS. 2019. Final Rule. https://www.govinfo.gov/content/pkg/FR-2019-09-30/pdf/2019-20732.pdf.
3. Agency for Healthcare Research and Quality (AHRQ). 2019. Readmissions and Adverse Events After Discharge. hhers://psnet.ahrq.gov/primers/primer/11/Readmisherns-and-Adverse-Events-After-Discharge.
4. LeadingAge. 2020. EHR Selection Matrix. https://leadingage.org/file/ehr-selection-matrix.

Chapter 17

Privacy and Security

Keith Weiner, PhD, RN-BC

Contents

DOI: 10.4324/9780429423109-17

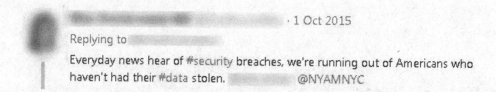

· 1 Oct 2015

Replying to

Everyday news hear of #security breaches, we're running out of Americans who haven't had their #data stolen. @NYAMNYC

Figure 17.1 Twitter post – author's night at New York Academy of Medicine for *Medical Informatics* 2nd edition book launch

Introduction

This chapter will introduce the reader to basic tenets of medical informatics privacy and security, relating fundamental security principles to thought-provoking case studies. A broad overview of an otherwise vast, complex subject will be explored in order to provide the reader with a basic understanding of the contemporary healthcare information security landscape. A mix of capers, challenges, and solutions will be used to demonstrate the current state of affairs in the industry. This chapter is neither a comprehensive guideline nor a blueprint for a developing or maintaining a security operation per se, but rather serves to provide a broad overview of healthcare information security and present-day topics of interest from which to deliver an executive primer. Note that any statistics and sensationalistic hacking escapades illustrated at the time of this text's draft are likely to quickly be outdated and overshadowed by even more profound incidents, perhaps even by press time. Health information security is a dynamic and evolving field in constant growth and development to address the challenges of both legacy and emerging threats. In other words, we have much work ahead for the foreseeable future and beyond.

Why Healthcare: Sutton's Law

Why is healthcare a target? Healthcare may at times be unintentionally attacked as part of a wide net of hacking cast by criminal enterprises, but this sector is still nonetheless intentionally targeted for some very specific reasons. Quite frankly, healthcare entities tend to have vast amounts of protected health information (PHI) and financial data that can be sold in the underground marketplace on the dark web. Some weaknesses endemic to the industry making this sector ripe for attack will be further explored as the current landscape of healthcare cybersecurity is discussed later in the chapter.

Criminal markets flourish on the dark web, a segmented internet accessible on the Tor Onion Network through special software applications. Healthcare and financial data are available for sale among a variety of products and services generally considered to be near-universally illicit. These may include recreational drugs, weapons, sensitive information, and driver licenses as well as services ranging from hacking to assassinations. Visiting these dark corners of the internet are typically not advisable. This author strongly cautions against exploring these areas so as to avoid any unanticipated consequences.

Criminal enterprises use various methods to find their way into health system networks and obtain sensitive information. Hacking may have historically been the most prevalent form of breach incidents to date, according to research that this author has performed, but it certainly accounts for the most significant large-scale exploits in recent years and for a disproportionally large number of patient records affected. Stolen health information is typically sold off in bundles of data, whereas financial information is often separated into pieces, but these structures can vary. Published quotes for the value of such information vary widely. The reason for fluctuations and variations in price is that the underground economy is not regulated in the same manner in which we find many commodities to be valued. For instance, $25 per "fullz" US record containing essential financial data of an individual is a rough ballpark figure. This amount has been diminishing in recent years due to a large supply inventory available for the demand. In other words, criminals have been so successful in obtaining data that they've driven down the market. This should be a sobering indicator of the current state of affairs in healthcare information security.

A more blatant and direct form of exploitation is the use of ransomware, a method of locking systems and/or vast quantities of the network, rendering them inoperable and inaccessible until the demands for a monetary transfer to the criminals are fulfilled. Financial remuneration is typically in the form of cryptocurrency, a digital currency of which Bitcoin is seemingly the best-known offering. If a health system is not familiar with cryptocurrency transactions or runs into difficulty with the recovery process, the criminal enterprise may offer a helpdesk service for assistance. Anecdotally and somewhat ironically, these criminal helpdesks tend to provide outstanding professional service and are most supportive. Another tactic used by criminals involved in ransomware schemes is the threat of exposing sensitive data. This serves as further leverage and a strategy to exploit those institutions choosing to take a moral stand against paying the ransom in exchange for the return of system functionality. Business email compromise, also known as phishing, remains the primary vector for breaking into the network, including break-ins involving ransomware incidents. The email compromise concept will be explored further as a case study.

Perhaps the motive for hacking healthcare may best be exemplified by revisiting the nostalgic crimes of yesteryear. Asked why he robbed banks, the infamous William "Slick Willie" Sutton purportedly responded, "because that's where the money is." While he would later go on to deny having uttered those words, the attribution stuck, resulting in his namesake immortalized into Sutton's Law. The concept of this law is the recognition of what is expected to be apparent and obvious to most (Sutton and Linn, 1976). A more contemporary equivalent is the pop-culture reference of "Captain Obvious." In other words, healthcare data theft reaps financial rewards as healthcare entities, often with a variety of weak links in the chain of protection, hold the keys to the proverbial kingdom.

Fast forward to the early 21st century as we substitute hard currency for data and consider the banks of yesteryear as today's computing infrastructure. Enter the "Slick Willie" of today as a multitude of possible characters ranging from mischievous individuals to organized criminal organizations to nation state actors and all points in between. Using Sutton's Law as a starting point, we have set the stage for the protection from and response to a more contemporary type of caper. Next, we will explore the current landscape to understand the current paradigm.

Current Landscape: How We Got Here

Today's healthcare infrastructure in the United States is a collection of fragmented entities, including ever-expanding multi-hospital health systems, diminishing numbers of freestanding community hospitals, government-run systems, solo practitioners, medical groups, labs, insurance companies, billing services, a supply-chain of vendor products and services, and various types of outpatient entities, among many other facets.

Each entity is responsible for developing and maintaining their own cybersecurity posture. They operate under basic federal and local legislation along with direction from government agencies such as the United States Health and Human Services Department and the Food and Drug Administration as well as state and local government agencies. There are private government collaborations and various associations that facilitate the flow of information, offer resources, and help foster inter-institution cooperation. However, this patchwork paradigm leaves a lot of room for vast differences in the methodology, maturity, and efficacy of each entity's cybersecurity model.

To further complicate matters, health systems tend to have a mix of relatively contemporary computer systems and vast quantities of antiquated ones, sometimes spanning decades of use and counting. For example, many medical devices' clinical usefulness can span several decades, thereby exceeding both vendor and operating system support. According to research conducted by the security firm Palo Alto Networks, 83% of imaging devices with internet connectivity run unsupported operating systems, such as Microsoft Windows XP, which has not been in support since 2014 (Hautala, 2020). Why is this a problem? Well, lack of support means that updates to address cybersecurity threats are not be made available and attacks may leave the health system in a vulnerable position, with many systems reliant on whatever network defense systems may be in place. Houses typically have locks on the doors even though public safety apparatuses in society are in place Having large swathes of houses without locks would seem like insufficient security, and likewise so should antiquated operating systems. The WannaCry case study later in the chapter provides a real-world example of how outdated and unmaintained operating systems can contribute to catastrophic conditions.

Even non-critical systems and devices off of the security radar can still present risks to the network. Suppose clinical operations would not be impacted should a certain system go offline and the cybersecurity risk would be acceptable as there is no sensitive data for bad actors to exploit. These vulnerable yet non-critical systems may be used as a jumping-off point from which to attack a hospital network and the critical systems that may be exposed as vulnerable as a result. The only pathway for having system support for depreciated operating systems is often a complete purchase of a new system and sometimes additional systems associated with the product or products. This may be an expensive venture, depending upon the scope. Purchasing and implementing a resolution or the acceptance of such risk may involve multiple stakeholders as there are clinical, financial, infrastructure, and other considerations. Should such systems remain in use, there are cybersecurity measures that may be taken to partially mitigate the risk by applying certain controls such as network segregation or custom local firewalls. Network segmentation is the process of separating devices from other parts of the network or grouping them together so that commherca-tion between devices is theoretically tightly controlled or even not possible.

Some health systems have an integrated electronic health record (EHR) with modules for multiple ancillary systems such as laboratory and radiology alongside a multitude of other systems either functioning independently orheregrated with one another in some fashion. Others have a patchwork of interconnected and freestanding computer systems. Mher than a decade following the American Recovery and Reinvestment Act (ARRA) Health Information Technology for Economic and Clinical Health Act (HITECH), EHR systems have been adopted throughout hospitals and health systems to near-ubiquitous levels, and various other clinical, financial, and operational computer systems became interconnected with one another. In more modern times, as more systems become linked together and further dependent upon a cloud/internet infrastructure, the surface vector and reach for attacking healthcare's electronic assets has expanded.

Furthermore, non-clinical systems falling under the oversight of a facilities management, physical security, and others traditionally non-technology-based departments are increasingly becoming connected within the healthcare systems' network. A diverse set of devices commonly referred to as the Internet of Things (IoT), which include everything from voice assistants to smart lightbulbs to wearable physiological monitors, are increasingly connected to the vast, diverse network ecosystem residing within a healthcare entity. One security camera or temperature monitor could perhaps be an entry point from which to inadvertently introduce security incidents.

This current paradigm of an interconnected and diverse technology ecosystem illustrates the challenges and complexity with which information security professions in the healthcare space must contend to continuously addressing.

A Moral Argument

In all likelihood, your healthcare information and those of people you care about will end up in an electronic format if not already there. Safeguard with extreme care others' sensitive information as if it was your own. This "do unto to others" adage is somewhat culturally universal, ancient wisdom predating HIPAA that is applicable to the modern-day healthcare information security professional.

Moral obligation notwithstanding, legislation exists to mandate the implementation and use of safeguards to minimize the risk of unauthorized disclosures. The Department of Health and Human Services summarizes the HIPAA Privacy Rule as follows:

> The HIPAA Privacy Rule establishes national standards to protect individuals' medical records and other personal health information and applies to health plans, health care clearinghouses, and those health care providers that conduct certain health care transactions electronically. The Rule requires appropriate safeguards to protect the privacy of personal health information, and sets limits and conditions on the uses and disclosures that may be made of such information without patient authorization. The Rule also gives patients rights over their health information, including rights to examine and obtain a copy of their health records, and to request corrections.

Paper-based systems could be easily tucked away from prying eyes with little chance of exposure en masse. Traditionally, charts could be copied, faxed, tampered with, or viewed without the likelihood of access being tracked. While this modality seems safe contrasted against a backdrop of sensational cybersecurity headlines, large and small paper-based breaches have occurred and continue to remain a risk.

With the electronic health record, data is available via multiple sources, people, and systems. Along with this liberalization of information and massive accessibility come the mechanisms by which to track, restrict access, and monitor for inappropriate access. It's a brave new world with an increase in both benefits and risks.

The legislative section further in the chapter will touch upon the physical, administrative, and technical safeguard components required by the HIPAA Security Rule to protect the patient information. The implementation of a comprehensive information security program is beyond the scope of this chapter. However, reflect on the following selected list in consideration of access to ePHI:

- How is ePHI access logged? Is there remote access by healthcare personnel, vendors, and other business associates? Does anyone review or become alerted to potentially inappropriate access? Remember that even trusted employees have been known to have inappropriately disclosed information. Countless examples exist of information sold for a variety of reasons. People have been jailed even after making only a scant profit.

■ Is information segmented in a fashion that limits access based on job role or even physical location? Maybe one hospital unit should not have access to another's. Maybe a physician sees a different set of information than a clerk.

■ Is there an education program for the workforce to help in the understanding of legislation and organization policies to which they must adhere? Are there supplementary security awareness reminders? While ignorance is no excuse for the law, HIPAA does compel entities to keep its workforce informed.

■ Is there a limitation on administrative access or even any access that goes unlogged? Remember, the NSA has curtailed their system administrators in the wake of Eric Snowden's disclosures. Healthcare IT should learn from this lesson as well.

■ Can tampering of information be prevented or at least be discovered?

■ What mechanisms are in place to prevent leaks from nefarious sources? (i.e. viruses, hackers, scammers, etc. . . .)

■ How secure is the information against damage – physical or otherwise? Are there contingency plans in place for periods of inaccessibility?

■ Do you have a disaster recovery, business continuity, and backup plan? Have you tested these plans? Careers have been cut short in disaster scenarios when untested backups fail.

■ What mechanisms prevent accidental disclosure? Is there a data leak prevention system – either comprehensive through a vendor or otherwise piecemeal? Can employees send patient files over email – internally and externally – where they reside ad infinitum in wait for a potential hacker to come along? We see in this chapter how email has been captured by nefarious actors.

■ Do you encrypt all data at rest and in motion? An inadvertent disclosure could be as simple as a download to USB thumb drive that gets lost or an unencrypted stolen laptop. Stolen laptops are a huge source of breaches, by the way. Proper encryption means the would-be thief just inherited a brick-shaped laptop for all intents and purposes.

■ Are your security mechanisms reasonable to implement? If not, people will go around them. One company made everyone change their passwords every day. So, all employees would gather every morning to choose the group password. Only their username was different. In the case of extremely complicated passwords and different usernames for various systems, employees tend to place notes under their keyboards or tape them to their monitors.

■ Do you have an identity and access management solution in place? In the first edition of this book, Dr. Jonathan Leviss outlines several solutions. While this topic is complex, consider how you ensure that only those with authorization obtain access. Sometimes the solutions are technological in nature (single sign-on, self-service password resets) and some are administrative (activation and termination notification).

Legislative Considerations

This section covers some of the basic legislative elements but merely scratches the surface of a rather vast subject. The purpose is to provide some background on the basic legal framework for healthcare cybersecurity. Healthcare information technology (IT) and cybersecurity are such dynamic topics that one must pursue the most contemporary material to stay current, and this includes emerging legislation.

For legislative resources in specific areas, commence any review by exploring the official source or agency responsible for the legislation. A few primary examples of agencies and their home pages are listed next. Specific information may also be found through a search engine query and then selecting official government source from the results.

- Health and Human Services – http://www.HHS.gov
- Centers for Medicare and Medicaid Services – http://www.CMS.gov
- US Government Printing Office – http://www.gpo.gov (Federal Register)
- US Cybersecurity and Infrastructure Security Agency – https://us-cert.cisa.gov

The federal government has established rules to guide covered entities, a term to describe the wide scope to whom these rules apply, in an effort to promote the safeguarding of patient information. Accompanying these rules are the potential for penalties due to infractions. Furthermore, state and local governments may have their own legislation, which may extend or add to requirements, guidelines, and penalties. Sanctions resulting from infractions do not necessarily preclude further legal action taken by others, including government entities.

Stemming from the 1996 Health Insurance Portability and Accountability Act (HIPAA), the Security Standards Final Rule was produced by the United States Health and Human Services Department (HHS) in 2003 to provide guidance on physical, administrative, and technological measures to safeguard protected health information (PHI) in any medium, whether electronic or in print. In 2013, HHS combined various security and privacy rules into one large "Omnibus Rule." Protecting healthcare information is more than an honorable and ethical endeavor, but rather a legal responsibility.

Florence Nightingale's 1860s "Notes on Nursing" discusses the concept of privacy long before HIPAA and provides a principle for the ages.

> And remember every nurse should be one who is to be depended upon, in other words, capable of being a "confidential" nurse . . . she must be no gossip, vain talker; she should never answer questions about her sick except to those who have a right to ask them.
>
> (Nightingale, 1860, p. 70)

PHI is broadly defined as individually identifiable protected health information while the federal government offers granular criteria in its definition. The term ePHI refers to PHI in an electronic format. Traditional paper-based charting systems have always carried a risk of breaches such as theft or loss. However, the pervasive introduction of the electronic health record to near omnipresent levels in the United States has significantly increased both the likelihood and impact of breaches and losses.

Government programs and grant opportunities as outlined in other chapters have incentivized healthcare entities and providers to adopt and implement EHRs. Suffice it to state that adoption and implementation of EHRs are now fundamental and essential parts of operating the healthcare business. These technological advancements come bundled with a significantly increased risk for data breaches. The burden is ultimately on the healthcare entities to take on the additional responsibility of safeguarding PHI. In other words, health systems and practitioners must have electronic records, which increase their risk, and then must solely be responsible for mitigating and controlling such risk else facing incidents and sanctions.

Below is some relevant legislation:

- HIPAA – Health Insurance Portability and Accountability Act (1996) – includes the protection of patient information and confidentiality.
- HIPAA Privacy and Security Rules (2003) – HHS published standards to safeguard PHI.
- HITECH Act – Health Information Technology for Economic and Clinical Health Act (2009) – enacted as part of the American Recovery and Reinvestment Act to promote health information technology.
- Omnibus Rule (2013) – HHS final rule – implements components of HITECH and strengthens HIPAA privacy and security protections.

Health and Human Services' Omnibus Rule
http://www.gpo.gov/fdsys/pkg/FR-2013-01-25/pdf/2013-01073.pdf
Security Rule Education Paper Series ***highly recommended***
http://www.hhs.gov/ocr/privacy/hipaa/administrative/securityrule/securityruleguidance.html
American Recovery and Reinvestment Act (including HITECH)
http://www.gpo.gov/fdsys/pkg/BILLS-111hr1enr/pdf/BILLS-111hr1enr.pdf
HITECH Enforcement Interim Final Rule
http://www.hhs.gov/ocr/privacy/hipaa/administrative/enforcementrule/hitechenforcementifr.html
Health and Human Services' Security Rule
https://www.hhs.gov/hipaa/for-professionals/security/
Health and Human Services' Privacy Rule
http://www.hhs.gov/ocr/privacy/hipaa/administrative/privacyrule/

Public Awareness

Cybersecurity had long been little more than a science fiction, pop culture phenomenon represented in movies such as *War Games*, *The Terminator*, and *The Matrix*. Legendary hackers possessed magical powers to break into government systems and banks with a few keystrokes or control the city's closed-circuit cameras. They even managed to thwart an alien invasion to save humanity in the film *Independence Day*.

Aside from cybersecurity professionals and corporate asset stakeholders, the general public has historically given data protection little more than a passing thought. The occasional virus, pop-up advertisement, or email from a Nigerian prince promising a secret fortune would present themselves more as an annoyance to the average computer user than a genuine threat.

More recently, data security has at times been front and center on the news and in the minds of the general public. Headline after headline, we are reminded of the potential pitfalls of living in a connected world. We have had disclosures of National Security Agency mass surveillance activities, massive breaches at Equifax and Yahoo, and multiple federal agencies being hacked, as well as reports of foreign interference in elections, to name a few. In this connected age of well-publicized data breaches, the general public has become ever more aware of the threat to their privacy, sacred health information, and finances.

Case Study: WannaCry

Prior to diving into the methodology and lending a sense of purpose to the field of cybersecurity, we will examine a case study showing how lapses in security protections can lead to potential devastating effects on healthcare delivery systems. This case study illustrates an extreme and uncommon example intended to exemplify not only how quickly the entire world can be blindsided but also what our industry could have done to potentially prevent the ensuing calamity.

Imagine all major computer systems in your hospital and many area hospitals suddenly and nearly simultaneously go completely offline without forewarning. Imagine you are either a clinician, information technology (IT) staff member, hospital administrator, or hold any number of roles that depend upon these systems in order to deliver care to patients. Imagine patients no longer being accepted for treatment, ambulances diverted to other hospitals, procedures delayed or cancelled, and those quality mechanisms to deliver care safely and efficiently are all suddenly vaporized. Would the quality of care be affected? Would patients be harmed directly or indirectly as a result? As an information security professional, would you not do everything reasonably possible to minimize the likelihood and impact from such a disruption? Later, we will discuss some possible preventative measures, including the augmentation of classic risk-based approaches to cybersecurity to address emerging and evolving cybersecurity threats to clinical operations.

In the days following May 12, 2017, an estimated 300,000 computers worldwide were rendered completely inoperable, requiring replacement, restore from backup systems, or complete rebuilding in some manner to restore the functionality to impacted computer systems and devices. In the interim, industries across the globe reeled from the effects of this attack (*Tribute Express*, 2017). These included Fortune 500 companies and the healthcare industry, including whole United Kingdom (UK) Trusts (i.e. healthcare systems). Simply put, large swaths of the UK health system's informatics infrastructure were taken offline, and many other industries suffered similar fates.

This attack was considered by some measures to be the largest cybersecurity incident in history at the time. While no standard ordinal scale may be used to qualify such a declaration, it is generally agreed upon in the industry that this event was catastrophic to a degree not yet realized at the time, serving to reshape perspectives about risk and mitigation preparation. Just like large patient record breaches that can be quantified on an ordinal scale, the potential for future incidents to knock this one from the monumental top spot remains almost an inevitability.

The Shadow Brokers, a group thought to act on behalf of the Russian government, had stolen hacking secrets from the United States National Security Agency. As a result of the theft, some powerful hacking utilities had been published on the internet and made freely available to the general public, whereas other, even more formidable tools were offered for a fee. Included within this stolen package was the means to exploit a depreciated Windows "service" (function) for which Microsoft had already produced a patch several months prior to the attack. In pandemic terms, the world already had a readily available vaccine in wide distribution free of charge for months but hesitancy to accept treatment left the world nowhere even close to having enough inoculation to create herd immunity from the virus. The elusive Lazarus Group, thought to be a North Korean state-sponsored organization, packaged the exploitation as a "worm" that can spread from computer to computer by itself (US Treasury Department, 2020). They were able to insert this code into the legitimate update services of a niche payroll software package that was used primarily in Ukraine. Naturally, this update quickly made its way into computers that downloaded and executed software from a seemingly trusted source. Upon infecting the host computer, this worm (virus) would propagate itself to susceptible computers on the network and then throughout internet to quickly reach across the globe. Each affected computer would also have its hard drive encrypted, a method of completely scrambling all of the computer's information. A ransom message would appear to make this attack look like a common criminal act known as ransomware, whereby the computer may be returned to a normal state once requested funds have been delivered. This attack was not actually ransomware but more like a massive indiscriminate drive-by attack. In other words, this was a virus intended to transmit itself far and wide while quickly killing off every single infected host in its path.

Using this example as a lesson learned, we can explore basic security principles that may have provided some protection to and resiliency from such an attack. There are circumstances specific to the healthcare industry that have made such preventative and responsive measures historically challenging to invoke. These measures may have been in place, in part or in whole, but no cyber-security program should be considered as completely impervious. Details not typically disclosed to the public could also shed light on the series of unfortunate events. To be fair, we have the benefit of hindsight while dissecting the aftermath for the purpose of illustrative standard security methods. In brief, the solution includes sound principles of patch management, network segmentation, operating system hardening, using supported operating systems, antivirus mechanisms, and layers of security through various modalities.

Case Study: Pentagon Down

On December 13, 2020, a major infiltration affecting multiple United States federal government agencies and other entities around the globe, including the Pentagon, nuclear labs, various intelligence agencies, and potentially the bulk of the Fortune 500 companies (Sanger et al., 2020). The true extent of the hacking may never be known, as discoveries and disclosures are being made public. This nefarious operation was thought to have been conducted by the Cozy Bear group, backed by the Russian SVR, a contemporary version of the KGB. They had been infiltrating sensitive, information-rich systems undetected over the course of many months until a private security firm provided notification to American intelligence agencies. This private security firm was itself also a victim.

Was this the worst attack in history to date? Again, this depends on the metrics employed and how one weighs the complex multitude of implications beyond sheer quantity of affected devices and the quality of the systems impacted. Conversely, WannaCry was certainly pervasive with seemingly indiscriminate targets around the globe. In contrast, this particular operation by Cozy Bear was an ongoing targeted act of espionage by a foreign rival who silently gained access to many sensitive systems by the United States, its allies, and businesses worldwide. Given that the United States had just conducted an election following documented Russian interference the previous cycle, and this nation's top security official had declared the election to be the most secure in history, it may have been embarrassing to note that the Department of Homeland Security was one of the agencies that had been the target of a months-long ongoing hack. While there is no evidence that this hack in any way affected the election outcome, the revelation of its discovery took place in between the bookends of a sitting president having declaring election fraud and a failed insurrection having taken place at the US Capitol building weeks later.

Like the WannaCry attack, a seemingly legitimate software update source was compromised. As security professionals, we are inclined to patch systems regularly and with increasing expediency to meet evolving threats. Installing updates from trusted sources is a natural tendency. A major difference is that WannaCry targeted a niche software package in a specific region and then quickly spread to computers across the globe, causing mass destruction. The Cozy Bear attack involved a software update in SolarWinds, an IT systems management solution commonly used in government agencies and corporations worldwide. Once this Trojan Horse type of software was installed, the hacker group may have obtained entry points into a plethora of computer networks and their computers. The implications are vast, as Russian-backed hackers had supposedly gained access to intelligence agencies and businesses for months without being detected.

Healthcare entities are among the many industries commonly known to use SolarWinds. While the target may have been government agencies, many other entities fell victim as collateral damage. Healthcare entities offer not only a treasure of patient health and financial data but also business information that can be quite valuable to interested parties. Such information could include business practices, research data, access to partners' information, and much more.

In addition to the consequences of data breaches, the mitigation strategy itself can prove to be quite disruptive. When the news of this massive breach was revealed, security experts were tasked with assessing the impact and enacting their incident response plans based upon relatively scant information. As a result, many computer systems had to be taken offline for forensic purposes, quarantine, or in some cases to be completely reconstructed before returning to operation.

Case Study: Barbie and Hot Wheels

Mattel, known for toys as such as Barbie dolls and Hot Wheels, had just hired a new Chief Executive Officer (CEO) when a certain financial executive received an email request from her new CEO boss to submit payment to a new vendor. Mattel typically requires two executives to complete the transfer, but this particular one was authorized by the "CEO." After verifying that this qualification indeed provided authorization, the executive made a transaction worth over $3M to internet scammers impersonating the CEO with an account in an area of China known for having money laundering operations operating in the region. Fortunately, this transaction took place on a banking holiday, and by luck the caper was thwarted (CBS News, 2016). This case stresses the importance of having measures to prevent such exploits, including workforce training on the basics of cybersecurity, periodic reminders, tools that support sound email practices, and security systems that help to thwart business email compromise attempts.

How is Hot Wheels relevant to healthcare information security? Business email compromise, also known as phishing, remains a major vector for which nefarious actors may attack or gain entry into networks and computer systems. Phishing is a broad term for deceptive activities using email for a variety of intents, including the immediate transfer of funds, harvesting credentials to gain access to particular systems and/or entire networks, or to persuade victims to install malicious code to compromise systems. Healthcare entities are subject to similar tactics and are often subject to custom, industry-specific techniques in attempts to gain access to the crown jewels of these organizations.

While there are technology solutions that can be implemented to prevent such emails from reaching inboxes, the human factor is key to safeguarding the healthcare entity's network. Strategies to thwart such evasive tactics include education, as humans may be both a weak link in the chain and the main guardian. These can include various traditional education measures as well as undeclared simulations involving carefully crafted deceptive, yet harmless emails often delivered as part of a service from contracted security vendors. Limitations on the use of personal email on company networks among other filtering service provide some mitigation as well as providing some sense of protection and authentication validation on personally owned devices accessing company resources. In brief, a combination of human and technical mechanisms is essential to mitigate the risk of business email compromise.

Building the Security Program

If you choose not to decide, you still have made a choice.

(Peart et al., 1980)

Building and supporting a comprehensive security program is necessary to protect both the organization and the patients. Security should be part of an organization's governing structure. Both a security official and privacy official should be named as curators of their respective areas of responsibility. This could be one individual in a dual role or kept separate. Individuals in these roles must be capable of either carrying out or overseeing security and privacy functions for the organization. Naming these officials is actually a requirement per HHS rules.

Most of this chapter foregoes explaining the minutia of IT security items such as antivirus, firewalls, vulnerability scans, and web filtering and intrusion detection devices. Those and other items are a necessary part of a comprehensive program in monitoring, detecting, and providing protection against threats. This chapter also does not discuss key elements such as operating system fortification or technically intricate facets such as firewalls or intrusion detection systems. These are tools of the trade, whereas the scope of this chapter is that of a broad overview. More in-depth and specific information is outside of the scope of this chapter, whereas one may explore such details in training and other texts more geared toward running security operations.

While much of this chapter is geared towards larger organizations with sufficient personnel and other resources, even the solo practitioner or small office must have a security program scaled to their circumstances. There are third-party organizations and services that could help to develop and manage the security program. Physician and hospital groups may provide some resources, services, or direction. Figure 17.2 displays some of the factors that serve as the foundation for the security program's building blocks.

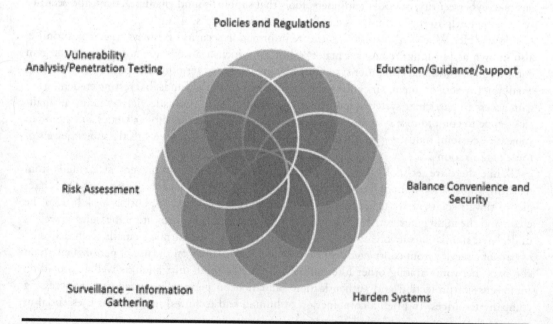

Figure 17.2 Security program building blocks

Incident Reporting

All suspected breach incidents must be logged and tracked. There are potential legal considerations and as such every instance should be handled meticulously.

The 2013 HHS Omnibus Rule replaces the "harm" standard as to qualify damage as a marker for determining the declaration of a breach with a more objective, self-conducted risk assessment, as previous determinations were more subjective and speculatively underreported. The covered entity or business associate has the burden of proof to determine that any unauthorized disclosure is not considered a breach. Under these new guidelines, contractors known as "business associates" enter into agreements that shift the burden of responsibility to a contractor who caused any such breach. Likewise, contractors do the same with subcontractors, who in turn are liable for breaches that they themselves may be responsible for causing or permitting to take place. This is a chain of responsibility. Regardless of legal and financial liability, it is the healthcare entity that may be prominently featured in the news and suffer reputational loss in the event of a significant incident resulting from contractors' or subcontractors' action. Therefore, the healthcare entity would be wise to have safeguards and evaluation of risk when employing contractors.

Exemptions to the breach notification requirement exist, such as the unintentional use in good faith used within the scope of their authority and without any further impermissible disclosure. There may be an inadvertent disclosure to an authorized person or an unauthorized person who could not have easily retained such PHI. In other words, HHS offers reasonable exemptions from declaring less risky episodic interactions as incidents where applicable.

If PHI is disclosed in a manner not otherwise exempt by the Omnibus Rule, then a breach may be considered presumed unless the healthcare entity can determine that a low probability of breach exists based on a risk assessment containing the following elements according to HHS:

- **Nature/Extent.** Determine how much information was involved, how it could be used in a manner adverse to the individuals affected, and how it could possibly be used by the person or people it was disclosed to. Was the patient information identifiable or did it contain particularly sensitive data?
- **Determine who accessed or received the data.** Are the individuals obligated to protect and secure this PHI? Was this information disclosed inappropriately to an employer?
- **Actually used or acquired.** Can you determine if the information was viewed or there was just an opportunity for viewing? Was information sent to the wrong address? Could information on a stolen laptop or lost hard drive actually be acquired?
- **Mitigation.** Has a confidential or other agreement provided assurances that the information will no longer be used or disclosed?

Where notification of a breach is required, all affected individuals must be notified by the covered entity within 60 calendar days since the discovery of the breach. Please note the word "discovery," as one cannot be expected to start the countdown for a breach of which one is unaware.

Notice to the HHS Secretary must occur via a web form within 60 days from the end of the calendar year for breaches of fewer than 500 individuals. For breaches of 500 or more individuals, notification to the Secretary of HHS occurs within 60 days along with a notification to the media. If ten or more individuals cannot be contacted, a post to a website or local media is required. See current regulations for details as these are subject to change.

The HHS website featuring details of breaches involving the records of 500 or more individuals is commonly referred to in the healthcare IT industry as the "Wall of Shame." This author implores readers to view this website and study common pitfalls and how they could be avoided. Go to the HHS website or do a search for the exact website URL. While hacking incidents are increasingly responsible for large-scale breaches in recent years, a large number of historical breaches have resulted from the loss of theft of systems or media. Breach settlement documents often cite lack of encryption, lack of training, lack of policy, and lack of a risk assessment in the text. Certainly, addressing these factors could go a long way to avoiding the pitfalls of the past.

Retaining expert services in advance of any severe incidents can not only help to prevent unfortunate occurrences and mitigate risks but also help with incident response activities should such incidents ever arise.

Patch Management: Closing Exploits

Months prior to what was the world's more expansive cyber-attack, Microsoft had released a patch to close the security hole. In other words, the means to prevent such a calamity was readily available. However, millions of computers were left unprotected.

Consider a boat that may have apparent leaks or discovered weaknesses in the hull. Some may pose a higher risk than others. Nonetheless, the boat should have patching considered as to

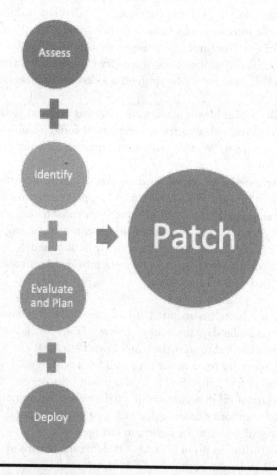

Figure 17.3   Patch management process

prevent an incident while afloat. Remediation of risks may occur during scheduled maintenance intervals and others may require more immediate attention. These should be patched to maintain the integrity of the hull and thus lower the risk to both boat and its passengers.

Similarly, information technology software and hardware may have known weaknesses that emerge over time. Likewise, these flaws must be patched to protect the integrity of the technology in question, adjacent systems in the network that may be affected, and the function that would be impacted as a result of such a flaw being exploited.

According to Microsoft's "Patch Management Process Model" (Figure 17.3), the four phases in the cycle are to assess, identify, evaluate/plan, and deploy (Wolenik, Marc, 2013).

In order to assess the risk, one must be made aware that a risk exists. Many consumers simply have their computers set to automatically download and install updates. The general public may cede any consideration of risk to vendors such as Apple, Microsoft, or Google. In the industry, risk must be assessed. More so than to the consumer, indiscriminate patching itself may pose a risk to the functionality of a computer system or device, and therefore a patch management strategy is typically followed. With systems purchased from vendors, the ability to patch may require either sanctioning or servicing from the vendor, which further complicates the process and may extend the time by which patches may be applied. A system of routine patching may be performed at a cadence determined by the organization or through vendor recommendation. For more urgent matters, patching may occur outside of these routine periods to address more critical emerging and imminent threats.

Security risks may be disclosed by the vendor, government, or industry group through distributed bulletins, postings, and other delivery formats. The software itself, operating system, or third-party management system may also provide such information on which IT or security personnel may act.

Vulnerability Scanning: Hunting Weak Links

Another method of finding weaknesses to patch is through the use of a vulnerability management strategy. A vulnerability scanning system from a vendor such as Nessus or Tenable may be used to scan systems across a network for weaknesses for which a patch or other measure may be considered. Conversely, protective measures against known or discovered weaknesses may not be feasible, and therefore the evaluated risk may be accepted by the organization's stakeholders.

These scanning systems are similar to a popular 1960s sci-fi television show, *Star Trek*, which had spaceships scan one another's defensive shields for weaknesses and other tactical information. This same show had a medical scanner that could diagnose a host of ailments in a non-invasive manner. Consider these as analogous to our modern-day vulnerability scanning systems that catalogue systems on a network and discover potential risks.

Typically, an organization should consider employing vulnerability scanning as a routine method of discovering risks, prioritizing risks, and then selecting those identified elements that should be addressed for patching, otherwise fixing, or simply relegating to acceptance of such risks by the organization's stakeholders. Such measures can help tilt the scales of security more in favor of the organization. Certainly, such an endeavor may have provided a distant early warning of a risk of exploitation such as the massive attack in our WannaCry example. Whether it would have been prioritized for remediation in a timely fashihero avoid falling victim to such an attack remains speculative (Figure 17.4).

Part of risk management and mitigation is identifying vulnerable points on the network and, where applicable, demonstrating the ability to actively exploit them or at least the likelihood of

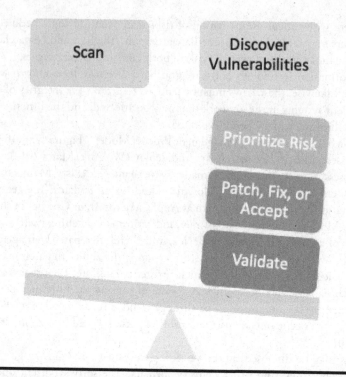

Figure 17.4   Vulnerability scanning: tipping the scales toward security

such exploitation taking place. A vulnerability detection and mitigation program, as part of an overall security program, can be performed through either specialized products, a third-party service, or a combination thereof.

A vulnerability assessment finds weak points and may provide recommendations for remediation. These procedures should be performed on a regular basis. Be prepared, as the initial results may be shocking and overwhelming should this be the first time one is conducted. However, the magnitude of results should eventually diminish over time as they are either categorized as not slated for remediation or are remediated.

Penetration testing is where trophies are sought. This is important in demonstrating that the keys to the castle may be obtained. Some methodologies involve exploiting computer systems directly, while other means can involve rather deceptive procedures or a multitude of steps to success. A security professional may try to dupe employees or use some reconnaissance to piece together a break-in method. A phishing email may be used to steal passwords. Please remember that this process is best done by the good guys before the bad guys get their chance, and no harm or disruption should result from such exercises.

Case Study: Government Penetration Testing

Security experts were sanctioned to test the defenses of a government agency that deals with cybersecurity. Using social media and a photo of a reportedly attractive female, they were able to build an identity and ultimately online friendships with government personnel in this agency.

The "woman" provided these employees with a virtual Christmas card containing malicious code, thereby duping employees who bypassed antivirus mechanisms to view it. Having carte blanche to the agency's computer systems, the security experts discovered the birthday of the agency's head of security, who was then given a virtual birthday card. Upon opening, these experts had the keys to the castle – including information about foreign leaders as well as knowledge of state-sponsored attacks. This is an excellent, albeit extreme, example of why security awareness training is so important. Even highly intelligent, knowledgeable individuals with expert security abilities should not be exempt from education programs.

Risk Assessment: Understanding Threats

The United States Department of Health and Human Services (HHS) released an Omnibus Rule in 2013 to finalize several key healthcare privacy and security regulations (HHS, 2013). Consistent with prior regulations, healthcare entities (i.e. hospitals, clinics, etc.) are required to perform annual and periodic security risk assessments on a cadence and schedule that is suitable to their circumstances. Much can be written about the concept of risk and the intricacies of risk assessment. In a nutshell, organizations have a methodology by which to comprehend, evaluate, prioritize, remedy, and accept risk. This concept is not exclusive to cybersecurity risks but is applied to this field for the protection of clinical, financial, and other operations. These annual risk assessments may address not only the electronic systems but also the people, processes, procedures, and other factors throughout the enterprise that may either be subject to or mitigate risk. On a tangential note, this author surveyed high-profile breaches in the United States in the course of research and found that the lack of an adequate risk assessment was a commonly cited theme in breach settlement documents. Could this risk assessment have exposed risks from organizations' patch management or other strategies that may have contributed to their exposure to the exemplified cyber-attack?

Classic risk management models examine two major factors in the calculation of risk: likelihood of occurrence and impact (degree of exposure) (Figure 17.5). In other words, how likely is it that something going to happen, and how bad will it be? Traditionally, equal weighing of likelihood and exposure have yielded a quantifiable measurement of risk. While this model may facilitate routine risk management activities, unanticipated catastrophic events have shaped the industry mindset toward an increased consideration of impact. The industry's assessment and appetite to accept risk has evolved as the result of unanticipated and unlikely events resulted in broad and catastrophic outcomes. Consider the impact that the events of September 11, 2001, have had on security measures. How likely was it to predict that a shadowy group would obtain National Security Agency spy tools that would find their way into state actors on behalf of North Korea, into legitimate software in the Ukraine, and ultimately wipe out millions of computer systems worldwide? What was the likelihood prior to the year 2020 that the US, among the entire world's nations, would be infected with a pathogen rapidly causing fatalities measured in the hundreds of thousands? While these types of incidents are not daily occurrences, shades of them, to varying degrees, certainly are. Therefore, providing equal weights to likelihood and impact in the classic calculation of risk must be revisited in the context of the contemporary paradigm of an increasingly connected world, with rising stakes accompanying the increasing prevalence and complexity of unanticipated profound incidents. Simply producing a quantitative value based upon the equal weighing of likelihood and impact is no longer considered a sound method of calculating risk in an era of increasingly complex and evolving threats among a vast array of confounding variables.

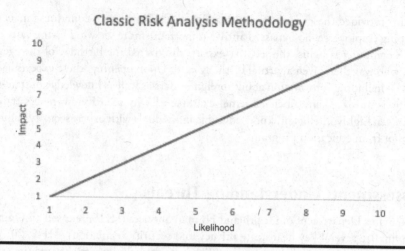

Figure 17.5 Classic outdated risk model: calculate impact and likelihood

A comprehensive risk assessment should be performed at least annually or where required by regulations and programs taken part in by the organization (such as meaningful use). Please note that in numerous breach incidents, the lack of a risk assessment is noted in the incident settlement statements.

According to the HIPAA Security Rule:

■ **Risk Analysis § 164.308(a)(1)(ii)(A)**
"Conduct an accurate and thorough assessment of the potential risks and vulnerabilities to the confidentiality, integrity, and availability of electronic protected health information held by the covered entity."

■ **Risk Management § 164.308(a)(1)(ii)(B)**
"Implement security measures sufficient to reduce risks and vulnerabilities to a reasonable and appropriate level to comply with § 164.306(a) [(the General Requirements of the Security Rule)]."

A security professional or vendor may lead or wholly conduct a risk assessment if sufficient resources are not available within the organization or if an independent surveyor is preferred. Commonly, variants of a National Institute of Standards and Technology (NIST) may be used as a framework for the exercise. There could be separate assessment efforts for elements within the organization and one specific to the IT department. Every clinical, financial, or other application housing, transmitting, or processing sensitive information should be assessed individually in detail. The assessment is not simply a one-time event, but rather a cycle of assessment, identifying risks, and implementing controls. As illustrated in Figure 17.6, the circle continues ad infinitum. This process may require multidisciplinary input and action depending on the makeup of the organization. Be vigilant in selecting or hiring your security professionals or services. Get past the smoke and mirrors of marketing and seek a reputable service or one that comes recommended from a trusted source. A risk assessment is more than placing marks in a spreadsheet or attestations from staff members – although that may be part of the process. Rather, the concept of seeking evidence that processes are followed and a detailed remediation plan with anticipated due dates should be constructed.

Risk Lifecycle

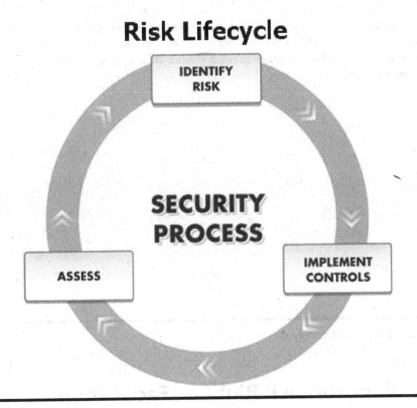

Figure 17.6   Risk lifecycle

Think of the organization as a patient, with the purpose being to diagnose, treat, and prevent illness and maintain health. Come clean with the doctor and be willing to take the good and the bad news. Objective lab tests such as vulnerability scanning and penetration testing can be most telling. How is the patient's immune system when it comes to viruses and other nefarious agents? Depending on the skill of the assessors and the condition of the patient, you may need to sit down for the results. Bad news can be constructive as an organization learns something of its risk. Once the diagnosis has been accepted and the bitter pill swallowed, the healing begins.

Surviving an Audit

The HITECH Act requires HHS to provide for periodic audits. These are conducted by the Office for Civil Rights (OCR), whose authority has increased under the Omnibus Rule. They may commission a third party to act on their behalf. The risk assessment is considered an essential component of the audit. Furthermore, government financial incentive programs may require a risk assessment to have been conducted per specifications. Anecdotally, an estimated 25% of all such financial incentive audits have resulted in failure due to the lack of a proper risk assessment. Common pitfalls include the lack of a remediation plan with dates in response to findings and simply not having performed an assessment at all.

Figure 17.7 outlines some factors to be mindful of when preparing for the organization's eventual audit. Think of an audit as an inevitable "when," not "if," scenario. Prepare accordingly. Figure 17.8 shows how OCR facilities covered entities in safeguarding PHI above and beyond enforcement activities.

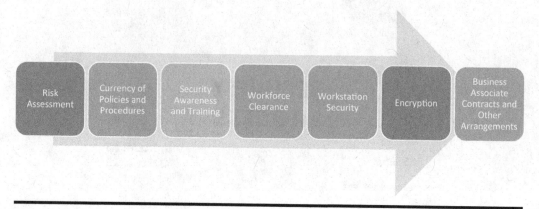

Figure 17.7   Likely audit coherents

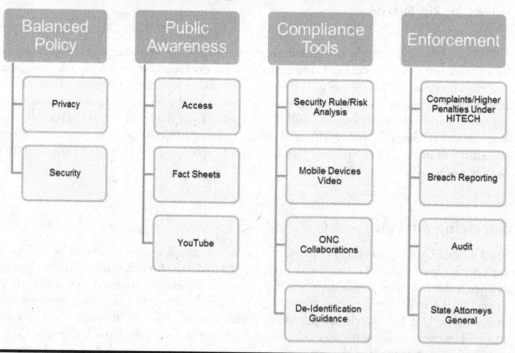

Figure 17.8   Office for Civil Rights – facilitating the safeguarding of PHI

Medical Devices and IoT

As the EHR increased in prevalence, so did interoperability with medical devices, and more recently the Internet of Things (IoT). These devices include a mix of antiquated equipment with outdated operating systems that no longer receive security updates and may not have been configured or even designed with today's cybersecurity risks in mind. A system may have clinical usefulness far exceeding its support, with the only vendor solution being an expensive upgrade. Also included in healthcare use are various emerging IoT devices such as wireless patient monitors. All of these may reside on the hospital network adjacent to systems that are clinically critical and may contain sensitive information. Any risk to these systems must be considered a risk to other networked computer systems and devices as such threats can traverse the network.

The US Food and Drug Administration (FDA) clears devices for the market but does not bear the responsibility of testing them for cybersecurity readiness. This agency has a scope of practice and levers of power that it cannot exceed. That limits its involvement in the cybersecurity process. They have produced pre- and post-market guidance for manufacturers indicating that their recommendations are not legally binding. Therefore, consumers of these medical devices must bear the burden of assessing risk when making purchases and typically responsibility for ensuring a sound cybersecurity posture with implementation and operation. In other words, the cybersecurity state of medical devices set by manufacturers is primarily based upon market forces rather than legislation. Having a dedicated medical device security program in healthcare institutions is highly recommended.

Case Study: Pacemaker and Insulin Pump Hack Example

Barnaby Jack was a security researcher famed among other things for presenting the ability to hack into ATMs and dispense bills as if he'd won the jackpot at a slot machine. He was influenced by an episode of the television program *Homeland*, in which a terrorist could remotely hack the pacemaker of the Vice President of the United States. In 2012, he demonstrated the means by which to send a high volt shock to a pacemaker from 50 feet away with lethal results. He also found a way to send the entire batch of insulin through an insulin pump, which, again, could be fatal. Barnaby Jack died under mysterious circumstances in 2013, one week before his scheduled presentation of medical device vulnerability findings at the Black Hat Conference in Las Vegas, a renowned cybersecurity forum attracting professionals from across the globe.

Encryption

If only one principle is learned in this chapter, it is that you must encrypt everything wherever possible. The 2013 Omnibus Rule summarizes encryption as a potential get out of jail free card.

> We encourage covered entities and business associates to take advantage of the safe harbor provision of the breach notification rule by encrypting limited data sets and other protected health information pursuant to the Guidance Specifying the Technologies and Methodologies that Render Protected Health Information Unusable, Unreadable, or Indecipherable to Unauthorized Individuals (74 FR 42740, 42742). If protected

health information is encrypted pursuant to this guidance, then no breach notification is required following an impermissible use or disclosure of the information.

(HHS Omnibus Rule – Modifications to the Breach
Notification Rule Under the HITECH Act)

Encryption is the process of scrambling data, making it completely incomprehensible to anyone other than intended parties. The National Institute of Standards and Technology guidelines calls for the use of an Advanced Encryption Standard (AES) algorithm to be used wherever possible. Generally speaking, 128-bit and 256-bit power of encryption implementations are used by the NSA for secret and top secret information respectively. The 256-bit encryption would take longer to hack with present-day technology than the time the universe has existed – including the recently discovered extra 100 million years. By comparison, 128-bit encryption only requires 31,536,000 years – so get cracking. Brute force hacking is an automated system of password attempts as a last-ditch effort to bust through password security. As outlined in prior examples, clever social engineering methodologies can thwart all this technology. Of course, encryption must be properly implemented to be effective. Encryption is a major part of the security program, not the whole picture.

Many data breaches could have been avoided if encryption were used. The stolen laptop, the lost USB thumb drive, the errant email, the missing smart phone – are all considered non-issues if protected with properly implemented encryptions. Basically, unencrypted data is not safe. Encrypted data is considered safe and protected under the safe harbor provision quoted earlier. Unencrypted data is an accident waiting to happen. Properly encrypted devices in the wrong hands are considered as electronically useful as a brick.

Encryption is need for data at rest for devices such as a laptop, desktop (yes, those too), smart phone, backup tape (commonly overlooked), and USB thumb drive. Encryption must also exist for data in motion. Data travels through the network to reach healthcare workers, but also other systems as well. This information might also be transmitted to a vendor facility or government organization. Whether the data resides on a piece of equipment or while in transit, encryption must be used. Contrary to common belief, a wireless device using wireless encryption on a network is not considered to be fully have encryption in motion. Once on the network wire, the data is not automatically encrypted just because a device is wireless. Wireless devices should also be considered for implementing encryption in motion where applicable.

A common misconception is that ePHI does not exist on the local computer or that a particular device does not contain sensitive information. Nothing could be further from the truth, and the assumption should be that healthcare systems have sensitive data flowing through them at some point in time. Even once a file is erased and removed from the trash container, someone with the right tools and expertise can recover the file – and recreate the ePHI. The skill level required is relatively rudimentary. The assumption cannot be that any lost or stolen items would likely not fall into capable hands. Sanctioning authorities may not agree. Even if a file with sensitive information was accessed but not residing on the computer itself, a cached copy could reside on the hard drive in one form or another while the end user would be otherwise unaware. Assume that every computer, server, and device can contain sensitive information and protect the organization accordingly.

Part of a comprehensive data leak protection program includes minimizing the ability to store data on a local computer, transmit data to a USB thumb drive, or even email sensitive information inappropriately or without secure mechanisms. There are products that make certain that USB drives are either not used or at least safeguarded. Email may be filtered and encryption may occur either through manual or automated processes.

The concept of BYOD (Bring Your Own Device) is a rapidly emerging phenomenon that is pervasive in the healthcare industry. With these devices comes a new set of risks. Healthcare practitioners expect to use such devices without necessarily securing the information. Having a mobile device management software solution in place will mitigate the risks while still affording convenience. One can impose access restrictions and enforce security protocols such as device encryption and strong passwords. As an added bonus, lost devices may sometimes be traced and recovered. In other cases, the information can be completely wiped clean. Moreover, the same technology used to secure personal devices is also commonly used for mobile assets owned and operated by healthcare entities.

Viruses, Malware, and Other Malicious Code

> Let's immunize hospital computers. Hackers are making better viruses, so we need to have better shots.
>
> – Beth Weiner

The HIPAA Security Rule states covered entities must have "procedures for guarding against, detecting, and reporting malicious software." Healthcare entities are expected to take all reasonable measures to prevent malicious software from entering the network and causing security incidents.

Organizations typically have antivirus systems in some form or another. These are typically centrally managed and may have next-generation sensor technology over traditional endpoint software. Servers and workstations should have configurations that consider their operating systems to be "hardened" with future-proofing by removing potential areas of vulnerability. Think of it as proactively surgically removing an appendix. Security updates are done in a timely fashion with a comprehensive patch management system.

Viruses will almost certainly make their way into a network, just as humans will be infected with viruses. Safe technology practices, having a healthy immune system, and an effective response to infection is key to maintaining a safe network. This includes automated detection, alerting, and response mechanisms. Persistent intrusion detection mechanisms can detect when a computer is communicating or otherwise behaving inappropriately when traditional virus mechanisms fail. Patch management and operating system hardening guidelines should be followed to minimize the risk of infection.

Viruses exist in all four corners of the globe – and beyond. The International Space Station has been attacked by "virus epidemics." Malware spread from infected devices while in orbit, proving not even computers in space are safe from viruses. One infection came from a Russian USB drive. Another came from a laptop infected with a virus used to steal gaming passwords. Perhaps no one can hear you scream in space, but systems can still get infected.

A virus is more than just an annoyance that slows down a computer and causes pop-up advertisements. They can be used to steal sensitive information, obtain ransoms, destroy computer systems, perform a host of illicit activities, and attack other systems. "Botnets," a network of infected computers, can "zombify" many computers hooked up to command and control centers just waiting for instruction to collectively commit a crime – such as knocking a government website offline. In other cases, infected computers' web traffic is rented by the day, week, or month on the underground market. Internet traffic now connects and passes through the renter agent. Directing hospital internet traffic to a criminal organization is a particularly dangerous scenario.

Protocols outlined earlier in addition to best practices by a security professional are warranted to safeguard a health system network.

Social Engineering

According to security expert and felon Kevin Mitnick,

> A company can spend hundreds of thousands of dollars on firewalls, intrusion detection systems and encryption and other security technologies, but if an attacker can call one trusted person within the company, and that person complies, and if the attacker gets in, then all that money spent on technology is essentially wasted. It's essentially meaningless.

Humans are indeed the weakest link in the chain and must be eliminated – the weakness, not humans, of course.

In a lecture on cybercrime, this author mentioned how one can simple call an employee and say, "This is Johnny calling from the helpdesk and I'm going to need your password." An exasperated participant slammed her hand on the table in self-disappointment and exclaimed that she would have just given up her password in such a scenario. There are those waiting in the wings to exploit our trust and have carefully crafted methods to do so. Sometimes, an exploit is just that easy, though. Aside from education, technology such as two-factor authentication can reduce such incidents. That often requires a code from a phone application or text message along with a password to authenticate outside of the hospital network. In other words, something that a user possesses is also used to double check the authentication of a password. Therefore, someone external to the organization would have some barriers to using a stolen password. This is not airtight, but is nonetheless a powerful tool to mitigate such risks.

Another example of social engineering is the impersonation of hospitals over the phone by overseas organizations preying on the vulnerable. These groups can spoof hospitals' phone numbers, cold-call victims, and attempt to extract details to steal identities and much more. As with many social engineering campaigns, perpetrators cast a wide net to gather whatever they can find. This is a numbers game. The more they play, the greater the odds of a significant cash-out. While not affecting the hospital directly, patients may be victimized and the hospital may have public relations issues to contend with.

The common thread in social engineering examples is that human intervention can inadvertently cause breaches. Solid security mechanisms can be completely undone by human error. Part of a comprehensive security program is to have an educated workforce. Staff needs to understand regulations, policies, and have an awareness of security. Annual training should be provided and reminders should be distributed periodically. Workforce training is a legislated requirement and also a sound practice for mitigating a major risk factor. Education may come from qualified staff or from a contracted service. The need for a well-informed staff cannot be overstated.

Conclusion and Key Takeaways

This chapter has served as a general overview of privacy and security considerations for a healthcare organization. Rather than providing a blueprint for a sound security model, this synopsis has served to provide a foundation of knowledge and familiarity with an essential component of medical informatics. The fundamentals of information security principles and case study examples should help to foster an appreciation for the ever-present and emerging challenges organizations face in the endeavor to safeguard their patients' ePHI.

Here are some key takeaways from this chapter to guide you through your journey:

- Risk assessment and remediation is a continuous process.
- Think of an audit as a matter of if, not when, and prepare accordingly.
- Healthcare security is a specialized field requiring qualified personnel with expertise in the field and its subspecialities.
- A solid program will protect both the business and the patients who put their trust of confidentiality in our hands.
- Safeguard data as if it is your own.
- Business associates' agreements must be current and constructed to protect the organization's interests, which also include their clients' interests.
- Encrypt everything – period.
- Policies should reflect both legislation and sensible safeguards while compliance comes from a well-informed workforce.
- Along with policies come associated procedure documents, which are subject to evolution in response to conditions and developing practices.
- Breaches are anticipated to occur. Be prepared responsibly and respond appropriately. Have a tested playbook. Seek the assistance of industry experts and the guidance of government agencies.
- Train the workforce on matters of security and privacy. Provide updates periodically.
- Keep up to date with current events, legislation, programs, and technology.
- Learn from the mistakes and close calls of others.
- Accept the results and findings of the risk assessment diagnosis and comply with the treatment regimen. That sometimes-bitter pill can improve the overall health of an organization.

The last but not least important takeaway – is the method of integrating privacy and security into informatics in lieu of a concurrent integration with business processes. Build sound security principles into solutions from the inception. Security and functionality do not have to be mutually exclusive notions but rather can become symbiotic companions. A comprehensive security program that remedies the ills of the past, fortifies defenses, protects, and responds to incidents in a manner that evolves to meet the challenges of emerging threats is a requirement to ensure the integrity and maintain the operation of a clinical program. So, last but not least, bake the aforementioned concepts into the mix very early and very often as the recipe's prime ingredients. Although an acquired taste for some, the organization should find the results of these efforts to be palatable.

About the Author

Keith Weiner, PhD, RN-BC, is a cybersecurity professional, researcher, and professor with 20 years of informatics experience including a decade in information security leadership positions.

He serves on several boards and committees in an effort to help improve health through informatics.

He is also a fellow of the New York Academy of Medicine and active member of HIMSS.

Keith continues to present at research and industry conferences. A contributing author of several textbooks and publications, he has also served on an editorial board and peer reviewer for scientific journals.

In his spare time, Keith plays several musical instruments and is constantly exploring new technologies.

References

2020. Govinfo.Gov. Retrieved from https://www.govinfo.gov/content/pkg/FR-2013-01-25/pdf/2013-01073.pdf.

"45 CFR Parts 160 And 164 Modifications to the HIPAA Privacy, Security, Enforcement, and Breach Notification Rules Under the Health Information Technology for Economic and Clinical Health Act and the Genetic Information Nondiscrimination Act; Other Modifications to the HIPAA Rules; Final Rule." 2020. *Govinfo.Gov.* Retrieved from https://www.govinfo.gov/content/pkg/FR-2013-01-25/pdf/2013-01073.pdf.

"Mattel vs. Chinese Cyberthieves: It's No Game." 2016. *CBS News.* CBS Interactive. November 27, 2020. Retrieved from https://www.cbsnews.com/news/mattel-vs-chinese-cyberthieves-its-no-game/.

"U.S. Department of the Treasury." Treasury Sanctions North Korean State-Sponsored Malicious Cyber Groups | U.S. Department of the Treasury, August 14, 2020. Retrieved from https://home.treasury.gov/news/press-releases/sm774.

Clarke, E. (2013, November 18). The Underground Hacking Economy is Alive and Well. Retrieved from SecureWorks: http://www.secureworks.com/resources/blog/the-underground-hacking-economy-is-alive-and-well/.

CNN. (2005, October 13). *CNN.com.* Retrieved from A Convicted Hacker Debunks Some Myths: http://www.cnn.com/2005/TECH/internet/10/07/kevin.mitnick.cnna/.

Constantin, L. (2013, October 31). Fake Social Media ID Duped Security-Aware IT Guys. Retrieved from CIO.COM: http://www.cio.com/article/2381282/security0/fake-social-media-id-duped-security-aware-it-guys.html.

The Express Tribune. (2017). Shadow Brokers Threaten to Release Windows 10 Hacking Tools. *The Express Tribune*, May 31, 2017. Retrieved from https://tribune.com.pk/story/1423609/shadow-brokers-threaten-release-windows-10-hacking-tools.

Greater New York Hospital Association. (2014). Retrieved from Greater New York Hospital Association: http://gnyha.org.

Hautala, Laura. (2020). Hospital Devices with Unsupported Operating Systems Exposed to Hacking. *CNET*, March 10, 2020. Retrieved from https://www.cnet.com/news/hospital-devices-exposed-to-hacking-with-unsupported-operating-systems/.

Nightingale, F. (1860). *Notes on Nursing: What It Is and What It Is Not.* London: Harrison and Sons.

Peart, Neil, Alex Lifeson, and Geddy Lee. (1980). *Freewill.* Mercury Records.

Sanger, David E., Nicole Perlroth, and Eric Schmitt. (2020). Scope of Russian Hacking Becomes Clear: Multiple U.S. Agencies Were Hit. *The New York Times*, December 15, 2020. Retrieved from https://www.nytimes.com/2020/12/14/us/politics/russia-hack-nsa-homeland-security-pentagon.html.

Scarfone, K. S. (n.d.). Guide to Storage Encryption Technologies for End User Devices. Retrieved from Computer Security Resource Center: http://csrc.nist.gov/publications/nistpubs/800-111/SP800-111.pdf.

Sutton, W. (1976). *Linn E: Where the Money Was: The Memoirs of a Bank Robber.* Viking Press, p. 160. ISBN 067076115X.

U.S. Department of Health and Human Services. (2003, February 20). Health Insurance Reform: Security Standards; Final Rule. Retrieved from Federal Register: http://www.hhs.gov/ocr/privacy/hipaa/administrative/securityrule/securityrulepdf.pdf.

U.S. Department of Health and Human Services. (n.d.). Health Information Privacy. Retrieved from HHS.GOV: http://www.hhs.gov/ocr/privacy/hipaa/administrative/securityrule/securityruleguidance.html.

U.S. Department of Health and Human Services. (n.d.). Health Information Privacy. Retrieved from HHS.GOV: http://www.hhs.gov/ocr/privacy/hipaa/administrative/privacyrule/.

U.S. Department of Health and Human Services. (n.d.). HHS.GOV. Retrieved from Breaches Affecting 500 or More Individuals: http://www.hhs.gov/ocr/privacy/hipaa/administrative/breachnotification rule/breachtool.html.

Wolenik, Marc J. (2014). *Microsoft Dynamics CRM 2013: Unleashed*. Indianapolis, IN: Sams. https://www.mitnicksecurity.com/in-the-news/the-five-steps-for-managing-cyber-security-threats

Chapter 18

Blockchain Primer

Paul Quigley, MBA

Contents

DOI: 10.4324/9780429423109-18

> The most profound technologies are those that disappear. They weave themselves into the fabric of everyday life until they are indistinguishable from it.[1]

Introduction

This blockchain primer seeks to establish a common understanding of the blockchain, describe the logical building blocks of the technology, and explain why the healthcare industry structure lends itself to broad horizontal adoption of blockchain technology. While blockchain will not be the solution for all the industry's problems, it provides a framework and a set of scalable options as we critically reexamine the entire system from a trust, privacy, cost, safety, and transparency perspective, and it has the potential to return the patients and the providers of care to the center of this ecosystem.

We review the underlying technology and why it offers so much promise in healthcare's heavily regulated siloed ecosystem. We will examine some of the innovation, adaptation, and improvements that are transpiring as this technology matures. Policy issues are inevitable, but they are beyond the scope of this chapter with the cognizance that technology does not operate independently of the industry it serves.

Blockchain is a general-purpose technology innovation.[2,3,4,5] that is both elegant in its simplicity and remarkable in its fungibility. At its most basic, a blockchain is an encrypted, publicly distributed, digital ledger or database. Its very structure facilitates greater collaboration and transparency; it also presents new opportunities to reestablish trust using computational finality, not organizational models. We will use the Bitcoin blockchain to illustrate the mechanisms of blockchain, as it was the first, but there are now hundreds of different blockchains advancing the original design. All blockchains are commonly referred to by their broader technical name of distributed ledger technology (DLT). The true power in blockchain is multifactorial in its design as a cryptographic software protocol and as a disruptive technology for public or shared databases of digital information. Its greatest power, however, may ultimately lay in its ability to create an institutional or social technology for coordinating people and digital assets.[6] Blockchain collaboration and transparency bring real opportunities to reduce costs, improve transparency, and reduce miscommunication, because blockchain fundamentally changes the rules of information/

---

[1] Weiser, Mark. "The computer for the 21st century." *ACM SIGMOBILE Mobile Computing and Communications Review* 3.3 (1999): 3–11.

[2] Kane, Ethan. "Is Blockchain a General-Purpose Technology?" *SSRN 2932585* (2017).

[3] Davidson, Sinclair, Primavera De Filippi, and Jason Potts. "Economics of blockchain." *SSRN 2744751* (2016).

[4] Wellman, William, Quigley, Paul, Private Correspondence, Babson College, 2014- ongoing, Harvard University (2017, 2018, 2019, ongoing)

[5] https://hbr.org/2017/01/the-truth-about-blockchain

[6] Davidson, Sinclair, Primavera De Filippi, and Jason Potts. "Economics of blockchain." *SSRN 2744751* (2016).

data stewardship.[7,8] This shift in data stewardship inspires a critical discussion of trust, decentralized governance, and the return of data provenance to its creators; this self-sovereign concept is revolutionary in healthcare. Although self-sovereignty has been discussed in many government and regional forums, as of this writing it has not been adopted on a large scale.

In March 2020, the US Department of Health and Human Services (HHS) finalized a set of historic rules, the 21st Century Cures Act (Cures Act)[9] and the MyHealthEData Initiative.[10] These two historic federal healthcare data–sharing policies involve both the public and the private sectors and provide patients more control over their information. Herein lies the challenge and the opportunity to achieve the goals that a person's individual data needs to be identified and made sharable while simultaneously protecting the security of that information. Decentralized technology like blockchain or blockchain-inspired technology may offer the consumer the best assurance of access, traceability, and security.

All sectors in healthcare need to be examined if we are to really reduce costs, reduce risks, and improve communication, not just transfer risk from one sector to another. The consumer also needs to be involved and move back into the center of this process. The complete healthcare ecosystem is considered in this chapter, including consumers, pharmaceutical firms, medical device firms, and the entire care delivery system (hospitals, ambulatory care, physicians, pharmacies, and post-acute providers), as well as data aggregators, software companies, and the broad group of payers that includes insurance companies, self-insured employers, government payers, and regulators. The use cases for blockchain in each sector vary; however, there are common themes of decentralization, cryptographically secured trust, and data provenance incorporated into each of the business cases. Some sources report the healthcare system generates approximately a zettabyte (a trillion gigabytes) of data annually, and this is doubling every two years;[11] that may be a conservative estimate, but it does substantiate that any solutions must be considered at scale.

After establishing the foundational building blocks of blockchain, we will transition to critical transformational themes and general use cases to highlight why the current state needs to change. To prevent this primer from becoming onerous, public domain links have been included in the footnotes so you can explore specific areas of interest by industry sector.[12] This primer will provide an approach to consider the business problems, understand how blockchain was used, what elements of the technology were incorporated into these solutions, and what adaptations, if any, were made for healthcare.

When we describe blockchain as a disruptive phenomenon reshaping entire industries, it manifests through a range of business-technology schemes, if not through blockchain-complete[13] projects, then certainly though blockchain-inspired initiatives. Data transparency and data provenance are being testing in existing and novel corporate governance models and nonprofit governance

---

[7] Ølnes, Svein, Jolien Ubacht, and Marijn Janssen. "Blockchain in government: Benefits and implications of distributed ledger technology for information sharing." *Government Information Quarterly* (2017): 355–364.

[8] Davidson, Sinclair, Primavera De Filippi, and Jason Potts. "Disrupting governance: The new institutional economics of distributed ledger technology." *SSRN 2811995* (2016).

[9] https://www.congress.gov/114/plaws/publ255/PLAW-114publ255.pdf.

[10] HHS-agency-financial-report, 2019, Department of Health and Human Services, page 293.

[11] Olivia Bryant. "Data in UK's national health service." *Harvard Technology Review*, May 11, 2020.

[12] Coravos, Andy and Warner, Sofia, Blockchains and health care: promising and moving quickly, though no silver bullet, Stat, 12/27.2017, updated 1/28/2019. Center for Biomedical Blockchain Research as of 4/15/2020 http://biomedicalblockchain.org/

[13] A term and a concept first seen and credited to David Furlonger and Christophe Uzureau of Gartner, Inc. *The real business of blockchain.* Harvard Business Press, 2019.

models. These governance changes are challenging for even the most committed organizations. There are some difficulties in describing exactly what today's blockchain represents because of rapid innovation cycles, emerging industry standards, and evolving nomenclature, as well as the competitive narrative that includes contested vocabulary used in the market today. Technical blockchain standards and smart contract standards[14,15,16,17,18] are emerging as blockchain enters the mainstream; innovation in and integration with legacy systems is inevitable.

As blockchain use cases are implemented, they are stimulating development of new forms of governance and new economic models. Blockchain use cases cross traditional business boundaries and bring organizations into situations where narrowly defined collaboration is necessary to solve problems; this creates angst for existing stakeholders, challenges and redefines their perception of value, and certainly redefines their traditional locus of control. These multidimensional challenges are often at the root of resistance and slow adoption. These use cases include public, permissioned, and hybrid blockchain networks operating with different consensus models while retaining the core principles of the blockchain: trust, immutability, transparency, and provenance. We will conclude this chapter with a brief introduction to some emerging post-blockchain innovations and their application. These include new consensus algorithms used to independently verify data integrity and much faster blockchains designed for gaming, sensors, medical devices, and the machine-to-machine (M2M) economy, also called the Internet of Things (IOT). Healthcare is very dependent on technology to deliver secure, less centralized clinical care, telehealth, and to monitor patients in less centralized environments. This expanding care delivery model has the same, if not higher, standards of data reliability and provenance, as if the person were in the examination room. This emerging segment of blockchain-secured healthcare IOT is called the Internet of Medical Things (IOMT). Chapter 19 is dedicated to the IOMT.

What Is a Blockchain?

The blockchain is a combination of technologies that have been present for decades; the innovation is in how those technologies are combined. The blockchain is unlike traditional rational databases where data is stored in one central database with centralized access control. On the blockchain, each node (computer) has a complete, immutable replica of a distributed digital database that includes all immutable and verified transactions ever made among participating parties. This data is organized into blocks that are cryptographically linked together (hashed) to each other in a chain. The blocks and the chain are the database, and the database is decentralized across all the nodes, so there is no single point of failure in the network. The cryptographic hashes are arranged in a one-way, hierarchical Merkle tree structure. The owner of that record has entered

[14] Anjum, Ashiq, Manu Sporny, and Alan Sill. "Blockchain standards for compliance and trust." *IEEE Cloud Computing* 4.4 (2017): 84–90.

[15] Al-Jaroodi, Jameela, and Nader Mohamed. "Blockchain in industries: A survey." *IEEE Access* 7 (2019): 36500–36515.

[16] Liang, Xueping, et al. "Integrating blockchain for data sharing and collaboration in mobile healthcare applications." In *2017 IEEE 28th annual international symposium on personal, indoor, and mobile radio communications (PIMRC)*. IEEE, 2017.

[17] Zhang, Peng, et al. "Metrics for assessing blockchain-based healthcare decentralized apps." In *2017 IEEE 19th international conference on e-Health networking, applications and services (Healthcom)*. IEEE, 2017.

[18] Griggs, Kristen N., et al. "Healthcare blockchain system using smart contracts for secure automated remote patient monitoring." *Journal of Medical Systems* 42.7 (2018): 130.

their cryptographic public key into the transaction, so ownership or the provenance (chain of trust) is maintained across owners and over time; this transaction record is compiled with other similar records and they are hashed into a data block and added to blockchain.

The term "blockchain" has been popularized as a single word since 2016. The blockchain and the elements of what constitutes a blockchain have been debated since its inception. As has been pointed out by several other authors,[19] the term blockchain is evolving from the public, cryptographically enhanced distributed digital ledger that underprops Bitcoin to now embrace entire private interbank transaction systems and entire private supply chain applications. The blockchain is a software protocol that consists of a time-based transaction record, a mechanism that assembles those transactions to an encrypted, sequential time block and then hashed to verify any evidence of tampering, a mechanism to bind the blocks together into an organized chain (Merkle tree), and then distributes this verified chain across the internet to nodes for fault tolerance and Miner verification (consensus). We will explore each of these in some detail so you have a firm understanding of how a blockchain works; then you will have a comparative reference to other blockchains. The regulatory and legal definitions are lagging the technology. The term "block" first appeared in 1991 when Haber and Stornetta[20] were trying to link cryptographically secured data into blocks, and then resurfaced in 1998 as Szabo was working on decentralized digital currency. The most notable mention of "block+chains" was in the pseudonymous authored 2008 white paper by Satoshi Nakamoto[21] describing a decentralized peer-to-peer cash payment model without a central authority using "block+chain." In 2009, the first block, also called the genesis block,[22] was issued, as the public ledger for transactions now known as Bitcoin was created. For many, this is when blockchain and Bitcoin came into the community consciousness.

With the launch of Ethereum, another public blockchain, and the creation of Ethereum smart contracts in 2014, the comingled Bitcoin currency and the Bitcoin technology became more clearly identified as blockchain technology. This is generally considered the time frame in which blockchain 2.0 was born; since then, the number of different blockchain protocols and the issuance of altcoins (alternative asset coins) have rapidly proliferated.

We are using the public Bitcoin blockchain for illustration but will also examine some important innovations/modification since the peer-to-peer Bitcoin blockchain premiered in 2008 and was first implemented in 2009.[23] These innovations expand the use of blockchain technology into other industry sectors, including healthcare, and make improvements on its transaction processing speed but retain the critical cryptographic security, transparency, and immutability tenets. We will also lay the foundation for next-generation blockchains with different consensus mechanisms more effective for M2M transactions and the Internet of Things (IOT).

Let us review the essentials and establish a common vocabulary to understand the blockchain's core components. There are six core components of the Bitcoin blockchain: transactions, blocks, a decentralized ledger, nodes, Merkle trees, and consensus mechanisms. The transaction data and their hashed blocks are organized using a hierarchical hashed tree structure called a Merkle tree. Merkle trees are an efficient mechanism to search and to detect tampering. We will examine each

---

[19] Adrianne Jeffries. "The blockchain is meaningless." *The Verge*, May 17, 2018.

[20] Haber, Stuart, and W. Scott Stornetta. "How to time-stamp a digital document." In *Conference on the theory and application of cryptography*. Springer, 1990.

[21] Nakamoto, Satoshi. *Bitcoin: A peer-to-peer electronic cash system*. Manubot, 2019.

[22] Genesis Block is the first block of any serial blockchain protocol. It is the base block from which all other blocks in the chain link. It is also often called Block 0 (zero).

[23] Nakamoto, Satoshi. *Bitcoin: A peer-to-peer electronic cash system*. Manubot, 2019.

of these components in depth so you will have a complete understanding of what constitutes a blockchain and how it operates.

One of the hallmark attributes of a blockchain is its value creation within an ecosystem. Some of the promises of blockchain when compared to traditional database systems include:

- Immutability. Once records are placed into a block, they cannot be changed (write once, read many). This creates resistance to censorship.
- Transparency.
- Improved auditability and verification.
- Decentralization of record keeping.
- Fault tolerance (no single point of failure).
- Security through cryptographic encryption.
- Distributed digital ledger of all transactions.
- Tokenization.

This leads to the following business benefits when the same information is available to all the participants:

- Decreased costs
- Pseudonymous (not anonymous) transactions
- Reduced influence of centralized entities
- Reestablishment of trust
- Reduced counterparty risk (or simply risk)
- Elimination of double spend.

Supporting Capabilities of a Blockchain: Encryption and Hashing

One of the central concepts in the blockchain is cryptographic encryption. Encryption is a mathematical process used to convert data into a code to protect and make confidential sensitive information that can only be viewed if the user has a private key to decrypt the data. If someone were to view encrypted data without a private key, it would appear to be a collection of letters and numbers. The most common algorithm in current use on the blockchain is Secure Hash Algorithm 256 (SHA256),[24] developed by the National Security Agency (NSA) and published in 2001. The encryption process is called "hashing." Hashes are one-way, deterministic, fixed-length cryptographic codes created by special algorithms. "One-way" means a transaction is easy to compute but very hard to reverse. "Deterministic" means if the underlying data remains unchanged, the hash will always return the same fixed-length code. That means if any data changes and the hash is rerun, the fixed-length hash code will change. These accumulated verified transactions are then assembled into a block up to the size limitation of the chain, and the SHA256 hash is applied again to each block of transactions. This results in a deterministic hash that halts any further

---

[24] Mukhopadhyay, U., A. Skjellum, O. Hambolu, J. Oakley, L. Yu, and R. Brooks. "A brief survey of cryptocurrency systems." In *2016 14th annual conference on privacy, security, and trust (PST)* (pp. 745–752). IEEE, 2016, December.

additions or changes to that entire block of transactions and provides tamper detection. This block hash is also fixed length and deterministic. This means, assuming no data has change within the block, that no matter how many times you run the function on the same input, the output will always be the same. Because the output is always the same, vast amounts of data can be uniquely identified and confirmed to be tamper proof solely through a single hash. This has the potential to create sizable storage savings and increase efficiency.

Blocks and Transactions

We will start with a single transaction, describe a block of transactions, and then explain how the network becomes an essential element of the security model as it connects a sequential string of blocks together into a blockchain. A time-stamped transaction is the smallest unit of the blockchain (Figure 18.1). Transaction records are accumulated and hashed into individual blocks based on a date-time stamp. Transactions are verified every ten minutes through miners and full nodes. The physical equivalent of accumulating transactions is the manual recording of data on the lines of a paper ledger book. A set of transaction lines fills the page in the ledger; that ledger, once filled, is hashed and presented to a full node as a block. When someone uses or sends bitcoin anywhere, it is called a transaction. Transactions are compiled into blocks by miners so they can be verified. A transaction is not finalized until the block in which the transaction has been placed is finalized by the full nodes. Finalization of a block requires two unrelated parties to agree; several miners must agree on the proof-of-work used by the claiming miner for that miner's block to be passed to a full node and to receive a block reward (Bitcoin reward); simultaneously, the full node must agree that the block

Bitcoin Block Structure (example) Block 655376	
Hash	0000000000000000000a42df2842db16c5e6f4c55c72a9df1f634a71c5e75f30
Confirmations	17,318
Timestamp	2020-11-23 14:25
Height	658376
Miner	Unknown
Number of Transactions	2,706
Difficulty	17,345,948,872,516.06
Merkle root	C068d9d123d8fc70035308ce34f720ee8aa5e668c38e3be71d718f1c65846b63
Version	0x20000000
Bits	386,939,413
Size	1,391,016 bytes
Nonce	1,684,209,302
Transaction Volume	6885.95554392 BTC
Block Reward	6.25000000 BTC
Fee Reward	0.91594469 BTC

©Paul Quigley, Bloclab,LLC 2020

Figure 18.1   Bitcoin block structure

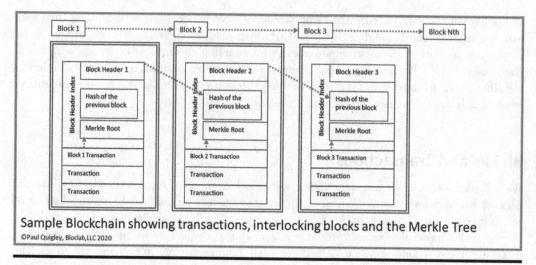

Figure 18.2 **Simplified blockchain showing transactions, interlocking blocks, and the Merkle tree**

produced and offered by that miner to the unbroken blockchain is valid by enforcing the consensus protocol. If a party tries to send a Bitcoin transaction to two differenhercipients at the same time, this is called a double spend. The consensus protocol eliminates the risk of a double spend. Once a Bitcoin transaction is confirmed, it is nearly impossible to double spend that transaction.

The more confirmations a block accumulates over time, the more difficult it is to introduce a fraudulent transaction, because the accumulated transactions and the accumulated blocks on top of that block would have to be individually altered, recompiled, and rehashed, and the rehashed blocks would have to be reinserted into the Merkle tree without changing the Merkle tree chain. We will examine this further when we discuss the blockchain network as part of the security model of the Bitcoin blockchain.

Bitcoin Block Structure

Bitcoin transactions (Figure 18.1) include a date-time stamp, the amount of a purchase, the parties participating in the transaction (represented by a cryptographic public key), a unique digital signature, and a hash. There is also a record of the block reward and a fee reward – the amount paid in Bitcoin to the miner for solving the nonce (See the next section).[25]

The hashes are then organized into a chain (Figure 18.2) and stored in a hierarchical tree structure called a Merkle tree (Figure 18.3).

Chain Assembly

The average Bitcoin transaction block size (2020) is 1.4 MB; however, when the metadata for the indexes are added, the block size increases to 2 MB. Transactions, once "blocked," are immutable

[25] https://support.blockchain.com/hc/en-us/articles/213276463-Bitcoin-Glossary

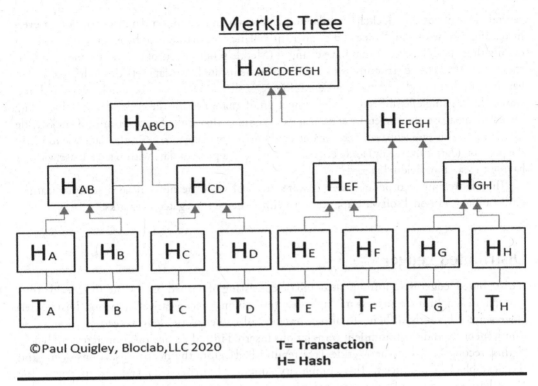

Figure 18.3   Merkle tree

and cannot be changed. Incorrect transactions can be appended, but the original, incorrect transaction will reside in a previous block.

All blockchains have multiple blocks. The initial block in the blockchain is called the "genesis block" or "block (0) zero," and the attachment of additional blocks is called "block height." As of this writing, the Bitcoin blockchain has surpassed 658,376 in block height. Each block contains a 32-bit, randomly generated whole number called a "nonce." This nonce is created by the protocol, once for each block, and it generates the block header hash (Figure 18.2). The SHA-256 hash is a 256-bit number that is unique based on the transactions in that block. These three elements constitute one block in the blockchain (see Figure 18.2).

Once a block has been accepted by a full node into the blockchain, all transactions become immutable. The Bitcoin network can process about one transaction every seven seconds and produces a block approximately once every ten minutes.

Merkle Trees

A Merkle tree[26] is a tamper-evident binary tree that acts as a navigational tool across the blockchain architecture. This hierarchical structure provides an efficient and secure form of verification of the underlying data structures without boundary to the number of data sets. This is one of the

---

[26] https://blockonomi.com/merkle-tree/

central elements of the blockchain, allowing it to scale and maintain data integrity of an ever-increasing data set. Compliance and tamper surveillance are maintained by exception processing of only those hash functions that have changed (Merkle proofs). One of the most important benefits of the Merkel tree structure is its ability to authenticate large data sets through a consistent hashing mechanism that delivers a deterministic hash code that can be efficiently stored and searched. This single hash becomes the tamper-proof guarantee for the entire data set, including the entire database and the entire state of a blockchain at that time. So, practically, if the Merkle root (an index) is publicly available, anyone could do a key value lookup in the database to verify the position (date-time stamp) and verify the integrity of a piece of data within a database without having to search individual records.

The blockchain incorporates the software protocol with the network as a security feature, unlike more traditional software applications with *N*-tiered segregated networks.

Distributed Ledger

A distributed ledger is an immutable database consisting of hashed blocks and the Merkle tree, shared and synchronized across multiple sites (nodes) on a decentralized network. Distributed ledgers are inherently difficult to attack because all copies of the ledger need to be attacked simultaneously and the fraudulent transactions inserted into the same position across all blockchains, recompiled, and the Merkle Tree republished before the next transactions occur and the next block is produced. This complexity supports both security and transparency. The blockchain sits on top of the internet – it is not a new internet;[27] it uses the internet to transport data back and forth between nodes. Decentralization of these ledgers eliminates any single point of failure and overtaking control of the ledger.[28] The database is public, although the data in the database is encrypted. Any changes or additions made to the ledger are shared with all the nodes immediately. Humans have been using ledgers for centuries; however, most of those ledgers have been centralized, paper-based, and not transparent, making them more susceptible to fraud.

Shared ledgers facilitate the flow of information, which make audits easier and improves operational efficiency because common data can be shared across parties.

Blockchain is a horizontal technology and has the potential to address some of the more complex technical interoperability challenges faced in healthcare. Sharing a consent-based ledger across a healthcare organization or multiparty network can facilitate critical information like patient identity and provider credentialing. It also has the very real potential to uniformly address technical standards required to empower interoperability with all stakeholders so they can securely share electronic health records (EMRs), wearable sensor data, and behavioral data.

The largest healthcare operational and technical opportunities are in the areas of standardization, interoperability, and horizontal integration across disparate legacy systems, including electronic health records (EHRs). Blockchain companies and providers should expect resistance from legacy software system companies because a decentralized blockchain threatens their business

---

[27] https://hbr.org/2017/01/the-truth-about-blockchain
[28] Sayeed, S., and H. Marco-Gisbert. "Assessing blockchain consensus and security mechanisms against the 51% attack." *Applied Sciences* 9.9 (2019): 1788.

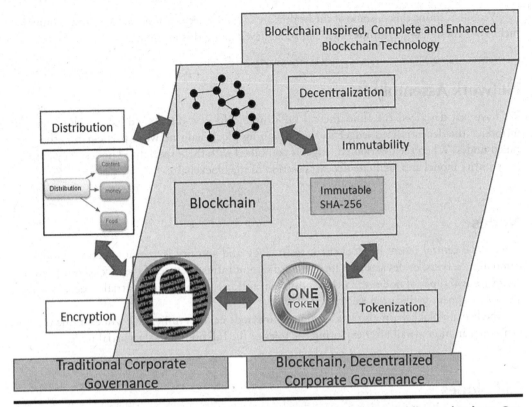

Figure 18.4 Traditional corporate governance provides the basis for enabling technology. Corporate governance needs to include strong data stewardship to support blockchain-inspired, blockchain-complete, and enhanced blockchain capabilities.

model, and it also disrupts the entire business model of insurance companies who could be replaced by smart contracts and new business innovations.

In 2019 Furlonger and Uzureau of Gartner, Inc.[29] proposed an elegant, four-phased approach to look at the market upheaval and innovative blockchain projects being creating across the economy. They recognized the difficulty of taking today's understanding of a business (enabling technology and blockchain inspired) and envisioning a fully decentralized blockchain future (enhanced blockchain). In some situations, it may not be practical or even feasible to implement a blockchain-complete solution; however, in healthcare—an industry wrought with information asymmetry and miscommunication—considerable risk could be reduced if these principles were applied. We believe it is too early to claim healthcare will get to the point of being an enhanced blockchain, but there are a lot of governance changes, structural changes, and process redesign opportunities that could move the industry along a predictable path. Value can be created today (Figure 18.4) with innovative governance changes even if the industry cannot envision a fully enhanced blockchain future.

---

[29] Furlonger, D., and C. Uzureau. "The real business of blockchain: how leaders can create value in a new digital age." *Harvard Business Review Press, Boston* (2019): 11.

We will examine this in some of the healthcare use cases because there are significant improvement and redesign opportunities that can be achieved along this journey.

Network Assembly

We have just described the fundamental building blocks of a distributed ledger. Next, we will introduce the decentralized ledger to the remaining blockchain network participants; these are called nodes. When the distributed ledger is combined with these specialized nodes, they amplify the security model and facilitate decentralization of the blockchain.

Nodes

One of the central tenets in blockchain technology and security is decentralization. Nodes are computers, servers, or devices that form the validation infrastructure of the blockchain network. There are two types of nodes each with a different role: a full node and a partial node, also called a simple payment verification (SPV) node.

The Bitcoin blockchain also has a unique third node called a miner. We will examine the role of a miner in more detail after exploring the roles of the full node and the partial node.

Full Nodes

Full nodes hold a single copy of the entire blockchain distributed ledger history including transactions, time stamps, and all verified blocks. Full nodes store all information, however old, on a blockchain and are the core servers across a decentralized network. Each block in a blockchain is verified, authenticated, and stored by all Full Nodes in the network. Because of this role, full nodes require more advanced computing power and are more expensive to operate than a partial node. It is estimated that the Bitcoin network has over 10,000 operational full nodes. Full nodes are often run by volunteers or stakeholders committed to further decentralized blockchains. Unlike miners, full nodes do not generally receive rewards.

Full nodes are essential to the overall security and validity of the blockchain network and have two responsibilities that differentiate them from other types of nodes. A full node inspects and validates each digital signature in every transaction to authenticate the transaction. A digital signature is usually the private key the sender of the transaction uses to sign each transaction. Full nodes are not miners, which is a common misconception.

A full node is also the key decision enforcer of the consensus protocol. Full nodes have the decision-making authority to reject any new transactions or new blocks. This includes blocks from other nodes on the network. Full nodes accept or reject a block based on a set of parameters or signatures dictated by their decentralized consensus protocol. They can reject newly formed transactions because they maybe incorrectly formatted; or they are a duplication of an already settled transaction, which could be potentially fraudulent; or they violate a consensus rule. Once the node accepts the block, it saves, stores, and places it on top of the chain of blocks it already has. This node then broadcasts (Chain ($N + 1$)) this change to the rest of the network nodes, which then update their copy of the chain with the new, longer chain, and the process is repeated about every ten minutes. In the public, trustless blockchain (Bitcoin blockchain), no one country, organization, mining pool, or computer network owns the blockchain. This makes the network and the ledger fault tolerant to destruction or corruption and maintains the provenance of the data on that blockchain.

Partial Nodes

Partial nodes, also called light or simple payment verification (SPV) nodes, are fractions of the entire blockchain and are typically downloaded wallets connected to full nodes to further validate information stored on the blockchain. They are much smaller in size and only hold information about partial blockchain histories, usually the block header supporting queries and validation of previous transactions. As shown in Figure 18.2, the block header is a detailed summary of a specific block including reference information to the previous blocks it is connected to. Light nodes (SPV) are totally reliant on full nodes to refresh and provide them validated data (Figure 18.5). These partial nodes require far fewer resources to operate and are often included on desktops or online wallets. The role they play in the overall blockchain ecosystem is to take transaction burden off the full nodes and further decentralize the network.

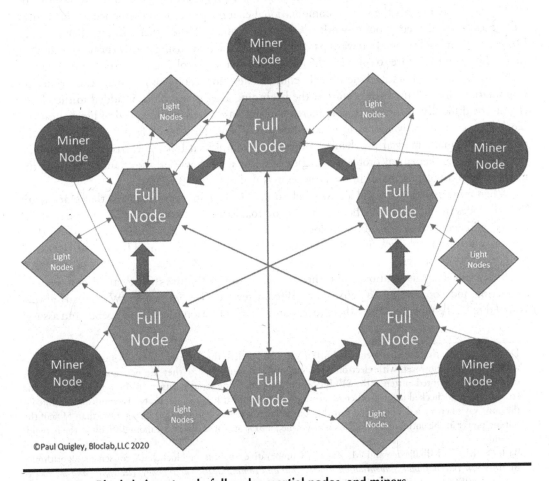

©Paul Quigley, Bloclab,LLC 2020

Figure 18.5 Blockchain network: full nodes, partial nodes, and miners

Mining Nodes

The third specialized node in the Bitcoin blockchain network is a mining node, which is often called a "bitcoin miner"; these are unique nodes that produce blocks for the blockchain. These nodes are also essential for the execution of the game theory underlying the proof-of-work consensus protocol.

Miners are a computer entity or a pool of computer entities that process transaction records on the public bitcoin ledger. Miners have a complete copy of the most current blockchain and perform the work of mining (compiling the transaction records and solve the mathematical puzzle called a nonce). When a Miner receives a transaction, they confirm it is not a duplicate transaction (double spend – a unique problem with electronic transactions).[30] Simultaneously, they compete to try to solve a highly complex computation in search of a nonce A nonce is randomly generated 256-bit string of numbers and letters produced by the bitcoin protocol. The difficulty of that random number increases and or decreases based on the rate of block production. The goal of the bitcoin protocol is to keep block production at about 10 minutes per block; when the rate of block production increases, the difficulty of the nonce increases to slow block production, and when block production is longer than ten minutes, the network difficulty decreases.

This computational work to solve for the nonce is a consensus protocol called proof-of-work (POW), and it represents the sum of computational energy used to find the nonce. If the miners are successful, and their proof-of-work (POW)[31] is verified by the other Miners, that winning Miner or Miner pool receives a reward paid in Bitcoin. Miners are using highly specialized graphical hardware and software to solve for the nonce. The chance of solving the correct mathematical problem is 1 in 13 trillion. Each new block requires a new nonce, none is repeated. This means the computation effort of the miners start at the beginning after a new block is added to the blockchain. The difficulty of the nonce may increase or decrease based on the speed of block creation. Block creation is directly related to bitcoin rewards. Therefore, if block formation is faster than expected, the mathematical problem becomes more complex; if block formation is slower than expected, the mathematical problem becomes easier to solve; however, the chance of solving the mathematical problem remains in the target range of about 1 in 13 trillion.

When miners attempt to add a new block to the blockchain, they broadcast that block to all the full nodes in the network. The first miner to broadcast a successful solution must have their results validated as they contribute a block of transactions to the full nodes; if successful, their block is added to the blockchain, and they receive a reward of newly minted Bitcoin for the use of their computer resources.

The elegance in this solution is that there is coopetition with miners. They are simultaneously competing and cooperating to achieve the Bitcoin reward. The longest POW chain is always assumed to be the most accurate. This process prevents duplication (the double spend) and assures

---

[30] Double Spend: with printed currency say $10 if you hand a clerk the $10 you cannot spend that same $10 in another location; however, with electronic transactions you must be sure they are not duplicate. if you were duplicating the printed currency the $10 bill would have the same serial number. In the Bitcoin network the serial number is checked against other serial numbers to confirm it is not duplicate. Theoretically, in Bitcoin the only way to create a double spend is if the counterfeiter was successful in overtaking more than 51% of the mining power in the entire network. This is also called a 51% attack and is much more difficult as the network expands,

[31] Bach, L. M., B. Mihaljevic, and M. Zagar. "Comparative analysis of blockchain consensus algorithms." In *2018 41st International convention on information and communication technology, electronics and microelectronics (MIPRO)* (pp. 1545–1550). IEEE, 2018, May.

	Able to send new transactions	Ability to propose new blocks	Holds wallet balance information	Holds the complete blockchain data and history
Mining Nodes	No	Yes	No	No
Full Node	No	No	Yes	Yes
Partial Nodes	Yes	No	Yes	No

©Paul Quigley, Bloclab, LLC 2020

Figure 18.6   Key blockchain node features by node type

the network of a single redundant chain. Trust is then mathematically confirmed using cryptography, tamper-proof hashes, and mathematical consensus.

Mining Nodes are only responsible for creating blocks to add to the blockchain; they are not responsible for the maintenance or validity of future blocks (unlike full nodes). Mining nodes offer a network opportunity to pool resources and work with others to increase the rate of receiving more rewards over time. It is worth mentioning that the process of mining consumes significant energy, and miners typically have high capital start-up costs and high operating costs to power their computers. These costs have led to the development of mining pools so the hash rate can be derived from multiple sources and users.

There are several key differences between mining nodes and full nodes.

When discussing the role of full nodes, we mentioned that users who run full nodes are not rewarded. Instead, they have incentives to preserve and further decentralize the blockchain. This is a different incentive than miners, who are typically rewarded through direct token rewards, such as Bitcoin.

Another key difference between mining and running a full node is that a miner is also required to run a full node to identify the consensus criteria for valid transactions. Without this information, a miner would be unable to deliver properly configured blocks to a network and be rewarded. On the other hand, a full node does not require a miner to exist. A full node device (such as a computer or server) can store and receive data without being able to propose new blocks.

We have explored the roles played by different types of nodes as part of the core infrastructure of a blockchain. Nodes can validate a blockchain and follow strict criteria for new blocks to join. In the blockchain, the software protocol, cryptography, and the network contribute features to amplify network and data security.

Figure 18.6 outlines core features of each of the node types and the characteristics that make them an essential part of the blockchain network.

Consensus Algorithm[32, 33] (The Heart of the Blockchain)

A consensus mechanism is an automated decentralized protocol that assures all nodes (computers), also called miners, are synchronized with each other and agree on the legitimacy of transactions

---

[32] "Different Blockchain Consensus Mechanisms." *Hackernoon, Blockgenic*, November 10, 2018.

[33] Bach, L. M., B. Mihaljevic, and M. Zagar. "Comparative analysis of blockchain consensus algorithms." In *2018 41st International convention on information and communication technology, electronics and microelectronics (MIPRO)* (pp. 1545–1550). IEEE, 2018, May.

that are being added to the blockchain. Consensus mechanisms are critical for the blockchain to function correctly and securely.

Consensus is simply a multiparty agreement that a value or that facts are the same. In the case of software protocols and mathematics, consensus was achieved when different parties were able to confirm the same computational result. The magnificence of using mathematics is that it transcends language, culture, and time. The blockchain protocol is open-source software that uses a consensus algorithm to independently verify results claimed by a miner; each result can be reproduced and verified. In a trustless, decentralized network, the parties do not know each other but are able to verify transaction integrity.

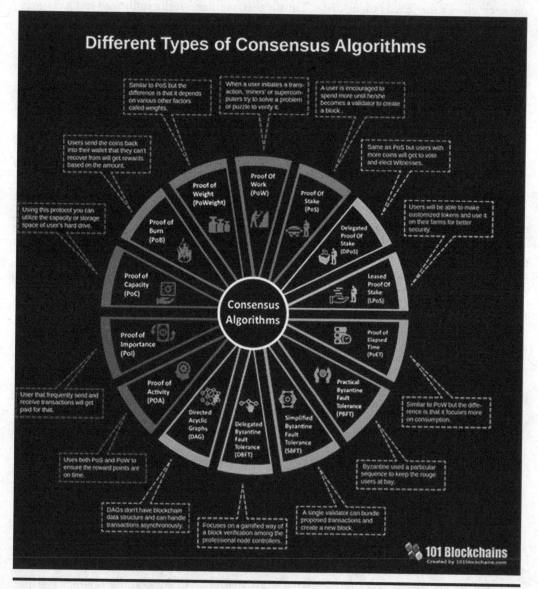

Figure 18.7   Different types of consensus algorithms

The Bitcoin consensus protocol or algorithm (POW) is the program that solves for the nonce so the winning miner can claim the Bitcoin reward. This algorithm is a source of some environmental concern because of the energy requirements to operate the Bitcoin[34] protocol; however, that assertion can be debated if one understands the energy production and distribution model of the present electrical grid. The energy intensiveness and the relative "slowness" of the Bitcoin network has inspired the development of faster protocols and faster, less energy-intensive algorithms. Some of those newer protocols will be described at the end of this primer and provide a segue into the emerging field of M2M blockchains and the IOT. IOT data management and security are one of the emerging use cases for blockchain and are very relevant in the healthcare blockchain. In these use cases, the blockchain becomes the validation mechanism for devices and maintains network awareness and immutability, laying the foundation for oracles and the use of artificial intelligence for predictive analytics.

The following diagram, from 101 Blockchains[35] (Figure 18.7), shows the range of different consensus algorithms. These are relevant metrics for certain use cases and the selection of a specific consensus algorithm has direct impact on the speed of the blockchain.

Smart Contracts

Smart contracts[36] are software programs that add layers of information onto the digital transactions being processed on the blockchain. Smart contracts are binary computer programs stored inside a block or blocks on a blockchain. These agreements stipulate terms and conditions that are fully executed without human interaction.

Smart contracts are a new development on the blockchain since 2014; they are open source, originally developed on the Ethereum protocol. The term "smart contract" is a misnomer: they are not smart, and they are not contracts in the legal sense of contract law, although the latter is evolving quickly. Smart contracts are not Ricardian agreements;[37] however, smart contracts can be supplemental to Ricardian contracts when using the blockchain to record date-time stamped digital signatures.

There is work underway to make smart contracts more commercially enforceable across jurisdictions. The first-generation smart contracts were single-layer programs; this means that all the information involved in a transaction – the identity of the buyer, the identity of the seller, the timing and value of the transaction as well as other key attributes—are all recorded at the same time. It became quickly apparent that transaction speed would be slow, and scaling would be difficult. The second- and third-generation smart contracts have learned from these mistakes and have created multilayered contracts to overcome these constraints.

Smart contracts may have conditional parameters to take alternative action based on the values and terms of the agreement. When smart contracts are stored and activated on a decentralized public blockchain, no third party is unable to stop the contract, because if they are well designed, they do not require a middleman to execute. Examples of smart contracts include the program

---

[34] Ghosh, Eshani, and Baisakhi Das. "A study on the issue of blockchain's energy consumption." In *International ethical hacking conference*. Springer, 2019.

[35] Different Types of Consensus Algorithms, 101 Blockchains.com

[36] Franco, Pedro. *Understanding bitcoin: Cryptography, engineering, and economics.* John Wiley & Sons, 2014.

[37] Grigg, Ian. "The Ricardian contract." In *Proceedings. First IEEE international workshop on electronic contracting, 2004.* IEEE, 2004.

used to determine Bitcoin halving, the decentralized determination that the miner reward will be reduced by 50%. The Bitcoin rewards for miners are set within the body of the Bitcoin core code. Smart contracts may receive (external) real-world data through trusted oracles, as the smart contract cannot "leave the blockchain" to obtain conditional data; it needs to be fed into the program. Smart contracts and oracles are another exciting and emerging area of the blockchain.[38]

Shared Governance Is Critical to the Success of Any Blockchain

Governance is important in any organization and technology project but the need for blockchain governance[39] and clear stakeholder responsibilities is even more important when using DLT because stakeholders are decentralized. In healthcare, where organizational governance is already complex, decentralized governance is a new endeavor, and this can be particularly disruptive to existing stakeholders; however, the needs are compelling. Underlying principles of decentralized governance include the doctrines of patient identity and patient rights to their data, and this impacts clinical workflow, billing, data attestation, and data liquidity. This is a complex area for any healthcare organization when simultaneously operating within the guidelines of HIPAA and a patchwork of state and federal privacy laws. We believe the US healthcare system should follow the lead of other jurisdictions, particularly the European Union's General Data Protection Regulations (GDPR)[40] statutes and the California Privacy Rights Act[41] and examine adaptations made by the financial services industry regarding data rights and data access. The financial services industry has already spent close to $1.4 billion and had several years of direct experience working with DLT in the financial sector.[42,43]

Types of Blockchains

Now that you know what the original blockchain is and how it operates, we will expand the definition to include the four general classifications of blockchains: public and private blockchains. The private blockchains divide further into private, consortium, and hybrid blockchains. Healthcare blockchain innovators are more attracted to the permissioned blockchains, because the industry structure lends itself more to ecosystems, the data structures are more complex than the Bitcoin blockchain, and transaction speed is a higher priority (Figure 18.8.)

A *public blockchain* is a permissionless distributed ledger system. Anyone with internet access can sign in to a public blockchain and see all transactions. This is the most transparent and decentralized of the blockchains, all transaction data is encrypted. Public blockchains are the most secure, most transparent, and least scalable (due to decentralization and rigorous consensus mechanism); they also have the slowest transaction speeds.

---

[38] https://chain.link/education/blockchain-oracles#:~:text=Blockchain%20oracles%20are%20entities%20that,legacy%20systems%2C%20and%20advanced%20computations.

[39] Bevir, Mark. *Key concepts in governance.* Sage, 2008. Pages 29–30.

[40] https://gdpr.eu/

[41] https://www.jdsupra.com/legalnews/as-california-enacts-new-data-privacy-71714/

[42] Paech, Philipp. "The governance of blockchain financial networks." *The Modern Law Review* 80.6 (2017): 1073–1110.

[43] https://www.weforum.org/reports/the-future-of-financial-infrastructure-an-ambitious-look-at-how-block-chain-can-reshape-financial-services/

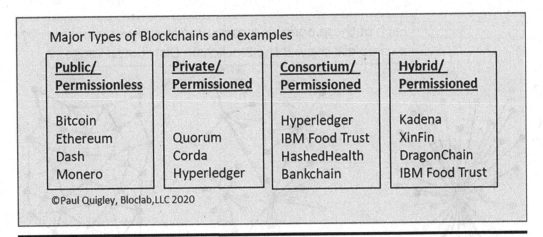

Figure 18.8   Major types of blockchains and example chains

Private blockchains: Permission and consortium blockchains are private, closed networks. They can be single organization or industry specific, with different governance guidelines for security permission and access. The network of nodes maybe smaller because these blockchains do not need to protect from a 51% attack, and they maybe more centralized. They generally have much faster transaction speeds (transactions per second [TPS]) than public blockchains, can scale quickly, and based on their governance model, they may not be as transparent as public blockchains. Government organizations and bank networks are good examples of consortium blockchains.

Hybrid blockchains: The hybrid blockchain is a combination of a private and public blockchain. In these networks, sections of the blockchain are private, whereas permission in other sections of the blockchain or permission lists are viewable by the public. Hybrid blockchains tend to have more nodes than private blockchains to increase transparency and security of the network.

Cross-chain interoperability is an area of ongoing development, especially in private or permissioned chains where some data is private and other segments of data are public.

There is an aspirational organization structure in the blockchain universe called a distributed autonomous organization (DAO). This is a non-human, automated entity that has no hierarchical structure and is governed by a series of nested smart contracts that have considered every possible combination of events. The DAO been theorized since the peer-to-peer model of Bitcoin showed one could remove the friction of a middleman in financial transactions. Healthcare is a human industry. We can certainly augment diagnostic decision-making and population health surveillance capabilities through IOT and artificial intelligence (AI), but that would not be a DAO. We have substantial near-term improvement opportunities using blockchain in lower value or in financial interactions across the healthcare system. Blockchain will also play an important role in protecting privacy, reducing cost, increasing transparency, and reestablishing trust, but care is still a human-to-human experience.[44,45]

---

[44] Wang, Shuai, et al. "Blockchain-powered parallel healthcare systems based on the ACP approach." *IEEE Transactions on Computational Social Systems* 5.4 (2018): 942–950.

[45] Zhang, Peng, et al. "FHIRChain: Applying blockchain to securely and scalable share clinical data." *Computational and Structural Biotechnology Journal* 16 (2018): 267–278.

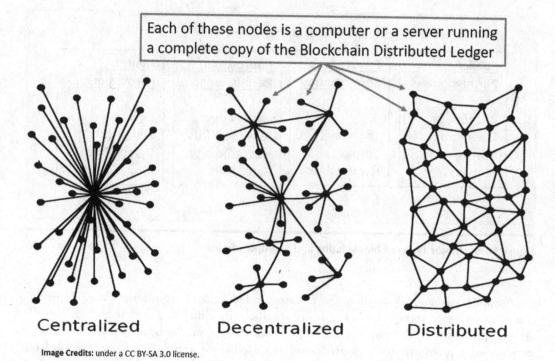

Figure 18.9 **Illustrations of different network configurations: centralized, decentralized, and distributed**

What Is a Decentralized Network?

A decentralized network is a trustless network that has no single point of failure. The nodes on this network are not dependent on any single server, and each node holds the entire copy of the network configuration. These are the most common network configurations (Figure 18.9); there is a hybrid network, but it is a combination of two or more of these three primary options.

Three types of networks in the healthcare environment, including mobile, are[46]

a. Centralized systems
b. Decentralized systems (newest)
c. Distributed systems.

Blockchain Programming Languages

Most blockchain development occurs in the following programming languages. Some of these languages are blockchain specific, and others are more general languages used across industries. New job growth for people learning these languages is high in healthcare as well as other industries (Figure 18.10).

Healthcare is ready for blockchain.

---

[46] https://www.geeksforgeeks.org/comparison-centralized-decentralized-and-distributed-systems/

Top 15 programming languages for blockchain		
C++	Ruby	C#
Python	Simplicity	GO
Java	Scilla	PHP
Rust	Vyper	JavaScript
Solidity	CX	Rholang

Source: © Quigley, Bloclab 2021.

Figure 18.10   Top 15 programming languages for blockchain

Now you should understand the blockchain how it operates and the role of consensus mechanisms and the basic structure that improves security. Blockchain governance is predicated on community engagement; that community may be a supply chain ecosystem, or it may be a healthcare delivery network. As the industry and consumers understand how a blockchain operates, we expect to see a rapid increase in consumer use cases as well as industry use cases.

Decentralization combined with this trust-but-verify mechanism creates the foundation for an entirely new ecosystem that exists outside of a corporation or government. As faster M2M networks (medical devices and personal wearable devices) emerge with the IOT, new, faster, and more energy-efficient consensus mechanisms and blockchain designs are emerging. These blockchains retain the essential building blocks of transaction security, decentralization, and encryption but have introduced new consensus mechanisms with transaction speeds that rival the credit card processing metrics of global financial networks.

We are on the cusp of the Fourth Industrial Revolution, where automation and horizontal platform solutions will threaten siloed vertical software systems. Healthcare has a very expensive fragmented vertical technology stack with a portfolio of highly specialized, disconnected systems; the only questions are how quickly and how deeply these horizontal platforms will extend into these vertical technology stacks. While some software solutions are clinically sophisticated, much of the administrative data and the charge data are commodities and could be shared across the entire system. Both administrative and charge modules can be simplified using application programming interfaces (APIs).[47] Data unification and interoperability have been the holy grail of healthcare for decades, but progress has been slowherd by stakeholder self-interests, lack of standards, and failure to enforce existing standards; the blockchain can change that and keep stakeholder data secure.

The problem of incomplete, paper-based records has been replaced by incomplete EHRs. Development of a unified common person identity remains a work in progress and needs to move into the application layer to make more than an incremental impact on miscommunication and reduce errors. There have only been a few consistent examples of complete patient information delivered to the desktops of the physicians; this is an important area of focus for blockchain and blockchain-enabled EMR projects.[48] Blockchain's greatest innovations may be the forced

---

[47] API are Application Program Interfaces. Most often APIs allow one application to access the features of another application. Also, if the source/ target systems are cloud-based then RESTful API are used because they use less bandwidth and are more suitable for efficient internet usage.

[48] www.BurstIQ.com and www.HashedHealth.com are two examples of blockchain companies and consortia focused in this area. Please see the public domain site http://biomedicalblockchain.org/ for a more complete and updated list of blockchain companies and associated projects.

modernization of data governance and data provenance, enhanced transparency, and greater consumer control of their own information; only a small fraction of that is directly related to development of the software protocols.

Market Size of Blockchain in Healthcare

Healthcare spending is now more than 20% of US GDP (2019), but we continue to slip lower in the rankings of health outcomes.[49,50] There are several directional indicators that we can use to estimate the size and the potential impact blockchain could have on the healthcare market. While we will focus predominantly on the US healthcare market, these orders of magnitude are comparative. The efficiency of healthcare services is heavily dependent on the ability to record, store and share information easily and securely between disparate applications and systems. It is interesting to note that BisResearch claims that "only 10% of healthcare organization regularly share medical information with providers outside their organization."[51] This would suggest that somewhere between 70% and 90% of a patient's information is stored within the healthcare organization; why, then, is miscommunication identified as one of the largest reasons for medical error?[52,53] This same group has forecasted that the use of blockchain technology across the healthcare ecosystem could save upwards of $100 billion per year by 2025. These recurring saving are in the areas of data breach–related costs, IT costs, operational costs, support functions and personnel costs, counterfeit related fraud, and insurance fraud. Two industries singled out to gain disproportionately through investment in blockchain include pharmaceutical companies, which are purported to lose $200 billion to counterfeit drugs per year, and health insurance companies, who stand to reduce insurance fraud by $10 billion per year.

Gminsights projects the US healthcare blockchain market to be $1.6 billion by 2025, with an annual forecasted CAGR of 65% between 2019 and 2025 with the following segmentation.[54]

Cybersecurity risks and data privacy will also be strong drivers for this growth. Several of the constraints on this industry growth are a very limited number of people with these combination skills.

Gartner's much followed Hype Cycle had blockchain as part of their emerging technologies graph until 2018, at which time they deemed blockchain to be enough of a phenomenon that it became its own Hype Cycle. Blockchain has started to make steady progress over the top of the hype curve, and the financial payments area leads that development.

---

[49] www.cms.gov

[50] https://www.commonwealthfund.org/publications/issue-briefs/2020/jan/us-health-care-global-perspective-2019

[51] https://bisresearch.com/industry-report/global-blockchain-technology-market-report-forecast.html Executive Summary and Description

[52] Carver N, Gupta V, Hipskind JE. Medical Error. [Updated 2020 Feb 16]. In: StatPearls [Internet]. Treasure Island (FL): StatPearls Publishing; 2020 Jan-. https://www.ncbi.nlm.nih.gov/books/NBK430763/

[53] Other locations patient information can be stored outside the healthcare organization include post-acute care locations, home care, laboratories, and pharmacies. There were no estimates for each of these locations.

[54] https://www.gminsights.com/industry-analysis/blockchain-technology-in-healthcare-market

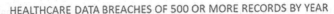

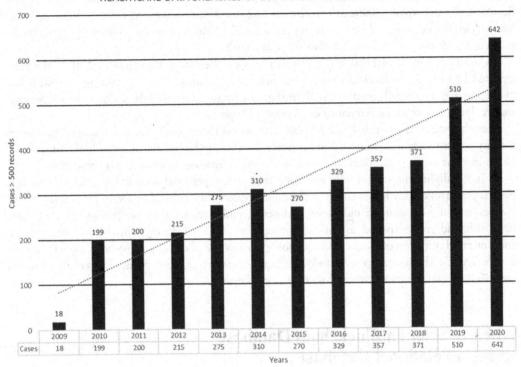

HEALTHCARE DATA BREACHES OF 500 OR MORE RECORDS BY YEAR

Years	2009	2010	2011	2012	2013	2014	2015	2016	2017	2018	2019	2020
Cases	18	199	200	215	275	310	270	329	357	371	510	642

Figure 18.11   Healthcare data breaches of 500 or more records

The Battle to Rebuild Trust

The Pew Research Center[55] has been tracking the American perception of trust with data security. In a 2017 study, they identified that 64% of people had online accounts for financial, healthcare, and sensitive personal information. In the same period, 64% experienced or had been notified of a significant data breach (Figure 18.11) pertaining to their personal data or accounts. More than 50% of the public feel their data are less secure. Many Americans expressed a lack of confidence in institutions – most notably, the federal government and social media platforms – to safeguard and protect their personal information. This has very important implications for a feeling of trust and the rate of innovation diffusion and adoption of blockchain or other personal data security strategies.

In 2018, the healthcare sector saw 15 million patient records compromised in 503 breaches[56,57,58,59] – three times the number seen in 2017, according to the Protenus Breach Barometer.[60] Data for 2020,

[55] Anderson, J., and L. Rainie. "The future of truth and misinformation online." *Pew Research Center* 19 (2017).

[56] https://www.protenus.com/resources/protenus-2019-breach-barometer/

[57] U.S. Department of Health and Human Services, Office for Civil Rights Breach Portal: Notice to the Secretary of HHS Breach of Unsecured Protected Health Information, April 2020

[58] https://healthitsecurity.com/news/the-10-biggest-healthcare-data-breaches-of-2019-so-far

[59] https://www.hipaajournal.com/healthcare-data-breach-statistics/

[60] https://www.protenus.com/resources/2020-breach-barometer/

the latest information available from the US Department of Health and Human Services Data Breach Reporting website, indicates more than 642 new breaches were reported.[61] These breaches have eroded public trust and negatively impact the entire industry's ability to keep a person's medical record information available but also safe and secure.

In the Department of Health and Human Services Report to Congress in 2018,[62] the HSS reported 12.1 million individual records were breached. Although there is a timing issue with formal reporting, the overall trend line is alarming. The fragmentation of data, system heterogeneity, and the lack of clear data governance exacerbates this problem.

Health systems need to balance reliable data access (horizontal demand requirements) with security across the delivery system and insurers – blockchain has immediate and high-value application in these areas, specifically in the areas of identity management and data protection.

This highlights the reason why solutions that secure personal identifying information and place the control of that information in the hands of consumer would be a very attractive option, independent of the healthcare industry's readiness to embrace such technology. Consumers understand this and are motivated to embrace protection of their information; this has opened the door for rapid diffusion of blockchain technology across the healthcare ecosystem, especially with mobile devices. The consumer will probably drag the healthcare industry into blockchain in much the same way the consumer dragged retail into e-commerce.

When to Select a Blockchain Database versus a Relational Database

When considering your technology options (Figure 18.12), it may make sense to build a business case for your technology platform. Blockchain is not the solution for every problem, and there are some very real costs in operating a blockchain network with high availability and transaction speed. However, there are principles like "blockchain inspired" parameters, previously described by Furlonger, that may create an acceptable IRR (internal rate of return)[63] to the organization.

Who Are the Dominant Companies in the Healthcare Blockchain Industry?

Identifying the most prominent companies exclusively focused on blockchain or companies with blockchain project experience would be too numerous to mention and would depend, in large part, on your area of focus. Blockchain is a horizontal technology solution, so part of its value is in bringing partners together into an ecosystem. To that end, there are open-source technology platforms, such as the Linux Foundation: Hyperledger Project,[64] which brings blockchain capability across

---

[61] U.S. Department of Health and Human Services, Office for Civil Rights Breach Portal: Notice to the Secretary of HHS Breach of Unsecured Protected Health Information, 2021

[62] HSS, Annual Report to Congress on Breaches of Unsecured Protected Health Information for Calendar Year 2018, page 4

[63] Hartman, J. C., and I. C. Schafrick. "The relevant internal rate of return." *The Engineering Economist* 49.2 (2004): 139–158.

[64] https://www.hyperledger.org/

Key Attribute to Consider	Blockchain	Relational Database
Cryptography	Yes	No
Authority	Decentralized	Centralized
Architecture	Peer-to-peer	Client Server/ Cloud
Cost	Costly	Less Expensive
Data Handling	Write once, read many	Read, Write, Update, Delete
Data Integrity	High	Low
Transparency	High	Limited to No transparency

Source: © Paul Quigley, Bloclab Enterprises, LLC 2020.

Figure 18.12   Business case considerations: blockchain technology versus relational databases

industries such as healthcare; the horizontal technology firms (Amazon,[65] Google,[66] IBM[67]) and the professional services firms (Accenture,[68] Deloitte,[69] Ernst & Young,[70] as well as regional and specialty advisory firms), that are a good start. There are some emerging platform solutions like BurstIQ,[71] Philips Healthcare,[72] and Consortium companies like Hashed Health[73] – with more than 50 companies in its network – for the reader to explore further. Open-source consortia like Hyperledger present an innovative opportunity to collaborate within the same industry ecosystem. Healthcare innovation has been siloed and limited by existing market participants seeking profit maximization over collaboration; some of that entrenched behavior is beginning to shift as consumers and employers demand greater transparency and accountability. A public domain link has been provided to give you are more up to date list of projects, funding, and areas of focus.[74]

Healthcare Blockchain

After describing the key elements of the blockchain and some of the unique issues facing the healthcare industry we are more informed and can now look at areas in the healthcare ecosystem where blockchain could make a high-value impact. This is by no means an exhaustive catalog of companies and projects; that is beyond the scope of this primer. Several links have been provided to facilitate answers to those questions. In healthcare blockchain, the structure of the blockchain may vary but the key elements remain the same.[75] Blockchain use cases are clustered into five major

[65] https://aws.amazon.com/health/
[66] https://health.google/
[67] https://www.ibm.com/industries/healthcare
[68] https://www.accenture.com/us-en/digital-health-index
[69] https://www2.deloitte.com/us/en/industries/life-sciences-and-health-care.html
[70] https://blockchain.ey.com/
[71] https://www.burstiq.com/
[72] https://www.usa.philips.com/healthcare
[73] https://hashedhealth.com/
[74] http://biomedicalblockchain.org/
[75] Agbo, C. C., Q. H. Mahmoud, and J. M. Eklund. "Blockchain technology in healthcare: A systematic review." *Healthcare* 7 (2019): 56.

challenges in the healthcare ecosystem: identity management, interoperability, patient engagement, supply chain, and financial.

As mentioned previously, one of the most disruptive influences of blockchain may not be technology but could be the network effect on organizations. When several parties can share and trust the same information, inconsistencies are reduced and operational efficiency is inevitable. This is some of the promise of blockchain as an interoperability strategy for health systems.

Logically, it makes sense that blockchain could solidify the industry's infrastructure, but that would miss the multilevel disruptive opportunity this represents. The United States sponsored an ambitious Nationwide Interoperability Roadmap (v1.0)[76] in 2005. From that came several key initiatives to secure, extend, and prioritize critical healthcare infrastructure and included named initiatives to solve problems around identity, authorization, and access as well as permission and patient consent with electronic health information. It recognized gaps in the data schema, data semantics and incomplete data, identity, and interoperability standards. Satoshi's Bitcoin white paper was released three years after the roadmap was released and was quickly added to the technology toolbox. In March 2020, the global COVID-19 pandemic began, and the US Department of Health and Human Services and the Cybersecurity Infrastructure and Security Agency required blockchain be used to track and confirm the provenance of critical infrastructure, including the entire healthcare supply chain.[77]

The Identity Use Case

One of the most vexing administrative problems in healthcare remains the issue of identity management. The goal is to establish an immutable, portable, reliable, and accurate identity management of a person as they move through the healthcare system. The healthcare delivery system has a myriad of integrated but not interoperable computer systems. Integration with non-government insurance/payment systems are primarily focused on eligibility and benefits payment, but the turnover rate of employees in employer-sponsored[78] insurance is directly tied to the business cycle or, most recently, the pandemic. Re-enrollment of a person in another employer sponsored health plan or government program creates another unique identifier without the benefit of historical medical and encounter information. We will focus on the technical challenges of data unification under the proper identity, not the policy or financial implications. The need for absolute accuracy is directly proportional to the harm of inaccurate data placed under the wrong person or retrieval of incomplete data upon demand. Meanwhile, advances in mobile computing, secure APIs, and blockchain security have put into the hands of consumers solutions that would retain and allow authorized sharing of their medical record, genomic data, and financial/insurance information; as they engage the health system, this puts even more pressure on seamless interoperability. The consumer healthcare experience is not keeping up with the consumer retail experience, and over the last 11 years, with HIPAA breach reporting (2009 was the first mandatory reporting year),

[76] https://www.healthit.gov/sites/default/files/hie-interoperability/nationwide-interoperability-roadmap-final-version-1.0.pdf

[77] "Memorandum on Identification of essential critical infrastructure workers during COVID-19 Response" https://www.cisa.gov/sites/default/files/publications/CISA-Guidance-on-Essential-Critical-Infrastructure-Workers-1-20-508c.pdf, March 2020.

[78] Buchmueller, T. C., and A. C. Monheit. "Employer-sponsored health insurance and the promise of health insurance reform." *Inquiry: The Journal of Health Care Organization, Provision, and Financing* 46.2 (2009): 187–202.

public awareness and concern has increased in response to a series of high-profile medical record, identity, insurance, and credit card data breaches. Cybersecurity and preservation of trust have moved to the top of the already crowded priority list for healthcare technology. The United States still lacks a national single person identity standard with flexible permission layers; a permissioned blockchain or several permissioned blockchains may offer solutions to that problem.[79]

Interoperability Use Cases

The cost of data integration and interoperability is high. This is due to unclear data standards[80,81] including nonstandard customized development and minimal software vendor incentives to be interoperable. We believe interoperability should be one of the high-priority requirements after functionality for all software purchases and should weigh heavily in the total cost of ownership (TCO) models of any healthcare contracting process.

The Health Level 7 International Standards Organization (HL7) recognized the need to move faster on the issues of interoperability and launched the fast healthcare interoperability resource standard (FHIR, pronounced "fire"), building on the previous data formats that had been the primary method of data integration across systems.[82] This API-based approach was faster, easier to use, and more extensible.[83] Rapid progress is being made in the evolution of the FHIR standards, including expansion into medical applications and research.[84] In 2018, Apple announced that its health application would be FHIR compliant for medical records.[85] Blockchain should be added to these standards.

Consistent with the hype cycle of emerging technologies, we have seen over the last several years that blockchain solutions or blockchain use cases were presented to solve every problem in healthcare. Discipline and healthy skepticism should be employed when evaluating use cases for blockchain. It has been our experience that many of the use cases proposed can readily be solved using traditional database structures and not the blockchain. There are some unique areas within healthcare, such as identity, credentialing, claims payment, and interoperability, where the combination of a blockchain network and smart contracts can be combined to create a high-value solution.

A systematic industry meta-analysis review of the ongoing research in the application of blockchain technology healthcare conducted by Agbo et al.[86] in 2019 revealed that several studies have proposed different use cases for the application of blockchain in healthcare; however, there is a lack of adequate prototype implementations and studies to characterize the effectiveness of these proposed use cases.

[79] Yaga, Dylan, et al. "NISTIR 8202 blockchain technology overview." *National Institute of Standards and Technology. Recuperado de: https://nvlpubs. nist. gov/nistpubs/ir/2018/NIST. IR 8202* (2018).

[80] Massimo Ferrara, F. "The CEN healthcare information systems architecture standard and the DHE middleware. A practical support to the integration and evolution of healthcare systems." *International Journal of Medical Informatics* 48.1–3 (1998): 173–182.

[81] Brandt, Mary D. "Health informatics standards: A user's guide." *Journal of AHIMA* 71.4 (2000): 39.

[82] Spyrou, S. S., et al. "Healthcare information standards: Comparison of the approaches." *Health Informatics Journal* 8.1 (March 2002): 14–19. doi:10.1177/146045820200800103.

[83] Peterson, Kevin et al. "A blockchain-based approach to health information exchange networks." *Proc. NIST Workshop Blockchain Healthcare* 1 (2016).

[84] Gordon, William J., and Christian Catalini. "Blockchain technology for healthcare: Facilitating the transition to patient-driven interoperability." *Computational and Structural Biotechnology Journal* 16 (2018): 224–230.

[85] Zhang, Peng et al. "Metrics for assessing blockchain-based healthcare decentralized apps." In *2017 IEEE 19th international conference on e-Health networking, applications and services (Healthcom)*. IEEE, 2017.

[86] Agbo, Cornelius C., Qusay H. Mahmoud, and J. Mikael Eklund. "Blockchain technology in healthcare: A systematic review." In *Healthcare*. Vol. 7. No. 2. Multidisciplinary Digital Publishing Institute, 2019.

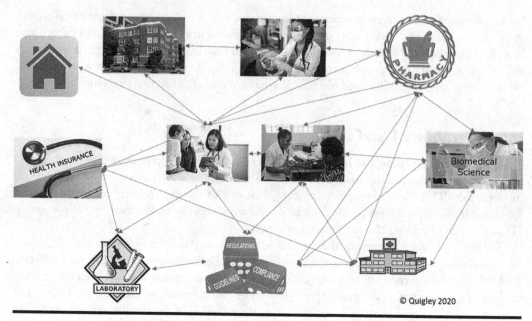

Figure 18.13 Fragmented communication and information siloes across stakeholders

Medical Records Decentralization

In healthcare, everyone is keeping their own version of the truth – their own system of record. Ledgers have existed for centuries, the most common being accounting and transaction ledgers for goods and services. A medical record is really nothing more than a composite of ledgers comprising identification, scheduling, visits, services, inventory, and charges. A patient's medical information and longitudinal healthcare information can also be considered a ledger and can be the basis for the development of a composite EHR and personal health record (PHR). The problem that would need to be resolved would be provider billing and coding, but that could be on a separate permissioned-based practice ledger. The challenge is to create a shared, permissioned, multilevel ledger as the source of truth for a consumer's healthcare services.

If designed properly, there is an opportunity to deploy a blockchain layer across medical records to improve operational efficiency (Figure 18.13) and deliver a robust patient-centric consent model. Health systems today, even those operating at HIMSS Level 4 interoperability,[87] struggle to provide the consumer an audit report of who accessed their health information over the previous year.[88]

What is revolutionary about the design of distributed ledger technology is that it is diametrically opposed to how most healthcare data is presently stored (centralized, minimally distributed applications). The technology design holds tremendous promise in making critical clinical data access (e.g., allergies, medications, diagnosis data) while at the same time democratizing data sharing, consumer control, consent, and time-limited data sharing.

---

[87] Walker, J., E. Pan, D. Johnston, J. Adler-Milstein, D. W. Bates, and B. Middleton. "The value of health care information exchange and interoperability: There is a business case to be made for spending money on a fully standardized nationwide system." *Health Affairs* 24(Suppl 1) (2005): W5–10.

[88] Laric, M. V., D. A. Pitta, and L. P. Katsanis. "Consumer concerns for healthcare information privacy: A comparison of US and Canadian perspectives." *Research in Healthcare Financial Management* 12.1 (2009): 93.

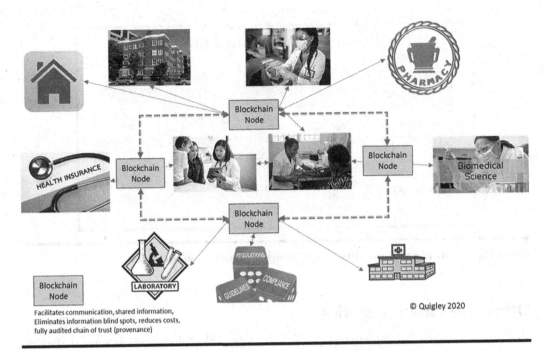

Facilitates communication, shared information,
Eliminates information blind spots, reduces costs,
fully audited chain of trust (provenance)

© Quigley 2020

Figure 18.14   Improved health information exchange managed by a blockchain identity layer

Innovation of blockchain-based medical records is underway;[89,90] however, the United States maybe a laggard in this area because of entrenched existing first-generation EHR companies, generational provider fatigue converting paper-based records to electronic records, and the fragmented profit maximization motivation of existing stakeholders.

The development of ACOs, where networks of providers have aligned incentives to managing a population of patients, would be good incubators for these use cases. Also, payer/provider partnerships – including Medicare and the Veterans Administration health system – allow sharing across entities through shared access, an audit trail, and authorization/authenticity confirmations of the clinical records.

Operational Efficiency and Redesign Use Cases

The healthcare communication process is fragmented and inefficient. The cost of this inefficiency results in medical errors, duplicate tests, and adverse outcomes. Figure 18.14 depicts the communication flow in across the healthcare system for one patient and includes post-acute care and the pharmacy. Electronic prescribing has been an outbound workflow improvement in all EHRs: the orders get to the pharmacy, but there is no confirmation the order was ever picked up and consumed as ordered. This is a lost opportunity for the physician and other caregivers to obtain any insight on the patient's medication consumption through the pharmacist.

---

[89] Liu, P. T. S. "Medical record system using blockchain, big data and tokenization." In *International conference on information and communications security* (pp. 254–261). Springer, 2016, November.

[90] Shahnaz, A., U. Qamar, and A. Khalid. "Using blockchain for electronic health records." *IEEE Access* 7 (2019): 147782–147795.

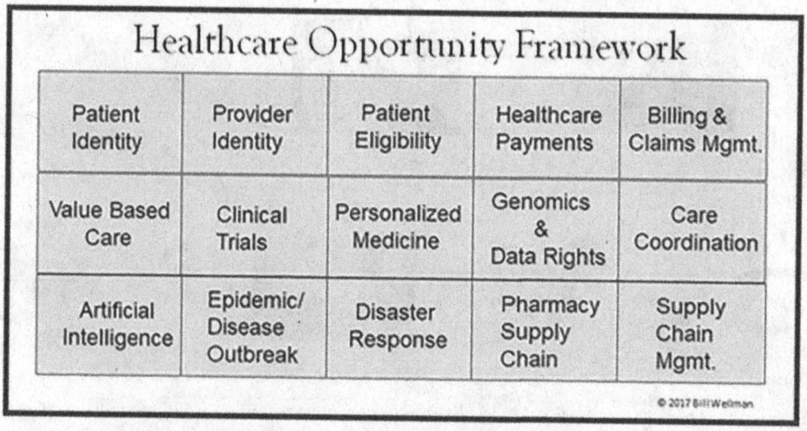

Figure 18.15   Healthcare opportunity framework for blockchain use cases

Other Use Case Categories

There have been several attempts to capture the wide range of blockchain projects across the health-care ecosystem. This has been a challenge for several reasons, as many projects are internal pilots and much of the work. If it were to extend into mainstream operation of a company, it would fundamentally challenge its corporate governance model. Represented here is a self-reported GitHub open source blockchain placemat layout[91] of the healthcare ecosystem across eight key areas.[92]

This site includes the name of the project and the company and if there have been any venture or private placement funds to support the project. Another way to look at the healthcare opportunity framework is to look at the operational framewok presented by Wellman (Figure 18.15).

There are additional projects underway inside most large insurance companies, pharmaceutical firms, and supply chain firms. Claims processing has been identified as a target for blockchain disruption or enhancement, inclusive of streamlining preauthorization submissions, health insurance claims adjudication, and eligibility management.[93,94]

These are being conducted internally and or being conducted with large integration partners such as IBM, Google, Amazon, and enterprise protocol solution providers such as Hyperledger and Oracle. Figure 18.16 presents already existing healthcare-related blockchain projects clustered around specific functional areas of the healthcare ecosystem.

With an industry consuming nearly 20% of US GDP, there are many opportunities to improve customer service, reduce operating costs, and increase communication efficiency between

[91] https://github.com/acoravos/healthcare-blockchains.

[92] Coravos, Andy and Warner, Sofia, Blockchains and health care: promising and moving quickly, though no silver bullet, Stat, 12/27,2017, updated 1/28/2019. Center for Biomedical Blockchain Research as of 4/15/2020 http://biomedicalblockchain.org/

[93] Kuo, T. T., H. E. Kim, and L. "Ohno-Machado. Blockchain distributed ledger technologies for biomedical and health care applications." *Journal of the American Medical Informatics Association* 24.6 (2017): 1211–1220.

[94] Roman-Belmonte J. M., H. De la Corte-Rodriguez, and E. C. Rodriguez-Merchan. "How blockchain technology can change medicine." *Postgraduate Medical* 130.4 (2018): 420–427.

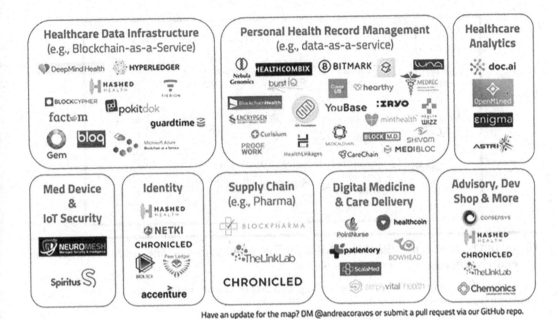

Figure 18.16 Healthcare-related blockchain projects

stakeholders. This will require political resolve and probably some national embarrassment to catch up with some of the innovations already underway in other countries. Independent of the catalyst – including a global pandemic – blockchain could be an important element in improving our technical infrastructure and improve the delivery of healthcare services.

The Blockweb: The Post-Blockchain Era

There is a convergence occurring in healthcare with blockchain: the IOT, also called the Medical Internet of Things (MIoT), and AI. It also includes the model of M2M communication and learning. Medical devices, wearables, sensors, and other pieces of hardware connected to the internet or a network are classified as IOT. Network and security monitoring using blockchains for device authentication and validation of device integrity may become cost-effective[95] input data to AL alert and event platforms.

Medical and nursing students are already using AI-assisted learning diagnostic programs, and some subspecialty areas in medicine are successfully using M2M "over-reading" of radiologic, pathology, and laboratory results. Most inpatient and some ambulatory EHR systems have ongoing sepsis detection, drug-to-drug interaction, and cardiac risk surveillance programs running in the background, which are programmed to deliver clinical alerts to physicians and nurses. All

---

[95] Mackey, Tim K., et al. " 'Fit-for-purpose?' – challenges and opportunities for applications of blockchain technology in the future of healthcare." *BMC medicine* 17.1 (2019): 68.

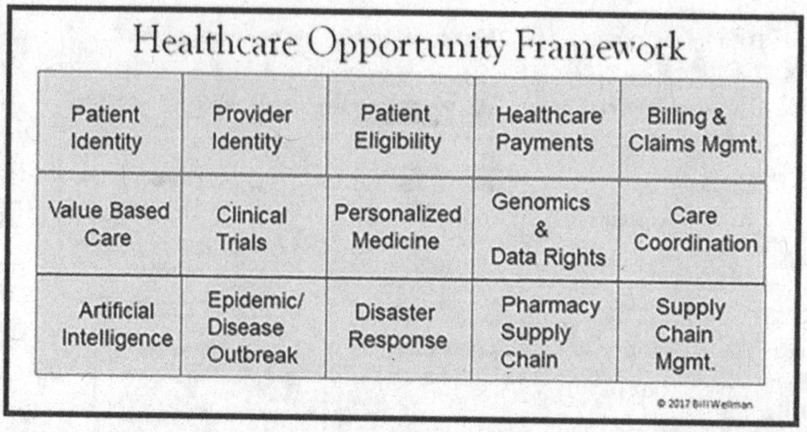

Healthcare Opportunity Framework

Patient Identity	Provider Identity	Patient Eligibility	Healthcare Payments	Billing & Claims Mgmt.
Value Based Care	Clinical Trials	Personalized Medicine	Genomics & Data Rights	Care Coordination
Artificial Intelligence	Epidemic/ Disease Outbreak	Disaster Response	Pharmacy Supply Chain	Supply Chain Mgmt.

© 2017 Bill Wellman

Figure 18.17   Next-generation blockchains for the machine-to-machine (M2M) economy will use entirely different consensus protocols

Source: Max Thake, Blockchain vs DAG Technology, with permission. https://101blockchains.com/consensus-algorithms-blockchain/

these programs operate in closed, permissioned systems where operating a clinical blockchain application would be unnecessarily expensive and deliver limited value.

When data gathering extends beyond the perimeter of a clinic, medical office, or a hospital into a less controlled environment (including telehealth, remote sensors, and other behavioral data), provenance of the data source is a prudent risk mitigation strategy.[96]

Beyond the identity challenges addressed in prior sections of this chapter, a host of practical issues need to be overcome in IOT, including the limited programmable/BIOS capacity of an IOT device, network latency, and the speed of the consensus protocol to verify the sensor and its data.

This places unique design requirements (Figure 18.17) on any M2M network and will exceed the traditional blockchain-based (Figure 18.2) capacity of block-based networks. Most healthcare IOT uses cases will find commonality in the industrial market and smart cities. However, healthcare has a different risk threshold, additional regulatory oversight, and possibly direct consequences from the US Food and Drug Administration (FDA) if subject to distributed denial of service (DDoS) attacks.[97] As more and more clinical care is being delivered at home, post-acute care monitoring and care management will need to be triaged so the limited capacity of clinicians can be prioritized by trustworthy monitoring systems.[98,99]

The speed requirement for M2M consensus requires a different approach than the proof-of-work consensus model. The decentralized ledger remains the same; the original blockchain model is very robust and secure but inherently slow, handling a limited number of transactions at a time.

[96] Kuo, Tsung-Ting, Hyeon-Eui Kim, and Lucila Ohno-Machado. "Blockchain distributed ledger technologies for biomedical and health care applications." *Journal of the American Medical Informatics Association* 24.6 (2017): 1211–1220.

[97] Banerjee, Mandrita, Junghee Lee, and Kim-Kwang Raymond Choo. "A blockchain future for internet of things security: A position paper." *Digital Communications and Networks* 4.3 (2018): 149–160.

[98] Griggs, Kristen N., et al. "Healthcare blockchain system using smart contracts for secure automated remote patient monitoring." *Journal of Medical Systems* 42.7 (2018): 130.

[99] Gupta, Rajneesh. *Hands-on cybersecurity with blockchain: Implement DDoS protection, PKI-based identity, 2FA, and DNS security using blockchain.* Packt Publishing Ltd, 2018.

Public blockchains (Bitcoin and Ethereum) are operating in the range of 8–20 transactions per second. This is not even usable when the sensor data feed rates could be thousands of data points reporting per minute, so a different approach is required. There are several innovations using entirely different structures, loosely termed post-blockchain solutions; these are permissioned blockchain that use a directed acrylic graph (DAG) system instead of a "chain." The DAG maybe best described as a block web instead of a blockchain.

Examples of these post-blockchain directed acrylic graphs are Hashgraph and IOTA, Byteball Bytes, and Nano Block Lattice. We will examine these post-blockchain use cases in another chapter.

Conclusion

In this chapter, we have introduced an entirely new disruptive innovation called blockchain technology that is beginning to have an impact across the entire healthcare industry. This technology is ideally suited to heavily regulated, information-intensive siloed industries; healthcare is uniquely qualified, and its costs have now exceeded more than 20% of US GDP. Cost containment measures and policy changes have had very little impact on changing the cost trajectory; the per capita cost in the United States continues to rise without a measurable improvement in quality. This requires that we look at the fundamental structural elements of the industry and explore new forms of collaboration that will reduce cost, measurably improve quality, and improve communication while remaining committed to improving security and privacy. We believe the blockchain can provide a decentralized platform for this information sharing and consent-based control at a lower cost.

We explored each critical element of the blockchain, using the Bitcoin blockchain as a model, while acknowledging the proliferation of several different blockchains and different consensus mechanisms. The development of specialized blockchains including public trustless and private blockchains are inevitable, but the basic design principles remain the same. Project-based blockchain initiatives were identified as well as the projected growth of blockchain across the industry. Several use cases were examined in detail specifically around identity, interoperability, and operational improvement. Several blockchain frameworks were provided to examine new blockchain opportunities. This chapter concluded with an introduction to the post-blockchain web and the emerging blockchain solutions that could be used for the emerging MIoT and the M2M economy. This is very important, as care within the healthcare system is becoming more decentralized, and data acquisition, monitoring, and security must be conducted in less controlled environments. The reader is encouraged to examine the footnotes for more information if they choose to pursue any of these topics in greater detail.

About the Author

Paul Quigley, MBA, is the CEO/CTO/co-founder of www.Liberado.io, a Wyoming-based start-up digital asset custody solution-as-a-service (SaaS) platform designed to support merchant, bank, and credit union partnerships. Paul is a serial entrepreneur with leadership, strategic, operating, and technical experience in eight start-up companies, one IPO, and two private exits. He has domestic and international experience in more than 20 high-growth and complex turnaround environments across several industries, including banking and healthcare. He was an early adopter (2012) of the blockchain and the use cases for interoperability, cryptocurrency, and identity management.

Paul spent more than 10 years at the international consulting firms of Ernst & Young and Accenture as a senior manager in their emerging technology practices. He was a founding member of the International Blockchain Lab for Philips Healthcare in the Netherlands, examining the global impact of Blockchain across all of Philips' product lines. He is presently a member of several Hyperledger (Linux Foundation) workgroups.

Paul is an Adjunct Professor at Harvard University's Graduate School of Arts and Sciences and co-teaches a graduate course about disruptive innovation, blockchain, and artificial Intelligence (ME-4508).

Paul recently completed a term as a governor-appointed (2018–2019) member for the Colorado Council for the Advancement of Blockchain Technology, which brought new legislation to Colorado for Open Blockchain/Utility Token/Virtual Currency Money Transmitter Exemption Bills to Colorado. He speaks regionally, nationally, and internationally (World Economic Forum) on the uses of blockchain in banking, financial services, and identity.

He was an active participant in the Wyoming Blockchain Coalition and helped bring 13 landmark pieces of legislation into Wyoming, and into the United States for an open blockchain, the definition of a utility token and SPDI (Special Purpose Depository Institution). This legislation has been adopted across more than 17 other states. This legislation is creating new space and a stable legal framework for digital asset innovation.

Paul is an honors graduate of the Massachusetts Institute of Technology (MIT) Fintech/Blockchain Certificate Program, has an MBA in entrepreneurship and finance from the F. W. Olin Graduate School of Business, Babson College, and is an honors graduate of Northeastern University, College of Health Sciences.

He earned a PhD in health services administration, an MBA from the University of Alabama at Birmingham (UAB), and an MS in information and communication sciences from Ball State University. He has published research articles in academic journals (e.g., *Health Care Management Review, Preventive Medicine, Journal of General Internal Medicine*, and *Studies in Health Technology and Informatics*) and presented at a number of conferences (e.g., Healthcare Information and Management Systems Society, Academy of Management, American Medical Informatics Association, and Academy Health).

Chapter 19

IoT Is Watching You

Salvatore G. Volpe, MA and
Paul Quigley, MBA

Contents

> The telescreen received and transmitted simultaneously. Any sound that Winston made, above the level of a very low whisper, would be picked up by it, moreover, so long as he remained within the field of vision which the metal plaque commanded, he could be seen as well as heard. There was of course no way of knowing whether you were being watched at any given moment.
>
> George Orwell, 1984[1]

Introduction

Some of the greatest advancements in technology were predicted by authors of science fiction decades before they ever made their way into our homes. One such invention is the telescreen of George Orwell's dystopian novel, *1984*. The telescreen, in many ways, is reminiscent of Skype or the now-ubiquitous Zoom, but it most frighteningly mirrors the voice-activated assistants taking over households across the world. Is your watch listening to everything you say? If you forget to turn off the camera on your webcam, will hackers be able to see into your house? These are all questions we ask now because of the fear instilled by entities like Big Brother, which used inanimate

DOI: 10.4324/9780429423109-19

objects to know everything about everyone. These inanimate objects, or smart objects, are all connected through the Internet of Things (IoT), which has been used in healthcare since 1997.[2]

This chapter is a brief survey of the vast landscape that is the IoT, its role in today's healthcare, and the role it will likely play in the future. First, we will discuss what exactly IoT is and why we should embrace it with open arms. After we establish a baseline for understanding IoT, we will review its applications in healthcare, which fall under two major categories: clinical services and operational support. There is a wide range of clinical services that benefit from IoT, such as patient monitoring, wearable devices for complementary physiological data collection, and artificial intelligence (AI)–facilitated clinical decision support (CDS). As for operational support, IoT helps facilitate asset tracking, warranty repair and recall compliance; remote data gathering to help organizations monitor product supply chains; environmental and temperature monitoring; GPS localization; asset protection; and potential fraud or tampering. Then, equipped with a clear definition of IoT and tangible examples, we will take a step back to acknowledge the importance of provenance, a data governance framework, and organizational governance to the success of IoT-enabled technologies in healthcare and globally. Finally, we will conclude by reviewing some open issues to consider in the hopes that we do not end up in Orwell's Oceania.

Internet of Things

We are all familiar with the internet, but what makes IoT so special? Well, the term "Internet of Things" began as a title for a presentation at Procter & Gamble in 1999 regarding linking supply chains using radio frequency identification (RFID).[3–4] Kevin Ashton, known as the Father of IoT, initially used the phrase to signify the need to use all of the things that exist in the world that help us capture information. Human time and attention are limited by population, skill, and availability; however, computers are not limited by the same constraints. If computers are taught to digest "things" in the form of bits rather than human-processed ideas, the potential could be limitless. Fast-forward 20 years, and we end up with a revolutionary new principle that is making its way into newspaper headlines, viral videos from Bosch,[5] and even your informatics primer. Now, IoT has become "a world-wide network of interconnected objects uniquely identifiable, based on standard communication protocols."[6]

These interconnected objects, commonly referred to as smart devices, are quite literally everywhere and could be almost anything (Figure 19.1). From your cell phone to your refrigerator, a smart device is any physical device with a unique identity (ID) and an "address" (a serial internet protocol [IP] address), which broadcasts a defined set of data about itself, position, activity, or environment. The devices tend to utilize simple digital or analog sensors that perform one or two operations. Because simplicity lies at the heart of the IoT device, any smart-enabled object can collect a wide variety of data from the physical world, from acceleration and geopositioned tilt on an axis plane to chemical composition of gas in the air, and convert it to digital data (Figure 19.2).

Smart devices transmit a very limited amount of information at tremendous speeds – some as fast as 10,000+ transactions per second, in comparison to the 8–20 transactions per second of public blockchains like Bitcoin and Ethereum. IoT requires a very different computing and data management paradigm because, unlike public blockchains, IoT devices are often static once deployed and, if they are remote sensors (e.g., active RFID tags), they are constrained by battery life. To put this in perspective, the magnitude of difference between transaction rates of a IoT network and a public blockchain is the top velocity of an F-16 fighter jet (IoT) and a garden snail (public blockchain). IoT blockchains achieve almost frictionless transmission rates thanks to their

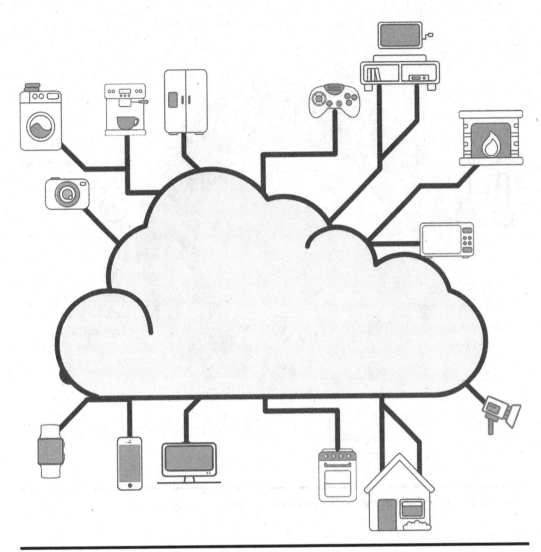

Figure 19.1 Various devices that can be smart enabled

underlying directed acyclic graph (DAG) architecture (Editor's note: see chapter 18 Blockchain). Rather than facilitating a human-to-machine consensus model, IoT operates under a machine-to-machine (M2M) model. We have just shown you what happens at the device level, but now let us consider what happens when we view M2M architectures at a macro scale, one example of which is the smart city[7-8] (Figure 19.3). Think about how many people use resources every day in a major city like New York City, with a population of 8.4 million (2020). Using industrial IoT, every instance of usage for a particular service can be collected as a data point and distributed through smart-enabled technology. Smart cities can employ machine learning (ML) and AI technologies to verify, manage, and analyze the deluge of data generated by the city to improve transportation signals, energy efficiency, foster economic growth, and improve the quality of life for its citizens. Such information can also be of great benefit to healthcare systems and public health organizations for ongoing initiatives – as well as during pandemics.[9-11]

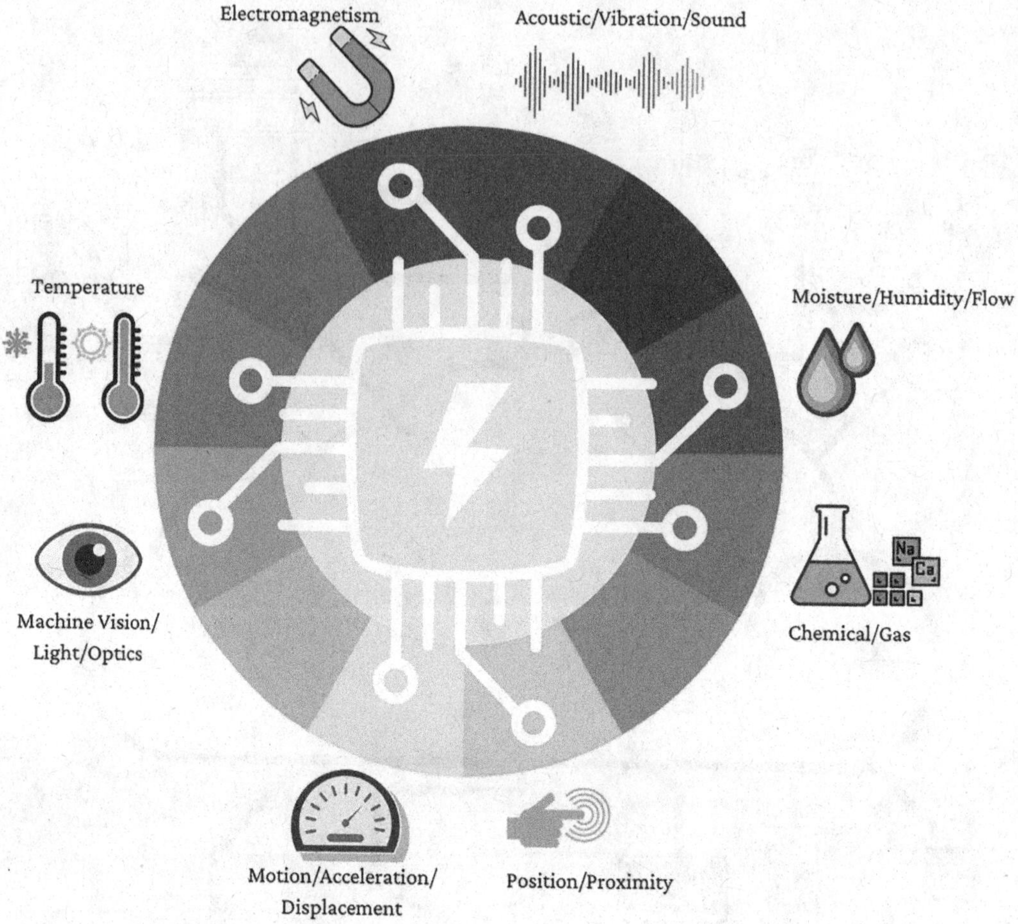

Figure 19.2   Sample of data modalities processed by smart devices

Medical Internet of Things

Now that we have introduced you to the IoT and have shown you actual examples of IoT devices, we will narrow the rest of this discussion to IoT in healthcare. We will begin with the first "smart" medical devices brought into healthcare: the smart inhaler.[12] Inhalers are used to deliver medications to treat asthma, chronic obstructive pulmonary disease (COPD), and other respiratory conditions. The device was a plastic container that replaced standard inhaler canisters. The smart inhaler recorded dose actuations and could be connected to a computer to graph them against time on a regular basis. Though the technology was not wireless, devices like the smart inhaler led to the development and widespread use of other smart medication adherence devices, such as smart pill bottles, smart pill organizers, smart injectable devices, and "true" smart inhalers.[13] The groundwork has already been laid for IoT across the healthcare industry, but now we finally have a label we can use to define this whole category of innovations: healthcare or medical IoT (MIoT).

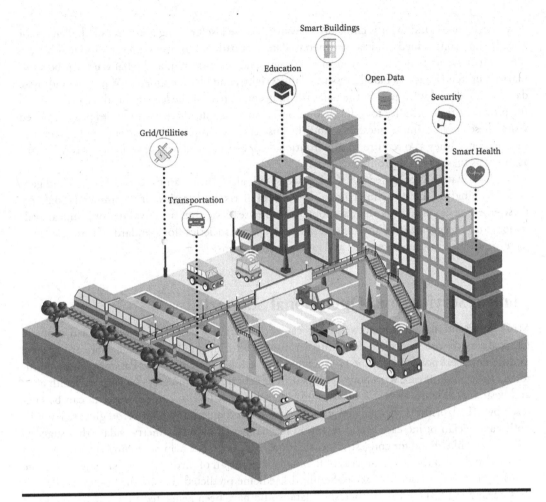

Figure 19.3   Processes that can connect in a smart city

MIoT enables tracking, sensing, and (when validated through the blockchain) immutable data validation[6] and has the potential to yield immense economic, security, and quality of care benefits.[14] By connecting these unique devices to a unique person at a verifiable location and time, we can capture a more complete digital representation of a patient's health in their own environment. We can also gain important insight into a person's physiological response to treatment outside the simulated environment of an exam room, clinic, or hospital. The patient and provider no longer need proximity to each other to assess and observe findings thanks to the incorporation of smart devices in telehealth.

Smart devices can be programmed based on physiological parameters, direct activation orders, or as part of an integrated telehealth visit.[15] In these scenarios, physiological, observational, and verbal datherwhich are generally encrypted, are securely collected about the patient in their home and then transmitted to the provider's electronic health record (EHR). This new capability, while offering both consumers and providers a new access channel to healthcare service, prompts us to now ask a new set of questions we did not have the perspective to ask before: what information do we really need, and what is clinically relevant? We are also creating a new set of challenges for already time-constrained clinicians related to data overload and information starvation. What are the seminal events that require clinical evaluation and intervention, and what data can be summarized in trends, such as blood pressure, daily weights, and blood oximetry? Where should these data be stored, and what part of the data stream becomes part of the legal clinical record? What is the provider's responsibility for data that becomes available outside the boundaries of a scheduled visit? These are not simple questions, and the answers have implications for both physicians and their patients. They also require an organizational commitment to data governance and risk management as these systems proliferate.

As information is collected by MIoT devices, ML algorithms can process these data and generate meaningful CDS for clinicians in the form of alerts, odds ratios, or recommendations. All these emerging access points and data sources require security attestation/validation, clinical evaluation, and endorsement by their respective professional societies (for standard of care and treatment protocols), risk management, and cybersecurity teams.

Clinical Services and Operational Support

MIoT interventions fall under two broad categories: clinical services and operational support. Clinical services can be broken down further into monitoring and CDS, which more or less serve as different checkpoints along the chronological timeline of care delivery. Patients can be monitored at the point of care with body sensors or remotely through integrations with mHealth apps and wearables (Figure 19.4).[14,16] Once transmitted by an IoT sensor node, the data can be analyzed by ML algorithms that may prompt an alert about dangerously high blood glucose levels or notify a clinician of increased fluid retention or changes in blood oximetry – data that suggests an increased likelihood for congestive heart failure. ML and CDS help to circumvent information overload and avoid the costly process of manually labeling all of medical data that enters from the MIoT system.[17] For a sense of scale, Stanford Medicine predicted that by the end of 2020, over 2,314 exabytes (2,314 × 10^9 gigabytes) of data would have been generated from the health sector globally.[18] CDS tools have the capacity to send and receive information from patients as well as clinicians. There is a growing community of patients who are leveraging the bidirectionality of MIoT systems in open-source technologies for diabetes self-management (OpenAPS)[19] or other chronic conditions such as HIV and COPD.[20]

With respect to operational support, the biggest concerns center around fraud prevention, supply chain management, and data integrity. Smart devices are founts of much more information than you would expect and could betray you in the blink of an eye.[21] Penetration tests, which are performed to determine the quality of security in many smart devices, have proven that you could steal someone's Wi-Fi password and – with some coding knowledge and a Google search[22] – plot a map of every person who bought a particular tea kettle. The company that designed the product has since improved their security protocols, but this serves as an example of how easily these devices can be manipulated if we are not too careful. When it comes to medical devices, the US Food and Drug Association (FDA) now requires devices to provide monitoring compliance with warranty services, upgrades, and BIOS upgrades.[23–24] Device notifications (push or pull) now save providers and manufacturers considerable time and expenses in compliance monitoring.

The pharmaceutical industry has a sizable investment in IoT for fraud prevention as well as supply chain management and verifying product integrity.[25] Pharmaceutical companies employ the IoT to enable preventive maintenance of equipment, control the drug manufacturing environment,

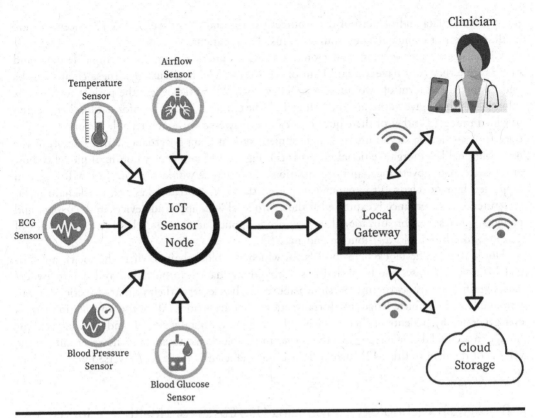

Figure 19.4 MIoT e-health environment

and facilitate monitoring of the supply chain through RFID tagging and GPS tracking. For example, if someone were to tamper with an IV pump, the machine can send information to the appropriate database from the system BIOS. After receiving the valid notification, a software probe will return to the pump to change the BIOS, and the pump will perform database updates behind a firewall to verify that it works properly.

Provenance, Data Governance, and Organizational Governance

IoT has been on the US government's radar since 2008, when it was labeled by the National Intelligence Council as one of six disruptive civil technologies to have potential impacts on US interests by 2025.[26] Since then, a number of regulatory bodies have paid particular attention to IoT and its associated technologies, including the FDA,[27–28] the Federal Trade Commission (FTC),[29] the Environmental Protection Agency (EPA),[30] and the European Union General Data Protection Regulation (GDPR).[31–32] These organizations, whose purviews had previously been siloed, now have to work in collaboration as IoT imposes new connections between them and introduces jurisdictional data concerns on a global scale. We have a responsibilher when handling IoT and MIoT to apply the same degree of provenance, governance, and privacy protection that we would employ for information generated from claims data or from the EHR. The only difference with MIoT is the volume of data and breadth of data sources. At the end of the day, MIoT advancements are producing new or complementary sources of insight on patients.

Clinicians are relying more and more on MIoT to provide them with actionable data, and they assume that they have a clear chain of trust and a chain of custody. These chains can be understood in the form of two questions: "How do I, the clinician, get the patient to trust the information that I give to them?" and "How do I, the clinician, trust the information that is being provided to me?" Neither of these questions can be answered without a reliable history of data to trace (provenance), a secure internal management system (data governance), and support at the organizational level (organizational governance). Figure 19.5 provides an optimal model of how provenance, data governance, and organizational governance would play out in a MIoT system supported by blockchain. Provenance is achieved through the data lakes and blockchain infrastructure; data governance is expressed at the micro level with apps and devices in the patient and provider spheres; and organizational governance is applied at the macro level from the point of data creation through its distribution and analysis.

Unlike the public blockchain models, in which the blockchain itself is the focus, an optimal MIoT system uses the blockchain as a ubiquitous data transportation and data/network/device verification infrastructure. As shown above, the blocks serve their primary function (i.e., an immutable and complete ledger of all transactions that are made). All of the information that is ever generated by patients or their clinicians is encrypted, digitally signed, and then indexed for storage in a data lake. We recognize the power in the blockchain networks; however, due to the volume of the data in this M2M network, it is most efficiently managed/traversed with a web of

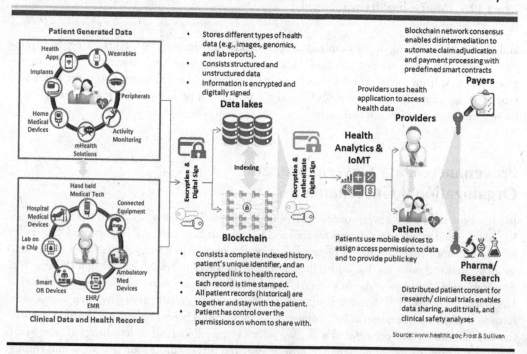

Figure 19.5   Blockchain technology use cases with MIoT

Source: Frost and Sullivan (www.healthit.gov).

blocks rather than a series of chains. A web of blocks relies on a different consensus mechanism than blockchains, and there are a number of options in the financial sector that rely on DAG systems, such as Hedera Hashgraph,[33] Tangle from Eclipse and IOTA,[34–35] and Obytes.[36] The distributed environment of MIoT requires decentralized security rather than a centralized environment because numerous parties are included on every transaction. If we assume that every transaction is a penetration risk into the network (bad actors feeding false information to a network), then we need to have a reliable model to incorporate known devices and their corresponding data stream service in place. High-speed, network-aware blockchain technology may be a viable lightweight solution because it helps to facilitate provenance fairly well, and its security and encryption requirements are also useful in data governance.

Within any MIoT system, there is bound to be a network of devices that need to be managed securely. As previously mentioned, IoT systems through the last decade have been susceptible to attacks because of limitations in engineering, authentication architecture, and direct connection to the cloud.[37–38] Developing systems that rely on smart contracts and blockchains help to preserve security and hold the data to a higher privacy standard. There have already been some solutions proposed for the management of MIoT networks using Ethereum smart contracts,[39] as well as additional cryptographic privacy and security measures imposed on blockchains.[40] With regard to managing open-source technology, the current model in healthcare prioritizes compliance and policy rather than governance, which is part of what makes the use of those solutions simultaneously enticing and dangerous. Individuals have the capacity to fork (i.e., generate local instances) of entire directories of open-source code and derive their own implementations. The availability of these open-source applications, however, generally is accompanied by a call for standardization.

The need for standards is to be expected with any informatics intervention but maybe not standardization. The call for standardization generally occurs not because no one has created a standard, but it is more likely that standards are not being enforced or implemented. Standards are less likely to be implemented at the device level (except perhaps for security)[14,41] than at the data level. Semantic interoperability between datasets and ontologies facilitates data processing and yields more meaningful ML results without stifling the innovation of engineers. For this reason, governing bodies and regulatory organizations often create unintended obstacles when they intervene in the name of standardization.

Conclusion

We have come quite a long way since Orwell's original predictions in 1948, despite taking a bit longer than the 35 years he had imagined. From creating secure whole-body sensor networks[40] to using IoT and blockchain technology to fight the COVID-19 pandemic,[42] MIoT has revolutionized the study and delivery of healthcare. Despite this progress, there are several challenges that must be addressed before MIoT reaches its peak efficacy and is ubiquitous in the healthcare system. There needs to be the development of a clear business case, including insight about the actual life of end users (the patients and their environment). This will be critical for the development of business, financial, and operating models of any company or project. These entities need a clear cybersecurity and data security operating plan as well as a clear, consent-based permission model to use the data. Further, any model they develop must be interoperable with other systems to share data with clear provenance or immutable reference to provenance. As you can see, much of the model needs to function within a principle-based governance and operational framework; these parameters apply to any company, stand-alone project, or additional partners in the healthcare system.

Moreover, the healthcare system needs to bring attention to financial incentives for clinicians and hospital systems to introduce MIoT technology into their infrastructure. The current fee-for-service (FFS) model, which sets a maximum fee, does not compensate providers for wellness in visit-based services. Economically, FFS exists as a proxy for workflow and the cost/complexity burden and operates exclusively within the bounds of visit-based codes. Without a means for reimbursement, as cost of equipment and integration in hospitals can be possibly as high as $60,000,[43] many providers have been hesitant to incorporate virtual care technologies. According to the Deloitte Center for Healthcare Solutions 2018 surveys of US health care consumers and physicians,[44] 50% of consumers use technology to track their health information, and 53% of consumers share this information with their healthcare provider. Only 9% of providers, however, have implemented remote monitoring and/or integration of data from wearables, with just 27% having intended to add this capability by the end of 2020. Alternatively, the value-based care model, which has gained increased traction over the last decade, offers reimbursement based on health outcomes and patient wellness and presents greater incentive to providers and health systems to implement more MIoT devices and CDS systems.[45-46]

This chapter is just a primer on IoT, but it does introduce you to some of the challenges, advancements, and possibilities of MIoT. We hope that this has awakened your interest to the power of MIoT, and we encourage you to explore our references to gain a deeper insight on the vast reaches of IoT in healthcare.

About the Authors

Salvatore G. Volpe, MA, is a medical student at SUNY Downstate College of Medicine pursuing a joint MD/MPH degree. He earned his MA in biomedical informatics from Columbia University, where he also received his BA in neuroscience with a concentration in computer science.

His areas of research include interoperability, quality improvement, user-interface design, patient-centered technologies, and health equity. Salvatore's graduate studies culminated in a thesis project developing a pipeline for transforming clinical trial data using Fast Healthcare Interoperability Resources (FHIR) protocols and standardized according to the Observational Medical Outcomes Partnership Common Data Model (OMOP CDM) for integration into translational research endeavors and clinical decision support. He has developed mobile applications for clinical and public use in collaboration with University of Colorado Anschultz, Cliexa, and the New York Health Artificial Intelligence Society. Salvatore has published research on COVID-19 in *Nature Communications* and has presented his research at the American Medical Informatics Association Annual Symposium.

When he isn't trying to become a medical multi-hyphenate, Salvatore is an avid musician and composer. He has written and produced songs for short films, stage plays, and full-length musicals.

Paul Quigley, is the CEO/CTO/co-founder of www.Liberado.io, a Wyoming-based start-up digital asset custody solution-as-a-service (SaaS) platform designed to support merchant, bank, and credit union partnerships. Paul is a serial entrepreneur with leadership, strategic, operating, and technical experience in eight start-up companies, one IPO, and two private exits. He has domestic and international experience in more than 20 high-growth and complex turnaround environments across several industries, including banking and healthcare. He was an early adopter (2012) of the blockchain and the use cases for interoperability, cryptocurrency, and identity management.

Paul spent more than 10 years at the international consulting firms of Ernst & Young and Accenture as a senior manager in their emerging technology practices. He was a founding member of the International Blockchain Lab for Philips Healthcare in the Netherlands, examining the global impact of Blockchain across all of Philips' product lines. He is presently a member of several Hyperledger (Linux Foundation) workgroups.

Paul is an Adjunct Professor at Harvard University's Graduate School of Arts and Sciences and co-teaches a graduate course about disruptive innovation, blockchain, and artificial Intelligence (ME-4508).

Paul recently completed a term as a governor-appointed (2018–2019) member for the Colorado Council for the Advancement of Blockchain Technology, which brought new legislation to Colorado for Open Blockchain/Utility Token/Virtual Currency Money Transmitter Exemption Bills to Colorado. He speaks regionally, nationally, and internationally (World Economic Forum) on the uses of blockchain in banking, financial services, and identity.

He was an active participant in the Wyoming Blockchain Coalition and helped bring 13 landmark pieces of legislation into Wyoming, and into the United States for an open blockchain, the definition of a utility token and SPDI (Special Purpose Depository Institution). This legislation has been adopted across more than 17 other states. This legislation is creating new space and a stable legal framework for digital asset innovation.

Paul is an honors graduate of the Massachusetts Institute of Technology (MIT) Fintech/ Blockchain Certificate Program, has an MBA in entrepreneurship and finance from the F. W. Olin Graduate School of Business, Babson College, and is an honors graduate of Northeastern University, College of Health Sciences.

He earned a PhD in health services administration, an MBA from the University of Alabama at Birmingham (UAB), and an MS in information and communication sciences from Ball State University. He has published research articles in academic journals (e.g., *Health Care Management Review, Preventive Medicine, Journal of General Internal Medicine*, and *Studies in Health Technology and Informatics*) and presented at a number of conferences (e.g., Healthcare Information and Management Systems Society, Academy of Management, American Medical Informatics Association, and Academy Health).

References

1. Orwell G. *1984*. Secker and Warburg; 1949.
2. Saffo P. Sensors: The next wave of innovation. *Commun ACM*. 1997;40(2):92–97. doi:10.1145/253671.253734.
3. Ashton K. *That "Internet of Things" Thing*. Published online June 2009:1.
4. Madakam S, Ramaswamy R, Tripathi S. Internet of things (IoT): A literature review. *J Comput Commun*. 2015;03(05):164–173. doi:10.4236/jcc.2015.35021.
5. *The Internet of Things Presents – #LikeABosch*. Accessed October 15, 2020. https://www.youtube.com/watch?v=v2kV6pgJxuo&list=PLToTXrdo6ZYFXnbQRx1a7OV_22jEZTYFE.
6. Atzori L, Iera A, Morabito G. The internet of things: A survey. *Comput Netw*. 2010;54(15):2787–2805. doi:10.1016/j.comnet.2010.05.010.
7. Gaur A, Scotney B, Parr G, McClean S. Smart city architecture and its applications based on IoT. *Procedia Comput Sci*. 2015;52:1089–1094. doi:10.1016/j.procs.2015.05.122.
8. Lai CS, Jia Y, Dong Z, et al. A review of technical standards for smart cities. *Clean Technol*. 2020;2(3):290–310. doi:10.3390/cleantechnol2030019.
9. Allam Z, Tegally H, Thondoo M. Redefining the use of big data in urban health for increased liveability in smart cities. *Smart Cities*. 2019;2(2):259–268. doi:10.3390/smartcities2020017.

10. Allam Z, Jones DS. On the coronavirus (COVID-19) outbreak and the smart city network: Universal data sharing standards coupled with artificial intelligence (AI) to benefit urban health monitoring and management. *Healthcare*. 2020;8(1):46. doi:10.3390/healthcare8010046.

11. Allam Z, Jones DS. Pandemic stricken cities on lockdown. Where are our planning and design professionals [now, then and into the future]? *Land Use Policy*. 2020;97:104805. doi:10.1016/j.land usepol.2020.104805.

12. Burgess SW, Wilson SSI, Cooper DM, Sly PD, Devadason SG. In vitro evaluation of an asthma dosing device: The smart-inhaler. *Respir Med*. 2006;100(5):841–845. doi:10.1016/j.rmed.2005.09.004.

13. Aungst T. The big list of digital health medication list companies. *Pharmacy Times*. Published November 2, 2018. Accessed October 16, 2020. https://www.pharmacytimes.com/contributor/timothy-aungst-pharmd/2018/11/the-big-list-of-digital-health-medication-list-companies.

14. Islam SMR, Kwak D, Kabir MDH, Hossain M, Kwak K-S. The internet of things for health care: A comprehensive survey. *IEEE Access*. 2015;3:678–708. doi:10.1109/ACCESS.2015.2437951.

15. How IoT is improving patient care. *Digital Health*. Published November 21, 2019. Accessed January 15, 2021. https://www.digitalhealth.net/2019/11/how-iot-is-improving-patient-care/.

16. Griggs KN, Ossipova O, Kohlios CP, Baccarini AN, Howson EA, Hayajneh T. Healthcare blockchain system using smart contracts for secure automated remote patient monitoring. *J Med Syst*. 2018;42(7):130. doi:10.1007/s10916-018-0982-x.

17. Yang Y, Nan F, Yang P, et al. GAN-based semi-supervised learning approach for clinical decision support in health-IoT platform. *IEEE Access*. 2019;7:8048–8057. doi:10.1109/ACCESS.2018.2888816.

18. Stanford Medicine. 2017. *Health Trends Report: Harnessing the Power of Data in Health*. Stanford Medicine, 2017. http://med.stanford.edu/school/leadership/dean/healthtrends.html.

19. Ragan SM. Medicine ignored this insulin problem. Hackers solved it. *Medium*. Published January 11, 2019. Accessed October 15, 2020. https://medium.com/neodotlife/dana-lewis-open-aps-hack-artificial-pancreas-af6ef23a997f.

20. Reeder B, Cook PF, Meek PM, Ozkaynak M. Smart watch potential to support augmented cognition for health-related decision making. In: Schmorrow DD, Fidopiastis CM, eds. *Augmented Cognition. Neurocognition and Machine Learning*. Lecture Notes in Computer Science. Springer International Publishing; 2017:372–382. doi:10.1007/978-3-319-58628-1_29.

21. Cronin A. Hitting the books: Hackers can convince your IoT devices to betray you. *Engadget*. Published March 26, 2020. Accessed March 28, 2020. https://www.engadget.com/2020-01-18-hitting-the-books-power-to-the-people-audrey-kurth-kronin.html.

22. *Internet of Things Security | Ken Munro | TEDxDornbirn*; 2018. Accessed October 17, 2020. https://www.youtube.com/watch?v=pGtnC1jKpMg.

23. Staff D. How to effectively meet FDA reporting requirements during a recall. *Deacom Blog*. Published October 22, 2018. Accessed January 14, 2021. https://blog.deacom.com/how-to-effectively-meet-fda-reporting-requirements-during-a-recall/.

24. Using a CMMS to comply with FDA regulations. *eMaint CMMS Software*. Published March 7, 2019. Accessed January 14, 2021. https://www.emaint.com/using-a-cmms-to-comply-with-fda-regulations/.

25. Shugalo I. The role of IoT in pharma manufacturing and distribution. *Pharma IQ*. Published February 26, 2019. Accessed October 15, 2020. https://www.pharma-iq.com/manufacturing/articles/the-role-of-iot-in-pharma-manufacturing-and-distribution.

26. National Intelligence Council. Six technologies with potential impacts on US interests out to 2025. Published April 2008:48.

27. Chacko A, Hayajneh T. Security and privacy issues with IoT in healthcare. *EAI Endorsed Trans Pervasive Health Technol Ghent*. 2018;4(14). http://dx.doi.org/10.4108/eai.13-7-2018.155079.

28. Health C for D and R. Artificial intelligence and machine learning in software as a medical device. *FDA*. Published October 5, 2020. Accessed November 14, 2020. https://www.fda.gov/medical-devices/software-medical-device-samd/artificial-intelligence-and-machine-learning-software-medical-device.

29. FTC report on internet of things urges companies to adopt best practices to address consumer privacy and security risks. *Federal Trade Commission*. Published January 27, 2015. Accessed October 16, 2020. https://www.ftc.gov/news-events/press-releases/2015/01/ftc-report-internet-things-urges-companies-adopt-best-practices.

30. The EPA has created a program for the smart home. Stacey on IoT | internet of things news and analysis. Published March 2, 2020. Accessed November 13, 2020. https://staceyoniot.com/the-epa-has-created-a-program-for-the-smart-home/.

31. Seo J, Kim K, Park M, Park M, Lee K. An analysis of economic impact on IoT industry under GDPR. *Mob Inf Syst.* 2018;2018:1–6. doi:10.1155/2018/6792028.

32. Wachter S. Normative challenges of identification in the internet of things: Privacy, profiling, discrimination, and the GDPR. *Comput Law Secur Rev.* 2018;34(3):436–449.

33. Baird DL, Harmon M, Madsen P. Hedera: A public hashgraph network & governing council. Published June 30, 2020:97.

34. McKendrick J. Enter the tangle, a blockchain designed specially for the internet of things. *ZDNet.* Published February 27, 2020. Accessed March 28, 2020. https://www.zdnet.com/article/the-tangle-or-blockchain-for-the-internet-of-things/.

35. Popov S. On the tangle, white papers, proofs, airplanes, and local modifiers. *Medium.* Published August 1, 2018. Accessed October 16, 2020. https://blog.iota.org/on-the-tangle-white-papers-proofs-airplanes-and-local-modifiers-44683aff8fea.

36. Churyumov A. Byteball: A decentralized system for storage and transfer of value. Published online October 1, 2016:49.

37. Yang Y, Wu L, Yin G, Li L, Zhao H. A survey on security and privacy issues in internet-of-things. *IEEE Internet Things J.* 2017;4(5):1250–1258. doi:10.1109/JIOT.2017.2694844.

38. Zhang B, Mor N, Kolb J, et al. The cloud is not enough: Saving IoT from the cloud. Published 2015:7.

39. Huh S, Cho S, Kim S. Managing IoT devices using blockchain platform. In: *2017 19th International Conference on Advanced Communication Technology (ICACT).*; 2017:464–467. doi:10.23919/ICACT.2017.7890132.

40. Dwivedi A, Srivastava G, Dhar S, Singh R. A decentralized privacy-preserving healthcare blockchain for IoT. *Sensors.* 2019;19(2):326. doi:10.3390/s19020326.

41. Miori V, Russo D. Anticipating health hazards through an ontology-based, IoT domotic environment. In: *2012 Sixth International Conference on Innovative Mobile and Internet Services in Ubiquitous Computing.*; 2012:745–750. doi:10.1109/IMIS.2012.109.

42. Huillet M. New blockchain solution to fight COVID-19 complies with EU data privacy regs. *Cointelegraph.* Accessed May 4, 2020. https://cointelegraph.com/news/new-blockchain-solution-to-fight-covid-19-complies-with-eu-data-privacy-regs.

43. Arndt R. Chief information officers roundtable: As technology drives consumerism, consumerism drives technology. *Modern Healthcare.* Published March 17, 2018. Accessed October 23, 2020. https://www.modernhealthcare.com/article/20180317/NEWS/180319929/chief-information-officers-roundtable-as-technology-drives-consumerism-consumerism-drives-technology.

44. Deloitte Insights. How do health care consumers and physicians perceive virtual care? Published June 14, 2018. Accessed October 23, 2020. https://www2.deloitte.com/us/en/insights/multimedia/infographics/virtual-health-care-survey-infographic.html.

45. Burrill S. *Physicians and Health Systems Could Be Left Behind.* Deloitte United States. Accessed October 23, 2020. https://www2.deloitte.com/us/en/pages/life-sciences-and-health-care/articles/health-care-current-june26–2018.html.

46. Burwell SM. Setting value-based payment goals – HHS efforts to improve U.S. Health care. *N Engl J Med.* 2015;372(10):897–899. doi:10.1056/NEJMp1500445.

Chapter 20

Case Study
New York City Department of Health and Mental Hygiene Uses of Public Health Informatics in Response to COVID-19

Contents

Introduction

Medical and public health systems face substantial challenges in responding to the COVID-19 pandemic, particularly in ensuring ongoing delivery of primary care and assuring equitable access to such care. Health information technology (IT) can facilitate tracking the impact of COVID-19 on healthcare delivery, identifying populations at risk for adverse outcomes from COVID-19,

DOI: 10.4324/9780429423109-20

and supporting engagement in ongoing primary care with at risk populations through telehealth and in-person services, as well as connecting them to resources to address needs related to social determinants of health, greatly exacerbated by COVID-19. The following case study describes how the New York City Department of Health and Mental Hygiene (NYC DOHMH) utilized health IT for these purposes.

Background Knowledge

The NYC DOHMH launched the Primary Care Informahern Project (PCIP) in 2006. The goal of PCIP was to improve the health of medically underserved communities through the herlementation of prevention-oriented electronic health record (EHR) systems. Through a competitive selection process, DOHMH selected eClinicalWorks to co-develop this prevention-oriented EHR, which is currently used by more than 640 healthcare practices across New York City, 589 of which were included in this analysis. DOHMH also worked with eClinicalWorks to create the Hub Population Health System (herein referred to as the Hub), which is a distributed query architecture that allows DOHMH to create and push queries to EHRs connected to the Hub and return aggregate count data to support quality measurement and feedback to providers, as well as public health surveillance. Additionally, DOHMH has a quality improvement team that works closely with practices participating in NYC REACH, the designated regional extension center for New York City through the former Office of National Coordinator for Health IT program. This team works with practices on implementing new clinical workflows that utilize their EHRs to drive improved prevention and chronic disease management. A critical aspect of this support is the creation and use of reports from EHRs that facilitate identification and outreach to patients with certain conditions.

Local Problem Being Addressed and Intended Improvement

The COVID-19 pandemic had a tremendous impact in New York City due to mortality and morbidity associated with COVID-19 infections, as well as reductions in healthcare seeking behaviors due to fear of exposure to the novel coronavirus at healthcare facilities. Considerable disparities were identified in the populations affected by COVID-19, with Black and Latino New Yorkers disproportionately burdened, which likely reflects longstanding policies and practices based on underlying racism that have resulted in adverse health outcomes already experienced by communities of color prior to the pandemic.[1-4] As a result, New York City designated 26 target neighborhoods for enhanced response to COVID-19, including efforts to ensure that healthcare delivery returned as quickly as possible to pre-pandemic levels. Neighborhoods were selected (see Figure 20.1) based on high COVID-19 mortality rates as well as prevalence of chronic conditions, such as diabetes, that increased risk of severe direct and related COVID-19 outcomes. Webinars were organized to help providers implement service delivery through telehealth and to offer practices help in outreach to patients in groups at higher risk for adverse outcomes from COVID-19. For practices that requested help, DOHMH reached out directly to patients in certain risk groups for serious COVID-19 disease to help connect them with their existing healthcare providers and ensure they were aware of key resources (e.g., medication refills, food, housing, health insurance, mental health support)[5-6] established therelp New Yorkers in need during the pandemic. In order to implement outreach to high-risk patients and monitor the rate of return to the healthcare delivery system, DOHMH relied heavily on EHR data.

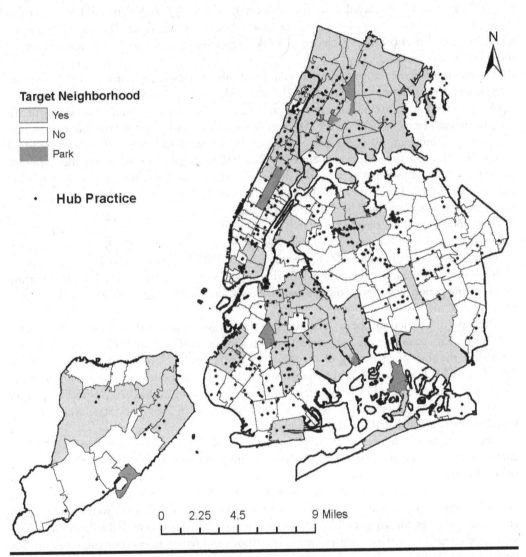

Geographic Distribution of 589 Small Practices Reporting Encounter Volumes to the Hub in Target and Non-Target Neighborhoods Across New York City

Figure 20.1 Geographic Distribution of 589 Small Practices Reporting Encounter Volumes to the Hub in Target and Non-Target Neighborhoods Across New York City

Design and Implementation

Monitoring Return to Ambulatory Care

DOHMH identified office visits and telehealth visits using evaluation and management (E&M) codes. DOHMH utilized the Hub to pull weekly ambulatory care encounter volume data in the form of aggregate counts, per practice. Data were collected and reported for 589 eligible practices on the Hub. Practices were considered eligible if they were categorized as a small practice, defined as having ten or fewer providers who each have a valid National Provider Index number and include titles such as MD, DO, or NP. Small practices were selected to complement other surveillance data from community health centers that DOHMH also monitored through other programs. Practices were excluded from weekly analysis and reporting if they did not meet this criterion or were missing data for any of the baseline or reporting weeks. Due to these requirements, the number of practices included in weekly reporting changed slightly depending on the success of data collection.

In order to track the return to normal volumes of care in ambulatory settings, weekly encounter volumes after the implementation of the statewide order to close non-essential businesses ("NYS on PAUSE")[7] were compared to a baseline average of weekly encounter volumes, calculated from the weeks preceding NYS on PAUSE in early 2020. The baseline period used for comparison began on December 29, 2019, the first Sunday of the first week in January 2020, and ended on March 14, 2020, the final Saturday before NYS on PAUSE began. Encounter volumes were collected for each week (Sunday to Saturday) during this time period. An average weekly encounter volume was calculated to create a baseline encounter volume against which subsequent weeks during the reporting period could be compared (See Table 20.1).

The reporting period started on March 15, 2020, five days in advance of NYS on PAUSE and coinciding with the announcement of school closures across NYC. Reporting of encounter volumes is ongoing as the DOHMH's response to COVID-19 continues, but for the purposes of this case study, the reporting period ends the week of August 23 to August 29, 2020. During the reporting period, encounter volumes were collected on a weekly basis and were presented as a proportion of the baseline encounter volume.

The reporting period can be divided into two sub-periods. The first sub-period coincides with NYS on PAUSE, spanning the announcement of school closures on March 15, to June 7, the last day before the start of reopening of non-essential businesses in New York State. The NYS on PAUSE period is characterized by the closure of non-essential businesses and more stringent social distancing measures across NYC. The other sub-period began on June 8, 2020 ("NYS Forward"),[8] and reflects the phased reopening of non-essential businesses in New York State and continues past the date range included in this case study.

Encounter data were further stratified by county and target neighborhood status to enable comparison of the return to baseline encounter volumes in targeted neighborhoods with return in neighborhoods that were not targeted. Additionally, encounter volumes for patients with chronic conditions, defined as having a diagnosis of diabetes, cardiovascular disease, chronic lung disease/COPD, or chronic kidney disease in their medical records were compared to encounter volumes for all patients in the general patient population. ICD diagnosis codes were used to identify patients with chronic conditions to further assess encounter data in this population.

Table 20.1   Time Period

Time Period	Baseline Period	Reporting Period	
		NYS on PAUSE	NYS Forward
Date Range	12/29/2019–3/14/2020	3/15/2020–6/7/2020	6/8/2020–Present

Technical Assistance Support to Accelerate Telehealth-Based Care Delivery in Independent Practices

Physical distancing measures to mitigate the spread of COVID-19, along with limited supplies of personal protective equipment, heightened the need for telehealth-based strategies to render ambulatory care early in the pandemic. Changes in policies by payers, along with the expanded range of acceptable technologies to deliver telehealth, were made swiftly. Rapid dissemination of information about these changes was therefore critical to ensuring provider awareness and implementation of telehealth services as quickly as possible. To that end, DOHMH launched a series of webinars directed at ambulatory care providers to communicate these important changes and address questions from providers.

A total of 13 webinars were provided over 18 weeks, with representatives from 203 provider practices participating in these webinars. Webinar content was designed to address the highest-priority needs identified by providers: billing and coding within the context of continuously changing regulations, obtaining HIPAA-compliant telehealth technology, documentation requirements, aligning with CDC guidelines to prioritize patients to engage in telehealth based on risk, and best practices for informing patients about accessing care via telehealth.

Webinar training was supplemented by a weekly email publication, which featured brief and actionable tips to enhance practices' telehealth programs, and by an email hotline where practices could submit questions. These resources were promoted within the NYC REACH provider network as well as to the greater NYC provider community through email announcements, the NYC Health Department website, and cross-marketing on citywide provider webinars.

A chief concern among practices was financial sustainability during the pandemic. Thus, the majority of the questions submitted by providers during webinars pertained to billing, coding, and reimbursement. Regulations for these changed, often weekly, in March and April. Maintaining up-to-date information on billing and coding for providers was critical to ensure they could maintain financial viability, as well as to ensure accurate coding to support DOHMH surveillance goals, which leveraged coding data to identify telehealth encounter volume. Other key issues included: barriers related to patients' access to technology like smartphones and computers, patients' comfort level using this technology, and sentiments from both provider and patient that telehealth visits came with inherent barriers like the inability to conduct a full physical examination.

Direct Patient Engagement With Individuals at High Risk for Severe COVID-19

DOHMH identified practices participating in NYC REACH that agreed to allow DOHMH staff to make proactive telephone calls to their patients who were at high risk for developing severe illness from COVID-19. A detailed script was developed for engagement with these patients, utilizing messaging on COVID-19 developed by DOHMH and other City agencies, including information on steps to take to prevent infection, what to do when experiencing symptoms, and how to access resources to address certain socioeconomic needs. In addition, details on the availability of care at these practices (in person, telehealth) were also incorporated. Persons at high risk were defined as individuals with one or more of the following chronic conditions: cardiovascular disease, diabetes, chronic lung disease, chronic kidney disease, and hypertension. Hypertension, while not directly implicated as a risk factor for severe COVID-19 disease, was selected due to its high prevalence, especially among older New Yorkers, and in order to help with self-management for these individuals. Specifically, to ensure adequate medication supplies and to prevent potential exacerbations that might result in the need for acute healthcare services (e.g., emergency department use, hospitalization). As part of practice facilitation, DOHMH staff routinely offer technical assistance to NYC REACH practices to generate lists of patients with specific conditions using health IT, and such assistance was offered during thhereffort.

The chronic diseases specified for this engagement effort were translated into their corresponding ICD diagnosis codes. Patients with one or more of these codes were identified using EHR registry reporting tools within the practice EHRs, and files including patient contact information derived from the patient record were created. These files were then transmitted via secure file transfer from the practice to DOHMH. DOHMH staff used these lists to contact patients. Given physical distancing measures and the fact that many practices were closed, DOHMH staff had to rely on virtual connections with these practices to run and securely export these reports.

Value-Derived Outcomes

Monitoring Return to Ambulatory Care

Trends in ambulatory care encounter volumes over the course of the initial COVID-19 pandemic phase are shown in Figures 20.2 and 20.3. Weekly encounter volumes during NYS on PAUSE (March 15 through June 7, 2020), expressed as a proportion of the baseline encounter volume, generally decreased and then gradually increased. During the NYS Forward period (June 8–August 29,

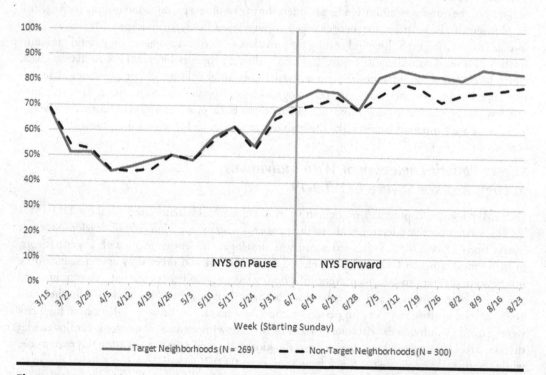

Figure 20.2 Weekly encounter volume as a proportion of baseline encounter volume across New York City

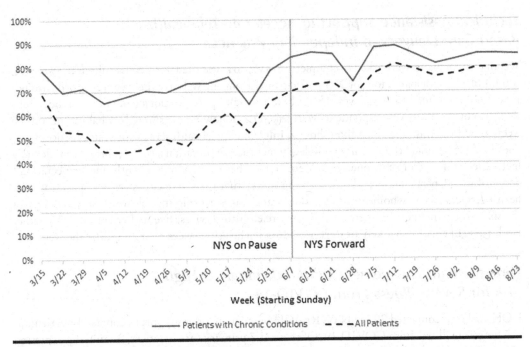

Figure 20.3   Weekly encounter volume as a proportion of baseline encounter volume, in patients with chronic conditions, across New York City

2020), weekly encounter volumes as compared to the baseline encounter volume increased week to week. In general, trends in weekly encounter volumes as compared to baseline encounter volume were similar in target versus non-target neighborhoods (Figure 20.2). These data helped inform DOHMH that, with regard to return to pre-pandemic ambulatory care volume, target neighborhoods were keeping pace with non-target neighborhoods, which include generally more affluent areas that have historically experienced better health outcomes. Similar trends were found when comparing patients with chronic conditions, defined previously, to the general patient population. However, patients with chronic conditions had consistently higher weekly encounter volumes, expressed as a proportion of baseline encounter volumes, compared to the general patient population at these practices from the start of NYS on PAUSE through NYS Forward periods (Figure 20.3). When stratified by target vs non-target neighborhoods, patients with chronic conditions continued to have higher encounter volumes compared to the general patient population.

DOHMH has previously reported on retrospective analyses that demonstrated the potential of the Hub to provide situational awareness during public health emergencies.[9–10] Here we describe prospective use of Hub data, to show how these data informed ongoing COVID-19 response efforts. Use of the Hub to enable support of ambulatory care was extremely valuable as it enabled DOHMH to implement healthcare utilization surveillance across several hundred practices in NYC with minimal commitment of resources. In the absence of the Hub, DOHMH would have had to coordinate direct data streams (automated or manual) with different practices in order to receive data to enable ongoing surveillance efforts. This would have entailed commitment of DOHMH staff and resources and would have required practices, which during the initial part of the COVID-19 pandemic were coping with urgent competing needs, to develop new data sharing agreements with DOHMH.

Technical Assistance Support to Accelerate Telehealth-Based Care Delivery in Independent Practices

Webinar participants were asked to complete a survey to assess their perspectives about the webinar. A total of 31 participants (out of 203 participants) from the webinars delivered in April through June 2020 responded to the survey. Using Likert scale response options (completely, moderately, slightly, not at all), survey respondents were asked the following question: To what extent did the webinar address your questions about how to implement telehealth services at your practice? Over one-third (35%) noted the webinar completely met their expectations, 61% reported it moderately met expectations, and only one respondent noted the webinar only slightly met expectations. Seven of the 31 participants had noted on the survey that they were currently not delivering telehealth services, six of whom noted that they wanted to start offering telehealth services. Out of the six participants noting interest in offering telehealth services, five had endorsed being either moderately likely or very likely to start providing telehealth services after attending the webinar.

Direct Patient Engagement With Individuals at High Risk for Severe Illness From COVID-19

DOHMH staff contacted 297 of NYC REACH practices to offer support in contacting patients at risk for severe illness from COVID-19. Of these 297 primary care practices, 29 initially expressed interest in the offer of direct patient engagement. DOHMH completed calls for 26 practices while four others identified staff or partners to conduct outreach.

A total of 9,272 patients with one of the chronic conditions selected and a valid telephone number were identified via EHR registry reports from the collaborating practices. The majority of patients called were female (57%) and were over 45 years old (91%) (Table 20.2). Over the course of 12 weeks, a multilingual team (Spanish, Cantonese, Mandarin, Bengali, Haitian Creole, French) of ten DOHMH staff placed calls to individuals on these lists. Forty-three percent of patients who were on these lists were successfully contacted, with no difference in the contact success rate by patient sex. Out of all patients reached, 26% expressed at least one or more needs (Table 20.3). Overall, support with medication (primarily refills) was the most common need elicited, with 59% of patients expressing needs noting this as an issue. Housing issues and food

Table 20.2   Age and Sex of Patients Called

	Called (n)	(%)	Reached (n)	(%)
Female	5326	57%	2309	58%
<45	407	4%	177	4%
45–64	2410	26%	1087	27%
65+	2509	27%	1045	26%
Male	3946	43%	1662	42%
<45	421	5%	170	4%
45–64	1937	21%	826	21%
65+	1588	17%	666	17%
Total	9272	100%	3971	100%

Table 20.3   Patients Who Expressed Any Need, and among Those, Type of Need Expressed

	Any Need (n)	(%)	Food (n)	(%)	Health Insurance (n)	(%)	Housing (n)	(%)	Medication (n)	(%)
Female	672	29%	218	32%	59	9%	219	33%	368	55%
<45	58	33%	18	31%	8	14%	19	33%	31	53%
45–64	362	33%	127	35%	33	9%	131	36%	190	52%
65+	252	24%	73	29%	18	7%	69	27%	147	58%
Male	390	23%	91	23%	29	7%	123	32%	255	65%
<45	34	20%	5	15%	2	6%	10	29%	25	74%
45–64	207	25%	38	18%	16	8%	71	34%	143	69%
65+	149	22%	48	32%	11	7%	42	28%	87	58%
Total	1062	100%	309	29%	88	8%	342	32%	623	59%

insecurity were the next most commonly identified need, with 32% and 29% reporting these as issues, respectively. A small percentage noted health insurance as an area of concern (8%). Additionally, patients took information about mental health support hotlines in 4% of all completed calls. Patients were provided information on the available resources within New York City to support these needs.

Patients expressed a variety of issues engaging with healthcare and other critical resources during the initial weeks of the COVID-19 emergency. Some shared fears of seeking healthcare whether for routine or emergency services while others were struggling to adjust to not having in-person resources accessible. For example, a Cantonese-speaking patient was unsure how to renew their Medicaid without going to the office in person and expressed concerns about language barriers when encouraged to follow up via telephone. Other patients were passively waiting for their providers to follow up to renew refills, schedule appointments, or clarify whether they should proceed with non-COVID related lab work, imaging, or specialty care. Given the numerous challenges practices faced at this time, call center staff explained that practices were likely relying on voicemails more than usual and coached patients to leave detailed messages in order to ensure a proper response. Furthermore, patients were not always aware of telehealth services. Though some expressed barriers such as lack of access to video technology or concerns about the quality of telehealth services, call center staff reassured them that follow-up with providers by phone was an option. Patients who found telehealth information particularly useful included those who had temporarily relocated outside of the city or were unable to return from travel. In at least one case a patient outside the country expressed interest in utilizing telehealth.

Although referrals to mental health hotlines were documented for only 4% of calls, a number of callers noted that even patients who declined mental health information spent time on the call sharing stresses and concerns related to isolation, separation from loved ones, or loss of loved ones related to COVID-19. Another common stressor shared on calls was having or being an essential worker in the household while trying to protect others from SARS-CoV-2 exposure. For example, one essential worker who was also the primary caregiver for a frail relative was struggling to find support for him as she was afraid to visit him.

During the last few weeks of call center activity, staff incorporated information about the city's contact tracing program including what types of information a contact tracer would or would not ask and caller IDs associated with the program. Patients expressed concerns about fraudulent calls and responded positively to information about how to identify a legitimate contact tracer.

Conclusion

DOHMH has previously reported on retrospective analyses[9–10] that demonstrated the potential of the Hub to provide situational awareness during public health emergencies. Here herdescribe prospective use of Hub data, to show how these data informed ongoing COVID-19 response efforts. While the existing infrastructure at DOHMH (Hub, existing field teams familiar with running EHR reports) certainly enabled rapid implementation of these use cases to support situational awareness and direct engagement of at-risk populations, other jurisdictions without these resources might still be able to leverage health IT to support similar efforts by engaging other stakeholders. Health information exchanges that have central data warehouses, as well as larger health systems and independent practice associations, are examples of potential partners with the health IT capacity to provide data to guide situational awareness, as well as provision of targeted lists for direct engagement. The use cases described here represent relatively basic data requests that should not represent a considerable burden to create and provide. (Editor's note: see chapter 15: Health Information Exchange: An Overview and New York State's Model.)

References

1. New York City Department of Health and Mental Hygiene (DOHMH) COVID-19 Response Team. Preliminary estimate of excess mortality during the COVID-19 Outbreak – New York City, March 11–May 2, 2020. *MMWR Morb Mortal Wkly Rep.* 2020 May 15;69(19):603–5. doi:10.15585/mmwr.mm6919e5.
2. Gogia S, Newton-Dame R, Boudourakis L, et al. COVID-19 X-curves: Illness hidden, illness deferred. *N Engl J Med Catalyst.* 2020. Epub May 29, 2020. https://catalyst.nejm.org/doi/full/10.1056/cat.20.0231.
3. https://www.cdc.gov/mmwr/volumes/69/wr/mm6923e1.htm.
4. https://www1.nyc.gov/site/doh/covid/covid-19-data.page.
5. https://www1.nyc.gov/assets/dsny/contact/services/COVID-19FoodAssistance.shtml.
6. https://www1.nyc.gov/site/coronavirus/resources/resources-for-new-yorkers.page.
7. https://www.governor.ny.gov/news/governor-cuomo-signs-new-york-state-pause-executive-order.
8. https://www.governor.ny.gov/news/governor-cuomo-announces-new-york-city-enter-phase-1-reopening-june-8-and-five-regions-enter.
9. Plagianos MG, Wu WY, McCullough C, Paladini M, Lurio J, Buck MD, Calman N, Soulakis N. Syndromic surveillance during pandemic (H1N1) 2009 outbreak, New York, New York, USA. *Emerg Infect Dis.* 2011 Sep;17(9):1724–6. doi:10.3201/eid1709.101357.
10. Sebek K, Jacobson L, Wang J, Newton-Dame R, Singer J. Assessing capacity and disease burden in a virtual network of New York City primary care providers following hurricane sandy. *J Urban Health.* 2014 Aug;91(4):615–22. doi:10.1007/s11524-014-9874-7.

Acknowledged contributors to this case study:

Alexandra Bragg
Amanda Spence
Amita Kothari

Babi Bose
Barbara Zidek
Brendan Kerr
Brian Couch
Carlos Devia
Charlene Ngamwajasat
Chien Ting Chen
Christine Binder
Danielle Cohen
Dominique Gabriel
Don Bill
Donna Castelblanco
Eleanor Rogowski
Emily Carroll
Ernesto Fana
Evan Miller
Francisco Valbuena
Gabriella Ansah
Gila Stadler
Gloria Mesa
Hang Pham-Singer
Hanna Liriano
Indira Debchoudhury
Janice Magno
Jennifer De Leon
Jennifer White
Jill Linnell
Joanna Davis
Karen Wong
Katherine Kaye
Keisha Haynes-Leith
Krystal Austin
Kyla Dayer
Lauri Berrita
Margot Abrahams
Maria Fernandez
Maria Regalado
Marie Jean
Matt Gannon
Matthew Krco
Melissa Cheung
Natalie Polinsky
Natoya Worrell-Gooding
Patrick Powell
Patrick Wan Cheung Pun
Phoenix Maa
Pia Iribarren

Pritiza Paromita
Rachel Lima
Sabrina Chung
Sachel Somwaru
Samantha De Leon
Samantha Witchey
Sarah Mednick
Sarah Shih
Shelby Rorabaugh
Shivana Seeram
Sparkle Johnson
Sruthi Venigalla
Tahirah Ellis
Tessa Schneider
Tracey McGruder
Vita Tambone
Vitaliy Shtutin
Wendyann Moore
Winfred Wu
Yvette Acevedo

Chapter 21

Genomic Informatics in the Healthcare System

Chang-Hui Shen, PhD

Contents

Introduction

Next-generation sequencing (NGS) is a high-throughput methodology that enables fast sequencing of the base pairs in DNA or RNA samples. Because NGS is rapidly evolving and gradually becoming more accessible and inexpensive, NGS technology has brought us to the era of personalized genomic medicine. This is because patient NGS data are already being generated by large-scale projects, and this has demonstrated the critical role of clinical NGS in precision medicine. For example, the foundation of basic human genomic research in disease is the discovery and identification of "new" causative genes from cohort sequencing followed up by functional studies including omics strategies. This allows for the identification of disease modifiers and novel genomic variants. On the other hand, clinical genomic research endeavors to sequence ambiguous cases to identify the cause of disease by ensuring all known disease-causing genes are covered. The merger

DOI: 10.4324/9780429423109-21

of both basic research and clinical genomics laboratories to form the genomic informatics can facilitate the discovery of novel disease-causing candidate genes. As such, recent NGS technology advances are important to the innovations and merger in all areas of basic and clinical genomics and molecular diagnostics. Currently, there is a global trend to collect genomic data of patients in clinical practice through routine tests. Moreover, the NGS empowers clinical laboratories with unprecedented genomic sequencing capability, and health insurance for NGS-based diagnostic panels has been provided in several countries. Although bioinformatics and clinical informatics are separate disciplines with typically a small degree of overlap, they have been brought together by the enthusiastic adoption of NGS-derived genomic informatics in clinical laboratories. The result has been a collaborative environment for the development of novel informatics solutions. It is foreseen that the genomic informatics generated by NGS will play an essential role in medical diagnosis and treatment regimes in the future.

What Is NGS, and How Is It Important to Medical Informatics?

DNA is the code of all biological life on earth. Humans have sought to unravel its mysteries so that the origins of life itself may be revealed. The first sequencing methodology, known as Sanger sequencing, uses specifically manipulated nucleotides to read through a DNA template during DNA synthesis. This sequencing technology requires a specific primer to start the read at a specific location along the DNA template and record the different labels for each nucleotide within the sequence up to 1000–1200 base pairs (bps). Subsequently, an approach called shotgun sequencing was developed for longer read of sequences. In this approach, genomic DNA is enzymatically or mechanically broken down into smaller fragments and cloned into sequencing vectors in which cloned DNA fragments can be sequenced individually. The complete sequence of a long DNA fragment can be eventually generated by these methods by alignment and reassembly of sequence fragments based on partial sequence overlaps.

Shotgun sequencing is a significant improvement of DNA sequencing. In fact, the core concept of massive parallel sequencing used in NGS is adapted from shotgun sequencing. In general, the NGS sequencing process involves the preparation of a library of short DNA fragments through either enzymatic or sonication techniques. These short strands of DNA are then ligated to generic adapters in vitro. Polymerase chain reaction (PCR) amplification follows, performed using either emulsion PCR in oil-water emulsion micelles or bridge PCR on a solid surface coated with complementary primers. Subsequent sequencing of the amplicon (the portion of the DNA that has been replicated) is performed by either pyrosequencing, sequencing by ligation, or sequencing by synthesis. The large number of short reads generated from this process must then be aligned against a reference sequence. A plethora of software has been developed not only to align the reads but also to determine where deviations from a reference sequence exist. Many platforms, including the Illumina, Roche/454 FLX, the Solexa Genome Analyzer, and the Applied Biosystems SOLiD Analyzer, have been developed based on the aforementioned different methodologies in sequencing. These NGS platforms generate different base read lengths, error rates, and error profiles. NGS technologies have increased the speed and throughput capacities of DNA sequencing and, as a result, dramatically reduced overall sequencing costs and time.

Genomics is the systematic study on a whole-genome scale for the identification of genetic contributions to human conditions. Because NGS is a rapidly evolving technology and it has the ability to sequence the whole genome in a short period of time, it becomes possible to reveal all genetic information for medical purposes. Progress in our understanding of many fundamental biological phenomena has accelerated dramatically over the last decade driven by advances in genomic informatics. The advances in NGS genomic technologies have resulted in great achievements in genetic linkage, association studies, DNA copy number, and gene expression analysis. Furthermore, rapid advances in NGS have introduced inexpensive methods to acquire a large set of genetic data with potential applications across many specialties of medicine. Human genomic medicine is the use of broad-based genetic testing by patients and their healthcare providers to enhance routine clinical activities including diagnosis, risk assessment, tailored therapy, and more precise prognosis. Widespread marketing of genomic medicine services and health system implementations have increased the availability of testing to patients and their clinicians. In the future, the advances of NGS technologies can continue to contribute significantly to the personalized genomic medicine.

NGS Informatics Workflow

As mentioned earlier, the NGS technologies are designed to yield millions of relatively short sequence reads (50–400 bps) redundantly overlapping a specified genomic region of interest (targeted sequencing) or potentially extending across the whole genome (whole-genome sequencing). The portion of the targeted genome for which reads are actually generated during sequencing represents the extent of coverage provided by a sequencing run. A typical NGS bioinformatics pipeline includes a series of complex and computationally expensive data analysis processes that derive a list of genomic alterations from raw NGS signal output followed by signal processing and alignment against a reference genome (Figure 21.1). The pipeline usually begins with proprietary, platform-specific algorithms generating sequential base calls from primary fluorescent, chemiluminescent, or electrical current signals. Each of the predicted nucleotide bases is assigned a quality score (Phred-like score or Q score), which reflects the degree of statistical confidence that the base call is correct. The sequence reads generated during this process are stored in one of the several file formats (FASTQ, XSEQ, unaligned BAM, or FASTA) with or without the base quality score information. Because of the platform-specific and proprietary nature of this portion of the pipeline, these Q scores are not comparable across different sequencing systems.

Subsequent demultiplexing analysis involves performing a quality control (QC) check on the sequenced data (typically FASTQ) to assess read-length distribution, quality scores, guanine-cytosine (GC) content, overrepresented sequences, and k-mer content. The purpose of these checks is to determine if the sequences generated have indicators of poor sequence quality. Additional steps, such as adapter and poor-quality sequence trimming, may be required depending on the QC results and pipeline configuration. The QC check phase is followed by alignment of the overlapping reads in a FASTQ file against a reference human genome. Under the sequencing alignment stage, good alignment algorithms have code designed to overcome ambiguities of repetitive sequence and sequencing errors. The aligned reads, which are tagged with several metadata, including alignment scores, are outputted in a sequence alignment map (SAM) or binary form of SAM (BAM) format.

The aligned reads in a SAM/BAM file form an input for a variety of applications that detect single-nucleotide variants (SNVs), short insertions or deletions (indels), large structural alterations, copy number variations, and gene fusions. Generally, local sequence realignment, duplicate marking, and adjusted base quality score thresholds are employed to enhance the discrimination of variant callers directed at SNV and Indels. However, structural variants and copy number aberrations require different processing pipelines. The list of sequence variants is typically rendered in

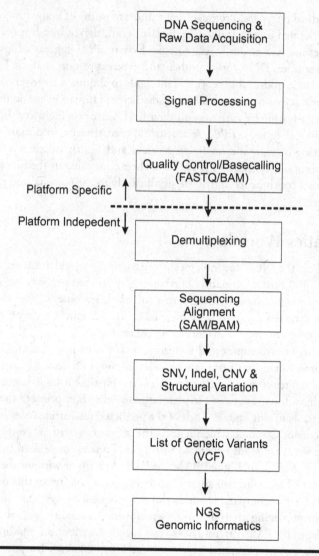

Figure 21.1 A schematic diagram of bioinformatic workflow for NGS. The bioinformatics algorithms employed in the signal processing and quality control (base calling) steps are usually platform specific and often proprietary. The variant detection process is variable, and a variety of software applications are available for different requirements. CNV, copy number variation; SAM/BAM, sequence alignment/map format (BAM is a binary format of SAM); SNV, single-nucleotide variant; VCF, variant call format.

Source: Adapted from Zhang et al. (2011).

one of the many variant call formats, such as variant call format (VCF) and genomic VCF (gVCF). Of the three file types generated in NGS (FASTA/FASTQ, SAM/BAM, and VCF), VCF takes up the least amount of memory and is the easiest to read computationally. Therefore, it can be the ideal candidate file to use to transmit and store genomic data on patients between NGS instruments, laboratory information systems (LISs), and electronic health records (EHRs). The detected variants are further annotated with metadata, such as Human Genome Variation Society annotations, predicted effect on transcription and translation, pathway analysis, genotype-phenotype correlation data, clinical features, therapeutic trials, and outcome data.

Introduction of a new test into a clinical environment requires significant interoperability with the existing informatics infrastructure for successful implementation. However, NGS is rapidly evolving, and limited resources have been devoted to developing informatics solutions to adapt to the magnitude and complexity of NGS data or to seamlessly integrate it into the existing clinical informatics infrastructure such as LISs and EHRs. Because of this, it is very challenging for the use of genomic informatics in the medical field. For example, little attention was paid to the downstream aspects of laboratory workflow, such as interoperability with existing information systems, patient and sample information integration with sequence data, report synthesis, data storage and transmission, and quality assurance. These elements, which are both upstream and downstream of an NGS sequencing run, are crucial for the successful establishment of genomic informatics in a clinical environment. It would be essential to develop an efficient integration mechanism for the validated genomic informatics and patient's health history.

Medical informatics workflow in a laboratory performing NGS-based molecular testing has similarities and unique attributes compared with any standard laboratory workflow, which includes pre-analytic, analytic, and post-analytic phases. A well-designed and tightly monitored laboratory workflow ensures that efficiency and accuracy in test results and data management related to genomic informatics should follow pre-analytic, analytic, and post-analytic components of laboratory workflow including data acquisition, data validation, data analytics, and data reporting. As such, upstream sample and patient information management, pre-sequencing wet bench processes, and downstream variant annotation, interpretation, and reporting are central to personalized genomic medicine. The utility of NGS-based testing can be widely adopted by precision genomic medicine and brings in revolutionary medical treatment, although we still face challenges include new analytic pipelines, image management systems, patient privacy concerns, and laboratory regulations. These challenges will continuously emerge as the technology in this field evolves. NGS and the data derived from these tests, if managed well in the clinical laboratory, will redefine the practice of genomic medicine. In order to sustain the rapidly progressing field of clinical molecular diagnostics, adoption of smart computing technology and introduction of the NGS informatics training will become essential.

Challenges of NGS Diagnostics

With the generation of large amounts of NGS data and identification of many variants, we face new challenges to determine genic (gene-related) or intergenic variant effects and their associations with genomic disorders. These challenges are primarily relevant to the relationship between the genomic sequence information and clinical phenotypic diagnosis. Here, we discuss several critical concerns that have to be resolved for the future personalized genomic medicine to be successful.

Challenge in Increased Finding of Variants of Uncertain Significance

With the massive amounts of NGS data, the number of variants of uncertain significance (VUSs) also increases. This causes a burden on variant classification, disease association, follow-up diagnosis, and therapy options. The American College of Medical Genetics and Genomics (ACMG) provides guidelines to clinical diagnostic laboratories for interpreting and annotating variants from NGS data to classify them as benign, likely benign, pathogenic, likely pathogenic, or as a variant of uncertain clinical significance. An uncertain finding can be frustrating for clinicians and patients, but it may occur when there is insufficient information to determine whether a variant is benign or pathogenic. Reports with uncertain findings can result in additional medical costs and a continued diagnostic process when a provider lacks sufficient information to rule in or rule out a diagnosis.

Initial interpretation requires caution, because many databases include misclassified variants, particularly benign variants classified as pathogenic. VUS can sometimes be reclassified when additional information becomes available. If this occurs after a VUS has been reported to a patient, laboratories have the obligation to re-contact the provider to communicate the revised classification. Although much has been written about the duty to re-contact, there is very little consensus reached on the specifics of how and when to do so. In theory, re-contacting patients and providers with updated information is optimal. However, it is the best practice to provide accurate and complete information as early as possible to minimize the re-contact. VUS are unavoidable results in clinical genetic testing, whether a single gene is sequenced by traditional methods or whether a large gene panel or exome is produced by NGS. As such, it is very important to make every effort to minimize uncertain findings and provide conclusive results to as many patients as possible.

Challenge in Genomic Locus Heterogeneity and Allelic Heterogeneity of the Genes with a Broad Spectrum of Detected Variants

Besides the high prevalence of VUSs, the diagnostic challenges are more complicated in cases of genetically and phenotypically heterogeneous disorders. In the early development of molecular biology, it was commonly agreed that a single gene affected a single phenotype. However, recent research indicates that a single gene can associate with multiple disease phenotypes (locus and allelic heterogeneity). For example, the *RET* (MIM# 164761) gene can cause both Hirschsprung disease and multiple endocrine neoplasias, and the *RYR1* (MIM# 180901) gene is associated with both malignant hyperthermia and central core disease. As the use of NGS for the diagnosis of diseases in the clinical setting is increasing and more genotype-phenotype heterogeneity is found, further comprehensive second-tier tests, such as whole-exome sequencing (WES) or whole-genome sequencing (WGS), should be included to uncover the novel variants in genes known to cause disease as well as variants in novel genes. The rationale for the use of WES is based on the finding that the majority of pathogenic variants causing Mendelian diseases that have been identified to date are located in protein-coding regions. On the other hand, because of the nature of WGS, it is also important to examine the introns and intergenic regions and to detect copy number variants through complex bioinformatic analysis. Both strategies raise the possibility of detecting an incidental finding that has implications for the health of the individual and their family. Because of these unexpected findings, it would be important to establish a standard protocol to report these results.

Challenge in Broad Phenotypic Overlap of Diseases and Disease Sub-types

It is challenging to understand the phenotype-genotype correlation and phenotypic variability of individuals with a specific genetic variant. Many alternative explanations for differing phenotypes among cases with the same genetic variant have been proposed. One consideration is the presence of another genetic variant that affects disease presentation. A true digenic disorder requires the inheritance of a distinct heterozygous mutation in two genes that, when inherited separately, do not cause a phenotype. The broader term of epistasis refers to possible interactions between genes. Determining genetic epistasis is complex and requires an appropriate pedigree, which includes more than one gene mutated in a single pedigree, a range of genetic permutations, and at least one member with wild type (WT) alleles in both genes.

Another possible explanation for the phenotypic heterogeneity among cases is epigenetic differences. Epigenetic processes such as DNA methylation, histone modifications, chromatin remodeling, and non-coding RNAs can alter the activity of a gene without changing the DNA sequence. To further understand and identify the detail of the heterogeneity, a strategy such as the chromatin immunoprecipitation sequencing (ChIP-Seq) or RNA-Seq can be used. Exploring factors that can account for the phenotypic variability may provide insight into the pathways involved in disease. Furthermore, the comprehensive genetic evaluation and investigation of various individuals with these conditions will likely enlighten the fields of genomic locus heterogeneity and allelic heterogeneity of the genes with a broad spectrum of detected variants.

Challenge in Pathogenic Variants with Varying Clinical Consequences

Pathogenic variants of variable clinical consequences are also a challenge for the molecular NGS diagnosis. Although the vast majority of genes reported as causally linked to monogenic diseases are true positives, false assignments of pathogenicity can have severe consequences for patients, resulting in incorrect prognostic, therapeutic, or reproductive advice. For the research enterprise, false assignments of pathogenicity can result in misallocation of resources for basic and therapeutic research. As the volume of patients' NGS sequencing data increases, it is critical that candidate variants are subjected to rigorous evaluation to prevent further mis-annotation of the pathogenicity of variants in public databases.

For NGS data, it is very important to focus on how to classify the evidence relevant to the implication of sequence variants in disease (Table 21.1). Assessment of evidence for variant implication should have statistical and computational algorithms that predict the effects of genomic variation. The overall evidence for implication of a gene should be considered, focusing primarily on the statistical support for implication from genetic analyses, potentially supplemented by ancillary data from bioinformatic sources and functional studies. Furthermore, a combined assessment of the genetic, experimental, and bioinformatic support for individual candidate variants should

Table 21.1   Classes of Evidence Relevant to the Implication of Sequence Variants in Disease

Evidence Level	Evidence Class	Examples
Gene level	Genetic	Gene burden: the affected gene shows statistical excess of rare (or de novo) probably damaging variants segregating in cases compared to control cohorts or null models.
	Experimental	Protein interactions: the gene product interacts with proteins previously implicated (genetically or biochemically) in the disease of interest.

(Continued)

Table 21.1   (Continued)

Evidence Level	Evidence Class	Examples
		Biochemical function: the gene product performs a biochemical function shared with other known genes in the disease of interest, or consistent with the phenotype.
		Expression: the gene is expressed in tissues relevant to the disease of interest and/or is altered in expression in patients who have the disease.
		Gene disruption: the gene and/or gene product function is demonstrably altered in patients carrying candidate mutations.
		Model systems: non-human animal or cell-culture models with a similarly disrupted copy of the affected gene show a phenotype consistent with human disease state.
		Rescue: the cellular phenotype in patient-derived cells or engineered equivalents can be rescued by addition of the wild-type gene product.
Variant level	Genetic	Association: the variant is significantly enriched in cases compared to controls.
		Segregation: the variant is co-inherited with disease status within affected families, and additional co-segregating pathogenic variants are unlikely or have been excluded.
		Population frequency: the variant is found at a low frequency, consistent with the proposed inheritance model and disease prevalence, in large population cohorts with similar ancestry to patients.
	Informatic	Conservation: the site of the variant displays evolutionary conservation consistent with deleterious effects of sequence changes at that location.
		Predicted effect on function: variant is found at the location within the protein predicted to cause functional disruption (e.g., enzyme active site, protein-binding region).
	Experimental	Gene disruption: the variant significantly alters levels, splicing or normal biochemical function of the product of the affected gene. This is shown either in patient cells or a well-validated in vitro model system.
		Phenotype recapitulation: introduction of the variant, or an engineered gene product carrying the variant, into a cell line or animal model results in a phenotype that is consistent with the disease and that is unlikely to arise from disruption of genes selected at random.
		Rescue: the cellular phenotype in patient-derived cells, model organisms, or engineered equivalents can be rescued by addition of wild-type gene product or specific knockdown of the variant allele.

Source: Adapted from MacArthur et al. (2014).

be performed. Such assessments should be performed even if the genes or variants have been previously reported as confidently implicated. In this way, prior evidence can be continuously re-evaluated with newly available information, and we can reduce the false assignments of pathogenicity.

Integrating NGS Data into Healthcare

The NGS technology can sequence an entire human exome or genome and provides vastly more information of potential relevance to a person's current and future health than was possible previously. As the relationship between sequence variation and disease management becomes better understood, personalized precision medicine – the use of genomic information from an individual's genome in the diagnosis and management of their condition – is becoming increasingly relevant to a broad range of health practitioners. Therefore, an effective integration of NGS data into a healthcare system is necessary, and the process requires system-wide change.

Figure 21.2 presents an example for integrated genome sequencing data processing, variant filtration, annotation, and interpretation combined with functional assays for the future of

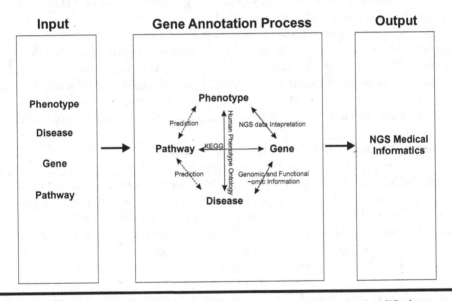

Figure 21.2   Gene annotation process through NGS genomic data. A simplified structure by which genes can be annotated using an integrated approach and their disease associations and functions can be searched by the medical community using patient phenotype, the disease diagnosed, the gene itself, or the possible pathways that might be affected. Genetic and phenotypic relationships can be inferred through NGS data. Curated genomic informatics and functional omics studies (including transcriptomics, proteomics, and metabolomics) databases at the downstream functional levels should give specific and sensitive information about genetic associations with diseases. Furthermore, pathway analyses using databases such as the Kyoto Encyclopedia of Genes and Genomes (KEGG) can also be used for information on genes that may be involved in a disease phenotype. All of this information should be compiled to generate consistent data and terminologies for gene annotations, which will lead to an integrated output for clinical diagnostics and genomic medicine.

Source: Adapted from Chakravorty and Hegde (2017).

understanding all disease-causing variants to facilitate the personalized medicine. The genome informatic pipeline involves a complex, tiered analysis of an extensively validated, disease-associated gene slice based on clinician's initial diagnosis, plus genes associated with disease, deep intronic and promoter pathogenic variants, genomic CNV and intragenic deletions and duplications, followed by genes of unknown clinical significance or currently not known to be associated with disease and finally analysis of noncoding sequence regions. This genome sequencing and its combination with other omics and functional analysis can be integrated into a healthcare database, and this process can be used to discover variants, especially rare variants in human diseases; this can lead to uncover of the genetic information unrelated to the original matter of concern. This generates challenges for the process of obtaining informed consent and pre- and post- test genetic counseling.

The introduction of genomic informatics into a health system is complex. This is because diverse barriers require change across many of its interacting component. For example, health systems are not generally amenable to change. Transformation of the experience of framework implementation is also very difficult. Furthermore, the barriers to widespread clinical implementation span diverse domains, including data integration and interpretation, workforce capacity and capability, public acceptability and government engagement, paucity of evidence for clinical utility and cost effectiveness, and ethical and legislative issues.

Several approaches have been taken to address the challenges inherent in genomics. For example, large-scale NGS sequencing initiatives and discovery-based research projects address gaps in understanding the clinical significance of genetic variation. Global collaborations aim to accelerate progress by fostering the sharing of genomic data and implementing research to identify strategies that assist the adoption of genomic informatics by clinicians. Each effort contributes to ensure that a genomic test is available for clinical use and that clinicians apply the test and its results in practice.

A widespread change and targeted support is necessary to ensure that patients' health is improved by using genomic informatics in their medical care. Figure 21.3 presents a model to deliver personalized precision medicine through the implementation of genomic informatics in medical practice. The model contains core elements for data analysis and its transmission to participants with the provision of variable components to modify and enhance delivery over time. For translation into practice, this model adopts a flexible learning framework to allow for adaptation to unanticipated challenges faced in real-life clinical settings. In addition, the implementation strategies can be monitored and adapted over time.

Governments and organizations considering the implementation of genomic informatics need to design a high-level, holistic model for how genomic informatics will be delivered in the future, based on their own unique context. For example, implementing genomic informatics requires considerable investment in infrastructure, personnel, and change management. Since 2013, the governments of at least 14 countries have invested over US$4 billion in establishing national genomic-medicine initiatives to address implementation barriers and transition testing from centers of excellence to mainstream medical practice (Table 21.2). In countries such as the UK, France, Australia, Saudi Arabia, and Turkey, workforce and infrastructure development have been coupled with testing large numbers of patients with rare diseases and cancer, and this is anticipated to have immediate clinical benefits. These "proof-of-principle" programs are driving change and fostering adoption among stakeholders under real-life conditions. Meanwhile, these programs also gather evidence for wider implementation. Other countries such as the United States, Estonia, Denmark, Japan, and Qatar have invested in population-based sequencing projects with return of results to participants. National initiatives in Switzerland, the Netherlands, Brazil, and Finland

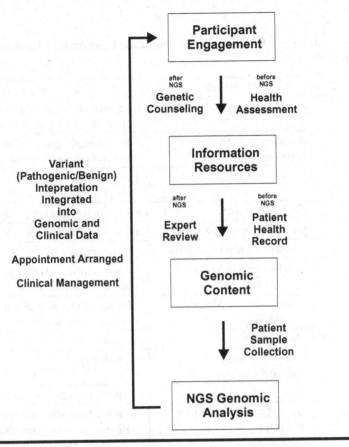

Figure 21.3 Genomics implementation process to describe the delivery of the genomic data into medical practice

Source: Adapted from Bylstra et al. (2019).

are primarily focusing on the development of infrastructure, such as common standards and data-sharing policies and platforms. Although it is a time-consuming process to integrate research evidence into clinical practice and to implement policy guidance, governments' initiatives to enable timely realization of the benefits of genomic informatics for individual patients, families, and healthcare systems can accelerate the implementation of genomic medicine. They can also play an important role in strengthening an international collaborative network and creating a global learning healthcare system to enable rapid translation.

Impact of Genomics Informatics on Health Outcomes

Genomic informatics is evolving from individual gene or single nucleotide polymorphism variant testing to exome or genome testing by the use of NGS technologies. The discovery of both rare and common variants has increased exponentially in the past few years. As we discussed above, many variants can confidently be designated but often have uncertain pathogenicity. In fact, only a few novel variants are sufficiently understood, and they can be considered for reporting to patients.

Table 21.2   Summary of Currently Active National Government-Funded Genomic Medicine Initiatives

Country	Initiative	Focus Area
Australia	Australian Genomics	Infrastructure and clinical cohorts, rare diseases, cancer, infectious disease
Brazil	Brazilian Initiative on Precision Medicine	Infrastructure, population-based cohort, rare and common disease cohorts
Denmark	Genome Denmark	Infrastructure, population-based cohort, FranceFranceject
	FarGen Project	Infrastructure and population-based cohort
Estonia	Estonian Genome Project	Infrastructure and population-based cohort
Finland	National Genome Strategy	Infrastructure
France	Plan France Médecine Génomique 2025	Infrastructure and clinical cohorts, rare diseases, cancer, diabetes
Japan	Japan Genomic Medicine Program	Infrastructure, clinical and population-based cohorts, drug discovery
The Netherlands	RADICON-NL	Rare diseases
	Health Research Infrastructure	Infrastructure
Qatar	Qatar Genome 2015	Infrastructure and population-based cohort
Saudi Arabia	Saudi Human Genome Program	Infrastructure, clinical cohorts (rare and common genetic conditions), and population-based cohorts
Switzerland	Swiss Personalized Health Network	Infrastructure
Turkey	Turkish Genome Project	Infrastructure, clinical cohorts (rare disease, cancer, neurological disease), and population-based cohort
United Kingdom	Genomics England	Infrastructure and clinical cohorts, rare diseases, cancer, infectious disease
	Scottish Genomes Partnership	Infrastructure, clinical cohorts (rare disease and cancer), population-based cohort
	Welsh Genomics for Precision Medicine Strategy	Infrastructure, clinical cohorts (rare disease and cancer), population-based cohort
	Northern Ireland Genomic Medicine Center	Infrastructure, clinical cohorts (rare disease and cancer), population-based cohort
United States	National Human Genome Research Institute	Infrastructure and clinical cohorts
	Precision Medicine Initiative (All of Us)	Population-based cohort

Source: Stark et al. (2019).

For example, ACMG recommends that pathogenic variants in 59 genes be returned to tested patients regardless of the indication for sequencing. The association between variants within these genes and specific medical conditions in cardiology, oncology, and many other medical specialties are well established and should contribute to individual risk assessments or to justify additional screening (Table 21.3). Different outcomes are expected, and these are dependent on whether the NGS information and variants are returned to individuals or family members.

Potential outcomes of interest span the individual, their family, and their healthcare system. Outcomes in each of these three domains can then be captured across three phases: return of genetic results, the application of the data to clinical decision-making, and longitudinal follow-up (Table 21.4). Given that much of genomic medicine will be assessed in the context of large observational studies and implementation strategies rather than in clinical trials, linking clinical outcomes to the return and application of genetic results will be particularly important to establishing causality. The scope of reportable outcomes will also depend on whether the focus is on a small panel of genes or a larger sequencing effort, such as genome or exome, the time frame over which outcomes are assessed in sequenced patients, the perspective of the study (societal, health system, or patient-centered), and whether clinical data from family members is sought and captured.

For the individual outcome, NGS sequencing results could lead to changes in a patient's understanding of genetic findings and clinical risks, anxiety or decisional conflict about the results, changes in health behaviors or lifestyle, and increased information-seeking and healthcare use. Any of these psychological effects or behaviors could have a substantial effect on downstream clinical outcomes. For example, a woman who learns of increased breast cancer risk due to a *BRCA1* gene variant might react by engaging with her healthcare provider or a genetic counselor and follow through with accelerated breast cancer screening. Conversely, she might avoid additional follow-up due to anxiety or perceived futility of efforts to prevent a poor outcome. Under this circumstance, the addition of mental health counselors to the treatment team is vital to address the psychological ramifications of results that could impact not just the target patient but family members as well. The application of NGS results to clinical risk prediction, additional screening tests, and receipt of individualized intervention are key process outcomes that link return of genomic informatics to patients and potential improved health.

One unique feature of genomic medicine studies is the potential for genetic risks identified within an individual to affect the care of family members through cascade testing of relatives. For the family outcome, clinical outcome studies would test first- and second-degree family members of study participants with a pathogenic variant and track family members with the consent of the patient and family member for changes in healthcare delivery and clinical outcomes. Given that family members are much more likely than average to also have the variant, cascade testing will increase the efficiency of the study and health effect of the original finding. This increased efficiency has been shown in the context of screening patients with colorectal cancer to identify Lynch syndrome. In practice, investigators need to plan to overcome logistical and health policy hurdles to cascade testing.

One of the most important mediators of individual outcomes is the context in which the NGS test results are obtained and applied to clinical care. Testing that is done within an established clinician-patient relationship and in a healthcare environment where results are interpreted, and clinical decision support is provided to both patients and clinicians, can have a substantially different effect than testing done in other contexts, such as direct-to-consumer or outside a traditional health system. The availability of services, such as genetic counselors and medical geneticists, could predict improvements in process outcomes such as effective delivery of results and

Table 21.3   Examples of Process, Intermediate, and Clinical Outcomes Potentially Resulting from Sequencing Studies by Generic Syndrome(s)

	Associated Genes	Pathogenic Variant Rate Among Unselected Population	Process Outcomes	Intermediate Outcomes	Clinical Outcomes
Hereditary breast and ovarian cancer	BRCA1, BRCA2	0.5%	Breast cancer screen modality and schedule	Breast biopsy findings	Prophylactic mastectomy or oophorectomy; diagnosis of breast or ovarian cancer an presenting stage
Lynch syndrome	MLH1, MSH2, MSH6, PMS2	0.4%	Colorectal cancer screen modality and schedule	Colonoscopy findings, polypectomy	Bilateral salpingo-oophorectomy; incidence and presenting stage of colorectal cancer, ovarian cancer, or endometrial cancer
Familial hypertrophic and dilated cardiomyopathy	TTN, TNNT2, LMNA, MYH7	0.2%	Echocardiogram screening; creatine kinase measurement	Left ventricular wall thickness; implantation of defibrillator or pacemaker	Diagnosis of cardiomyopathy; incidence and presenting stage of congestive heart failure

Source: Adapted from Peterson et al. (2019).

Table 21.4 Potential Clinical Outcomes for Personalized Precision Medicine

Phases	Individual Health Domain	Family Health Domain	Health System Domain
Return of results	■ Individual understanding ■ Perception of disease risk ■ Psychological adjustments ■ Behavioral changes	■ Collection of family health history ■ Family communication ■ Family understanding	■ Accessibility of results and interpretation ■ Clinician understanding ■ Genetic counselling capacity
Application to clinical practice	■ Application to risk prediction ■ Additional screening for genomic diagnosis ■ Receipt of individualized intervention	■ Cascade testing of at-risk family ■ Screening for genomic diagnoses ■ Receipt of individualized intervention	■ Clinician response to clinical decision support
Longitudinal follow-up	■ Diagnosis of individual genomic Syndromes ■ Drug response ■ Mortality, morbidity, and quality of life	■ Diagnosis of familial genomic syndromes ■ Reproductive decision-making	■ Health-care utilization ■ Cost-effectiveness

Source: Adapted from Peterson et al. (2019).

recommendations to patients but also incur costs to the system in the form of increased healthcare use, which could reduce overall cost-effectiveness.

As the use of genomic informatics in personalized genomic medicine increases, patients in various clinical contexts are likely to be recipients of genetic findings that were not related to the indication for testing. Clinical outcome studies in these patients is crucially important to developing evidence-based policies around the return of secondary findings and guidelines for genome-informed care. Although randomized clinical trials would provide the strongest evidence for clinical benefits or harms for returning specific types of variants, the uncommon frequency and latency of genetic variation strongly associated with disease make such trials expensive, impractical, or preempted by compelling observational data. In the future, large cohort studies that return results to participants and follow up participants over time will gradually inform the use of genomic informatics in clinical practice.

Development of publicly available, standardized outcome measures can rapidly expand knowledge. Offering cascade testing to families of proband study participants will increase the efficiency of identifying carriers. For example, if these family members are also followed up with clinically, the pace of determining outcomes will be greatly amplified. Finally, national and international consortia, similar to the ClinVar and Clinical Genome Resource (ClinGen), could accumulate evidence-based algorithms for managing secondary findings, just as existing resources catalog the clinical relevance of genes and variants.

The practice of genomic informatics in personalized precision medicine is expected to expand from the identification and care of patients with single-gene Mendelian disorders to more common conditions with complex genetic associations. The development of polygenic risk scores to predict the onset of cardiovascular disease in adult patients is an extant example. As these disorders have multifaceted causes with established clinical risks, high-dimensional genomic risks involving thousands or millions of variants, and potential epigenetic risks, outcome evaluations will need to compare clinical-to-clinical genomic strategies at a scale that can differentiate the incremental benefit of adding genomic data to a standard clinical risk model. Building evidence for genomic informatics to individualize preventive care strategies can improve early diagnosis of diseases and therapeutic plans. Increased emphasis on implementation of genomic informatics will help achieve the necessary scale and identify sustainable strategies for accelerating the adoption of personalized precision medicine practices.

About the Author

Chang-Hui Shen, PhD, is a professor and Chair of Biology at the College of Staten Island, City University of New York. He is also affiliated with the Graduate Center and Institute of Macromolecular Assemblies, City University of New York. Dr. Shen completed his doctorate at the University of Edinburgh (UK).

He previously was a visiting fellow of the National Institutes of Health (USA) before taking a position at the College of Staten Island. Dr. Shen's research interests lie in the area of the regulation of gene expression, with an emphasis on the roles of epigenetic factors and transcription factors in gene activation. He also pursues topics such as the regulation of programmed cell death through major cellular signal transduction pathways, as well as the use of next generation sequencing in microbiome and genomic analysis. He supervises the Medical Laboratory Science program at the College of Staten Island and works closely with hospitals to provide clinical training for medical laboratory science students. Recently, he is funded to establish the CSI Genomic Facility for NGS training and genomic research.

References

Belkadi A., Bolze A., Itan Y., Cobat A., Vincent Q.B., Antipenko A., et al. (2015) Whole-genome sequencing is more powerful than whole-exome sequencing for detecting exome variants. *Proc. Natl. Acad. Sci. U.S.A.* 112, 5473–5478.

Bell C.J., et al. (2011) Carrier testing for severe childhood recessive diseases by next-generation sequencing. *Sci. Transl. Med.* 3, 65ra4.

Birtel J., Gliem M., Mangold E., et al. (2018) Next-generation sequencing identifies unexpected genotype-phenotype correlations in patients with retinitis pigmentosa. *PLoS One.* 13 (12), e0207958.

Botstein D. and Risch N. (2003) Discovering genotypes underlying human phenotypes: Past successes for mendelian disease, future approaches for complex disease. *Nat. Genet.* 33, 228–237.

Bylstra Y., et al. (2019). Implementation of genomics in medical practice to deliver precision medicine for an Asian population. *NPJ Genomic Medicine,* 4, Article number 12.

Chakravorty S. and Hegde M. (2017) Gene and variant annotation for mendelian disorders in the era of advanced sequencing technologies. *Annu. Rev. Genom. Hum. Genet.* 18, 229–256.

Cirulli E.T. and Goldstein D.B. (2010) Uncovering the roles of rare variants in common disease through whole-genome sequencing. *Nat Rev Genet.* 11, 415–425.

Consortium APG, AACR (2017) Project GENIE: Powering precision medicine through an international consortium, *Cancer Discovery.* 7, 818–831.

Cooper D.N., Chen J.M., Ball E.V., Howells K., Mort M., Phillips A.D., et al. (2010) Genes, mutations, and human inherited disease at the dawn of the age of personalized genomics. *Hum. Mutat.* 31, 631–655.

Cordell H.J. (2002) Epistasis: What it means, what it doesn't mean, and statistical methods to detect it in humans. *Hum. Mol. Genet.* 11, 2463–2468.

Gaff C. L., Winship I. M., Forrest S. M., Hansen D. P., Clark J., Waring P. M., South M. and Sinclair A. H. (2017) Preparing for genomic medicine: A real world demonstration of health system change. *NPJ Genom Med.* 2 (16).

Gazzo A., Raimondi D., Daneels D., Moreau Y., Smits G., Van Dooren S., et al. (2017) Understanding mutational effects in digenic diseases. *Nucleic Acids Res.* 45, e140.

Genomic Common Data Model for Biomedical Data in Clinical Practice Seo Jeong Shina, Seng Chan Youb, Jin Rohc, Yu Rang Park d, Rae Woong Park MEDINFO 2019: Health and Wellbeing e-Networks for All L. Ohno-Machado and B. Séroussi (Eds.) © 2019 International Medical Informatics Association (IMIA) and IOS Press

Zhang, Jun, Chiodini, Rod, Badr, Ahmed, and Zhang, Genfa. (2011) The impact of next-generation sequencing on genomics. *J Genet Genomics.* 38, 95–109.

Lupski J.R. (2012) Digenic inheritance and Mendelian disease. *Nat. Genet.* 44, 1291–1292.

MacArthur D.G., Manolio T.A., Dimmock D.P., et al. (2014) Guidelines for investigating causality of sequence variants in human disease. *Nature.* 508, 469–476.

Majewski J., Schwartzentruber J., Lalonde E., Montpetit A. and Jabado N. (2011) What can exome sequencing do for you? *J. Med. Genet.* 48, 580–589.

Meienberg J., Bruggmann R., Oexle K. and Matyas G. (2016) Clinical sequencing: Is WGS the better WES? *Hum Genet.* 135, 359–362.

Moghaddas F. and Masters S.L. (2018) The classification, genetic diagnosis and modelling of monogenic autoinflammatory disorders. *Clin Sci (Lond).* 132, 1901–1924.

Narravula A., Garber K., Askree S., et al. (2017) Variants of uncertain significance in newborn screening disorders: Implications for large-scale genomic sequencing. *Genet Med.* 19, 77–82.

Peterson J.F., et al. (2019) Building evidence and measuring clinical outcomes for genomic medicine. *Lancet.* 394, 604–610.

Roy Somak, LaFramboise William A., Nikiforov Yuri E., Nikiforova Marina N., Routbort Mark J., Pfeifer John, Nagarajan Rakesh, Carter Alexis B. and Pantanowitz Liron (2016) Next-generation sequencing informatics: Challenges and strategies for implementation in a clinical environment. *Arch Pathol Lab Med.* 140, 958–975.

Stark Z., et al. (2019) Integrating genomics into healthcare: A global responsibility. Am J Hum Genet. 104 (1), 13–20.

Sudlow C., Gallacher J., Allen N., Beral V., Burton P., Danesh J., Downey P., Elliott P., Green J. and Landray M. (2015) UK biobank: An open access resource for identifying the causes of a wide range of complex diseases of middle and old age. *PLoS Med.* 12, e1001779.

Chapter 22

Managed Care Organizations Leverage Health Information from Multiple Sources to Drive Value

Michael Renzi, DO and Owen Moss, MPH

Contents

Health Information

To managed care proponents, data is essential to drive strategy and mission. As a pillar of organizational effectiveness, the successful conversion of insights gained from data aggregation and analysis into sustainable cost of care reductions and reproducible five-star quality ratings is rare. Cost control efforts seldom result in a downward trend; instead, success is defined by stabilizing the year-over-year increases.[1] Furthermore, less than 5 percent of managed care organizations (MCO) achieve the highest quality rating.[2] The purpose of this discussion is to lead to an honest review of your organization's analytic approach and its translation to strategy and outcomes.

DOI: 10.4324/9780429423109-22

Data Alignment with Strategy

MCOs aggregate data into gigantic warehouses and then dredge for opportunities to direct their clinical and business strategies. These analytic conclusions ought to drive programmatic and operational improvements, but the best intended value programs often result in disappointing quality outcomes and cost reductions.[3] These platforms are administratively burdensome to health plans,[4] and they often leave the member in a traditional episodic care model.

Professional fees occupy 20 percent of the overall health care spend, grow at a rate of 5.4 percent per year, and have outpaced global healthcare spending.[3] The payment of value-based health care dollars must promote plan-aligned provider behavior. Additionally, provider work effort is directly related to service reimbursement rates. The clear and frequent communication to provider regarding the financial benefit of this high-value care is critical to large-scale adoption.[4]

Data Management and Governance

To build a data infrastructure that delivers value, an MCO must first clearly define its data management governance model. The goals of this process are the delivery of timely and actionable information to the clinical and business teams. This cyclical process of clinical and analytic collaboration drives better outcomes to the value program. The analytic team is just as responsible for quality outcomes as the business and clinical groups. The quality of the analytics is a joint responsibility between technical and clinical stakeholders.

Data management leadership should consist of both subject matter–specific individuals and clinical expertise. Internal stakeholders will not receive value from data analytic products unless key clinical leadership provides guidance and feedback along the way. These relationships will also help facilitate external value when data analytics is utilized for value-based contracting and care delivery by network practitioners.

Data governance should be clear to every internal stakeholder within the MCO, and leadership and staff should prioritize the need to understand the processes and procedures behind data management and data delivery. This will allow for organizational transparency around data analytics within the MCO and encourage participation and cooperation in the process.

Data and Execution

MCOs will receive internal organizational value from data analytics by aligning their goals and strategies to the products and analyses created through the data infrastructure. The data management and governance model identifies the leadership, stakeholders, and structure to facilitate value delivery, but execution of this process, in the form of working sessions and dedicated project resources and staff, is critical to ultimate success. Near-constant communication between data analytics staff and clinical leadership, facilitated by operational teams, is necessary to achieve the level of value that impacts and drives outcomes. It is common for data analytics products and outputs to sit on the shelf or rarely be utilized because of an execution failure. Either clinical leadership is not effectively conveying its goals throughout the process, data staff is not appropriately responding to clinical or business needs, or operational staff is not facilitating communication channels between all parties.

The success of internal teams for operational and strategic progress and a productive and efficient data infrastructure will then feed external success in developing and facilitating effective value-based models for network practitioners and members. There are several core components of data analysis for value-based models: timely and accurate practitioner progress, concise and reliable information on key quality metrics and program goals, and digestible reports on incentivized clinical actions that impact payment and outcomes. MCOs must share valuable cost and quality information with practitioners and groups to help drive performance. Data on individual and regional medical loss ratios (MLRs), for instance, is not typically reviewed by participating providers but can be immensely valuable when trying to measure performance and improvement.

Ultimately, successful data analytics for MCOs, both for internal stakeholders and external partners in value-based contracts, must translate into health care improvement for membership. If data analytics cannot impact downstream costs and network performance, members will never perceive "value" to their own health. Operational and strategic success hinges on the MCO's ability to translate disparate raw data elements into action and success in the clinical setting. This, at its core, is about execution.

Data and the Last Mile

Many organizations fail to derive value from their data analytics and data infrastructure because they fail in the "last mile" of execution. The difference between data analysis sitting on the shelf versus driving operational and strategic success is small. The MCO might have established proper data analytics teams and processes but failed programmatic implementation and adoption. Or possibly, communication channels between the groups – subject-matter experts, clinical leadership, and operation staff – were weak or non-existent.

Failure in the last mile may also imply data analysis that is sufficient for operational tracking and reporting but insufficient for strategy development or value-based care implementation. This type of data analytics is even more about the collaboration between teams and the organizational infrastructure established around data management than it is about the data or dashboards or reporting.

Data-Driven Organizational Change

If an MCO is serious about data analytics, then it will implement full-scale organizational change to support a powerful data infrastructure. First, leadership – from data analytics, medical management and overall organization management – must be willing and open to publicly discuss the organization's performance, and to do so often. Large stakeholder-run meetings should occur frequently, and they should begin with detailed data presentation and subsequent discussion that is driven from data elements that are shown. The organization needs to constantly level-set around the data that it possesses and be transparent with teams, all the way down to frontline staff, concerning the significance of trends and how they impact the MCO. These sessions will fuel an internal data revolution that will subsequently fuel tremendous external progress, as those data are utilized to develop value-based contracts and programs. Next, data should be accessible and frequently updated: organizational stakeholders should have daily access to dashboards, reports, and analysis. They should incorporate these outputs into their daily workflows and consistently drive team meetings with this information. This level of data analysis will create something of another language at the organization and become ubiquitous with progress. At the end of the day, leaders should ask themselves – "if meetings are not driven by analytics, why not, or how can they be?" Finally, the MCO data analysis infrastructure should support frequent and repetitive sharing of data with external stakeholders. One of the most common failures of value-based contracting in many markets is the lack of timely data to participating practitioners and practices. Performance evaluations at the end of measurement cycle assist metric improvement plans. Organizational analytics foundationally underpin strategy, mission, and performance. Invest in provider behaviors that promote quality and MLR sustainability while fostering deepening provider relationships and member satisfaction.

About the Authors

Owen Moss, MPH, is the Director of Healthcare Delivery at CDPHP in Albany, NY. He's been at the organization for over eight years and helps operationalize CDPHP's healthcare delivery strategy. He specializes in healthcare policy, primary care and specialty value-based reimbursement models and healthcare business operations. He began his career at Booz Allen Hamilton, driving quality improvement and innovation efforts for large federal healthcare agencies. He is currently completing his master's in public health at the Yale School of Public Health. He graduated from Williams College with a BA in Political Economy. He lives just south of Albany with his wife, Julia, and their son, William.

Michael Renzi, DO, joined CDPHP in 2019 as medical director for population health development, and currently serves as president of healthcare delivery. As a fervent proponent of aligned member payer-provider value, Dr. Renzi leads CDPHP in network development, sustainable MLR, reproducible five-star quality and next-generation care delivery. Additionally, Dr. Renzi oversees CDPHP technology, analytics, and clinical data aggregation.

Dr. Renzi received his bachelor's degree at Lafayette College and earned his doctor of osteopathic medicine degree at Philadelphia College of Osteopathic Medicine. He spent 25 years as a primary care internist while developing several multi-specialty physician groups. Over the last 15 years, Dr. Renzi pioneered and built population health ventures with the sole intent of aligning payment and value for everyone who finances, delivers, and receives medical care.

For Dr. Renzi, the best part about working for CDPHP is the single-focus, matrixed, and collaborative culture that extends from the boardroom to the mailroom: provide members what they need.

References

1. PWC Health Research Institute analysis of medical cost trend compared to 2020 consumer price index reported through "Congressional Budget Office Budget and Economic Outlook: 2019 to 2029," January 2019, https://www.cbo.gov/system/files/2019-03/54918-Outlook-3.pdf.
2. 2020 Star Ratings Fact Sheet. https://www.cms.gov/Medicare/Prescription-Drug-Coverage/PrescriptionDrugCovGenIn/PerformanceData.
3. *JAMA Netw Open*. 2020, 3(2), e1920500. doi:10.1001/jamanetworkopen.2019.20500.
4. Kuipers, S.J., Nieboer, A.P., & Cramm, J.M. (2020). Views of patients with multi-morbidity on what is important for patient-centered care in the primary care setting. *BMC Fam Pract*, 21, 71. https://doi.org/10.1186/s12875-020-01144-7https://www.cms.gov/Research-Statistics-Data-and-Systems/Statistics-Trends-and-.
5. Reports/NationalHealthExpendData/Downloads/highlights.pdf.
6. Xiaoyu, Xi, Wang, Ennan, Lu, Qianni, Chen, Piaopiao, Wo, Tian, & Tang, Kammy (2019). Does an economic incentive affect provider behavior? Evidence from a field experiment on different payment mechanisms. *Journal of Medical Economics*, 22:1, 35–44. doi:10.1080/13696998.2018.1539399.

Chapter 23

Workforce Application of Informatics to Target Initiatives

William D. Myhre, MPA

Contents

The Staten Island Performing Provider System (SI PPS) engaged more than 50 local healthcare and healthcare affiliated partners (higher education, organized labor, etc.) in a workforce needs analysis in 2015.

Our partnership represents a healthcare workforce of more 22,700 people, according to the Office of the NY Comptroller (2017 data). In addition to the local healthcare labor market, the Bureau of Labor Statistics predicted, in 2016 that we will need 11.6 million healthcare workers by 2026, necessitating the creation of 3.5 million new jobs and the replacement of 8.1 million individual who leave the healthcare sector or retire.

The data gathered created a gap analysis that allowed the SI PPS to work with partners and external providers to create skills training to help staff meet the demands of a changing healthcare landscape. The SI PPS created new programs with an annual budget of $4 million under the New York State Medicaid redesign program.

In addition to needed training, a number of emerging jobs were discovered during the data gathering. Community health worker, care manager, and certified recovery peer advocate job titles required recruitment and development. Regarding short-term training programs, the SI PPS has provided training to more than 15,000 partner staff, exceeding 45,000 hours in training with more than 50 partners accessing the training – a truly island-wide acceptance. The next part of this chapter will concentrate on specific programs and outcomes associated with our Workforce Development Program.

Both training and new job development were connected to the SI PPS strategic initiatives to improve health outcomes on Staten Island. One clear example of this merging of skills training

DOI: 10.4324/9780429423109-23

and improved health outcomes was our sepsis program in nursing homes. The SI PPS was able to bring together all ten nursing homes on Staten Island to review the way they treated the onset of sepsis in each facility. From this discussion came agreement to adapt a new clinical approach to be implemented in all ten nursing homes. The SI PPS then arranged to engage a training vendor to provide the staff the necessary training to implement the new common clinical approach across all ten partners. More than 100 registered nursing staff were trained. From a data outcomes perspective, the common approach to sepsis management resulted in a 22% reduction in the number of nursing home patients referred to local hospitals for treatment. In addition, this joint employer approach to staff learning demonstrated a shift away from single-employer approaches with varying processes to address common industry problems.

Scholarships are also an important part of our hiring pipeline development process. Along with the College of Staten Island (CSI; part of the City University of New York), 84 economically disadvantaged students who were studying social work or mental health counseling were provided scholarships (in excess of $240,000) with funds from the SI PPS. With the first 21 graduates, we found 18 went from their internships to employment with our local partners. This program has been a successful way to both improve the talent pipeline for needed positions and help students complete their studies while relieving the financial burden of college costs.

Lean process redesign has also been a valuable tool in helping our partners redesign their workflows to improve patient outcomes. One successful project was the merger of the Richmond University Medical Center and the Staten Island Mental Health Society. As part of the merger process, Lean was used to examine current work processes and design a streamlined process to benefit both organizations. The results of this redesign led to improvements in decreased patient time from entering the clinical to see a provider, standardization of equipment used in the clinics, staff training/upskilling, and transitioning paper processes to connected electronic record keeping.

In partnership with CSI, the SI PPS and partners also created longer-term training programs through the Adult Education Department of CSI. One program, the Community Health Worker (CHW) program, graduated more than 30 candidates. All 30 candidates were from existing employers, and the training was required to permit the organizations to redeploy these staff into the newly created CHW jobs. These positions are critical community-facing positions that help educate patients about appropriate community healthcare services. Through proper education of patient options, we have been able to reduce emergency department (ED) use as a stop for primary care. In addition to the skills learned from the CHW program, 3 of the initial 11 students entered into degree programs the next fall with the college, which was another added benefit. We have developed three additional CHW tracks since then. One program was a concentrated weekend program, another was with a specific focus upon behavioral health populations, and a third was developed with the New York City Housing Authority to train housing residents to serve as healthcare resources for their fellow residents. One of the CHW programs was also created to reskill employees facing layoff. By reskilling, these employees were able to move into existing jobs with their home organization and the organization eliminated unemployment costs and retained employee loyalty.

A community navigator program was also created to help link local residents to healthcare services. The navigator helps uninsured and Medicaid recipients access primary care services across the Island. Our initial group of navigators consisted of 16 people who reviewed the needs of more than 15,400 people in conjunction with hospital EDs and community-based organizations.

Table 23.1 Success of Scholarships Leading to Jobs

Scholarships Provided 82–2015–2018	Percentage of Scholarship Graduates Working for SI PPS Partners: 88%

In an effort to address the opioid crisis on Staten Island, the Certified Recovery Peer Advocate (CRPA) position was developed and staff were hired to provide one-to-one counseling to those in crisis and connect them to immediate care options. The CRPA position located in hospital EDs, community partners, and law enforcement now provided the ability of a person in crisis to speak with someone who is in recovery. The CRPA can discuss real lived experiences and paths to seek recovery and do so in a way that is compassionate for the person in crisis. Originally there were two CRPAs on Staten Island, and in the intervening years we have grown that number to more than 75 trained and functioning advocates. The CRPA program has helped to again provide a common curriculum, revised and enhanced by seeking the feedback from both employers and prior CRPA graduates. The program was also recently certified by ASAP of New York State, the New York Certification Board.

Data for 2019 demonstrated a 45% decrease in total overdoses, a 35% decrease in fatal overdoses, and a 49% decrease in naloxone saves compared to 2018.

Federal funding continues to support the growth of our programs, with a $650,000 grant secured from the US Health Resources and Services Administration to train more than 240 CRPAs and CHWs between 2019 and 2022.

In 2020, the Staten Island Performing Provider System and Community Cares of Brooklyn began developing a regional partnership to expand the Certified Peer Recovery Program to overlay the Staten Island PPS model in the borough of Brooklyn. The two groups are proposing to New York State a three-year demonstration project that will train an additional 300 CRPAs and CHWs.

In 2019, the SI PPS launched a federally approved registered apprentice program using a learn-and-earn model. Employer leaders in our nursing home partnerships told the SI PPS they faced challenges in recruiting and retaining staff for certified nursing assistant positions. The learn-and-earn model combines classroom learning through our local higher education partner, the College of Staten Island, and on-the-job learning with our employer partners. Each apprentice works with an experienced mentor while on the job to provide direct feedback and review of how the apprentice is applying the skills they learn. Apprentice results to improve the hiring pipeline are provided in Table 23.3.

Additional apprentice class details are provided in Table 23.4.

In the two certified nursing assistant apprentice classes we have noted, nearly 50% of students in our second class were hired from outside healthcare, helping to expand our recruitment

Table 23.2　Growth of CRPA Workforce—New Training Fills New Jobs

Initial CRPA Supply: 2–2017	CRPA Supply After 18 Months: 90

Table 23.3　New Training Improves Hiring Pipeline

Pre-training Program	Post-Training Program
Staffing issues facing nursing homes.	Desired outcomes: Improved retention, wider recruitment pool, improved quality and staff morale.
Turnover in excess of 24%.	Reduced turnover
Retraining of new hires; longer time to provide service on clinical unit.	Better trained staff and quicker time to provide care on the clinical unit.
Overtime costs created by turnover.	Reduce overtime and boost employee morale and staff retention.

Table 23.4 Success of Newly Created Apprentice Training Programs

Class	Additional Details
Initial Apprentice Class—2018	9 with 100% complete pass rate- state exam and a three-credit college course.
Second Round of Class	16 students in both classes 2019/2020.

pipeline. We also were able to recruit a number of home health aides, who used the program to build a career ladder for themselves. During the COVID-19 pandemic, a number of the apprentice learners were able to provide significant help to the licensed staff. Their classroom learning and on-the-job training created a ready-made supply of additional hands on deck.

The SI PPS convened nursing home partners, organized labor, and the College of Staten Island to conduct a deep dive discussion about the recruitment/retention impacts upon the nursing homes. This initial discussion process is integral to the success of programs such as these. A major finding of our analysis was the lack of such skills as conflict resolution, team building, and understanding disease management as part of a healthcare team. We then rebuilt a new curriculum to meet these training needs and received recognition from the US Department of Labor to launch a federally approved apprentice learn-and-earn program. The apprentice is a learn-and-earn program, with a combination of classroom and on-the-job learning. On-the-job staff are mentored by seasoned staff who have demonstrated excellence in their work habits. Classroom funding for the program is through federal and SI PPS dollars. Our first class had nine participants, and we have been asked by our partners to create a second class with 20–24 slots. Employers have been pleased by the deliberate process of learning by the apprentices, and the mentors indicate that they believe the apprentices will enter their job role well prepared, which should help improve retention and teamwork. We also included a three-credit college course on sociology designed for the nursing home population. Every one of the apprentice students passed this college course. Partner organizations and the SI PPS are now in discussion to explore additional apprentice learning, particularly in the occupations of licensed practical nurse and lab technician. A growing apprentice program, designed with employer and labor input, creates career pathways for internal staff and new opportunities for the community. The input or data permits the creation of a focused curriculum that addresses the future employers' needs and helps fast-track the onboarding process. Our first class saw two-thirds of apprentices come from home health aide positions. The home health aides now would earn a federally recognized certificate and see an increase in their wages. This new class of recruits also created a new hiring pipeline for the nursing homes.

In a September 26, 2019, article in *Modern Healthcare* titled "Health Systems Redefine Training to Re-energize Employees," the following important points were made:

- "The healthcare industry lags behind other sectors' training practices and many providers will need to adapt their internal development programs to remain competitive."
- New research indicates that healthcare workers spend 25.5 hours on training a year, which is about a third less than the average 34.1 hours for other industries. Healthcare organizations spend less money on training, too: $602 compared to $1,296 per employee per year, according to the Association for Talent Development.
- Disengaged employees can drain the life out of an organization. Revenue drops along with productivity. Displeased employees displease patients, which can swing reimbursement.
- Employees will need to be tech savvy, nimble, and customer centric to keep up with the evolving healthcare landscape.

In 2018, Cornell ILR published a study resulting from its on-site research regarding the impact of our workforce transformations. The report was titled "Findings of the Cornell Research Team Regarding DSRIP-Promoted Change in the SI PPS." A summary of those findings follows:

Key Finding #1: Breadth and depth of organizational restructuring and workforce transformation

- The restructuring effort led by the SI PPS is a profound change in how frontline healthcare employees are working, supported by extensive training and a broadening in the roles that employees play.
- Workforce transformation is supported by promotion of work task integration within and between the 70 organizations in the SI PPS.
- Data and analytic based decision-making that is used to evaluate and reward performance.
- Extensive workforce preparedness providing both soft and hard skill development.

Key Finding #2: Breadth of organizational and clinical integration

- Integration of information systems.
- Occupation integration involving greater communication between different occupational groups.
- Integration of clinical practices within a facility.
- Within-unit and between-unit integration.
- Inter-facility integration.

Policy implications: With the impact of COVID-19, many training programs are now challenged with replacing what was a traditional classroom approach with the development of remote/ online learning. Consistent with this conversion is the need to balance the requirement of physically demonstrating certain job skills such as transferring a patient, administering medications, and applying medical devices with the online modification of didactic content.

Beyond the learning transformation are licensing and budget considerations. It may require that licensing/credentialing organizations review and approve the modifications required by the impact of COVID-19. The budget implications also will be reflected in funding sources both organizational and external for the future. The parameters adopted to fund the licensing/credentialing processes under the old method of classroom learning will need to be refashioned to accept the reality and utility of remote/online learning.

About the Author

William D. Myhre, MPA, (American University) has 30 years' experience in human resources leadership of non-profit organizations. His expertise is transforming human resources via mergers, new government programs, and consulting and governmental lobbying and testimony.

Recent recognitions include the President's Medal, College of Staten Island; an Award from the Richmond County Medical Society; and National Fund for Workforce Solutions: Emerging Champion of the Front Line Workforce.

Chapter 24

Patient-Centered Medical Home and Social Determinants of Health (SDoH)

Salvatore Volpe, MD FAAP, FACP ABP-CI,
FHIMSS, CHCQM and Rick A. Moore, PhD

Contents

Introduction

Much has transpired since the initial patient-centered medical home (PCMH) models became widely adopted by about 20% of practices in the United States:

1. Most experts would agree that we have moved from pilot stage to actual working models.
2. More payers and employers have accepted the need to modify reimbursement systems from the acute care model to one that helps cover the cost of managing populations and rewarding for positive outcomes and improved patient satisfaction.

DOI: 10.4324/9780429423109-24

3. Most studies now support that PCMHs have a positive impact on quality, though the degree of that impact varies widely.
4. There is a greater alignment between government programs and PCMH.
5. PCMH recognition programs are being offered to specialists.
6. PCMH recognition programs are also being offered by the Joint Commission, the Utilization Review Accreditation Commission (URAC), and the Accreditation Association for Ambulatory Health Care (AAAHC).

In this chapter, we will review the origins and philosophy of PCMH, the benefits of PCMH, details specific to the most widely used PCMH recognition program, and the impact of the COVID-19 pandemic, as well as emerging strategies to leverage PCMH as a foundational guide to move toward value-based versus volume-based healthcare.

Origin of the Patient-Centered Medical Home Model

There is a French saying, *"Plus ça change, plus c'est la même chose"* (The more things change, the more they stay the same). I am sure that there are few primary care providers (PCPs) who have not heard of the term "medical home." Compare that with awareness of the concept ten years ago, as American medicine was reaching its peak in dividing care into the maximal number of silos possible. The drive to sub-subspecialization, the inadequate reimbursement for anything other than acute procedure-driven healthcare, and rising medical liability led to many PCPs being little more than gatekeepers.

Fifty-four years ago, the Council of Pediatric Practice (COPP) had a prescient opinion regarding healthcare. At that time, they were trying to address children with special healthcare needs (CSHCN). The federal Maternal and Child Health Bureau defined CSHCN as "those who have or are at increased risk for a chronic physical, developmental, behavioral, or emotional condition and who also require health and related services of a type or amount beyond that required by children generally."[1] The American Academy of Pediatrics stated:

> For children with chronic diseases or disabling conditions, the lack of a complete record and a "medical home" is a major deterrent to adequate health supervision. Wherever the child is cared for, the question should be asked, "Where is the child's medical home?" and any pertinent information should be transmitted to that place.[2]

In 1967, there were no fax machines, no secure email, and no graphical user interface (GUI) electronic health records (EHRs). There was, however, the realization that without the coordination of care by all providers, the families of these children would suffer from gaps in care, redundant care, and skyrocketing expenses. Sound familiar?

The COPP made three recommendations:

> The first requirement is the teaching of all medical students that a medical home and a complete central record of a child's medical care are the sine qua non of proper pediatric supervision. Second, the concept must spread from physicians to all agencies and people caring for children – schools, child guidance clinics, well-infant stations, surgical specialists, emergency departments, and so forth. The third step is the indoctrination of parents.[3]

While the goals were laudatory, it was not until Dr. Calvin Sia took up the gauntlet that the concept gained the exposure and funding needed to be implemented. Between 1978 and 1979, Dr. Sia succeeded in having the term "medical home" incorporated in legislation passed in Hawaii.

> This was the birth of the medical home concept as we know it today. It stated that a medical home would be family centered; be community-based (geographically and financially accessible and available); offer continuity, comprehensive, and coordinated care; and use the resources of related services in the neighborhood.[4]

In 1998, Dr. Edward H. Wagner proposed the following model for chronic disease management based on his work at Group Health Cooperative (See Figure 24.1). Communities depend on healthcare delivery systems to have four key features:

- *Self-management support*: Patients and their families are given tools and resources to participate in management of their health.
- *Delivery system design*: The system to deliver healthcare has to take into account the multiple agents and facilitate communication.

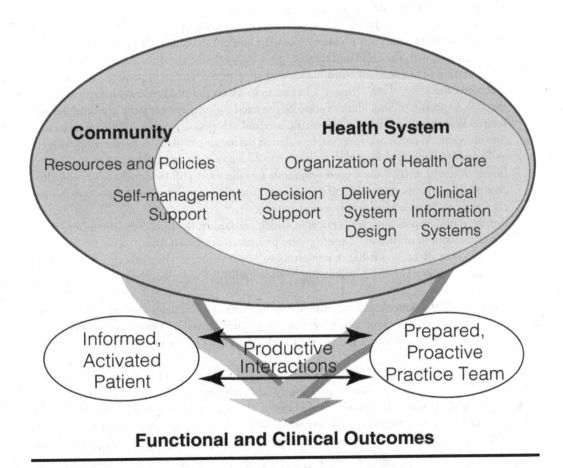

Figure 24.1   Edward Wagner's model for chronic disease management

■ *Decision support*: Evidence-based clinical support tools need to be available at the point of care.
■ *Information systems*: Information technology needs to be developed to facilitate communication between providers, patients, and the community.[5]

In 2002, the American Academy of Pediatrics (AAP) issued the following description of the medical home:

1. Provision of family-centered care through developing a trusting partnership with families, respecting their diversity, and recognizing that they are the constant in a child's life.
2. Sharing clear and unbiased information with the family about the child's medical care and management and about the specialty and community services and organizations they can access.
3. Provision of primary care, including, but not restricted to, acute and chronic care and preventive services, including breastfeeding promotion and management, immunizations, growth and developmental assessments, appropriate screenings, healthcare supervision, and patient and parent counseling about health, nutrition, safety, parenting, and psychosocial issues.
4. Assurance that ambulatory and inpatient care for acute illnesses will be continuously available (24 hours a day, 7 days a week, 52 weeks a year).
5. Provision of care over an extended period of time to ensure continuity. Transitions, including those to other pediatric providers or into the adult healthcare system, should be planned and organized with the child and family.
6. Identification of the need for consultation and appropriate referral to pediatric medical subspecialists and surgical specialists. (In instances in which the child enters the medical system through a specialty clinic, identification of the need for primary pediatric consultation and referral is appropriate.) Primary, pediatric medical subspecialty, and surgical specialty care providers should collaborate to establish shared management plans in partnership with the child and family and to formulate a clear articulation of each other's role.
7. Interaction with early intervention programs, schools, early childhood education and child care programs, and other public and private community agencies to be certain that the special needs of the child and family are addressed.
8. Provision of care coordination services in which the family, the physician, and other service providers work to implement a specific care plan as an organized team.
9. Maintenance of an accessible, comprehensive, central record that contains all pertinent information about the child, preserving confidentiality.[6]

In 2007, AAP, the American Academy of Family Practice, American College of Physicians, and American Osteopathic Association, representing approximately 333,000 physicians, developed the following joint principles to describe the characteristics of the PCMH:

■ *Personal physician*: Each patient has an ongoing relationship with a personal physician trained to provide first contact, continuous, and comprehensive care.
■ *Physician-directed medical practice*: The personal physician leads a team of individuals at the practice level who collectively take responsibility for the ongoing care of patients.
■ *Whole-person orientation*: The personal physician is responsible for providing for all the patient's healthcare needs or taking responsibility for appropriately arranging care with

other qualified professionals. This includes care for all stages of life: acute care, chronic care, preventive services, and end-of-life care.

- *Care is coordinated and/or integrated* across all elements of the complex healthcare system (e.g., subspecialty care, hospitals, home health agencies, nursing homes) and the patient's community (e.g., family, public, and private community-based services). Care is facilitated by registries, information technology (IT), health information exchange, and other means to assure that patients get the indicated care when and where they need and want it in a culturally and linguistically appropriate manner.

- *Quality and safety* are hallmarks of the medical home:
  - Practices advocate for their patients to support the attainment of optimal, patient-centered outcomes that are defined by a care planning process driven by a compassionate, robust partnership between physicians, the patient, and the patient's family.
  - Evidence-based medicine and clinical decision support tools guide decision-making.
  - Physicians in the practice accept accountability for continuous quality improvement through voluntary engagement in performance measurement and improvement.
  - Patients actively participate in decision-making, and feedback is sought to ensure patients' expectations are being met.
  - IT is utilized appropriately to support optimal patient care, performance measurement, patient education, and enhanced communication.
  - Practices go through a voluntary recognition process by an appropriate nongovernmental entity to demonstrate that they have the capabilities to provide patient-centered services consistent with the medical home model.
  - Patients and families participate in quality improvement activities at the practice level.

- *Enhanced access* to care is available through systems such as open scheduling, expanded hours, and new options for communication between patients, their personal physician, and practice staff.

- *Payment* appropriately recognizes the added value provided to patients who have a PCMH. The payment structure should be based on the following framework:
  - It should reflect the value of physician and non-physician staff patient-centered care management work that falls outside of the face-to-face visit.
  - It should pay for services associated with coordination of care both within a given practice and between consultants, ancillary providers, and community resources.
  - It should support adoption and use of health IT for quality improvement.
  - It should support provision of enhanced communication access, such as secure email and telephone consultation.
  - It should recognize the value of physician work associated with remote monitoring of clinical data using technology.
  - It should allow for separate fee-for-service payments for face-to-face visits. (Payments for care management services that fall outside of the face-to-face visit, as previously described, should not result in a reduction in the payments for face-to-face visits.)
  - It should recognize case mix differences in the patient population being treated within the practice.
  - It should allow physicians to share in savings from reduced hospitalizations associated with physician-guided care management in the office setting.
  - It should allow for additional payments for achieving measurable and continuous quality improvements.[7]

The COVID-19 Pandemic and Social Determinants of Health

COVID-19 has cast a light on the generations of health inequity in the United States. Social determinants of health (SDoH), as defined by the World Health Organization (WHO), are "the conditions in which people are born, grow, live, work and age." Despite US health expenditures, healthcare only accounts for 20% of health outcomes, and individual factors and health behaviors account for 10%–20%. Economic and social factors account for another 40% while the physical environment account for about 10%. "The Social Determinants of Health: Coming of Age" is an excellent review of the topic.[8] According to an article in the *Proceedings of the National Academy of Sciences of the United States of America*, overall US life expectancy in 2020 will decrease by 1.13 years, whereas the reductions for Black and Latino populations will be 3 to 4 times that of Whites.[9]

Organisation for Economic Co-operation and Development (OECD) nations on average spent about \$2 on social services for every dollar of healthcare spending, compared to only about 55 cents per dollar on social services in the United States, according to a study of 2009 data by Elizabeth Bradley of Yale University and Lauren Taylor of Harvard University. Factoring in these expenditures presents a new perspective: the United States 13th among OECD countries in total healthcare outlays.[10] Despite the US combined per capita spending on healthcare and social services exceeding that of any nation, the US lags in many measures of quality such as life expectancy at birth, adults with chronic conditions, and suicide rates.[11]

Practices espousing PCMH principles will not just focus on the "traditional" medical and behavioral issues, but rather will be working with an even greater expanded team as they help identify SDoH gaps (e.g., data interoperability gaps) and direct their patients to the appropriate resources. The team will include agents who can help address food, housing, transportation, connectivity, and environmental issues. For example, a patient who lives in a food desert will have difficulty managing his diabetes regardless of the medications prescribed. A mother living downwind of a refinery will have difficulty keeping her asthmatic children consistently in school and out of the emergency department (ED) regardless of the number of metered-dose inhalers prescribed. This new focus on social services will be necessary if the United States is to ever improve truly the health outcomes of all its citizens. Fair access to the explosion of devices and services that will connect our healthcare providers, educators, and employers can only be achieved by adding broadband to the list of necessary utilities such as heat, electricity, and water. (Editor's note: see chapter 15: Health Information Exchange: An Overview & New York State's Model.)

Figure 24.2 by artist Angus Maguire is one example that illustrates the difference between equality and equity. In this version, the idea of liberation is shown, represented by the removal of an obstacle that was previously assumed to be essential to the situation. With the artificially limited choice between *only* equality and equity thus disrupted, the reader is encouraged to reimagine further how relationships and power in the illustration might be further transformed in the fourth box.

In addition to shining a light on the inadequacies of our current delivery system with regard to health inequities, the COVID-19 pandemic has also shone a light on the inadequacies of health information systems, specifically the lack of data interoperability. These inadequacies in health data interoperability to deliver quality healthcare at scale were some of the root causes of the inadequate response to the global pandemic that ensued. Whether it be the lack of information at the bedside or in the exam room due to the lack of data sharing across the health system, each country fighting the pandemic was adversely affected by its inability to quickly detect and respond to this global crisis. While the PCMH model of care is focused on the delivery of accessible, affordable, and high-quality primary care, it (the PCMH) is the "home" or hub that will assist in the early

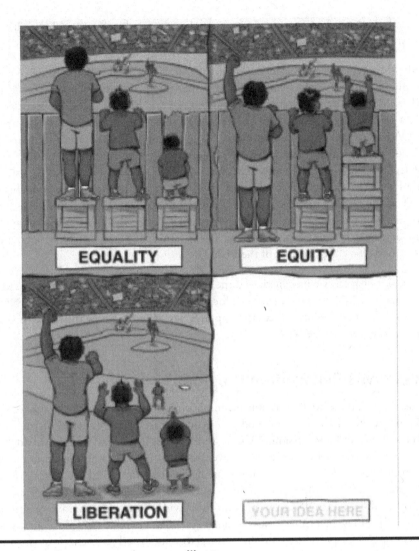

Figure 24.2   Equality versus equity versus liberty

Credit: A collaboration between the Center for Story-Based Strategy and the Interactive Institute for Social Change.

prevention (vaccines), detection (accessibility), and treatment (follow-up) of future pandemics that are sure to come our way. Now more than ever, we have a moment in time when the warning signal of COVID-19 will be viewed as the signal that prompted us into action for change, or the moment in time we squandered to only maintain the status quo.

Moving from Volume-Based to Value-Based Care

It's now been over a decade (2008) since the National Committee for Quality Assurance's (NCQA's) PCMH recognition model swept the country; as of this writing, about 20% of primary care practices (~13,000) and clinicians (~67,000) recognized by NCQA for having achieved

PCMH transformation. And over this time, much has occurred to further substantiate the model's importance to healthcare delivery reform:

■ While there remains an ever-increasing total cost of care in the United States – now at over $3 trillion – studies show that the PCMH model consistently decreases the utilization of higher cost care, such as avoidable hospitalizations and ED visits, and support that PCMHs have a positive impact on quality of care,herugh the degree of the impact still varies widely.
■ NCQA has extended the medical home neighborhood with the Patient-Centered Specialty Practice and Patient-Centered Connected Care recognition programs.
■ The Centers for Medicare/Medicaid Services (CMS) released the Comprehensive Primary Care Plus (CPC+) and Primary Care First (PCF) innovation programs, which are largely based on the PCMH model coupled with alternative/incentive payment models.
■ All of these have led to the federal government's planned shift from fee-for-service (FFS) reimbursement to value-based payment (VBP). This VBP accountability model of care is largely based on the principles of the PCMH.

So far in this chapter, we have reviewed the concepts and importance of team-based, patient-centered primary care. Now we will shift our focus to a specific recognition program (NCQA) and the latest research regarding implementation approaches, including how the model is shaping the healthcare delivery reform agenda.

NCQA's PCMH Recognition Program[11]

As previously stated, there are (at the time of this writing) four organizations that have operationalized the core tenets of the PCMH model of primary care delivery into evaluation programs: the AAAHC, the Joint Commission, NCQA, and URAC. The oldest and most widely adopted is operated by NCQA. Now in existence for over 30 years, NCQA (a not-for-profit organization) has built an industry reputation as a leading quality measurement and accrediting organization with its flagship quality measurement program called HEDIS (The Healthcare Effectiveness and Data Information Set). HEDIS is the nation's most widely used comparative quality measurement system. HEDIS is the primary measurement system in use by many federal and state quality improvement programs, particularly when it comes to value-based payment programs such as the CMS Medicare Stars. In addition, the CMS Quality Payment Program (QPP) uses the HEDIS measures as a foundation for their Merit-Based Incentive Programs (MIPS) for eligible providers. The HEDIS measures used in the CMS QPP/MIPS program are formatted into Electronic Clinical Quality Measures (eCQMs) for ease of implementation and reporting within and from EHRs. In addition, HEDIS is also used by NCQA to produce Health Plan Ratings, a program that crosses the delivery of care continuum and provides the ecosystem with a measurement system to help move from volume-based to value-based care. While the PCMH recognition programs do not currently require reporting of quality measures, the federal government has been piloting PCMH-like programs such as CPC+. And these PCMH-like programs are a signal that the federal government is likely to start incentivizing all primary care practices to transform and start reporting standardized quality measures. (Editor's note: see chapter 11: Promoting Interoperability and Quality Payment Programs: The Evolving Paths of Meaningful Use.)

Around 2006, NCQA collaborated with the founding organizations of the PCMH model of care to develop its first recognition program to assess a practice's transformation toward delivering whole-person, patient-centered care. That early program, called Physician Practice Connections (PPC), later evolved into the 2008 PCMH Recognition Program.

The 2008 NCQA PCMH Recognition Program was modeled after the NCQA Health Plan Accreditation evaluation model in terms of establishing a set of must-pass standards and scoring points to demonstrate a practice as conforming to the PCMH principles. The early (2008, 2011, and 2014) NCQA PCMH evaluation products compartmentalized the evaluation criteria into capability areas known as standards. Each standard has elements, and several elements have factors. This layeredhertion model allows for varying approaches in the transformation process of primary care delivery. The latest version of the model was released in 2017.

PCMH 2017 builds on and integrates concepts from PCMH 2014, such as providing 24/7 access to care, reinforcing the care team, integration of behavioral health, coordinating care transitions, and measuring improvement of quality measures. With the 2017 program, NCQA still has a layered framework but now uses the terms of concepts, competencies, and criteria.

- *Concepts* represent the core principles/tenets of the PCMH model of care.
- *Competencies* are areas of capability the practices must demonstrate.
- *Criteria* additional details of a competency – like a sub-competency.

NCQA PCMH 2017 Concept Areas

1. *Team-Based Care and Practice Organization (TC)*: Defines the leadership/governance structure necessary for an effective PCMH.
2. *Know and Manage Patients (KM)*: Defines the information management infrastructure needed (e.g., electronic medical record, clinical decision support) for an effective PCMH.
3. *Patient-Centered Access and Continuity (AC)*: Defines what practices provide to patients to ensure access to and continuity of care.
4. *Care Management and Support (CM)*: Defines for clinicians the care management/population health protocols needed.
5. *Care Coordination and Care Transitions (CC)*: Defines that primary and specialty care clinicians are to share information needed to manage the whole person as they go from one caregiver to the next in their medical home neighborhood.
6. *Performance Measurement and Quality Improvement (QI)*: Defines for practices to develop ways to measure performance and to set improvement goals.

No More Recognition Levels: A Practice Is Either Transformed or Not under PCMH 2017

There is no longer a three-tier recognition status with the latest iteration of the NCQA PCMH program. For a practice to attain recognition their recognition, they must (1) meet all 40 core criteria in the program and (2) earn 25 credits in elective criteria across 5 of 6 concepts. In addition, NCQA has moved from three-year renewal process of the recognition to an annual, two-phase approach: (1) transform (achieve recognition) and (2) sustain recognition.

New practices will follow a three-step process:

1. *Commit: Learn about Recognition Eligibility and the Recognition Process.* Practices complete a self-assessment and work with NCQA to develop a "custom" plan to achieve recognition.
2. *Transform: The Evaluation Process.* If determined to be ready to move forward from the commit phase, the practice candidate will submit data and documentation to NCQA's recognition system for an independent surveyor to review. All reviews are done via virtual interviews via web portal interfaces, like Microsoft Teams and Zoom.

3. *Sustain: Keeping Your Recognition*. Each year, the transformed practice is required to go through a subset of the standards for review, as well as demonstrate quality improvement progress.

CMS Demonstration Programs Related to PCMH[12]

Since its inception, each successive iteration of the NCQA PCMH recognition model has attempted to align with other programs seeking to attain similar outcomes, specifically related to reductions in cost and improvements in access to quality primary care. Other primary care evaluation models took their lead from the NCQA PCMH evaluation model, and just modified/incorporated a few standards to address specific criteria aimed at "testing" the model's impact on the select criteria. The most prominent model that adapted the majority of the NCQA PCMH criteria is the CPC+ program established by CMS in 2017.

CPC+ Model Details

This model, much like the PCMH model, seeks to improve quality, access, and efficiency of primary care. Practices that opt to enroll in this demonstration program will make changes in the way they deliver care, centered on five key CPC+ functions that are essentially the same as the NCQA PCMH Concept Areas:

1. Access and Continuity
2. Care Management
3. Comprehensiveness and Coordination
4. Patient and Caregiver Engagement
5. Planned Care and Population Health.

Unlike the NCQA PCMH recognition model, where there is no direct incentive from NCQA, the CPC+ includes two payment elements:

1. *Care Management Fee (CMF)*: Provides for a risk-adjusted (care intensity–based) non-visit-based CMF paid per beneficiary per month (PBPM).
2. *Performance-Based Incentive Payment*: Prospectively pays and retrospectively reconciles incentive payment based on specific measures.

PCMH Implementation Strategies

As alluded to earlier in this chapter, there has been much research done to measure the impact of several PCMH implementations across the United States. And while each study has its specific area of interest, most all conclude that the model does help practices transform into a more team based/whole person–centered model of care delivery. Yet, there are varying degrees of improvement attained by the numerous studies conducted. NCQA staff amassed most of these studies (specific to the NCQA PCMH recognition model), and compiled them in a report to assist practices, policy makers, and payers in their pursuits to understand the impact of the model in its various implementations across the United States.[13]

As with any intervention introduced into an ecosystem, there are many conflating environmental variables/factors that are in most cases challenging if not impossible to control. In most studies conducted, there was no "pre-assessment" of the practices to determine if they were or were not already delivering care as defined by the model, much less to the degree the practice had "transformed" prior to receiving recognition. So, most studies cite selection bias as a primary reason for the variation in the outcomes, where some studies indicate greater improvements versus others that show a modicum or varying level of improvement in comparison to the control group. However, one study took a novel approach at grouping practices together based not just on their before-and-after recognition level attainment or their points attained for recognition. David et al. clustered the practices that achieved NCQA PCMH recognition based on the groupings of capabilities they performed stronger.[14] This study formed about 100 practices into 1 of 3 clusters by which each cluster performed comparatively better than the other cluster. This approach to grouping practices based on their relative score of capabilities helped to better understand the heterogeneity of the practices in their approached to PCMH implementation. This heterogeneity is largely due to the design of the recognition model requiring must-pass elements and specific points to attain levels. As a result of this implementation heterogeneity, there are inaccurate signals being sent to the payers and practices. This study provides evidence to refine PCMH implementations more toward targeted capabilities, so that practices/payers would focus on those capabilities that benefit the patient and not just achieving an incentive and/or cost savings.

About the Authors

Salvatore Volpe, MD, FAAP, FACP, ABP-CI, FHIMSS, CHCQM, has achieved board certification in pediatrics, internal medicine, geriatrics and clinical informatics and he currently serves as the Chief Medical Officer working closely with the IT staff at the Staten Island Performing Provider System (SI PPS). The SI PPS is an alliance of clinical and social service providers focused on improving the quality of care and overall health for Staten Island's Medicaid and uninsured populations, which include more than 180,000 Staten Island residents, and was the highest performing group under the New York State Department of Health's Delivery System Reform Incentive Payment (DSRIP) program.

His practice was the first solo practice in the United States to achieve Level 3 2011 NCQA Patient Centered Medical Home Recognition. In addition to running a solo primary care practice for 30 years, Dr. Volpe has had many leadership roles outside the office. He served as physician champion for the NYC Department of Health and Mental Hygiene Primary Care Information Project (NYC DOH MH PCIP); president of Healthcare Information and Management Systems Society New York State (HIMSS NYS); president of the Richmond County Medical Society (RCMS); chairman of the HIT Committee for the Medical Society of the State of New York (MSSNY) and Richmond County; member of the board of directors of the New York eHealth Collaborative (NYeC); and member of the board of the Medical Liability Mutual Insurance Company.

Learning from others and sharing this knowledge has been another important aspect of his professional career. He has been invited to speak on health and technology topics locally and nationally. In addition to contributing to numerous journals, Dr. Volpe was a contributor for the PCMH chapter for the second and third editions of *Medical Informatics: An Executive Primer.*

Dr. Volpe and his practice have been recognized by many organizations. For work with the geriatric population and informatics, they were presented the Island Peer Review Organization

(IPRO) Quality Award and SUNY Downstate Medical School Geriatrics Medicine Award. Their focus on PCMH was acknowledged by the Patient-Centered Primary Care Collaborative (PCPCC) with the Patient-Centered Medical Home Practice (PCMH) Award. Due to the innovations introduced by Dr. Volpe and his executive board at HIMSS NYS, he was honored with the Chapter Leader of the Year Award.

Dr. Volpe received his bachelor of arts from Columbia University, his medical degree from SUNY Downstate and completed a combined pediatrics and internal medicine residency at Staten University Hospital (now a member of the NorthWell Health Network).

Rick A. Moore, PhD, FACHE, FHIMSS, CPHIMS, CISM, CCSFP, PMP. As NCQA's Chief Information Officer, Rick Moore is responsible for the vision and strategic direction of the Information Services, Information Technology and Information Products. The National Committee for Quality Assurance (NCQA) is a private, 501(c)(3) not-for-profit organization dedicated to improving healthcare quality. Since its founding in 1990, NCQA has been a central figure in driving improvement throughout the healthcare system, helping to elevate the issue of healthcare quality to the top of the national agenda.

Prior to joining NCQA in 2008, Rick was the director of health informatics at the National Association of Children's Hospitals, where he led the development of information services and products for over 200 member hospitals. He has also served the Office of the Secretary of Health Affairs at the Department of Defense, where he led the development of electronic health record (EHR) systems and was awarded the Information Technology Officer of the Year of the Joint Medical Information Systems Office in 2004.

References

1. McPherson, M., Arago, P., Fox, H., et al. A new definition of children with special health care needs. *Pediatrics*. 1998:102:137–140.
2. American Academy of Pediatrics. Council on pediatric practice. Pediatric records and medical home. In: *Standards of Child Care*. Evanston, IL: American Academy of Pediatrics, 1967:77–79.
3. American Academy of Pediatrics. Council on pediatric practice. Fragmentation of health care services for children. *News and Comment* (Suppl), April 1977.
4. History of the medical home concept. *Pediatrics*. 2004:113(5 Suppl):1473–1478.
5. Wagner, E. H. Chronic disease management: What will it take to improve care for chronic illness? *Effective Clinical Practice*. 1998:1(1):2–4.
6. The medical home. *Pediatrics*. 2002;110(1 Pt 1):184–186.
7. http://www.aafp.org/dam/AAFP/documents/practice_management/pcmh/initiatives/PCMHJoint. pdf. Accessed November 25, 2014.
8. Annual Review of Public Health Volume 32, 2011 Braveman, pp. 381–398, https://www.annual reviews.org/doi/full/10.1146/annurev-publhealth-031210-101218.
9. Reductions in 2020 US life expectancy due to COVID-19 and the disproportionate impact on the Black and Latino populations Theresa Andrasfay. *Noreen Goldman Proceedings of the National Academy of Sciences* February 2021:118(5):e2014746118; doi:10.1073/pnas.2014746118.
10. To Lower the Cost of Health Care, Invest in Social Services, Kenneth Davis. https://www.healthaffairs. org/do/10.1377/hblog20150714.049322/full/#:~:text=OECD%20nations%20on%20average%20 spent,Lauren%20Taylor%20of%20Harvard%20University.
11. U.S. Health Care from a Global Perspective, 2019: Higher Spending, Worse Outcomes? Issue Briefs January 30, 2020. https://www.commonwealthfund.org/publications/issue-briefs/2020/jan/ us-health-care-global-perspective-2019.

12. @CMSinnovates. *Comprehensive Primary Care Plus | CMS Innovation Center.* @CMSinnovates. 2021. https://innovation.cms.gov/innovation-models/comprehensive-primary-care-plus.
13. *PCMH Evidence – NCQA.* 2021. https://www.ncqa.org/programs/health-care-providers-practices/patient-centered-medical-home-pcmh/benefits-support/pcmh-evidence/.
14. David, G., Saynisch, P. A., & Smith-McLallen, A. The economics of patient-centered care. *Journal of Health Economics.* 2018:59:60–77. https://doi.org/10.1016/j.jhealeco.2018.02.012.

Chapter 25

eMOLST
Electronic System for Completing Medical Orders for Life-Sustaining Treatment

Patricia Bomba, MD, MACP, FRCP and Katie Orem, MPH

Contents

Advance Care Planning

Advance care planning (ACP) is a process that prepares a trusted individual to act as a health care agent and apply shared medical decision-making on behalf of a person who loses the capacity to make medical decisions. ACP conversations occur with a person, their health care agent, primary physician, nurse practitioner (NP) or physician assistant (PA), other members of the clinical team, and family and loved ones. The person's values, beliefs, goals, and what matters most are recorded in a state-specific advance directive. The ACP process allows for flexible decision-making in the context of the patient's current medical situation.

Advance Directives versus MOLST

Standard medical care means a patient receives all necessary medical treatment unless there is a medical order to withhold treatment.

DOI: 10.4324/9780429423109-25

Medical Orders for Life-Sustaining Treatment (MOLST)*

8-Step MOLST Protocol**

1. Prepare for discussion
   - Review what is known about patient goals and values
   - Understand the medical facts about the patient's medical condition and prognosis
   - Review what is known about the patient's capacity to consent
   - Retrieve and review completed advance directives and prior DNR/MOLST forms
   - Determine key family members and if the patient lacks medical decision-making capacity, identify the health care agent or surrogate
   - Find uninterrupted time for the discussion
   - Review the legal requirements under New York State Public Health Law, based on who will make the decision and where the decision is made
2. Begin with what the patient and family knows
   - Determine what the patient and family know regarding condition and prognosis
   - Determine what is known about the patient's values and beliefs
3. Provide any new information about the patient's medical condition and values from the medical team's perspective
   - Provide information in small amounts, giving time for response
   - Seek a common understanding; understand areas of agreement and disagreement
   - Make recommendations based on clinical experience in light of patient's condition/values
4. Try to reconcile differences in terms of prognosis, goals, hopes, and expectations
   - Negotiate and try to reconcile differences; seek common ground; be creative
   - Use conflict resolution when necessary
5. Respond empathetically
   - Acknowledge
   - Legitimize
   - Explore (rather than prematurely reassuring)
   - Empathize
   - Reinforce commitment and non-abandonment
6. Use MOLST to guide choices and finalize patient/family wishes
   - Review the key elements with the patient and/or family
   - Apply shared, informed medical decision-making
   - Manage conflict resolution
7. Complete and sign MOLST
   - Obtain verbal or written consent from the patient or designated decision-maker
   - Follow legal requirements under New York State Public Health Law, including Family Health Care Decisions Act (FHCDA)
   - Document conversation
8. Review and revise periodically

* Honoring patient preferences is a critical element in providing quality end-of-life care. To help physicians and other health care providers discuss and convey a patient's wishes regarding cardiopulmonary resuscitation (CPR) and other life-sustaining treatment, the New York State Department of Health has approved a physician order form (DOH-5003), Medical Orders for Life-Sustaining Treatment (MOLST), which can be used statewide by health care practitioners and facilities. MOLST is an approved Physician Orders for Life-Sustaining Treatment (POLST) Paradigm Program and incorporates New York State Public Health Law.

www.health.state.ny.us/professionals/patients/patient_rights/molst/
www.CompassionAndSupport.org

** Bomba, 2005; revised 2011 to comply with Family Health Care Decisions Act, effective June 1, 2010.

Figure 25.1   8-Step MOLST Protocol

Table 25.1 Differences between New York MOLST and Advance Directives (Authority and Accountability, as of June 17, 2020)

Characteristics	New York MOLST	Advance Directives
Population	For seriously ill individuals with advanced illness, advanced frailty	All adults
Time frame	Current care	Future care
Who completes the form	Physicians, NPs, PAs	Patients
Resulting form	Medical orders (MOLST)	Advance directives
Health care agent or surrogate role	Can engage in discussion if patient lacks capacity	Cannot complete
Portability	Physicians, NPs, PAs responsibility Physician only for Patients with IDD	Patient/family responsibility
Periodic review	Physicians, NPs, PAs responsibility Physician only for Patients with IDD	Patient/family responsibility

Source: Adapted from Bomba et al. (2012). © Patricia Bomba, MD.

Advance directives (like New York's health care proxy) are legal documents that identify a person who is entrusted by an individual to make medical decisions on their behalf, document the person's values, beliefs, goals, and what matters most. An advance directive, like the living will, documents future care preferences but is difficult to interpret and cannot be followed in an emergency. The Patient Self-Determination Act ensures all adults 18 years of age and older have a right to complete advance directives. Public health law varies in each state, and as a result, there are different state-specific advance directives. Like wills and power of attorney documents, advance directives are legal documents that should be reviewed periodically and updated as needed.

New York's MOLST is not an advance directive. MOLST is a set of medical orders that defines life-sustaining treatments the patient wants to receive and/or avoid today. A physician, NP, or PA reviews the current health status, prognosis, and goals for care, as well as the risks and benefits of each life-sustaining treatment with the patient if they have capacity and with the patient's health care agent or surrogate if they lack capacity. The 8-Step MOLST Protocol (Figure 25.1) was developed in 2005 to provide a standardized approach to MOLST discussions. All ethical and legal requirements must be followed, including special procedures when an individual with an intellectual or developmental disability lacks capacity to make these decisions. This may require a series of discussions to ensure well-informed medical decisions. Once MOLST is properly completed and signed by a physician, NP, or PA, MOLST must be honored by all health care professionals in all settings. Patients who are appropriate for MOLST should have an up-to-date health care proxy in the event MOLST orders need to be revised after the patient loses capacity. MOLST is not an advance directive.

A summary of the differences between advance directives and MOLST are outlined in Table 25.1.

Population Appropriate for MOLST/eMOLST

MOLST is not for everyone. Rather, MOLST is designed primarily for patients with advanced illness, including advanced frailty. Patients who are appropriate include:

1. Patients whose physician, NP, or PA would not be surprised if they die in the next 1–2 years
2. Patients who live in a nursing home or receive long-term care services at home or in assisted living

3. Patients who want to avoid or receive any or all life-sustaining treatment today
4. Patients who have one or more advanced chronic conditions or a new diagnosis with a poor prognosis
5. Patients who have had two or more unplanned hospital admissions in the last 12 months, coupled with increasing frailty, decreasing functionality, progressive weight loss, or lack of social support.

Origin of MOLST

New York was one of the first states to adopt a POLST or MOLST program and is a founding member of the National POLST Paradigm, now referred to as National POLST.

The MOLST program was one of several projects developed as a community initiative in Rochester to improve end-of-life care in 2001. MOLST was coupled with a complementary advance care planning program, the Community Conversations on Compassionate Care (CCCC) program, which launched in 2002 to support New York MOLST as part of the community initiative. From a population health perspective, the CCCC program supports early advance care planning discussions and completion of advance directives, particularly health care proxies, for everyone 18 years of age and older. After working from 2001 to 2003 on the creation of the MOLST form and program, MOLST was launched in the Greater Rochester Region in 2004, followed quickly by adoption in Syracuse and the surrounding areas in Upstate New York.

The New York State Department of Health (NYSDOH) approved use of MOLST in all health care facilities in 2005, prompting further spread and use in all counties. A change in New York State Public Health Law (NYSPHL) was required to permit emergency medical services (EMS) to use a MOLST to follow both Do Not Resuscitate (DNR) and Do Not Intubate (DNI) orders in the community. Legislation provided for a community pilot in Monroe and Onondaga counties, EMS quality data collection, and a three-year period to prove EMS could successfully follow the MOLST. The legislated community pilot was successful (2005–2008). As a result, MOLST was signed into NYSPHL as the alternate form to the Non-hospital DNR form. Indeed, the MOLST form is the only form tested and approved by NYSDOH for both DNR and DNI orders. NYSDOH approved MOLST for statewide use in all settings in July 2008 and directs all health care providers to follow MOLST orders in all settings, including the community.

MOLST became a NYSDOH form in 2010 on the effective date of the Family Health Care Decisions Act (FHCDA). This was a significant change in public health law that allows surrogates to make end-of-life decisions when a health care agent was not named or was not available.

Evolution to eMOLST

During the community pilot (2005–2008), quality data was collected in hospitals and nursing homes. Careful observation and community collaboration resulted in identifying essential elements and developing tools for proper implementation. The initial vision for eMOLST is a direct result of the rapid adoption of MOLST statewide after MOLST became part of the statute. Lessons learned during the successful community pilot affirmed the need for a standardized approach to thoughtful MOLST discussions and creation of MOLST.

The original eMOLST program began in 2008. A prototype was built with seed money from a health information technology Health Care Efficiency and Affordability Law (HEAL) grant secured by the Rochester Regional Health Information Organization (RRHIO). In collaboration with the RRHIO, Excellus BlueCross BlueShield (EBCBS) led a clinician planning group to develop the initial design of an electronic MOLST web-based completion system and registry.

In 2010, MOLST became a DOH form and FHCDA became effective. NYSDOH, together with the Office for People with Developmental Disabilities (OPWDD), created seven checklists to ensure the quality of the process and the ethical-legal framework for end-of-life decisions are followed. The ethical and legal requirements apply for any order to withhold or withdraw life-sustaining treatment in New York and is not specific to MOLST. These changes required significant modification of eMOLST.

In 2011, the authors, both employed at EBCBS, conducted site visits with physicians and other clinicians and representatives from long-term care facilities, hospitals, hospices, and EMS to understand the best methods to promote eMOLST adoption as part of their general practice. Based on clinician feedback, eMOLST was revised to include the 8-Step Protocol and the NYSDOH and OPWDD Checklists. By following the protocol and checklists, practitioners can complete the NYSDOH eMOLST form and the appropriate MOLST Chart Documentation Form, and these documents are automatically included in the registry.

By 2014, Dr. Pat Bomba and the eMOLST system were recognized by NYeC (the New York eHealth Collaborative) with a PATH Award for Promoting Advancement of Technology in Healthcare.

Description of eMOLST

New York's eMOLST system is the first operationalized web application for MOLST or POLST form completion and electronic retrieval in a registry nationally. The tools and features in the eMOLST system ensure a standardized process is used for end-of-life conversations. When the physician, NP, or PA electronically signs the eMOLST, a copy of the medical orders and the discussion automatically becomes part of the NYeMOLST registry and is available in all settings and across care transitions. eMOLST may be used with paper records, integrated in an electronic medical record EMR or hybrid system or a health information exchange (HIE), and allows for electronic signature for providers and for the form to be printed for needed workflow in the paper world, as illustrated in Figure 25.2. eMOLST serves as a risk management tool to provide access to properly completed eMOLST forms across care transitions statewide and ensure patients' preferences for care and treatment are honored in all care settings. eMOLST is free, available statewide, and accessed at NYSeMOLSTregistry.com.

Technology

Over the past decade, several key questions and issues were addressed and solved related to electronic form completion systems and registries, including how to best protect data, employing multiple tiers of validation, form versioning, and knowing how to successfully engage and integrate with EMRs in hospitals, nursing homes, and HIEs. Integration options include:

- *Single sign-on (SSO)*: Allows eMOLST user to log into eMOLST automatically when their login credentials are passed to eMOLST from an authorized source

Pathways for eMOLST Use

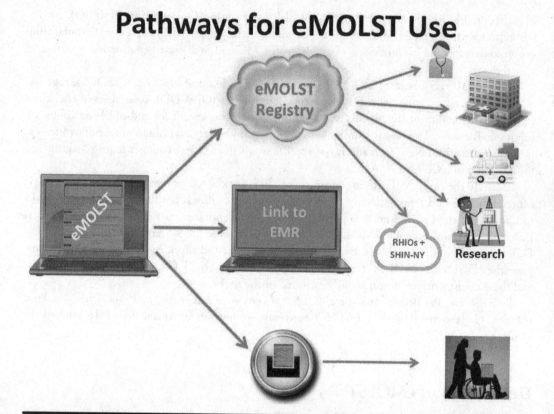

Figure 25.2   Pathways for eMOLST use

Source: © Patricia Bomba, MD.

- *Single sign-on with patient context*: Allows SSO and automates the search for a patient during the login process by incorporating patient details within the same action
- *Application programming interface (API)*: Allows a trusted system to query eMOLST for relevant information on a specific patient or group of patients, or to see if a patient matching those details even exist in the eMOLST registry. More granular information such as order status can also be retrieved.

eSignature functionality is available. Providers document the end-of-life discussion and selection of orders by logging into the eMOLST system, where they can view all data entered on a patient. They can then confirm the conversation and electronically sign eMOLST forms and all documentation by answering a security question and choosing a secret image that they configure on first login. The authorized provider's signature is then printed on all documents.

The eMOLST system is a mature product that has the capability to integrate industry-leading optical character recognition tools, such as ABBYY, to validate, remediate, and accept paper documents into the registry. Finally, eMOLST provides a form completion and storage solution that has been functioning well and growing in New York for nearly a decade, providing data to hospitals, nursing homes, hospices, physician practices, and HIEs with on-demand web services.

eMOLST has a sophisticated set of administrative tools that allows one person (the eMOLST administrator) to configure and manage all organizations and users across New York State. Currently, the eMOLST system has the capability to display simple reports regarding growth of patients, organizations, users, and so forth. The eMOLST team is building connections with a leading data visualization tool to allow administrators the ability to quickly see key metrics for their organization.

Introductory information is found at NYSeMOLSTregistry.com. A multidimensional approach is needed for successful implementation. Administrative support, including an array of implementation tools, educational resources, and detailed workplans, is provided to participants to support culture change and the other key elements needed for success.

Clinical Benefit

In August 2014, a frail elderly man with multiple medical problems, including chronic obstructive pulmonary disease (COPD), recurrent acute respiratory exacerbations, and recurrent hospitalizations, presented to the emergency department (ED) at a critical access hospital in the North Country in rural upstate New York. He was in acute respiratory distress and was treated aggressively with standard medical treatment without improvement. He lacked the capacity to make complex medical decisions regarding life-sustaining treatment. He had a health care proxy and MOLST that were unavailable at the time of evaluation. Before he was intubated and transported to a major academic medical center for further intensive respiratory support, the ED physician checked the eMOLST registry. Fortunately, the man had an eMOLST in the registry, which was created by his primary care physician. The eMOLST indicated how he wanted to be treated and the details of the discussion that led to his decision. His goals were to focus on functionality and die at home; he did not want resuscitation or respiratory support. As a result, the patient avoided an unwanted intubation and a 99-mile ambulance ride to a major academic medical center. The patient was admitted, treated conservatively, and discharged home, consistent with his preferences for treatment and care. He died peacefully at home two months later. This real-life case illustrates how eMOLST (1) improves the quality of discussion of patient values, beliefs and goals for care and shared decision-making to drive the choice of life-sustaining treatment; (2) honors individual patient preferences by providing MOLST orders and copy of discussion across care transitions; and (3) reduces unwanted hospitalizations, ED use, service utilization, expense.

About the Authors

Katie Orem, MPH, Katie Orem is the geriatrics and palliative care program manager at Excellus BlueCross BlueShield and the eMOLST administrator for New York State. She has worked on New York's MOLST program for more than ten years. She supports the expansion and evaluation of advance care planning, palliative care and end-of-life care initiatives internally, across New York State and nationally. She has assisted many organizations in improving their advance care planning and MOLST processes, complying with New York State Public Health Law, and implementing eMOLST.

Katie is a member of the New York State MOLST Team's Executive Committee, the National POLST Technology Committee and New York's National Healthcare Decisions Day Committee.

Katie graduated with her Master's in Public Health from the Yale School of Public Health, with a concentration in Health Policy & Administration. She received her undergraduate education at Cornell University and earned a BS in Biology & Society with a concentration in Community & Public Health.

Patricia Bomba, MD, MACP, FRCP, a nationally and internationally recognized palliative care/end-of-life expert, served as vice president and senior medical director of geriatrics and palliative care at Excellus BlueCross BlueShield (BCBS). Dr. Bomba founded the New York Medical Orders for Life-Sustaining Treatment (MOLST) and eMOLST programs. At the request of the commissioner of the New York State Department of Health, she developed and served as chair of the MOLST Statewide Implementation Team. Prior to working at Excellus BCBS, Dr. Bomba spent four years in academic medicine and nearly two decades in private practice focused on the care of frail older adults and patients with multiple co-morbidities.

She is a founding member of National POLST, serves on the Leadership Council and the Executive Committee of the Plenary Assembly, and chairs the Public Policy Committee. She served on the Institute of Medicine's Committee that produced *Dying in America: Improving Quality and Honoring Individual Preferences Near the End of Life*, the NASEM Roundtable on Quality Care for People with Serious Illness; NCQA's Geriatric Measurement Advisory Panel (GMAP); and the Medical Society of the State of New York Ethics Committee.

Dr. Bomba is author of several articles on issues related to advance care planning, palliative care, elder abuse, and end-of-life concerns. She has spoken extensively regionally, statewide, nationally and internationally to professionals, community groups, and professional organizations on issues related to advance care planning, MOLST, palliative care, pain management, elder abuse, and other geriatric topics. Dr. Bomba earned a bachelor's degree from Immaculata College and graduated from the University of Virginia School of Medicine. She completed her residency in internal medicine at the University of Rochester. Dr. Bomba is board certified in internal medicine, with added qualifications in geriatric medicine. She attended the Executive Development Program at the Wharton Business School.

Key Articles

Baharlou, S., Orem, K., Kelley, A., Aldridge, M., & Popp, B. (2020). Rapid Implementation of eMOLST Order Completion and Electronic Registry to Facilitate Advance Care Planning: MOLST Documentation Using Telehealth in the Covid-19 Pandemic. *NEJM Catalyst* link.

Bomba, P. (2017). Supporting the Patient Voice: Building the Foundation of Shared Decision-making. *Generations*, 41(1), 21–30 link.

Bomba, P., & Karmel, J. (2015). Medical, Ethical and Legal Obligations to Honor Individual Preferences Near the End of Life. *Health Law Journal*, 20(2), 28–33 link.

Bomba, P., Kemp, M., & Black, J. (2012). POLST: An improvement over traditional advance directives. *Cleveland Clinic Journal of Medicine*, 79(7), 457–464 link.

Bomba, P., & Orem, K. (2012). eMOLST and electronic health records. *NYSBA Health Law Journal*, 17, 77–83 link.

Bomba, P., & Orem, K. (2015). Lessons Learned from New York's Community Approach to Advance Care Planning and MOLST. *Annals of Palliative Medicine*, 4(1), 10–21 link.

Electronic End-of-Life and POLST Documentation Access through HIE. (2019). *The Office of the National Coordinator for Health Information Technology* (New York's eMOLST, pp. 14–19) link.

Chapter 26

Medical Liability Insurance Data Analytics

An Opportunity to Identify Risks, Target Interventions and Impact Policy

Thomas R. Gray, Esq.

Contents

Just as no two person's health issues are quite the same, facts at issue and allegations in each medical malpractice lawsuit are unique. Just as clear though, if a lawsuit was brought in medical malpractice, a patient is not happy with the outcome and blames the care and treatment for that outcome. Regardless of whether the care rendered was compliant with or deviated from the standard of care, the simple fact the that outcome was not optimal in each case pursued gives us a foundation for the utility of claims data analytics.

Since patients began suing health care practitioners, medical and legal data has been collected in methods and combinations peculiar to the process of defending the practitioner. While rules of procedure and evidence can differ from jurisdiction to jurisdiction, all medical malpractice lawsuits require a plaintiff to identify, with specificity, their allegations of how and when the defendant provider deviated from the standard of care, the nature and extent of injury, and how this damage is causally connected to the deviation. The defense is entitled to discovery testimony of the plaintiff patient which, along with other things, can identify the patient's specific demographic, personal and familial health history, treatment history and specific, current health/injury status. This deposition testimony takes place after collection of all pertinent medical records from each potentially relevant provider, reviewed by the defendant practitioner's attorney and, ideally, medical providers of the appropriate specialty. All this information is collected and stored, in some format, in a medical malpractice insurer's claim file.

DOI: 10.4324/9780429423109-26

The monetary toll that medical malpractice litigation takes on health care costs, in forms of insurance cost, excess exposure, and defensive medicine is undeniably significant, and the personal toll on the practitioner placed in a position of defending themselves is immeasurable. The theory of malpractice claims analytics application is equally evident. Identification of circumstances that lead to injury and thus lead to lawsuits can lead to changes in patient care. These changes, which should lead to fewer adverse outcomes, can reduce lawsuits, thereby allowing practitioners to focus on patient care, not spending substantial time and resources defending lawsuits. Continuing the dominoes, the related reduction in litigation will decrease expenses and indemnity paid by insurers, thereby reducing malpractice insurance premiums and ultimately, the cost of health care. In theory, the enhanced time and additional available resources will further enhance patient care, resulting in fewer adverse outcomes.

Recognizing all of this, in 1985, PIAA (now the Medical Professional Liability [MPL] Association) launched a collaborative database of information provided by member professional liability insurance carriers. Upon the closure of a claim file, from discontinuance, dismissal, settlement or verdict, the participating members provide 65 data points to identify the defendant practitioner's characteristics, the patient's characteristics, loss causation and location information, and case resolution, along with costs of defense. Analysis of this information is the basis for predictive modeling toward the direction of risk management programs. The MPL Association has used the data sharing project, and indicated trends, to identify and quantify topics for their quarterly, *Inside Medical Liability* magazine, their study on the drivers of professional liability claims, their breast cancer claims study, aortic diseases claims study and their specialty specific series, which provides national claims analysis for 21 medical specialties. In 2016, the program was expanded to incorporate hospital/health system claims.

Acknowledging how valuable this national data has proven to be, MLMIC, New York State's largest medical malpractice insurer, began their analytics project in 2017 to use their substantial data to identify risks peculiar to specific practitioners, practices, and healthcare organizations in New York. Put simply, MLMIC conducted a claim history analysis, beginning with its insured hospitals, largest to smallest. Data already submitted to MPL readily established some framework for the program. Claims professionals then reviewed and coded identified claims files and medical records to fill in gaps, enhance detail, and tailor the analysis to the hospital setting. Any commonalities or trends were scrutinized toward identifying the circumstances that led to litigation against that facility. Going beyond indications from the hospital's own litigation history, the data was then compared to that of substantially similar, de-identified MLMIC-insured facilities within New York State and to that of facilities nationally, using MPL data sharing information. This benchmarking process has proven invaluable toward identifying the department, specialty, diagnosis, and procedure within the facility that generates losses outside of the mean, which is then used by MLMIC's Risk Management Department, in collaboration with hospital RM/QA, to develop a comprehensive risk management plan. In one example, diagnostic error claims against one small hospital exceeded benchmarking numbers (See Figure 26.1). Risk management root cause analysis conducted in collaboration with the claims examiner revealed a consistent problem with documentation and use of the electronic health record, apparently connected to the diagnostic errors. Communication ensued with the electronic health record vendor, changes were implemented, and hospital staff was provided with focused education.

MLMIC continued with claims analytics studies for large practice groups and even small office practices, focusing on repetitive indications within a claim history and deviations from national and local benchmarking. Quantity of data is more than adequate for substantial analysis, with more than 243,000 cases defended by MLMIC since its inception in 1975 (See Figure 26.2).

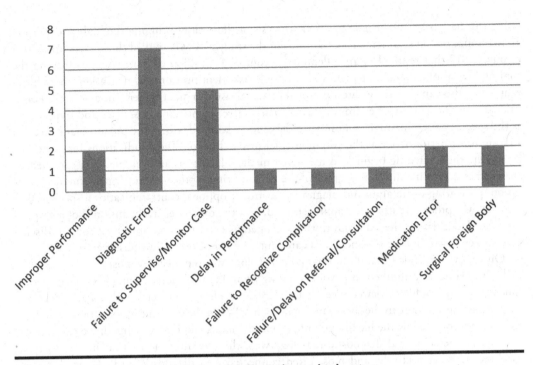

Figure 26.1   Subject hospital all events/claims/suits – misadventure

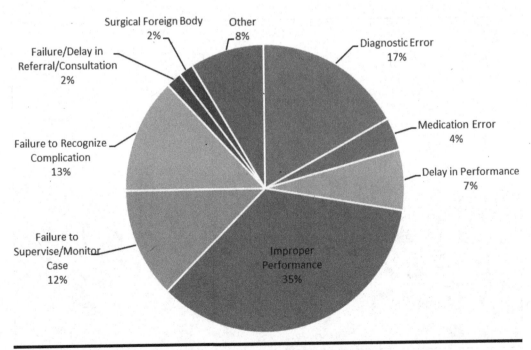

Figure 26.2   Combined MLMIC hospitals all events/claims/suits – misadventure

Using this data base, the next step was an analysis of those cases bringing the highest exposure. To maximize relevance and manage the scope of the study, MLMIC pulled those cases from 2013 through 2017 that resulted in an indemnity payout of $1 million or more. Acknowledging the continued goal of enhancing patient care through risk identification and education, these high-value cases also can pose the greatest personal financial risk to a practitioner. The almost 500 cases studied brought few surprises from a macro perspective, identifying obstetrics and gynecology as the specialty with the highest number of large loss claims, death as the predominant severity, and improper performance as the common chief medical factor. These indications form the surface where the scratching begins. To use "chief medical factor" as an example, data can then be analyzed to determine the demographic of the patient bringing the "improper performance" allegation, presenting complaints and diagnosis, treatment options, contraindications, specialty(ies) involved, the procedure itself, the approach used, and the outcome. In the instance of a surgical case, did the deviation alleged occur during the operative consultation, informed consent discussion, surgery itself, in the post-anesthesia care unit, or at some other time postoperatively?

Our findings revealed that obstetrics and gynecology was the specialty most frequently associated with claims that resulted in payouts totaling $1 million or more, having been identified in almost 1 of 4 (25%) files reviewed (See Figure 26.3). In the field of obstetrics, physicians are caring for two patients (or more in the case of multiple births). When the outcome is not anticipated, damages are compounded by the likelihood of multiple claimants and jurors' sympathy in such cases.

Internal medicine and diagnostic radiology were the specialties noted next in frequency, at 16% and 12%, respectively, and most often connected to a diagnostic error. General surgery rounds out our top four with 9% of total claims, with the most common allegation being an improperly performed procedure.

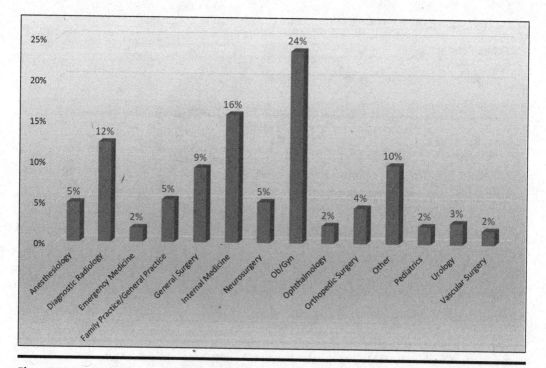

Figure 26.3   **Reviewed cases by specialty**

Given the skill set and expertise required to deliver care in each specialty, it was not unexpected that these four specialties were identified in our study as those claims or suits that generated indemnity payments of $1 million or more.

Improper performance is an allegation made any time the anticipated outcome does not meet the expectations defined by the patient.

Our analysis of this data indicates that over 2 of every 5 (42%) claims brought against an insured alleged improper performance. This is seen most frequently in surgery and in obstetrics, for example, when complications arise during labor and delivery (See Figure 26.4).

Diagnostic error is an allegation made any time a diagnosis is delayed, missed, or incorrectly identified.

Our data indicated that diagnostic error was alleged in more than 1 in 3 (35%) claims. It has been cited as one of the top five allegations made in the medical liability industry by the Medical Professional Liability Association (MPL Association). Diagnostic error is one of the top concerns of patient safety experts as identified by ECRI Institute, having first been named a healthcare issue in the groundbreaking report "To Err is Human" in 1999.

A closer look at the chief medical factor of improper performance shows that multiple specialties are involved, and different types of procedures are triggering lawsuits (See Figure 26.5). For example, in a surgical specialty, improper performance may be alleged during the operative consultation, the operative procedure itself, the management of a patient in the PACU immediately after surgery, or during the care rendered prior to discharge from the floor or ambulatory surgical center. Nearly 4 in 10 (39%) of our files reviewed involved a surgical procedure. Examples include:

- A laparoscopic procedure that required conversion to an open procedure (e.g., to repair a bowel perforation)
- A spinal fusion performed with or without instrumentation (e.g., resulting in nerve damage)
- An orthopedic procedure (e.g., a total knee replacement with postoperative sepsis, requiring joint removal and subsequent amputation above the knee)

Using specialty-specific data, and outside of the million-dollar study, MLMIC joined with the New York State Society of Orthopedic Surgeons and the American Joint Replacement Registry

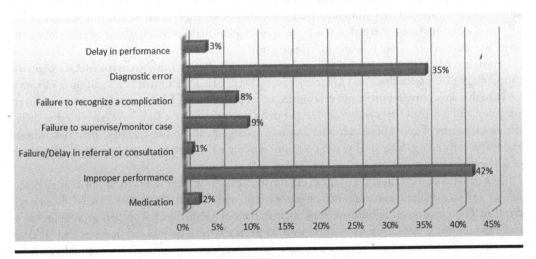

Figure 26.4 Reviewed cases by chief medical factor

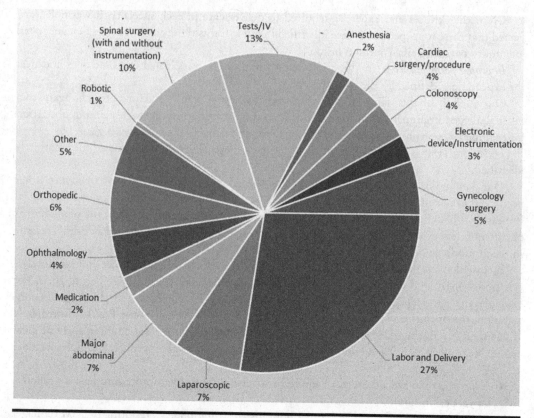

Figure 26.5   Improper performance: a breakdown by procedure/service

with the common goal of improving procedure outcomes, specifically to decrease the number of nerve injuries related to joint replacement surgery. This analysis of adverse outcome data and MLMIC claim data led to an exploration of potential risk factors, including history of anticoagulation use, nicotine and oral contraceptive use, history of sepsis or deep vein thrombosis, and on and on. Commonalities emerged that will be used to assist orthopedic surgeons to recognize patterns and develop strategies to limit adverse outcomes.

Similarly, MLMIC data is used to fuel its Joint Patient Safety Initiative with ACOG (American College of Obstetricians and Gynecologists) District II. Loss indemnity analysis confirmed catastrophic loss correlation to pre-eclampsia, eclampsia and HELLP (hemolysis, elevated liver enzymes, and low platelets) syndrome. Deeper dives into specific case facts have been used to drive the development of educational sessions and risk management tools to identify these risk factors and foster early recognition during pre-conception office visits, during pregnancy, and at the time of delivery.

The goal being identification of those circumstances that present opportunity to change practice to enhance patient outcome, it is apparent that malpractice claim data can be sliced and diced in countless ways. Should we look at instances of birth injuries occurring at acute care facilities in upstate New York to mothers over 35 years old with gestational diabetes and lacking prenatal care? Can we study adverse outcomes involving nurse midwives? Do we add cesarean section (C-section) versus normal vaginal delivery as a factor? Was the C-section emergent? Was it an attempted VBAC (vaginal birth after C-section)? What were the indications of fetal distress, Apgar score, chord gases, and so forth? The point is that data can lead us in different directions, much worth pursuing toward our goal. We have taken the time and spent resources to conduct analysis of a class of cases; that analysis may lead to some conclusions that identify a new or more specific class of cases, and that class may be worthy of analysis. Review of insurance carrier's case files and medical records each time another worthy query presents itself is beyond impractical for these deeper dives and cannot yield a satisfying risk management direction.

Consistent with the goals of protecting patients and providers from impacts of medical error, the Risk Management Foundation of the Harvard Medical Institutions was established in 1979 to apply a data-driven approach to claims management and patient safety. Originally available to the Harvard medical institutions, the CRICO Strategies Comparative Benchmarking System (CBS) membership includes medical centers and insurance organizations nationally.

Using data provided from Harvard Medical Institutions and member facilities and malpractice insurers, CRICO Strategies has released *Medical Malpractice in America, a 10-Year Assessment with Insights*. From the insurer's perspective, on a national level, the assessment identified trends in frequency of cases and costs of indemnity and expenses. Using frequency to prioritize, top procedures, top injuries, contributing factors, and other data was provided. Findings from this data are used to address a facilities concern and as a tool to develop and implement corrective action plans. CBS has also generated reports specific to surgery, obstetrics, the diagnostic process, emergency medicine, routine medical procedures, and communication failures, all based on trends identified in their national data and all toward mitigating clinical risks and patient safety vulnerabilities.

While there is no doubt that data storage for the more than 400,000 medical malpractice claims from more than 500 health care entities and 180,000 physicians that make up the CBS is an accomplishment, Strategies has accomplished much more in the processing and retrieval aspects of informatics. CRICO collects claims data provided through its membership claim management information technology system and uses its Clinical Coding Taxonomy code sets to classify and describe malpractice and patient safety events in a format that facilitates retrieval and analysis. Toward insuring good data in, good information out, data input is managed by registered nurses trained in CBS taxonomy, which is based on nested sets of codes. Top-level categories comprise subcategories and subcategories, which comprise detail codes. Data can be extracted and analyzed from a clinical description and by identified severity, co--morbidities, allegation, location, admitting or responsible service, device, medication, and so on.

The following chart illustrates findings from analysis of case frequency and average injury severity by service (See Figure 26.6 and Figure 26.7).

An enormous benefit of the properly coded taxonomy with a substantial database is the ability to conduct analysis on the micro level, to dive deeper without hitting bottom. The study of national trends in malpractice data can and does lead to better medicine, but what of the risk manager at a community hospital who suspects that quality in ambulatory care is substandard or that a physician group providing emergency services coverage is generating unacceptable losses? What of the physician in a small practice who wants to identify and ameliorate their risk? Data on a national level might not satisfy the need of the community or practitioner at issue. The current state of malpractice claims informatics allows for users with access to apply high, national-level benchmarking and then shrink the sample group, perhaps to region, type of practice, facility, practice group, practitioner, and so forth without the extraordinary time commitment of rereviewing claim files and without the inaccuracies generated by inconsistently entered data.

Perhaps not directly impacting patient care is the role malpractice data can play in public policy. There is a correlation between the frequency and severity of malpractice cases and the law of

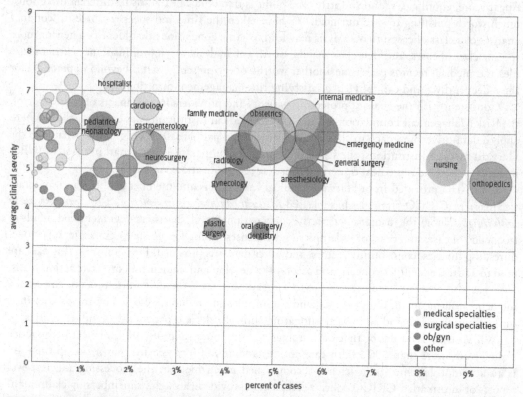

Figure 26.6   Responsible service details

Proportionate shifts among sub-specialty services are evident.

Over the 10-year study period, downward (blue) trends can be identified among medical and surgical sub-specialties.

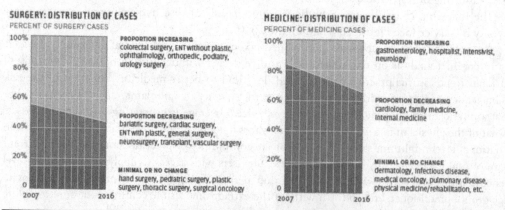

Figure 26.7   Proportionate shifts among sub-specialty services are evident

the land at issue. Affordability of professional liability insurance continues to drive up healthcare costs and can impact access to providers and institutions. Some states have enacted health care liability reforms that limit amounts recoverable for related pain and suffering and limit attorney contingency fees. Some also maintain practical statutes of limitations, whereas other states have none of these protections. A robust database, with the capacity to compare frequency of claims brought and extent of indemnity and expenses from one state to another, is fodder for lobbying efforts toward tort reform. Likewise, easily accessible claims analytics can be a resource in the inexact science of assessing malpractice case values. Claims adjusters generally base value on their own experience and judgment with assistance from past verdicts along with sustainable verdict values in similar cases, reported by the appellate courts. Acknowledging that each case is unique, because malpractice verdicts are infrequent, access to past settlement data that can be sliced and diced on the medicine, patient demographic, venue and even to the extent of identifying the plaintiff's attorney can provide substantial guidance in determining value and defense strategy.

About the Author

Thomas R. Gray, Esq., is a 1997 cum laude graduate of Albany Law School, admitted to practice in New York state and federal courts. Mr. Gray began his legal career representing defendants in civil litigation and ultimately complex civil litigation including labor law, products liability and medical malpractice. He has represented his clients through trial to verdict and argued in the Appellate Division.

In 2003 Mr. Gray joined the law firm that is now Fager Amsler Keller & Schoppmann, LLP, opening the Latham office to expand legal services to MLMIC and its insureds. While at FAK&S, he represented physicians, dentists, hospitals, and other healthcare providers in medical malpractice and professional licensing matters and provided legal counsel on risk management and health law issues.

Mr. Gray joined MLMIC Services, Inc. in 2014, overseeing upstate claims operations from the Latham office. He currently holds the position of Senior Vice President of Risk Management, working toward positive patient outcome through the identification and mitigation of risk in all healthcare settings.

Chapter 27

Medical-Legal
Attorney's Perspective

Joshua R. Cohen, J.D.

Contents

Background

Medical information has always been a cornerstone of good medical care. The Smith papyrus created in Egypt in the 17th century BC charted information for 48 patients. Each case included the following subheadings: "Introductory heading," "Significant symptoms," "Diagnosis," and "Recommended treatment." Most of the cases also include an additional subheading, "Explanation." While the original author is unknown, the document showed an organized method to approaching medical information even though therapies and treatments were extremely limited at that time. It did start an (albeit limited) method of describing disease and injury and started to form a knowledge database as to the effectiveness of intervention and progression of illness.

Hippocrates (4th century BC), widely considered to be the "father of medicine," wrote that records should accurately reflect the course of the disease and indicate possible causes. Since then, with the development of better medical equipment and knowledge, we now generate more information in one day than all of the papyruses in the past 5,000 years combined. In addition,

DOI: 10.4324/9780429423109-27

as medicine progressed with more specialties and healthcare professions, there were many more scribes entering data into a patient's chart. All of this information needed to be better organized and made more easily available to those caring for the patient.

Fortunately, like medicine, technology was also rapidly advancing. In the mid-1800s, the telegraph was used to for the two-way transmission of data over long distances. During the Civil War, the telegraph was used to order medical supplies and transmit casualty reports. By 1900, the telephone was used by healthcare providers, and it is still used today.[1] With the advent of computers, medical data could be collected and processed at greater speeds and larger volumes. Moreover, the data could more easily be shared among the healthcare team, and medical databases started growing.

It has often been said that the electronic medical record (EMR) is the panacea for all of the ills of the paper chart. Dr. Lawrence Weed published the first article on EMRs in the *New England Journal of Medicine*, titled "Medical Records that Guide and Teach."[2] By 1971, hospital computers were starting to be connected to local area networks (LANs) so that multiple computers in a hospital could access the same information in different areas. Wide area networks (WANs) soon allowed medical academics to collaborate from distant institutions. These are the foundations of medical informatics, which continues to grow exponentially through computers with ever-increasing processing speeds, greater connectivity, faster transmission speeds, massive storage of indexed data, and more uniform information input.

Current Benefits

Every day, millions of patients benefit from medical informatics. Physicians practice medicine because they are always learning new knowledge and developing innovative skills. Not only can healthcare providers quickly access patients' prior information, but medical informatics also allows healthcare providers to review current literature and search for articles and data to better care for patients. Information can be better organized in a searchable format to facilitate access. An example would be looking for information in a large textbook that has no index at the end. The reader would have to read through the book to see if it has relevant information and where it is located. Medical informatic databases are usually indexed to the information contained in it or multiple databases, which can quickly be located and reviewed. Most systems recall the data so that the most relevant information is at the top of the search results while still providing all potentially pertinent information for the clinician. To refine a search even further, searches can be done using controlled vocabularies such as a MeSH (Medical Search Headings) search that looks for search terms in the publication's heading. It is more specific and leverages knowledge and indexing.

Medical informatics also enhances the patient's experience for those who want to use features such as a patient portal to schedule appointments, send a message to their physician, review test results with comparison to prior results, refill medications, and follow set goals. When properly implemented, it brings the patient more into their medical information and care and provides better access to their healthcare provider. Patients can choose to have their medical information stored in a secure cloud-based service, so that if they need medical attention outside of their usual providers, that information can be accessed to better care for the patient.

---

[1] K. M. Zundel, Telemedicine: history, applications, and impact on librarianship. *Bull Med Libr Assoc.* 1996 Jan; 84(1): 71–79.

[2] *N Engl J Med.* 1968; 278: 652–657.

Electronic Health Records

On January 20, 2004, electronic medical records (EMRs) made their way into the State of the Union Address, when President George W. Bush announced that "By computerizing health records, we can avoid dangerous medical mistakes, reduce costs, and improve care." President Bush announced that by 2014, most Americans would have an electronic health record (EHR). The day after his address, President Bush signed an executive order establishing the Office of the National Coordinator for Health Information Technology (ONC) and directed the coordinator to develop a national health information technology (HIT) strategy to promote the adoption and use of interoperable EHRs. By 2020, 89% of physicians had implemented EHRs.

Of course, there are many improvements to be made, and as the software and technology improves, they will enhance patient care but will also absorb more of the healthcare provider's time; they are also one of the major causes of physician burnout. It is well known that the EMR, now often referred to as an EHR because they include data from multiple practices and hospitals, can interfere with the physician-patient relationship. Often the computer into which the data is being entered requires the healthcare provider to turn their back to the patient when entering data, making the patient feel that the provider is not paying attention to them. This can be cured by better implementation when possible by having the computer in a position where the provider can interact with the patient while entering data. If not, it is good practice for the provider to tell the patient that they are listening while they enter the data.

As for the physician, they are now spending much of the time during the patient encounter reviewing prior notes, including in an EHR notes of other physicians and test results, and then spending more time entering a note for the visit. In one study of emergency department physicians working a busy ten-hour shift, the physician made 4,000 clicks, accounting for 43% of the encounter time and 28% in direct patient care. The remaining time was reviewing test results and records and discussion with colleagues.[3] In addition to time away from direct patient care, there is potential liability for a physician reviewing an extensive EHR for a specific new issue not to see the prior consult sent to another physician recommending a diagnostic test, such as a mammogram or colonoscopy. The more data available, the greater chance of data overload. While EHR systems have been upgraded to flag items for follow-up, it has the potential to become similar to alarm fatigue.

EHRs often automatically carry over information from a prior note, such as the chief complaint or presumptive diagnosis. Providers need to learn how to discontinue the use of a carryover function when appropriate. It is also important that the provider document whether the original complaint or diagnosis has been resolved so that subsequent notes, whether during a hospital admission or months later in an office setting, are not auto-populated and do not accurately reflect the current complaints or diagnosis of the patient.

Not usually visible to the practitioner or included when the EHR is printed is the metadata generated by the EHR system. Metadata is "data about data." A simple example is a digital photograph. When viewed, you only see an image; however, behind that image is the metadata such as what camera took the image, the date and time the photograph was taken, the shutter speed and lens aperture, and (with most smartphones) the location of where it was taken. An EHR records far more metadata, including when and what data was accessed, medical record number, the patient's name, the user's ID, how long the data was accessed, and what the user did, with a

---

[3] Hill RG Jr, Sears LM, Melanson SW. 4000 Clicks: a productivity analysis of electronic medical records in a community hospital ED. *Am J Emerg Med.* 2013 Nov;31(11):1591–1594. doi: 10.1016/j.ajem.2013.06.028.

pointer back to the original data and the location of the computer terminal where the data was entered or accessed. Every time a user accesses an EHR, they leave a digital fingerprint in the form of metadata.

Metadata can be used to help defend a healthcare practitioner in litigation or be used as a weapon of mass discovery. Patient's attorneys frequently demand audit trails and access logs to determine when a note was entered and if it was modified or deleted. They also try to show that a note was entered from a computer in a location in a different area of the hospital from where the patient was located when the physician claims to have created the note contemporaneously with the evaluation of the patient. Metadata can call into question the entire note or parts of the EHR if there is a discrepancy between the notes and the audit trail.

Given the complexities of the EHR software and technology, glitches occur that can provide erroneous information to the providers and be exploited in litigation to question the authenticity and accuracy of the EHR. It can also be case dispositive (something that resolves a legal issue, claim, or controversy). In a published case, there was a malfunction of the vital sign monitoring for 93 minutes during a seven-hour neurosurgical procedure. The patient became quadriplegic following the surgery. Initially, the neurosurgeons were the target of a lawsuit. After the missing vital sign data was discovered, the plaintiff's theory shifted to hypotension during the surgery. Because the hospital's policy required vital signs to be recorded every five minutes during surgery, and there was a gap of 93 minutes, the cases was settled based on a violation of the hospital's policies.[4] Other examples are copying and pasting the exact same note from a prior provider – including the same typographical errors – in a subsequent provider's evaluation, making the note suspect; errors in medication orders involving similar names on a drop-down list and dosage; and improper templates for review of systems, where a cisgender male patient is noted to have no vaginal bleeding. It is often said in litigation that when you are the one doing the explaining, you are probably losing.

Medical Informatics Process

The DIKW Pyramid:[5] Data – Information – Knowledge – Wisdom.

Medical informatics begins with data. Today, almost all data is in electronic form in binary code, meaning it is simply many millions if not billions of 1s and 0s. For example, the binary code in bytes for JOSH is 01001010 01001111 01010011 01001000.[6] For example, the data size capacity of the original 5.25-inch floppy disk (which few remember) was 1.2 megabytes, which is 1.2 million bytes. To save a typical MRI study, you would need over 300 of these disks, and because the data would have to be broken up, it would take an inordinately long period of time to try to combine them, if at all. Today, the storage devices are exponentially larger, and peta drives are now commercially available.[7] As storage keeps expanding and multiple drives can be combined to increase capacity, storage is not an issue now with medical informatics.

Data is usually entered via a keyboard but can also be a scanned-in document with information from radiology, cardiology, laboratory, barcode, and so forth and then digitized into binary code. While raw data is unusable, computers, software, and other technologies are used to analyze

---

[4] *Anesth Analg.* 2006; 102: 1798–802.

[5] Jennifer Rowley, *Journal of Information Science.* 2007; 33(2): 163–180.

[6] Notice each byte is composed of 8 digits or bits.

[7] A peta drive is 1,000 gigabytes. A gigabyte is 1,000 megabytes. A megabyte is 1,000 kilobytes. It would take approximately 1 million 5.25 floppy disks to hold the same amount of data as a 1 petabyte drive.

the code, process it, and store it in an organized format that makes it functional. Using technology, the data can be analyzed, searched, compared with prior data, and shared.

The ultimate purpose of the raw data is to produce information for the clinician to better evaluate the patient. The EHR is often where the healthcare provider goes to review the data, including prior notes, medical history, consultations, prescriptions, tests, vital signs, and much more. The information should be organized to facilitate the healthcare provider's review of the relevant data and flag important findings that require follow-up. Physical exam findings, any current complaints or change in condition, testing, and consultations can be noted and requested, all at the EHR terminal. The patient portal can be updated either in the office setting or through a secure remote connection.

Information requires knowledge as to how to interpret it. For example, the EHR may return test values, but without knowing the normal range of values, the advantages of medical informatics would end here. While physicians know the normal values of most tests they order (and normal ranges are usually included with the results), specialty tests or studies may require additional knowledge. Medical informatics permit the physician to research to quickly access scholarly and peer-reviewed information to help interpret the information and enhance the physician's knowledge to help suggest appropriate care. Of course, the individual is not a patient of the computer but of the physician, who must use their information, knowledge, and experience (and perhaps a consult) to formulate a proper treatment plan.

Wisdom is the ability to increase effectiveness and adds value to enhance the clinician's judgment by combining experience and knowledge to better assess the patient and be prepared for a similar case that may present in the future. Wisdom can also be shared though medical informatics by combining knowledge and outcomes with other practitioners. It has been suggested that moving from data to information involves "understanding relations"; moving from information to knowledge involves "understanding patterns"; and moving from knowledge to wisdom involves "understanding principles."[8] Thus, the DIKW Pyramid is a hierarchy of how informatics moves data with no useful meaning into meaningful information for humans with context that can be combined with skill and experience to become wisdom for the individual physician and can be shared with others to be searched and found in the many databases.

Telehealth

Telehealth is the use of IT hardware, software, and telecommunications technologies to provide communications, remote care, and public health administration. While telehealth has always been evolving, the COVID-19 pandemic greatly accelerated it use. The two biggest drivers of this are (1) avoiding public healthcare practices and facilities to avoid exposure and (2) the increase in healthcare providers willing to pay for telehealth visits. Fortunately, the technology and most patients' internet bandwidths have increased over the past few years, permitting telehealth to become functional.

Telehealth also applies not just to telephonic or video conferences, but with additional equipment it can transmit blood glucose levels, blood pressure, simple ECGs, photographs taken with a smartphone of a skin condition, heart rate and heart sounds through a stethoscope, pulse, O_2, and

[8] Rowley, Jennifer. "The wisdom hierarchy: representations of the DIKW hierarchy." Journal of Information and Communication Science. 2007; 33(2): 163–1.

so forth. Some smartphones even have the capability to determine if it appears a patient has fallen, and if they do not respond to a phone call, GPS emergency services can be dispatched.

While there are many platforms today over which telehealth is being conducted, whichever one the practitioner selects needs to be HIPAA compliant and compatible with the practitioner's and patients' technology. If there is someone else at the patient's location who can hear the encounter, the provider should document the patient's consent to have them present; if consent is not given they should be asked to leave the area. The practitioner should also be cognizant that the patient may be able to use the telehealth technology to record the visit or use a separate device such as a smartphone to do so.

It is incumbent on the physician to determine if a telehealth visit is medically appropriate. Patients requiring in-person encounters or the need for higher-level care should be directed accordingly. Many states require a consent form for telehealth visits. If conducting a telehealth visit, usually the patient must agree to conditions and give consent. In addition, some states require the physician be licensed in the state to participate in a telehealth visit with a patient in the same state. Other states consider it a felony to have a telehealth visit with a patient from a state the physician is not licensed in. It is considered practicing medicine without a license.

Security

When asked many years ago why he robbed banks, William "Slick Willie" Sutton replied, "That's where the money is." Interestingly, the quote evolved into Sutton's law, which is often invoked to medical students as a metaphor for emphasizing the most likely diagnosis rather than wasting time and money investigating every conceivable possibility. As medical informatics seeks to expand interoperability and silo-sensitive data, healthcare systems have become increased target for cyber-crimes seeking to breach security and access vast troves of patients' data or hold the system hostage to ransomware. (Editor's note: see chapter 17: Privacy and Security.)

Healthcare data can sell for as much as $1,000, while a Social Security number or credit card number can sell for $1 and up to $100, respectively.[9] Medical records contain the full patient's name, address, often the Social Security number, health insurance information that can be used for others to pretend to be the patient to get medical care, family members, employment data, and other personal information that can be exploited. Furthermore, like a bank, once a hacker gets into a healthcare system, they can obtain thousands of patient records, making hospitals a prime target for hackers. The impact on the institution is not only the negative publicity but also substantial HIPAA breach fines, remedial measures, and extensive investigations with accompanying costs. In 2009 breach, burglars broken into a large health insurance company and stole 57 unencrypted disk drives containing more than 1 million patient records from a secured closet. In addition to a $1.5 million fine, the estimated cost for corrective actions was an additional $17 million.[10]

Another popular tactic employed by hackers to monetize healthcare data is to inject ransomware into a healthcare institution to secretly encrypt and then lock up the hospital's data so that the hospital computer network cannot function. There is no access to the EHR, no billing, no ability to care for patients, which usually results in a shutdown of the hospital until a hefty ransom is paid, with no guarantee the hackers will send back a key to unencrypt the data; attempting to

---

[9] https://www.advisory.com/daily-briefing/2019/03/01/hackers.
[10] https://www.insidearm.com/news/00008979-bluecross-blueshields-data-breach-leads-t/.

restore the data from backups (which may have also been corrupted) is time-consuming and likely will result in some loss of data. A recent study by Mimecast, a leading cybersecurity firm, found that 90% of healthcare facilities have been victims of an email-borne attack, such as phishing emails, and 72% of those organizations were negatively affected by those attacks.[11]

Every organization that maintains protected healthcare information must protect from loss of data and intrusions not only to avoid extremely expensive fines and costs but also to reassure patients that their data is protected and secure. This involves a multilayered approach of proper handling of data-containing devices, strong encryption, frequently changing passwords and ensuring they are not easily discerned, training staff to not click on hyperlinks even if they appear to be from a trusted sources, and working with IT to implement robust firewalls to filter out suspicious emails and secure ports to keep hackers out.

Artificial Intelligence

A heuristically programmed algorithmic computer (HAL) in Arthur C. Clarke's *2001: A Space Odyssey* appeared in the film in 1968 to show us what computers using artificial intelligence (AI) would be capable of by 2001, even though HAL turned out to be a computer antagonist. While real computers are not as sophisticated as HAL at machine learning (ML) and AI, computers are becoming more abundant in processing the vast amounts of data generated every day in healthcare and through the use of better algorithms and ML to provide increasing value in the care and treatment of patients. (Editor's note: see chapter 9: Artificial Intelligence and Hospital Automation.)

AI in health informatics has been around since the 1970s, when it was mostly based on knowledge-based decision support. It was not connected to the EMR and was limited to the knowledge bases loaded into the systems. It was more useful to teaching students and residents than for a clinical or hospital practice. Fast-forward to today: software and technology has exponentially increased since then, and computers are now capable of ML coupled with better algorithms and interfaces or are built into EHRs.

In a recent study of chest CT scans, a computer with learning capabilities was trained by providing it with many CT scans from patients with lung cancer. The researchers then programmed it with instructions and "pop quizzes" so that it learned to recognize the lung features consistent with cancer and those that were benign. The computer was then shown 6,716 CT scans with known diagnosis, and was 94% accurate at detection. Compared to six radiologists with no prior scans available, the computer performed better than the radiologists, with fewer false positives and false negatives. When earlier scans were available, the results were comparable.

This same technology is being applied to areas of medicine such as radiology, pathology, cardiology, text analysis of notes and reports, and other areas. Computer-assisted diagnosis has been in use in radiology for years. The physician is still responsible for the care and treatment provided to the patient, not AI. C3PO from Star Wars will not be getting hospital credentials or a license to practice medicine anytime soon. Healthcare computers will be required to obtain US Food and Drug Administration (FDA) approval as medical devices, although the FDA has taken the position that EHRs do not require approval or oversight. It is clear that as enormous amounts of data are generated in healthcare, the role of AI will continue to grow to harness this data to improve patient care.

---

[11] https://www.mimecast.com/blog/fbi-warns-of-healthcare-ransomware-what-hospitals-can-do/.

Conclusion

From bits to bytes, from vacuum tubes to microchips, from stand-alone to massive networks, healthcare informatics has become necessary to organize and manage the vast amounts of data being generated every day and stored for long periods of time. It encompasses a spectrum of multidisciplinary areas including medicine, information technology, software, interoperability, security, telehealth, EHRs, and law to improve patient care and efficiency. When properly implemented, it increases efficiency, productivity, and interoperability. Through technological innovations and improved software algorithms, healthcare informatics have affected the delivery of healthcare while advancing better communications between providers, patients, and consultants. It enhances a provider's access to information and expansion of knowledge.

While healthcare informatics has grown from its infancy, much development needs to be done for it to further mature and enrich the experience for both healthcare providers and patients. Current implementations are known for more time entering data than patient-centric care. It interferes with the physician-patient relationship, which is the cornerstone of every patient encounter. In an attempt to balance the competing demands of attention to the patient and documenting a visit in the EHR, the provider may resort to copying and pasting and other shortcuts that call into question the accuracy of the entire note. Even though the EHR is the core technology in patient care, it is generally not regulated by the FDA.[12] Therefore, it is the responsibility of the healthcare institution and vendors to structure health informatic systems to enhance care and sagacity of the professionals tending to the infirmed.

It has been said that "Not to be" was Hamlet's backup plan. Healthcare informatics continues to move forward with new improvements and expand connectivity. Through the use of faster computers, higher internet speeds, larger healthcare data silos, better search algorithms, and the ability to exponentially expand comprehension of evolving knowledge, health informatics will continue to progress. While data must be backed up, the momentum of health informatics moves forward on an accelerating continuum. With all technology, along with the benefits there will be kinks and adjustments; however, it is fair to say that health informatics is here to stay.

About the Author

Joshua R. Cohen, J.D., is a founding member of the law firm DeCorato Cohen Sheehan & Federico, LLP. He has been representing physicians, hospitals, and healthcare professionals for over 30 years. He has devoted his practice to innovative strategies on the cutting edge of law, including health informatics and technology. A frequent author and lecturer, he shares knowledge and experience on complex health litigation and risk management.

Mr. Cohen is a past president of the New York State Medical Defense Bar Association and was the chairperson for the Association of the Bar of the City of New York Committee on Medical Malpractice. He is listed in *Who's Who in American Law* and is A.V. Peer Review rated by Martindale-Hubbell, its top rating. He is also a fellow of the Litigation Counsel of America, an invitation-only honorary society representing less than one half of one percent of American lawyers. He is the Secretary of the Health Law section of the International Association of Lawyers.

---

[12] https://www.fda.gov/media/97567/download.

Chapter 28

Telehealth

Salvatore Volpe, MD FAAP, FACP ABP-CI, FHIMSS, CHCQM

Contents

The COVID-19 pandemic was a seismic event in many ways. Telehealth in the United States had been weighed down by multiple regulations and payment models that significantly limited its use. The need to provide care to patients in the face of multiple lockdowns affecting transportation and access to medical offices and hospital clinics led to a "relaxation" of regulations and more equitable payment for much needed services. (Editor's note: see chapter 1: HIMSS Value of IT.)

According to the American Medical Association (AMA), "telehealth, telemedicine and related terms generally refer to the exchange of medical information from one site to another through electronic communication." The Centers for Medicare and Medicaid Services (CMS) defines "telehealth as a two-way, real-time interactive communication between a patient and a physician or practitioner at a distant site through telecommunications equipment that includes, at a minimum, audio and visual equipment."[1]

DOI: 10.4324/9780429423109-28

In addition to the good old audio call, many patients with broadband access can now have a video session.

> During the first quarter of 2020, the number of telehealth visits increased by 50%, compared with the same period in 2019, with a 154% increase in visits noted in surveillance week 13 in 2020, compared with the same period in 2019. During January – March 2020, most encounters were from patients seeking care for conditions other than COVID-19. However, the proportion of COVID-19 – related encounters significantly increased (from 5.5% to 16.2%; $p<0.05$) during the last 3 weeks of March 2020 (surveillance weeks 11–13). This marked shift in practice patterns has implications for immediate response efforts and longer-term population health.[2]

At the time of writing, the use of telehealth visits has declined, while in-office visits approach pre-COVID-19 levels.

Examples of permitted video platform apps commonly used by patients were FaceTime, Google Meet, Skype, WhatsApp, and Zoom. The advantages of these platforms were that they were free and that the learning curve for the patients and medical providers was not steep. Among the problems with the apps is that off-the-shelf versions are not HIPAA compliant without a business associates agreement (BAA), and some did not initially have protections in place to prevent unintended "guests" to join, "bomb," or "raid" the call. By holding the session "outside" the electronic health record (EHR), there would be a need to separately document the visit within the EHR to preserve what transpired. Federal and state regulations are beginning to tighten, and thus it is recommended to use secure platforms, preferably integrated with the EHR.

There are three main types of telehealth visits: synchronous, asynchronous, and remote patient monitoring (RPM). Synchronous (live) visits have both the patient and the medical provider interacting "live." Asynchronous (store and forward) visits usually involve the sharing of information for later review by the medical provider. This could be done via patient portals or secure email and may include pre-visit questionnaires, medical status updates, or even photos for the evaluation of dermatological conditions.

RPM involves the review of patient data either synchronously or asynchronously. The patient could be located at home, an intensive care unit, a skilled nursing facility, or in an ambulance. The types of data include vital signs such as blood pressure, pulse, respiration, oxygen saturation, weight, blood glucose and ECG. Even mHealth apps could be a source of data. (Editor's note: see chapter 2: Personal Health Engagement and chapter 19: IoT Is Watching You.)

The AMA Implementation Playbook is an excellent guide to review, whether one is looking to set up a program or looking to refine what is already in place.[3] For ongoing updates and collaboration, consider the Healthcare Information and Management Systems Society (HIMSS) Telehealth Community and American Medical Informatics Association (AMIA).[4–5] We will now cover some of the topics mentioned in the playbook.

Pricing

There are many different pricing options available. Many EHRs now incorporate a virtual visit option either at a per-encounter fee or as an addition to an annual license fee.

Virtual Waiting Room

Whether you are in solo or group practice, there is an advantage to having a virtual waiting room. This "room" permits your staff to queue up the visit by collecting vital signs, chief complaint, updates to medications, and any pre-visit surveys. Many practices have pre-visit surveys associated with the chief complaint. Other pre-visit surveys could include a PHQ-9 depression screen and the PRAPARE assessment for social determinants of health (SDoH).[6] Please note that pre-visit data collection can also be done via patient portals, which are part of most EHRs.

Sandbox Access

It is imperative that as you compare different vendor platforms that you request access to a sandbox. This is an option that you should also request if you are shopping for an EHR. The sandbox gives you and your staff access to many of the features of the EHR/telehealth platform before you commit to a contract. Quite frankly, everyone on staff should be given an opportunity to sample the system: physicians, mid-level providers, medical assistants, clerical staff, and billing staff. They will give you the feedback you need to identify if the system will meet your needs.

Contact List of Customers with Similar Practices and Professional Organization Reviews

The vendor should not have a problem giving you the contact information of several practices that have been using the system for a while. Again, it is important to have different members of your staff either speak to their counterparts or generate a list of questions. Any issues shared by the other customer(s) could then be brought up with the vendor and explored in the sandbox.

Group Visits: Multiple Providers, Multiple Patients

This could be useful in several situations. First, a primary care provider may want to bring on a subspecialist for combined evaluation of the patient. Think outside the box. This could be an excellent way to introduce and perform a warm handoff to a community-based organization staffer who could help address SDoH issues. Identified inequities related to the social determinants of care will be part of the EHR, and referrals to address them will be part of the care plan. Individual factors and health behaviors account for 10%–20% of the plan, economic and social factors for another 40%, and the physical environment account for about 10%. The article "The Social Determinants of Health: Coming of Age" is an excellent review of the topic.[7]

Second, the provider could invite a live interpreter, if the practice often requires one to be present. Third, a patient's family member or close friend could be offered the opportunity to join the call. It is not uncommon for a geriatrician to have a son, daughter, niece, nephew, or friend participate in a face-to-face visit. A person that is trusted by the patient and is engaged can be a very valuable member of the care team. Where at one time some of these individuals could not attend the visit, as they might have been hundreds or even thousands of miles away, they could participate either by phone or asynchronously via the patient portal.

Transcription Services

For those of you who rely on transcription services, you may have at least three options: (1) via the telehealth application; (2) in conjunction with an EHR that has transcription as an option; and (2) via a free-standing transcription application, such as Dragon Medical One.

Data Exchange Options

If you are not using the EHR telehealth option, you and your staff may be put in a situation of performing significant double entry or maintaining multiple open screens between your EHR and independent telehealth solution. Other categories of data to consider include appointments, demographics, active problem list, medications, and allergies or, if possible, the continuity of care document (CCD).

Can the telehealth solution pull information from the local health information exchange (HIE)? This would provide updates regarding recent ED visits, hospitalizations, diagnostic tests, and so forth. If not, this could potentially be another screen that would need to be viewed during the visit. The EHR should be the final repository of all information generated during the visit. (Editor's note: see chapter 15: Health Information Exchange: An Overview & New York State's Model). Does the telehealth solution leverage fast healthcare interoperability resources (FHIR) or substitutable medical applications, reusable technologies (SMART) on FHIR?

Liability Issues: Part 1

The following is not meant to be an exhaustive list, and a review of the telehealth contract by legal counsel should be needed.

1. Request proof of liability insurance.
2. Request proof that you are indemnified for attack and breaches related to the vendor's services.
3. Confirm that the coverage is above is just the for the cost of using the service, such as fines and penalties.

Liability Issues: Part 2

Threats of a privacy breach are diminished using an encrypted and HIPAA-compliant platform. Please note that some of the commonly used platforms during the COVID-19 pandemic require a separate BAA to be exchanged. For example, with Zoom,

> A BAA needs to be in place for covered entities or business associates that wish to place PHI on the platform, but no manual configuration needs to occur to enable feature enhancements. Zoom's HIPAA offering allows you to leverage the Zoom platform, while still maintaining privacy, security, and compliance.[8]

Done properly, practice and patient communication is enhanced, reflecting better access to the healthcare provider. The audit capability, which documents the date and time of the interaction, may be of value during a deposition.

Workflow

Here are some highlights are more deeply detailed in the references:

1. Pre-visit questionnaire: The chief complaint, biometric data, and so forth can sometimes be done via the patient portal. This could be sent out several days in advance as the appointment is confirmed.
2. Before the scheduled appointment:
   a. Confirm the patient has the proper equipment and broadband access.
   b. Confirm the patient will be in a location that permits a private interaction.
   c. Consider having staff perform a "dry run" call prior to scheduled event.
   d. Have a back-up plan in place in case the patient has issues:
      i. Cannot login
      ii. Forgets password
      iii. Loses broadband access
   e. At the onset of the appointment:
      i. Confirm that the patient can see and hear the provider
      ii. Ensure privacy is addressed
3. During the appointment: Monitor for any cues that the patient is not engaged in the telehealth visit
4. At the close of the appointment:
   a. Summarize the visit and discuss next steps/plan
   b. Use teach-back for any education provided
   c. Allow for questions
5. Special case for patients with possible disabilities. For example, in the case of impaired hearing:
   a. Ensure the provider's face is visible.
   b. Make sure the office area is well lit.
   c. Avoid shadows on the provider's face so that facial expressions can also be communicated.
   d. Use non-verbal gestures to augment the spoken words.
   e. Encourage the use of headphones with the volume turned up.
   f. Minimize background noise.
   g. Use closed-captioning if your platform has this feature.
6. Triage: Once your staff has begun engaging with the patient, they may triage the patient just as they would with an in-person visit.
7. Engage an interpreter, if necessary.
8. Engage the caregiver, if necessary.
9. Engage the other consultant or SDoH resource.
10. Document the visit: Are multiple screens needed: EHR, telehealth, HIE?
11. Generate and transmit prescriptions.
12. Generate and transmit referrals.
13. Share patient education materials and links.
14. Schedule follow-up visit.
15. Bill for the visit.
16. Transfer items 10–14 into the EHR.

Patient Portals

As previously mentioned, patient portals that can be incorporated in the telehealth workflow can provide many benefits for the patient and the practice. Patients and caregivers can:

- Request an appointment
- Request a prescription renewal
- Request a referral to another physician
- Review bill balances and make payments
- Review medical visit notes
- Review diagnostic test results
- Review consultation notes.

Staff Buy-in

- A successful telehealth implementation begins with complete staff buy-in and enthusiasm.
- Review with the staff the advantages to the patient.
- Review with the staff the increased professional satisfaction of being more involved with patient care management (i.e., chronic care management).
- Staff incentives.

Enrolling Patients

- Location, location, location
- Posters in waiting room and exam room
- Staff buttons
- Kiosks in waiting room and/or exam rooms
- Website notice and social media notice
- Provide flyers and other instructional materials that review the benefits and address common questions. (See Figure 28.1)
- Date/time convenience
- Expense avoidance: transportation, babysitting
- Coordination with other specialists
- Coordination with care givers or other concerned individuals
- During pandemics, avoid risk of exposure to others.

TELEMEDICINE 101
for Patients and Family Caregivers

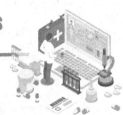

WHAT IS TELEMEDICINE?

- Telemedicine is a way to get health care from your doctor or other health care provider by phone, mobile app, or online video without going to a health care provider's office or hospital when your health care provider deems it appropriate.
- Telemedicine is sometimes called telehealth or virtual care.

WHAT DO I NEED TO GET TELEMEDICINE CARE?

- If your provider offers telemedicine, it could be through the telephone or by video, or both.
- For video visits, you will need a stable internet connection. You can use a computer, tablet or smartphone to connect with your doctor or other health care provider.
- Your health care provider will give you an app, website or phone number to call to start your appointment.
- Your health care provider may sometimes provide you with equipment to use at home to help you manage chronic conditions such as Asthma, Congestive Heart Failure, COPD, Diabetes.

WHY DO PATIENTS LIKE TELEMEDICINE?

- Telemedicine reduces the risk of COVID-19 transmission. It allows patients to get expert medical care without leaving their home. It keeps care providers and other patients safe, too.
- Telemedicine is convenient. It lets you connect with your provider when you need to from your home or wherever you are.
- Telemedicine means no driving and no waiting in the waiting room. You don't even have to get out of your pajamas if you don't want to!

WHY IS MY HEALTH CARE PROVIDER USING TELEMEDICINE NOW?

- COVID-19, also known as the coronavirus, is a very contagious virus.
- Telemedicine helps patients get care while staying home and keeping themselves safe.

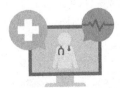

Figure 28.1   A sample "flyer" to share with your patients

HOW WILL MY HEALTH CARE PROVIDER USE TELEMEDICINE?

Your doctor or other health care provider can:

- Diagnose health issues such as a rash
- Discuss medicines with you and give you prescriptions
- Review diagnostic results and consultations with other healthcare providers
- Help you manage your health conditions such as high blood pressure
- Answer your medical questions, including about COVID-19

WHEN CAN I USE TELEMEDICINE?

Check with your health care provider on what they treat and what to do in the case of life-threatening emergencies. Telemedicine may be used for many health care issues including:

- Allergies, Asthmas and Sinus issues
- Arthritis pain
- Colds, Bronchitis and Flu
- Diarrhea
- Infections and Insect Bites
- "Pink Eye" and rashes

- Sore Throats
- Sprains & Strains
- Bladder Infections and UTIs
- Sports Injuries
- Vomiting

HOW MUCH DO TELEMEDICINE VISITS COST?

- Ask your health care provider or insurnace company about any copays.
- Most insurance plans include some coverage for telemedicine visits, including Medicaid and Medicare.

X4 HEALTH IS A PURPOSE-DRIVEN ORGANIZATION WORKING TO MAKE HEALTH CARE BETTER FOR PEOPLE.

WWW.X4HEALTH.COM

X4 HEALTH

Figure 28.1 (Continued)

Here are some current examples of telehealth beyond traditional ambulatory visits (See Figure 28.2):[9]

Digital emergency care
Digital stroke care
Home visits
Telehealth hubs
Identification of child abuse
Intensive care unit
Postoperative visits

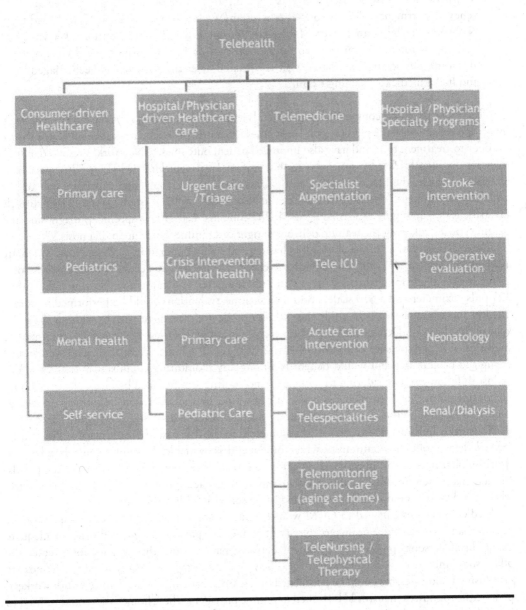

Figure 28.2   A sample telehealth ontology

Prenatal and postpartum
Skilled nursing facilities (SNFs)
Telepsychiatry (Editor's note: see chapter 12: Telebehavioral Health: Mental Health Landscape)

Here are some details on the above examples:

> Digital emergency care: "The innovative response of NewYork–Presbyterian and Weill Cornell Medicine was to create digital emergency department capability. One such example is the launch of the first Emergency Department-based Tele-health Express Care Service. Patients with minor complaints arriving at the emergency departments of NewYork–Presbyterian/Weill Cornell Medical Center and NewYork–Presbyterian/Lower Manhattan Hospital are given the option of a virtual visit through real-time video interactions with a board-certified Weill Cornell attending physician. The virtual visit is initiated after the patient has been triaged and had a medical screening exam."

"Telestroke programs connect regional hospitals with a neurologist who can rapidly evaluate a CT image and consult with the physician on-site on the best course of action. Telestroke programs reduce the door-to-treatment time and have also improved patient outcomes.[6,7] NewYork–Presbyterian took this care one step further by creating a Mobile Stroke Treatment Unit (MSTU). This specialized emergency vehicle, the first of its kind on the East Coast, has CT imaging capability onboard, is staffed by a neurologist, and is dispatched by the New York City 911 System via the FDNY directly to a patient showing signs of a stroke. The MSTU contains medications specific to diagnosing and treating strokes, allowing the team to deliver the right drug immediately upon diagnosis."[10]

The availability of a "home clinic" kits has opened many opportunities. These kits, which are available for as little as $199, can provide the clinician with remote access to a stethoscope, otoscope, tongue blade for evaluating the mouth, thermometer, and camera with a ring light. Add a $25 pulse oximeter and a $10 scale, and many routine evaluations could be performed remotely. The kits include apps that help guide the end user on device placement with or without the guidance of the clinician. Depending on the health coverage, many of these are covered items. Imagine the value of deploying such devices during the COVID-19 pandemic. Patients who were not ill enough to be admitted but would benefit from ongoing monitoring could stay at home and not be lost to follow-up. Considering the financial and staffing strains faced by hospitals, this should be considered during future emergencies. What would be the return on investment related to decreased ED room visits, hospital admissions, hospital readmissions and staffing burnout?

Telehealth hubs are a variation of the home clinic. In this case, the inexpensive kits can be located throughout the community where broadband is available. Examples could be places of worship, pharmacies, and libraries. Think of a comfortable telephone booth with privacy panels. In fact, many new medical facilities are incorporating space for this sort of "walk-in" service, which if necessary could lead to an escalated in-person visit within the center.

Medical practices engaged in CCM would certainly appreciate having access to more of the patient than just their voice or image from a cell phone. The pandemic logistical issues of adequate changing of personal protective equipment between patients and timing patients to enter the office, sometimes from parked cars near the office, would be obviated. Many in-person home care visits using remote devices could be performed by a team consisting of community health workers, paramedics, or nurses that would be linked to remote providers. These home visits could be used to not only provide medical support but also help provide healthcare and SDoH navigation services which are in high demand but not well addressed.

SNFs: CMS uses the patient-driven payment model (PDPM) to compensate SNFs. This is meant to prioritize patient needs over service volume. Because SNFs do not bill for each individual service provided, there is an incentive to be more efficient. In the US Northeast, the average cost to transport a patient to a specialist office for initial or follow-up evaluation could range between $300 and $500. The costs include staff and transport vehicle. Depending on the size of the facility and when clinically appropriate, 10–30 transports per month could be obviated by providing devices at the facility like those previously described. Often such devices can be linked to the SNF EHR. In addition to the significant financial savings and facility staffing efficiencies, patients could benefit by more timely evaluation and avoidance of an uncomfortable transport experience. Specialists could benefit by redirecting the time spent commuting to the SNFs to time with patients. On call clinicians would also benefit by having greater "access" to the patient than would be provided by phone. In many cases, whether the clinician was 18 inches or 18 miles away, an adequate exam could be performed. Taking a page from the digital emergency care example, a clinician working on the seventh floor could initiate treatment on a non-critical patent on the first floor with the assistance of such equipment. The net result is faster care with less staff stress.[11]

Identification of child abuse: A recent article in *Pediatrics Consultant* highlighted the issues with identifying and preventing child abuse during the COVID-19 pandemic. A telehealth visit could bring the provider "into the home," where certain telltale signs might be noticed. This could help fill the gap normally addressed by schoolteachers, after-school personnel, and sports and religious staff.[12]

About the Author

Salvatore Volpe, MD, FAAP, FACP, ABP-CI, FHIMSS, CHCQM, has achieved board certification in pediatrics, internal medicine, geriatrics and clinical informatics and he currently serves as the Chief Medical Officer working closely with the IT staff at the Staten Island Performing Provider System (SI PPS). The SI PPS is an alliance of clinical and social service providers focused on improving the quality of care and overall health for Staten Island's Medicaid and uninsured populations, which include more than 180,000 Staten Island residents, and was the highest performing group under the New York State Department of Health's Delivery System Reform Incentive Payment (DSRIP) program.

His practice was the first solo practice in the United States to achieve Level 3 2011 NCQA Patient Centered Medical Home Recognition. In addition to running a solo primary care practice for 30 years, Dr. Volpe has had many leadership roles outside the office. He served as physician champion for the NYC Department of Health and Mental Hygiene Primary Care Information Project (NYC DOH MH PCIP); president of Healthcare Information and Management Systems Society New York State (HIMSS NYS); president of the Richmond County Medical Society (RCMS); chairman of the HIT Committee for the Medical Society of the State of New York (MSSNY) and Richmond County; member of the board of directors of the New York eHealth Collaborative (NYeC); and member of the board of the Medical Liability Mutual Insurance Company.

Learning from others and sharing this knowledge has been another important aspect of his professional career. He has been invited to speak on health and technology topics locally and nationally. In addition to contributing to numerous journals, Dr. Volpe was a contributor for the PCMH chapter for the second and third editions of *Medical Informatics: An Executive Primer.*

Dr. Volpe and his practice have been recognized by many organizations. For work with the geriatric population and informatics, they were presented the Island Peer Review Organization (IPRO) Quality Award and SUNY Downstate Medical School Geriatrics Medicine Award.

Their focus on PCMH was acknowledged by the Patient-Centered Primary Care Collaborative (PCPCC) with the Patient-Centered Medical Home Practice (PCMH) Award. Due to the innovations introduced by Dr. Volpe and his executive board at HIMSS NYS, he was honored with the Chapter Leader of the Year Award.

Dr. Volpe received his bachelor of arts from Columbia University, his medical degree from SUNY Downstate and completed a combined pediatrics and internal medicine residency at Staten University Hospital (now a member of the NorthWell Health Network).

References

1. https://www.ama-assn.org/practice-management/digital/telehealth-resource-center-definitions.
2. Koonin LM, Hoots B, Tsang CA, et al. Trends in the Use of Telehealth During the Emergence of the COVID-19 Pandemic — United States, January–March 2020. MMWR Morb Mortal Wkly Rep 2020;69:1595–1599.
3. AMA Telehealth Implementation Playbook. https://www.ama-assn.org/system/files/2020-04/ama-telehealth-playbook.pdf.
4. https://www.himss.org/membership-participation/telehealth-community.
5. https://www.amia.org/.
6. https://www.nachc.org/research-and-data/prapare/.
7. Braveman, P., Egerter, S., & Williams, D. R. (2011). The social determinants of health: Coming of age. *Annual Review of Public Health*, 32(1), 381–398.
8. https://support.zoom.us/hc/en-us/articles/207652183-HIPAA-Business-Associate-Agreement-BAA-.
9. AMA return on health: Moving beyond dollars and cents in realizing the value of virtual care. https://www.ama-assn.org/system/files/2021-05/ama-return-on-health-report-may-2021.pdf.
10. Sharma, R., Fleischut, P., & Barchi, D. (2017). Telemedicine and its transformation of emergency care: A case study of one of the largest US integrated healthcare delivery systems. *International Journal of Emergency Medicine*, 10(1), 21. https://doi.org/10.1186/s12245-017-0146-7.
11. Mark Aaron Unruh, PhD, Dhruv Khullar, MD, MPP, Hye-Young Jung, PhD. The Patient-Driven Payment Model: Addressing Perverse Incentives, Creating New Ones. *The American Journal of Managed Care*. April 2020, 26(4), 150–152.
12. Repine, A., Macaulay, J., & Deutsch, S. A. (2021). COVID-19 and child abuse: Practical steps to address child safety. *Consultant*. Published online March 15, 2021. doi:10.25270/con.2021.03.000108.

Additional resources:

Regional Telehealth Resources Centers is a collaborative of 12 regional and 2 national centers that are dedicated to assisting those in rural and underserved communities. In addition to access to their experts, the site provides a multitude of tools and educational materials. https://telehealthresourcecenter.org/resources/

Chapter 29

Future Possibilities

Salvatore Volpe

Contents

In this final chapter, we will present one potential future state where much of what has been described in the previous 28 chapters has come together to work synergistically.

The Digital Twin

In a variation of the movie *The Matrix*, a digital twin would be "born" at the same time as their organic counterpart (real person).[1–4] Unlike the movie, the person will not be held in a cocoon but rather live and participate in all of life's activities as we do today. The digital twin's "initial genomic" and physiologic profile will be continuously updated. Recent research indicates that epigenetic, heritable modifications to our cells' machinery (DNA, RNA, etc.) occur over time that can predispose us to different illnesses as we get older.[5–6] As the years proceed, our exposures to different chemicals, emotional situations, and environmental exposures will also be added to our hypothetical digital twin's programming to keep track with our epigenetic changes. In this future state, an artificial intelligence (AI) guide, named B^^WELL*, would be available to help us make certain food or lifestyle choices based upon the ever-growing experience of our virtual selves. Our healthcare providers would be guided by their AI evaluation of our digital twin as to which medications would be best to manage our chronic conditions after having run multiple permutations to see which has the best long-term risk/benefit profile. Our opinions would also be added to the "equation" in a true personalized fashion.[7–8]

DOI: 10.4324/9780429423109-29

The Biometric Connection 24/7?

Commonly used devices such as wristbands and watches will provide a full set of vital signs, oxygen levels, glucose levels, electrocardiograms, and activity tracking (such as fall detection). A present-day example is DETECT (Digital Engagement and Tracking for Early Control and Treatment). This study uses an app to track patients with viral illnesses, including COVID-19, using over-the-counter smart wristbands and watches. [9]

Researchers at the Hospital for Special Surgery (HSS) have collaborated to use TESLASUIT which covers 95% of the muscle mass of the human body. These researchers are combining 157 years of accumulated HSS knowledge of musculoskeletal health with TESLASUIT smart technology, which integrates biometry, motion capture, and haptic feedback. [10]

Someday, power for some of these devices may be provided using kinetic charging as we move and heat or electrical conductivity from the skin. [11–12]

Artificial Intelligence: Benevolent Guardian Angel or Intrusive Big Brother?

Our biometric/wellness AI (B^^WELL) will be busy analyzing the information received from a multitude of wearable devices and external "monitors." Even now watches can ask, "How are you doing?" based upon our pulse rate and rhythm and will even call our emergency contacts if a fall is detected and one is unresponsive for one minute. [13–14] Can 911 calls be far behind?

Biometric panic values (results that are outside predefined normal range) that did not result in an emergent intervention would need to be tracked, trended, and evaluated in the proper context of our activity. Based upon pre-defined parameters, B^^WELL might recommend a virtual visit with a healthcare professional. In this case, upon receipt of my data, my healthcare provider AI might reach out to me for a dialogue or prompt my healthcare provider to initiate an in-person visit.

A Medical Visit in the Not-Too-Distant Future

The pre-visit questionnaire is auto-populated by B^^WELL and presented to me for review and any supplemental responses. B^^WELL uses TECFA (Trusted Exchange Framework and Common Agreement) to access information from the West Coast QHIN (Qualified Health Information Network) regarding medical care rendered while I was visiting a college friend. [15–17] Due to repair work being done in front of the usual office entrance, the medical office's AI might notify my navigation system and direct the self-driving vehicle to a different section of the building.

After the history is taken and physical examination is completed, the healthcare provider has decided to launch a virtual visit with my cardiologist so that the three of us could review the findings and agree upon a treatment plan. This would be done after multiple medication options are presented to my digital twin and the combination with the best future risk/benefit profile chosen. My daughter is sent a summary as a member of the care team. Part of the treatment plan will be managed by B^^WELL, which could schedule daily activities and short surveys supported by my cell phone. [18]

After the medical visit, I meet my daughter at a restaurant for dinner. My B^^WELL reviews the menu and presents me with recommendations based upon my current medical profile, my palate history, and nutritional composition of each meal. After a delightful dinner, I pay for my order using my blockchain-based financial account.

This parable can be viewed in many ways. Some may say that it uses some of the better implementations of informatics to improve one's quality of life. Others might be concerned about a darker Orwellian or Huxleyan dystopia. To paraphrase Isaac Asimov, "science gathers knowledge faster than society gathers wisdom." [19] Fortunately, there are advocates working to protect our privacy and freedom. Biometric laws are being written that prevent the sharing and sale of our data, give us the right to opt out and the right to sue as well as the right to specify the length of time the data could be used before its mandatory destruction.

In Conclusion

As my wife, Rachel, would say, "Thank you for your time."

Thank you for reading our book. May it spark your interest to collaborate with those outside your field of training or experience to develop a more holistic approach to improving the health and quality of life for us all. We encourage the reader to engage not just in the technological revolution but also in the societal evolution. By expanding the pool of participants in this endeavor, we can reduce errors and biases from selected points of view and increase the likelihood of more equitable outcomes.

Spread the word to get involved: this is one situation where we cannot have too many cooks!

Note: Regarding B^^WELL, please note this is a work of fiction. Any similarity to actual persons/entities, living, artificial or dead, or actual events, is purely coincidental.

References

1. IMDB. https://www.imdb.com/title/tt0133093/?ref_=fn_al_tt_1.
2. Openaccessgovernment. https://www.openaccessgovernment.org/digital-twins/93402/#:~:text=In%20the%20medical%20%EF%AC%81eld%2C%20the%20term%20digital%20twin,of%20granularity%20of%20metabolism%2C%20physiology%2C%20behaviour%20and%20morbidity.
3. Venturebeat. https://venturebeat.com/2021/07/04/21-ways-medical-digital-twins-will-transform-healthcare/.
4. Genomedicine. https://genomemedicine.biomedcentral.com/articles/10.1186/s13073-019-0701-3.
5. Bjornsson, H. T., Sigurdsson, M. I., Fallin, M. D., et al. (2008). Intra-individual Change Over Time in DNA Methylation with Familial Clustering. *JAMA, 299*(24), 2877–2883. doi:10.1001/jama.299.24.2877.
6. Breton, C. V., Landon, R., Kahn, L. G., Enlow, M. B., Peterson, A. K., Bastain, T., Braun, J., Comstock, S. S., Duarte, C. S., Hipwell, A., Ji, H., LaSalle, J. M., Miller, R. L., Musci, R., Posner, J., Schmidt, R., Suglia, S. F., Tung, I., Weisenberger, D., Zhu, Y., . . . Fry, R. (2021). Exploring the Evidence for Epigenetic Regulation of Environmental Influences on Child Health Across Generations. *Communications Biology, 4*(1), 769. https://doi.org/10.1038/s42003-021-02316-6.
7. FDAnews. https://www.fdanews.com/ext/resources/files/10/10-28-13-Personalized-Medicine.pdf.
8. Ginsburg, G. S., & Phillips, K. A. (2018). Precision Medicine: From Science to Value. *Health affairs (Project Hope), 37*(5), 694–701. https://doi.org/10.1377/hlthaff.2017.1624.
9. Radin, J. M., Quer, G., Ramos, E., et al. (2021). Assessment of Prolonged Physiological and Behavioral Changes Associated With COVID-19 Infection. *JAMA Netw Open, 4*(7), e2115959. doi:10.1001/jamanetworkopen.2021.15959.

10. HSS.edu. https://news.hss.edu/HSS-Innovation-Institute-and-TESLASUIT-to-Advance-Healthcare-with-Immersive-%D0%A5R-Training-Technology/.

11. Ren W, Sun Y, Zhao D, Aili A, Zhang S, Shi C, Zhang J, Geng H, Zhang J, Zhang L, Xiao J, Yang R. High-performance wearable thermoelectric generator with self-healing, recycling, and Lego-like reconfiguring capabilities. Sci Adv. 2021 Feb 10; 7(7), eabe0586. doi: 10.1126/sciadv.abe0586. PMID: 33568483; PMCID: PMC7875524.

12. Mohammed, Noor, Wang, Rui, Jackson, Robert W., Noh, Yeonsik, Gummeson, Jeremy, and Lee, Sunghoon Ivan. (2021). ShaZam: Charge-Free Wearable Devices via Intra-Body Power Transfer from Everyday Objects. *Proceedings of the ACM on Interactive, Mobile, Wearable and Ubiquitous Technologies*, *5*(2), Article 75 (June 2021), 25 pages. doi:10.1145/3463505.

13. González-Cañete, F. J., & Casilari, E. (2021). A Feasibility Study of the Use of Smartwatches in Wearable Fall Detection Systems. *Sensors (Basel, Switzerland)*, *21*(6), 2254. https://doi.org/10.3390/s21062254.

14. Abou, Libak, Fliflet, Alexander, Hawari, Lina, Presti, Peter, Sosnoff, Jacob J., Mahajan, Harshal P., Frechette, Mikaela L., & Rice, Laura A. (2021). Sensitivity of Apple Watch Fall Detection Feature among Wheelchair Users. *Assistive Technology*. doi:10.1080/10400435.2021.1923087.

15. Healthit. https://www.healthit.gov/topic/interoperability/trusted-exchange-framework-and-common-agreement.

16. Healthit. https://www.healthit.gov/sites/default/files/draft-trusted-exchange-framework.pdf.

17. Healthit. https://www.healthit.gov/sites/default/files/page/2019-04/FINALTEFCAQTF41719508 version.pdf.

18. Strauss, D. H., Davoodi, N. M., Healy, M., Metts, C. L., Merchant, R. C., Banskota, S., & Goldberg, E. M. (2021). The Geriatric Acute and Post-Acute Fall Prevention Intervention (GAPcare) II to Assess the Use of the Apple Watch in Older Emergency Department Patients with Falls: Protocol for a Mixed Methods Study. *JMIR Research Protocols*, *10*(4), e24455. https://doi.org/10.2196/24455.

19. Asimov, I. (1988). *Isaac Asimov's Book of Science and Nature Quotations*. Weidenfield & Nicolson.

Acronyms and Terms Related to Electronic Health Records[10]

Acronyms

ANSI	American National Standards Institute
APHL	Association of Public Health Laboratories
ARRA	American Recovery and Reinvestment Act of 2009
CAH	Critical Access Hospital
CDC	Centers for Disease Control and Prevention
CFR	Code of Federal Regulations
CLIA	Clinical Laboratory Improvement Amendments of 1988
CMS	Centers for Medicare and Medicaid Services
CQM	Clinical Quality Measure
DHHS	Department of Health and Human Services
EHR	Electronic Health Record
ELR	Electronic Laboratory Reporting
EMR	Electronic Medical Record
EP	Eligible Professionals
FACA	Federal Advisory Committee Act
FDA	US Food and Drug Administration
FHIMS	Federal Health Interoperability Modeling and Standards
FHIR	(Fast Healthcare Interoperability Resources) Specification, which is a standard for exchanging healthcare information electronically[11]
FR	Federal Register
HIE	Health Information Exchange
HIPAA	Health Insurance Portability and Accountability Act
HIT	Health Information Technology
HITECH	Health Information Technology for Economic and Clinical Health Act
HITPC	Health IT Policy Committee
HITSC	Health IT Standards Committee
HL7	Health Level 7
IT	Information Technology
LIS	Laboratory Information System
LOINC	Logical Observation Identifiers Names and Codes
LRI	Laboratory Results Interface (specifically in relation to an ONC workgroup)
LRR	Laboratory Results Reporting

MU	Meaningful Use
NIST	National Institute of Standards and Technology
NwHIN	Nationwide Health Information Network (formerly NHIN)
OCR	Office of Civil Rights
ONC	Office of the National Coordinator for Health Information Technology (also ONC-HIT)
ONC-AA	ONC-Approved Accreditor
ONC-ACB	ONC-Authorized Certification Body
ONC-ATCB	ONC-Authorized Testing and Certification Body
PHIN	Public Health Information Network
PHITPO	Public Health Informatics and Technology Program Office (at CDC)
PHR	Personal Health Record
PMR	Personal Medical Record
REC	Regional Extension Center
RHIO	Regional Health Information Organization
SMART on FHIR	SMART App Launch Framework connects third-party applications to EHR data, allowing apps to launch from inside or outside the user interface of an EHR system 12
SNOMED-CT	Systematized Nomenclature of Medicine–Clinical Terms
VLER	Virtual Lifetime Electronic Record

Terms

Certified Electronic Health Record – An EHR or module of an EHR that has been reviewed by an ONC-ATCB and determined to be compliant with the standards set forth in the Health Information Technology Standards and Certification requirements (45 CFR 170). MU incentive payments require participating hospitals and providers to use certified EHR systems.

Electronic Health Record (EHR) – (1) An electronic record of health-related information on an individual that conforms to nationally recognized interoperability standards and that can be created, managed, and consulted by authorized clinicians and staff across more than one health care organization (reference 1, p. 17). (2) A comprehensive, structured set of clinical, demographic, environmental, social, and financial data and information in electronic form, documenting the health care given to a single individual (reference 2, p. 8).

Electronic Health Record System (EHR-S) – An information technology system designed to store and manage EHRs.

Electronic Laboratory Reporting (ELR) – The transmission of data of public health importance (specifically notifiable diseases) from clinical laboratories to public health agencies using electronic format and data specifications defined by public health partners.

Electronic Medical Record (EMR) – An electronic record of health-related information on an individual that can be created, gathered, managed, and consulted by authorized clinicians and staff within one health care organization (reference 1, p. 16).

Federal Health Interoperability Modeling and Standards (FHIMS) – A federal initiative intended to coordinate the efforts of the partner agencies with respect to information and terminology standards.

Health Information Exchange (HIE) – The electronic movement of health-related information across organizations within a region, community, or hospital system and according to nationally recognized standards.

HIMSS – Health Information and Management Systems Society.

Interoperability – The ability of health information systems to work together within and across organizational boundaries in order to advance the effective delivery of healthcare for individuals and communities.

Laboratory Results Interface (LRI) Initiative – An initiative under the S&I framework tasked with addressing interface interoperability challenges associated with laboratory reporting to ambulatory primary care providers. Challenges include mapping, interface configuration, and harmonization of core subsets of LOINC codes.

Laboratory Results Reporting (LRR) – The transmission of laboratory results in an electronic format from a clinical laboratory to an EHR system (EHR-S) for association with a patient's EHR.

Meaningful Use (MU) – A federal incentive program and regulations administered by CMS defining the minimum requirements that providers must meet through their use of certified EHR technology in order to qualify for the payments.

Nationwide Health Information Network (NwHIN) – A federal initiative for the exchange of healthcare information that supports MU, being developed under the auspices of the US ONC. Formerly known as NHIN.

ONC-Approved Accreditor (ONC-AA) – An accreditation organization approved by the National Coordinator to accredit electronic health record certification bodies under the permanent certification program, namely, the National Institute of Standards and Technology (NIST).

ONC-Authorized Certification Body (ONC-ACB) – An organization or a consortium of organizations that has applied to and been authorized by the National Coordinator to perform the certification of complete EHRs, EHR module(s), and/or other types of health information technology under the ONC Permanent Certification Program.

ONC -Authorized Testing and Certification Body (ONC-ATCB): An organization or a consortium of organizations that has applied to and been authorized by the National Coordinator to perform the testing and certification of complete EHRs and/or EHR modules under the Temporary Certification Program.

Personal Health Record (PHR) – An electronic record of health-related information on an individual that conforms to nationally recognized interoperability standards and that can be drawn from multiple sources while being managed, shared, and controlled by that individual (reference 1, p. 19).

Personal Medical Record (PMR) – See PHR; the terms are used interchangeably.

Regional Health Information Organization (RHIO) – An organization that brings together healthcare stakeholders within a defined geographic area and governs health information exchange (HIE) among them for the purpose of improving health and care in that community. RHIOs are a component of the structure intended to implement the NwHIN.

Standards and Interoperability (S&I) Framework – A set of integrated functions, processes, and tools being guided by the healthcare and technology industry to achieve harmonized interoperability for HIE.

Surescripts – Private company authorized to test and certify EHR modules. One of six ONC-ATCBs; awarded a CDC grant, along with the College of American Pathology (CAP) and the American Hospital Association (AHA), to electronically link hospital laboratories and public health agencies to support MU.

Technology Transfer & Technology Transfer Office – Government agency function and office intended to support collaboration and transfer of federal technology to the commercial marketplace and/or research community.

Tiger Team – A group of experts assigned to investigate and/or solve technical or systemic problems, particularly in relation to security (reference 9).

Sources

1. The National Alliance for Health Information Technology Report to the Office of the National Coordinator for Health Information Technology on Defining Key Health Information Technology Terms, April 28, 2008.

2. Glossary, HL7 Electronic Health Record System Functional Model, Release 1, February 2007.

3. HL7 Version 2.5.1 Implementation Guide: Orders and Observations; Interoperable Laboratory Result Reporting to EHR (US Realm), Release 1, ORU R01, version 2.5.1, November 2007.

4. Office of the National Coordinator for Healthcare Information Technology, Harmonized Use Case for Electronic Health Records (Laboratory Result Reporting), March 19, 2006.

5. HL7 Version 2.5.1 Implementation Guide: Electronic Laboratory Reporting To Public Health (US Realm), Release 1, ORU R01, version 2.5.1, February 2010.

6. Electronic Reporting of Laboratory Data for Public Health: Meeting Report and Recommendations, November 23, 2007.

7. Standards and Interoperability website: http://jira.siframework.org/wiki/display/SIF/Introduction+and+Overview.
8. HIMMS Whitepaper: Interoperability Definition and Background, June 9, 2005.
9. http://en.wikipedia.org/wiki/Tiger_team.
10. Adapted from the CLIAC Fall 2011 meeting: https://ftp.cdc.gov/pub/CLIAC_meeting_presentations/pdf/Addenda/cliac0811/O_addendum_EHR_Related_Acronyms_and_Terms.pdf.
11. https://www.hl7.org/fhir/overview.html.
12. https://hl7.org/fhir/smart-app-launch/.

Index

[Note: numbers in **bold** indicate a table. Numbers in *italics* indicate a figure on the corresponding page.]

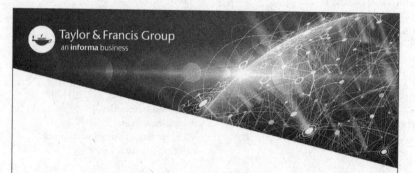

Printed in the United States
by Baker & Taylor Publisher Services

Printed in the United States
by Baker & Taylor Publisher Services